Reptile Medicine and Surgery in Clinical Practice

Reptile Medicine and Surgery in Clinical Practice

Edited by

Bob Doneley
University of Queensland
Queensland, Australia

Deborah Monks
Brisbane Bird and Exotic Veterinary Service
Queensland, Australia

Robert Johnson
South Penrith Veterinary Clinic
New South Wales, Australia

Brendan Carmel
Warranwood Veterinary Centre
Victoria, Australia

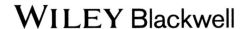

Registered Office(s)
John Wiley & Sons, Inc., 111 River Street, Hoboken, NJ 07030, USA
John Wiley & Sons Ltd, The Atrium, Southern Gate, Chichester, West Sussex, PO19 8SQ, UK

Editorial Office
9600 Garsington Road, Oxford, OX4 2DQ, UK

For details of our global editorial offices, customer services, and more information about Wiley products visit us at www.wiley.com.

Wiley also publishes its books in a variety of electronic formats and by print-on-demand. Some content that appears in standard print versions of this book may not be available in other formats.

Library of Congress Cataloging-in-Publication Data

Names: Doneley, Bob, editor. | Johnson, Robert, Dr., editor. | Monks,
   Deborah, 1972– editor. | Carmel, Brendan, editor.
Title: Reptile medicine and surgery in clinical practice / edited by Bob
   Doneley, Deborah Monks, Robert Johnson, Brendan Carmel.
Description: Hoboken, NJ : Wiley, 2017. | Includes bibliographical references
   and index. |
Identifiers: LCCN 2017033936 (print) | LCCN 2017035572 (ebook) |
   ISBN 9781118977682 (pdf) | ISBN 9781118977699 (epub) | ISBN 9781118977675 (hardback)
Subjects: LCSH: Reptiles–Diseases | Reptiles–Surgery. | MESH: Reptiles |
   Animal Diseases | Surgery, Veterinary
Classification: LCC SF997.5.R4 (ebook) | LCC SF997.5.R4 R466 2017 (print) |
   NLM SF 997.5.R4 | DDC 639.39–dc23
LC record available at https://lccn.loc.gov/2017033936

Cover Design: Wiley
Cover Image: Courtesy of Bob Doneley

Set in 10/12pt Warnock by SPi Global, Pondicherry, India

10 9 8 7 6 5 4 3 2 1

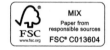

As always when producing a book like this, there are many people who have helped us along the way, often unnoticed. We would like to dedicate this book to those people: the authors who contributed their time and expertise; our veterinary colleagues and clients who, while not directly contributing to this book, taught us much about reptiles and their care, medicine and surgery; and our work colleagues who endured our distraction while we put this book together. Lastly, but by no means the least, we dedicate this book to our families who have patiently supported us in not just this book, but in all aspects of our lives and careers.

Thank you!

Contents

List of Contributors

Frances M. Baines MA, VetMB, MRCVS
UV Guide UK
Govilon
Abergavenny
United Kingdom

*Hamish Baron BVSc (Hons), MANZCVS
(Avian Health)*
Avian Reptile and Exotic Pet
Hospital
Faculty of Veterinary Science
The University of Sydney
Camden
New South Wales
Australia

*Brendan Carmel BVSc, MVS, GDipComp,
MANZCVS (Unusual Pets)*
Warranwood Veterinary Centre
Warranwood
Victoria
Australia

John Chitty, BVetMed, CetZooMed, MRCVS
Anton Vets
Andover
Hampshire
United Kingdom

*Bob Doneley BVSc, FANZCVS
(Avian Medicine)*
Associate Professor, Avian and Exotic Pet
Service
University of Queensland
Gatton
Queensland
Australia

Gary Fitzgerald BApSci (Veterinary Technology)
University of Queensland Veterinary Medical
Centre
University of Queensland
Gatton
Queensland
Australia

*Kimberly Vinette Herrin DVM, BA Biology, MS
(Biological Oceanography), MANZCVS
(Zoo Medicine)*
Taronga Wildlife Hospital
Taronga Conservation Society Australia
Mosman
New South Wales
Australia

Peter Holz BVSc, DVSc, MACVSc, Dipl ACZM
Faculty of Veterinary and Agricultural
Sciences
University of Melbourne
Melbourne
Victoria
Australia

*Tim Hyndman BSc, BVMS, PhD, MANZCVS
(Veterinary Pharmacology)*
Murdoch University
Perth
Western Australia
Australia

*Robert Johnson BVSc, MANZCVS (Feline),
CertZooMed, BA*
South Penrith Veterinary Clinic
Penrith
New South Wales
Australia

Michelle Kischinovsky DVM, MRCVS
Avian and Exotic Animal Clinic
Manchester
United Kingdom

Zdeněk Knotek DVM, PhD, Dip ECZM (Herpetology)
Faculty of Veterinary Medicine
University of Veterinary and Pharmaceutical Sciences
Brno
Czech Republic

Melinda L. Cowan BVSc (Hons), MANZCVS (Medicine Surgery of Unusual Pets), FANZCVS (Avian Medicine)
Small Animal Specialist Hospital
North Ryde
Sydney
New South Wales
Australia

Angela M. Lennox DVM, DABVP-Avian; ECZM-(Small Mammal)
Avian and Exotic Animal Clinic
Indianapolis
Indiana
USA

Stacey Leonatti Wilkinson DVM, DABVP (Reptile and Amphibian)
Avian and Exotic Animal Hospital of Georgia
Pooler
Georgia
USA

Adolf K. Maas III DVM, DABVP (Reptile and Amphibian Practice), CertAqV
ZooVet Consulting PLLC
Bothell
Washingon
USA

Rachel E. Marschang PD Dr.med.vet., Dip ECZM (Herpetology), FTÄ Mikrobiologie, ZB Reptilien
Laboklin GmbH & Co. KG
Bad Kissingen
Germany

An Martel DVM, PhD, Dip ECZM (WPH)
Department of Pathology, Bacteriology, and Avian Diseases
Ghent University
Merelbeke
Belgium

Paolo Martelli
Cert Zoo Med
Director of Veterinary Services
Hong Kong

Helen McCracken BSc(Vet), BVSc, MVS
Senior Veterinarian
Melbourne Zoo
Victoria
Australia

Michael McFadden BSc (Hons)
Curator, Native Fauna
Taronga Conservation Society Australia
Mosman
New South Wales
Australia

Sasha Miles BVSc (Hons), MANZCVS (Avian Health - Caged and Aviary Birds)
Veterinarian
Brisbane Bird and Exotics Veterinary Service
Queensland
Australia

Mark Mitchell DVM, MS, PhD, Dip ECZM (Herpetology)
Director, Veterinary Teaching Hospital
Professor, Zoological Medicine
Louisiana State University
School of Veterinary Medicine
Department of Veterinary Clinical Sciences
Los Angeles
California
USA

David Modrý MVDr, PhD
Department of Pathology and Parasitology
Faculty of Veterinary Medicine

University of Veterinary and
Pharmaceutical Sciences Brno
Brno
Czech Republic

Deborah Monks BVSc, CertZooMed,
FANZCVS (Avian Medicine), DECZM (Avian)
Brisbane Bird and Exotics Veterinary Service
Greeenslopes
Brisbane
Queensland
Australia

Bairbre O'Malley MVB, CertVR, MRCVS
Bairbre O'Malley Veterinary Hospital
Bray
Co. Wicklow
Ireland

Annabelle Olsson BVSc, MSc, PhD, MANZCVS
Boongarry Veterinary Surgery
Aeroglen
Quennsland
Australia

Frank Pasmans DVM, PhD, Dip ECZM
(Herpetology)
Department of Pathology, Bacteriology,
and Avian Diseases
Ghent University
Belgium

David N. Phalen DVM, PhD, Dip ABVP (Avian)
Associate Professor
School of Veterinary Medicine
University of Sydney
Camden
New South Wales
Australia

Timothy J. Portas BVSc, MVSc, MANZCVS, DACZM
Zoo and Wildlife Veterinary Consultancy
Queensland
Australia

Aidan Raftery MVB, CertZooMed, CBiol,
MRSB, MRCVS
Avian and Exotic Animal Clinic
Manchester
United Kingdom

Jane Roffey BVSc, BA, GCM(VP)
South Penrith Veterinary Clinic
Sydney
New South Wales
Australia

Alex Rosenwax BVSc(hons), MANZCVS
(Avian Health)
Bird and Exotics Veterinary Clinic
Waterloo
Sydney
New South Wales
Australia

Shivananden Sawmy BSc (Hons),
BVM&S, MRCVS
Avian and Exotic Animal Clinic
Manchester
United Kingdom

Catherine M. Shilton BSc, DVM, DVSc
Senior Veterinary Pathologist
Berrimah Veterinary Laboratories
Berrimah, Northern Territory
Australia

Mark Simpson BVSc, MANZCVS
Sugarloaf Animal Hospital
West Wallsend
New South Wales
Australia

Shane Simpson BVSc (Hons), GCM(VP)
Karingal Veterinary Hospital
Frankston
Victoria
Australia

Jan Šlapeta MVDr, PhD
Sydney School of Veterinary Science
Faculty of Science
University of Sydney
New South Wales
Australia

Tegan Stephens BVSc(Merit), MANZCVS
(Unusual Pets)
Bird and Exotics Veterinary Clinic
Waterloo

Sydney
New South Wales
Australia

Linda Vogelnest BVSc, MANZCVS, FANZCVS
Specialist Veterinary Dermatologist
Associate Lecturer University of Sydney
Small Animal Specialist Hospital
New South Wales
Australia

Emma Whitlock RVN BSc (Hons), VNSc, PgDip, MCAM
Hospital Manager
Veterinary Department
Currumbin Wildlife Sanctuary
Currumbin
Queensland
Australia

Preface

The word 'herpetology' is from Greek *herpeton*, 'creeping animal' and *-logia* 'knowledge'. It is the term used to describe the study of reptiles and amphibians. Some sources describe those who keep reptiles as 'herpetoculturists' and the hobby as 'herpetoculture'. It is a hobby that has been in existence for over 300 years, with an increasing focus and enthusiasm in the last 50 years. 'Herps', as these enthusiasts are known, keep an often bewildering array of snakes, lizards, turtles, tortoises, and crocodiles in conditions ranging from sophisticated to almost primitive. From a few enthusiasts breeding reptiles for a hobby, we now see reptiles commonly kept as children's pets.

In the last 40 years, the veterinary care of these fascinating animals has grown at an amazing rate. From a few pioneers seeing a handful of clients, we now see reptiles presented for veterinary care presented at many companion animal practices, as well as a growing number of specialist reptile hospitals and clinics. Reptile medicine and surgery, once unheard of in the veterinary curriculum, is now a growing subject area in most university veterinary courses.

We still have a long way to go, but our body of knowledge is growing exponentially.

Reptile medicine is one area where, on an almost daily basis, clinicians will see something that has either never been described, or only a handful of cases seen somewhere else. Given this, no textbook can hope to hold all knowledge, even for a brief period of time.

This book does not attempt to be an encyclopaedic reference encompassing all veterinary knowledge on reptile medicine. That task is beyond the scope (and word count) of this book. Rather, it is a handbook designed to assist busy clinicians in their day to day approach to the increasing flow of reptile patients, and as a study guide for veterinarians and veterinary students. To that extent we have gathered a team of veterinary experts from around the world and sought their input in their areas of expertise.

We hope that the reader finds this book a useful tool to assist them in their approach to reptile medicine and surgery. If it helps you to provide better care, or to help you solve a problem, we will consider this book a success.

Bob Doneley, Deborah Monks, Robert Johnson, Brendan Carmel

1

Taxonomy and Introduction to Common Species
Bob Doneley

Taxonomy

Class Reptilia is one of the largest groups of vertebrates, with over 10,000 species. It is also the oldest, evolving some 310–320 million years ago during the Carboniferous period. They share several common characteristics: all are covered with scales or scutes and are ectothermic. Most lay amniotic eggs (oviparity), although some are live bearers (viviparity, including ovovivaparity). They may be carnivorous, omnivorous or herbivorous.

Class Reptilia is made up of four orders: Squamata, Testudines, Crocodilia and Rhynchocephalia (Table 1.1). Each order is further divided into sub-orders, families, genera and species.

Squamata

Squamates are characterized by their scaled skin, which is shed periodically (ecdysis), and a moveable quadrate bone that allows the maxilla to open wide relative to the rest of the skull. The order is divided into three sub-orders: Lacertilia (the lizards), Serpentes (the snakes) and Amphisbaenia (the worm lizards), although some classifications place Amphisbaenia within Lacertilia.

Lacertilia has five infraorders based mainly on morphological similarities between family groups. These are the Diploglossa (including the glass lizards and the American legless lizards), Gekkota (the geckos, the blind lizards and the legless lizards), Iguania (including the agamids, chameleons, iguanas, anoles, collared lizards and the neotropical ground lizards), Platynota (varanids and Gila monsters) and Scincomorpha (including skinks, tegus, plated lizards and spiny-tail lizards). Most are omnivorous or carnivorous. They are primarily oviparous, although some are ovoviviparous.

Serpentes has two infraorders: Alethinophidia (including the boas, pythons, vipers, elapids, colubrids, file snakes and rattle snakes) and Scolecophidia (the blind snakes). All snakes are carnivorous. Most are oviparous, although some are ovoviviparous.

Amphisbaenia has five families found in the northern hemisphere, Africa and South America. They are largely legless squamates with rudimentary eyes capable of only detecting light (two species have rudimentary forelimbs). Their skin is loosely attached to the body, and appears to be their means of locomotion; the skin moves and 'drags' the body behind it. They are carnivorous, with strong jaws and interlocking teeth. Most species lay eggs, although some are known to be ovoviviparous.

Testudines

Testudines, sometimes known as Chelonia, are the turtles, tortoises and terrapins. They are characterized by a bony or cartilaginous

Reptile Medicine and Surgery in Clinical Practice, First Edition. Edited by Bob Doneley, Deborah Monks, Robert Johnson and Brendan Carmel.
© 2018 John Wiley & Sons Ltd. Published 2018 by John Wiley & Sons Ltd.

Table 1.1 Reptile orders.

Order and sub-order	Common name	Species (*n*)
Squamata	Squamates	9,671
Lacertilia	Lizards	5,987
Serpentes	Snakes	3,496
Amphisbaenia	Worm lizards	188
Testudines	Turtles, tortoises and terrapins	341
Crocodylia	Crocodiles, gharials, caimans and alligators	25
Rhynchocephalia	Tuataras	1

shell developed from their ribs. There is some confusion in the terminology. In North America, 'turtle' is used to describe the whole order, while in Europe and Australia it refers to freshwater and sea-dwelling chelonians, with 'tortoise' used to describe terrestrial, non-swimming species. 'Terrapin' is a term used to describe several small species of turtle living in fresh or brackish water. Terrapins do not form a taxonomic unit and are not closely related. There are two suborders of Testudines: the Pleurodirans (three families), also called the side-necked or long-necked turtles, have long necks that are folded sideways to align them with the shell; the Cryptodirans (eleven families), or short-neck turtles and tortoises, pull their neck straight back to conceal their head within the shell. Sea turtles are Cryptodirans, although they have lost the ability to retract their heads.

Crocodylia

Crocodylia, an order of large, predatory, semi-aquatic reptiles, is divided into three families: Crocodylidae (the true crocodiles), Alligatoridae (the alligators and caimans) and Gavialidae (the gharial and false gharial).

Rhynchocephalia

Rhynchocephalia is a primitive order of lizard-like reptiles that includes only one living species, the *Tuatara* (*Sphenodon punctatus*) of New Zealand. There is debate as to whether *S. guntheri* is a separate species. They are slow-growing, reaching sexual maturity at 10–20 years, and breed until they are at least 60 years old. It takes the female between one to three years to develop eggs and up to seven months to form the shell. It then takes between 12 and 15 months from copulation to hatching. Thus, reproduction occurs at two- to five-yearly intervals, the longest of any reptile.

Tuatara lack external ears and possess a parietal eye (a light-sensitive spot located on the top of the animal's head, thought to play a role in setting circadian rhythms). They are capable of autotomy and have only rudimentary hemipenes. *Tuatara* have unique dentition, namely two rows of acrodont teeth in the maxilla and one row in the mandible.

Commonly Kept Species

Key
The following abbreviations are used in this section: d, days G, gestation I, incubation m, months O, oviparous OV, ovoviviparous PBT, preferred body temperature y, years

Tables

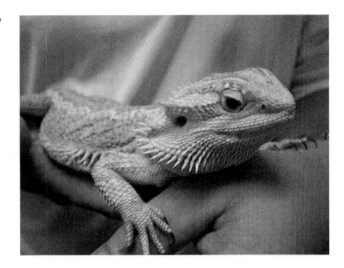

Figure 1.1 Bearded dragons (courtesy of Bob Doneley).

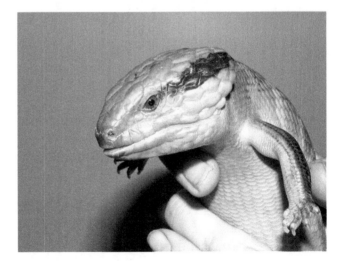

Figure 1.2 Blue-tongued skinks (courtesy of Bob Doneley).

Table 1.2 Lizards.

Reptile	Origin	Species	Habitat	Diet	Sexual maturity	Mode of reprod.	Incubation or Gestation	Thermal gradient (°C)	PBT (°C)	Relative humidity (%)	Longevity (years)
Bearded dragon (Figure 1.1)	Australia	Most common: inland or central (*Pogona vitticeps*) eastern (*P. barbata*) blacksoil (*P. henrylawsoni*) dwarf (*P. minor*) Others include: western (*P. minima*) northwest (*P. mitchelli*) Nullarbor (*P. nullarbor*) Kimberley (*P. microlepitoda*)	Terrestrial	Omnivorous, although the juveniles are initially insectivorous but will eat vegetables and flowers as they grow	9–24 m [a]	O	(I) 61–74 d at 30–31 °C (*P. vitticeps*)	28–40	35	25–40	10–15
Blue-tongued skink (Figure 1.2)	Australia	eastern (*Tiliqua scincoides scincoides*) pygmy (*T. adelaidensis*) centralian (*T. multifasciata*) blotched (*T. nigrolutea*) western (*T. occipitalis*)	Terrestrial	Omnivorous	18–36 m [b]	OV	(G) 3–5 m	28–32 (higher for inland species)	25–35	25–40	10–15
Shingleback	Australia	Also known as bobtail lizard (*T. rugosa*)	Terrestrial	Omnivorous	18–36 m [c]	OV	(I) 4–5 m	36–40	25–45	25–40	10–15
Frilled lizard	Australia	*Chlamydosaurus kingii*	Primarily arboreal	Primarily insectivorous but will accept some vegetables	12–18 m (male) to 2–3 y (female)	O	(I) 60–90 d	32–37	28–38	50–70	10–15

[a] Depending on species (small species mature younger than larger species).
[b] Male matures earlier than female.
[c] This species forms close pair bonding and should be paired before sexual maturity.

Table 1.3 Geckos.

Reptile	Origin	Species	Habitat	Diet	Sexual maturity	Mode of reprod.	Incubation or Gestation	Thermal gradient (°C)	PBT (°C)	Relative humidity (%)	Longevity (years)
Leopard gecko	Pakistan, northern India and Asian desert regions	*Eublepharis macularius*	Terrestrial	Insectivorous	1 y	O	(I) 45–60 d	21–32	26	20–40	6–10 (large males can live up to 20)
Tokay gecko	North-east India, Nepal, Indonesia and the Philippines	Two species: *Gekko gecko* and *G. g. azhari*	Arboreal	Insectivorous	1–2 y	O	(I) 60–100 d	27–28	25–31	55–80	10–20
Knob-tailed gecko	Australia	9 species; most commonly kept: three-lined (*Nephrurus levis*) central rough (*N. amyae*)	Terrestrial	Insectivorous	7–12 m	O	(I) 57–70 d (*N. levis*) 77–94 d (*N. amyae*)	20–30	26	Keep one end of the enclosure moist	7–8 (*N. levis*); 9–11 (*N. amyae*)
Crested gecko	New Caledonia	*Correlophus ciliatus*, also known as the New Caledonian crested gecko, Guichenot's giant gecko or eyelash gecko	Arboreal	Insectivorous	6–9 m (male) 12 m (female)	O	(I) 60–90 d[a]	21–29	Heat intolerant	50–70	15–20

[a] At room temperature; up to 120 days at cooler temperatures.

Table 1.4 Chameleons.

Reptile	Origin	Species	Habitat	Diet	Sexual maturity	Mode of reprod.	Incubation or Gestation	Thermal gradient (°C)	PBT (°C)	Relative humidity (%)	Longevity (years)
Veiled chameleon (Figure 1.3)	Saudi Arabia and Yemen	(Chamaeleo calyptratus), also known as the Yemen chameleon	Arboreal	Insectivorous but will take some vegetables and fruit	1 y	O	120–270 d	24–35 by day	–	50–60	4–8
Panther chameleon	Madagascar	Furcifer pardalis	Arboreal	Insectivorous	7 m	O	240 d	24–35	–	50–70	5–7
Green iguana (Figure 1.4)	Mexico, Central America and the Caribbean	Iguana iguana	Arboreal	Herbivorous	18 m	O	70–105 d	26–35	35	65–75	15–20
Chinese water dragon	China and Indochina	Physignathus cocincinus, also known as Thai water dragon, green water dragon, and Asian water dragon	Arboreal	Insectivorous, although they will eat some vegetables	1–2 y	O	55–65 d	29–33	–	40–80	15–25
Varanids	Australia, Africa, Asia and Indonesia	Currently 78 species recognized[a]	Most terrestrial but some semi-arboreal and some semi-aquatic	Carnivorous	3–5 y	O	170–265 d	30–40	35–36	60–80	10–20

[a] Some of the more common species include: Lace monitor (Varanus varius), Australia; Gould's monitor (V. gouldii, also known as the sand monitor), Australia; Merton's water monitor (V. mertensi), Australia; Savannah monitor (V. exanthematicus, also known as Bosc's monitor), Africa; Nile monitor (V. niloticus), Africa; Black-throated monitor (V. albigularis ionidesi), Africa.

Table 1.5 Snakes.

Reptile	Origin	Species	Habitat	Diet	Sexual maturity	Mode of reprod.	Incubation or Gestation	Thermal gradient (°C)	PBT (°C)	Relative humidity (%)	Longevity (years)
Carpet pythons	Australia	3 species, with 4 subspecies[a,b]	Semi-arboreal	Carnivorous	18–24 m (male); 24–36 m (female)	O	55–65 d when incubated at 31°C	20–32	29–30	40–80[c]	15–30
Green python (Figure 1.6)	Australia and Papua New Guinea	Also known as chondropython or green tree python (*M. viridis*)	Arboreal	Carnivorous	After 2.4 y (male); After 3.6 y (female)	O	50 d when incubated at 31°C	20–32	30–32	40–70[d]	15–20
Antaresia spp.	Australia	Spotted python (*Antaresia maculosa*); Children's python (*A. childreni*), pygmy python (*A perthensis*); Stimson python (*A. stimsoni*) – 2 subspecies: western (*A. s. stimsoni*) and eastern (*A. s. orientalis*)	Terrestrial	Carnivorous	2–3 y	O	55–60 d at 31°C	26–32	29–32	50–70	15–30
Aspidites spp.	Australia	Black-headed python (*Aspidites melanocephalus*) and the Woma python (*A. ramsayi*)	Terrestrial	Carnivorous	18–24 m	O	50–60 d at 31°C	28–36	28–32	40–50	15–25
Boa constrictor	Mexico, South America and the Caribbean	*Boa constrictor constrictor*, also known as the red-tailed boa	Semi-arboreal	Carnivorous	3–4 y	OV	100–120 d	27–33	–	50–70	20–30

(*Continued*)

Table 1.5 (Continued)

Reptile	Origin	Species	Habitat	Diet	Sexual maturity	Mode of reprod.	Incubation or Gestation	Thermal gradient (°C)	PBT (°C)	Relative humidity (%)	Longevity (years)
Rainbow boa	South America	*Epicrates cenchria*, also known as the slender boa	Terrestrial	Carnivorous	2.5–4 y	OV	150 d	21–30	–	70–90	15–20
Ball python	Africa	*Python regius*, also known as the royal python	Terrestrial	Carnivorous	11–18 m (male), 20–36 m (female)	O	50–60 d	27–32	50–60	–	20–35
Corn snake	North America	*Pantherophis guttatus*	Terrestrial or semi-arboreal	Carnivorous	2 y	O	70 d	24–30	–	50–60	20–25

[a] Centralian carpet python (*Morelia bredli*); South western carpet python (*M. ariegate*); Diamond python (*M. spilota spilota*); Jungle carpet python (*M. s. cheynei*; Figure 1.5); Coastal carpet python (*M. s. mcdowelli*); Murray/Darling carpet python (*M. s. metcalfei*); Darwin carpet python (*M. s. ariegate*).
[b] In addition to these, there are four other *Morelia* species: the scrub python (*M. amesthistina*), the rough-scaled python (*M. carinata*), the green python (*M. viridis*, see below) and the Oenpelli python (*M. oenpelliensis*).
[c] Varies with species but in this range.
[d] Avoid constant high humidity.

Table 1.6 Turtles.

Reptile	Origin	Species	Habitat	Diet	Sexual maturity	Mode of reprod.	Incubation or Gestation	Thermal gradient (°C)	PBT (°C)	Relative humidity (%)	Longevity (years)
Eastern long-necked turtle	Australia	*Chelodina longicollis*, also known as the snake-necked turtle	Semi-aquatic	Carnivorous	7–8 y (male); 10–12 y (female)	O	90–150 d	Water 24–26 Air 22–26	–	–	30–40 (possibly longer)
Broad shelled turtle	Australia	*C. expansa*	Semi-aquatic	Carnivorous	9–11 y (male), 14–15 y (female)	O	In response to low temperatures, embryos enter a diapause, which enables them to survive over winter in nests, resulting in a year-long incubation period	Water 22–26	–	–	30–40 (or longer)
Short-necked turtles (*Emydura spp*; Figure 1.8)	Australia	The genus *Emydura* is still taxonomically controversial[a,b]	Semi-aquatic	Initially carnivorous but become omnivorous as they get older	5–6 y (male), 10–12 y (female)[c]	O	45–60 d	25–28	–	–	15–20
Saw-shelled turtle	Australia	*Myuchelys latisternum*	Semi-aquatic	Predominantly carnivorous but will take some vegetables	10 y (male), 20 y (female)	O	60 d at 30°C	Water 24–28	–	–	Over 40
Mary river turtle	Australia	*Elusor macrurus*	Semi-aquatic	Omnivorous	25 y (male), 30 y (female)	O	47–64 d at 28–29°C	Water 24–28	–	–	75–100

(*Continued*)

Table 1.6 (Continued)

Reptile	Origin	Species	Habitat	Diet	Sexual maturity	Mode of reprod.	Incubation or Gestation	Thermal gradient (°C)	PBT (°C)	Relative humidity (%)	Longevity (years)
Pig-nosed turtle	Northern Australia and southern New Guinea	*Carettochelys insculpta*, also known as the pitted-shelled turtle or Fly river turtle	Semi-aquatic, verging on completely aquatic	Omnivorous	16 y (male), 18 y (female)	O	86–102 d	Water 26–30 Air 26–28	–	–	35–40
Red-eared slider	Southern United States and northern Mexico[d]	*Trachemys scripta elegans* or red-eared terrapin	Semi-aquatic, freshwater	Carnivorous as juveniles, becoming omnivorous as they get older	3–5 y	O	59–112 d, depending on temperature	Water 24–30 Air 24–32	–	–	30–50
Musk turtle	South-east Canada and eastern United States	*Sternotherus odoratus*	Semi-aquatic	Predominantly carnivorous but adults will eat some vegetable material	4 y (male), 10 y (female)	O	65–86 d	Water 20–23 Air 23–30	–	–	50
Painted turtle	Southern Canada, the United States and northern Mexico	*Chrysemys picta* with 4 subspecies: eastern (*C. p. picta*), western (*C. p. bellii*), southern (*C. p. dorsalis*), Midland (*C. p. marginata*)	Semi-aquatic	Omnivorous	2–4 y (male); 6–10 y (female)	O	72–80 d	Water 24–27 Air 27–32	17–23	–	25–30

[a] Accepted species are currently: Macquarie turtle (*E. macquarii*); Murray river turtle (*E. m. macquarii*); Krefft's turtle (*E. m. krefftii*); – Fraser island short-neck turtle (*E. m. nigra*); Cooper creek turtle (*E. m. emmotti*); Red-bellied short-necked turtle or Jardine river turtle (*E. subglobosa*); Red-bellied short-necked turtle (*E. s. subglobosa*); Worrell's short-necked turtle (*E. s. worrelli*); Northern yellow-faced turtle (*E. tanybaraga*); Victoria river red-faced turtle (*E. victoriae*).

[b] As well as the genus *Emydura*, other short-neck turtles include the Mary River turtle (*Elusor macrurus*) and the saw shell turtle (*Myuchelys latisternum*); see individual entries.

[c] Some species may have delayed onset of sexual maturity.

[d] This is an invasive species and has become established in the wild elsewhere in the world.

Table 1.7 Tortoises.

Reptile	Origin	Species	Habitat	Diet	Sexual maturity	Mode of reprod.	Incubation or Gestation	Thermal gradient (°C)	PBT (°C)	Relative humidity (%)	Longevity (years)
Mediterranean tortoises	North Africa, western Asia and Europe	Currently 5 species accepted. Likely that some will be reclassified based on DNA differences[a]	Terrestrial	Herbivorous	9–12 y	O	55–100 d, depending on species	21–32	–	30–50	30–100
Sulcata	Northern Africa and southern edge of the Sahara desert	Centrochelys sulcata, also known as the African spurred tortoise	Terrestrial; burrows into the ground to escape the heat	Herbivorous	5–8 y	O	90–120 d	29–40	–	Low	50–150
Leopard tortoise	Eastern and Southern Africa, from Sudan to the southern Cape	Stigmochelys pardalis	Terrestrial	Herbivorous	6–15 y	O	150–400 d at 28–32°C, often following a cooling period of 30 d at 18–24°C	24–38	–	Low	80–100
Box turtle	United States and Mexico	Genus Terrapene are terrestrial members of the American pond turtle family (Emydidae). Currently, 4 species are classified within the genus and 12 taxa are distinguished[b]	Terrestrial	Omnivorous	7–10 y	O	56–75 d at 29°C	24–32	–	60–80	50–100
Star tortoise (Figure 1.10)	India and Sri Lanka	Geochelone elegans, also known as the Indian star tortoise	Terrestrial	Herbivorous	6–8 y (male), 10–12 y (female)	O	90–170 d	24–32	–	<40	30–80
Red-footed tortoise	Northern South America	Chelonoidis carbonaria, also classified as Geochelone carbonaria	Terrestrial	Omnivorous	6–8 y (male), 8–12 y (female)	O	105–202 d	21–30	–	50–70	20–30

[a] Russian tortoise (*Testudo horsfieldii*), also known as Horsfield's tortoise; Hermann's tortoise (*T. hermanni*); Spur-thighed or Greek tortoise (*T. graeca*; Figure 1.9); Kleinmann's tortoise (*T. kleinmanni*), also known as the Egyptian tortoise; Marginated tortoise (*T. marginata*).

[b] Common box turtle (*T. carolina*); Florida box turtle (*T. c. bauri*); Eastern box turtle (*T. c. carolina*); Gulf coast box turtle (*T. c. major*); Mexican box turtle (*T. c. mexicana*); Three-toed box turtle (*T. c. triunguis*); Yucatán box turtle (*T. c. yucatana*); Coahuilan box turtle (*T. coahuila*); Spotted box turtle (*T. nelsoni*); Northern spotted box turtle (*T. n. klauberi*); Southern spotted box turtle (*T. n. nelsoni*); Ornate box turtle (*T. ornata*), also known as the Western box turtle; Desert box turtle (*T. o. luteola*).

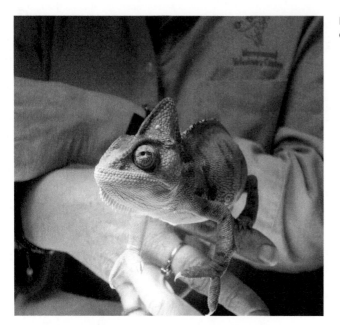

Figure 1.3 Veiled chameleon (courtesy of Brendan Carmel).

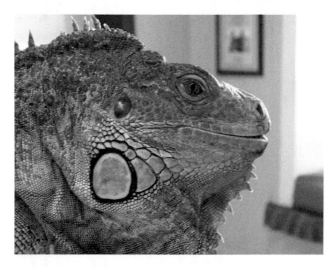

Figure 1.4 Green iguana (courtesy of Bob Doneley).

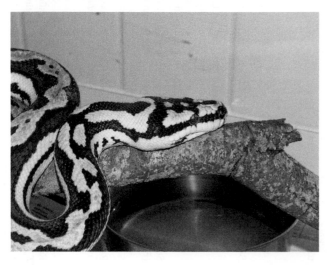

Figure 1.5 Jungle carpet python (*Morelia spilota cheynei*; courtesy of Bob Doneley).

Figure 1.6 Green python (courtesy of Bob Doneley).

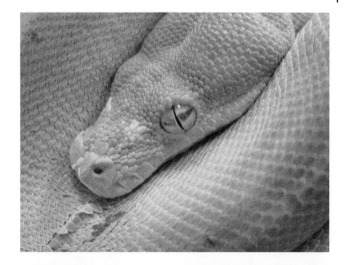

Figure 1.7 Corn snake (courtesy of Robert Johnson).

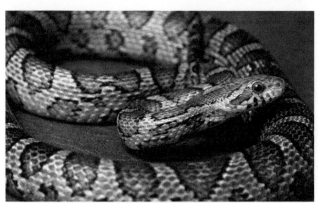

Figure 1.8 Short-necked turtle (*Emydura* spp; courtesy of Bob Doneley).

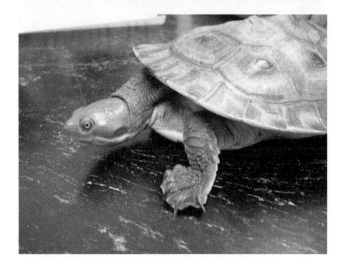

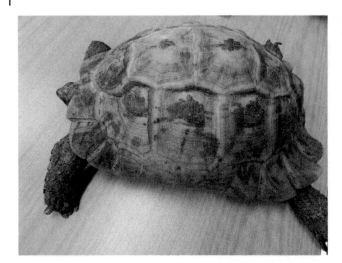

Figure 1.9 Spur-thighed or Greek tortoise (*Testudo graeca*; courtesy of John Chitty).

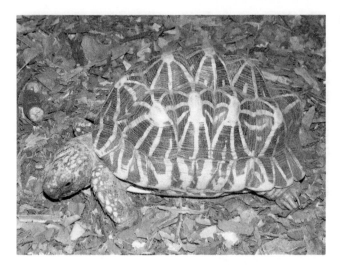

Figure 1.10 Star tortoise (courtesy of Bob Doneley).

2

Anatomy and Physiology of Reptiles

Bairbre O'Malley

Introduction

As a veterinary surgeon it is impossible to treat reptiles without a thorough understanding of their anatomy and physiology. For example, to anaesthetize a turtle we need to be aware of the challenges of a species with a large lung volume, no diaphragm or intercostal muscles and known to able to breath hold for many hours. When presented with an iguana for tail amputation, the veterinary surgeon needs to understand the importance of not always stitching the wound site as in many cases a new stump may regenerate. Likewise, therapeutic and enteral treatments will fail unless the vet understands ectothermy and the need to provide adequate temperature levels to allow drugs and food to be metabolized and digested. This chapter aims to help vets to gain a basic understanding of structure and function of chelonians, lizards and snakes and highlights their relevance to clinical practice.

Metabolic Rate

Reptile metabolism is slow, being one-fifth to one-seventh that of a mammal of equivalent size. Metabolic rate varies with temperature, diet, size and species. For example, the primitive New Zealand tuatara has one of the lowest metabolic rates while the varanid monitors have the highest metabolism of most lizards. In general, passive 'sit and wait' predators such as pythons and boas also have lower metabolism while active 'seek and hunter' insectivorous lizards have higher metabolic rates.

Thermoregulation

Reptiles are ectothermic: they are unable to generate their own body temperature. Unlike mammals that draw their heat from food, reptiles derive their heat from the environment. Ectothermy has some advantages in that reptiles do not need major food sources to meet energy demands. For example, a reptile of equivalent size as a mouse will have just one-tenth the energy requirement. This lower energy requirement and efficient food conversion has enabled reptiles to endure long hibernation and night cooling and to survive in arid deserts. Reptiles can use basking, changes in skin colouration and cardiovascular shunting to increase body temperature, and use shade seeking, soaking in water and gular fluttering to reduce body temperature.

The main disadvantage of ectothermy is that all activity is limited by ambient temperature, such that many reptiles become inactive and vulnerable at night and have to hibernate when temperatures drop. They have a much lower aerobic capacity than endotherms and need to switch rapidly to

Reptile Medicine and Surgery in Clinical Practice, First Edition. Edited by Bob Doneley, Deborah Monks, Robert Johnson and Brendan Carmel.
© 2018 John Wiley & Sons Ltd. Published 2018 by John Wiley & Sons Ltd.

anaerobic metabolism for any vigorous activity such as diving, chasing prey or escaping predation. Although anaerobic metabolism is independent of temperature, it drains energy reserves tenfold. As reptiles also rapidly build up lactic acid, they easily get fatigued so cannot sustain intense activity levels for more than two to three minutes.

Preferred Optimum Temperature Zone

The preferred optimum temperature zone is the temperature range of the reptile's natural habitat. It usually lies between 20°C and 38°C but can vary by 4–10°C, depending on the species. Within this range, each species has a preferred body temperature for each metabolic function such as predation, digestion and reproduction (Table 2.1).

Mechanism of Thermoregulation

Reptiles derive their heat via heliothermy or thigmothermy or a combination of the two. Heliothermy means obtaining radiant heat by basking in the sun and is used by chelonian and diurnal lizards. Thigmothermy is acquiring thermal heat via conduction with hot surfaces and is common in nocturnal or forest species. Reptiles also use physiological and behavioural means of thermoregulation. They raise their body temperature by increasing their heart rate to pump warm blood from the core to the periphery. Their three-chambered heart can also shunt blood from right to left, to the peripheral blood vessels bypassing the evaporative cooling of the lungs. Lizards also heat up by increasing melanin pigment in their skin or by selecting a dark background. Snakes coil up to conserve heat and uncoil to lose heat, while lizards angle their body axis perpendicular to the sun to heat up and face the sun to cool down. Many lizards cool down by panting or gular fluttering, which is when they hold their mouth open to vibrate their throat. They also cool down by shade seeking and plunging into water.

Table 2.1 Preferred body temperature (PBT) of commonly kept species.

Species	PBT (°C)
Turtles:	
Eastern long-necked turtle (*Chelodina longicollis*)	26
Box turtles (*Terrapine* sp.)	26–32
Snakes:	
Children's python (*Antaresia childreni*)	30–33
Ball python (*Python regius*)	c. 29
Carpet python (*Morelia spilota*)	29–33
Diamond python (*Morelia spilota spilota*)	29
Burmese python (*Python molurus*)	c. 29
Water python (*Liasis fuscus*)	34
Boa constrictor (*Boa constrictor constrictor*)	c. 29
Corn snake (*Elaphe guttata*)	25–29
Lizards:	
Eastern blue-tongued lizard (*Tiliqua scincoides scincoides*)	28–32
Shingleback lizard (*Tiliqua rugosa*)	33
Eastern bearded dragon (*Pogona barbata*)	35–39
Lace Monitor (*Varanus varius*)	35
Green iguana (*Iguana iguana*)	28–32
Tortoises:	
Most species	28–31

Sources: Carmel and Johnson 2014; Rossi 2006.

External Anatomy

Chelonia

The dome of the shell is called the carapace and the flat under part the plastron. The joint between is called the bridge. The shell is formed from dermal bone and consists of about 60 bones formed from the modified pectoral and pelvic limb girdles, trunk vertebrae, sacrum and ribs. These are covered by keratinized epidermal scales called scutes that are innervated and bleed if damaged.

Growth occurs by the addition of new keratin layers to the base of each scute. The limb girdles lie inside the fused shell and are attached by powerful fan shaped pectoral and pelvic muscles.

Anatomical modification depends on whether the species is terrestrial, marine or freshwater. Terrestrial species have a high-dome carapace with short stubby legs. Freshwater species have webbed feet and a smooth shell. Marine species are very streamlined with a flat soft shell and their metacarpus/tarsus and phalanges are elongated for swimming, similar to flippers. Aquatic species can hold their breath for long periods and use anaerobic and non-pulmonary respiration through skin, pharynx and cloaca.

Lizards

Although lizards are modified for swimming, flying and climbing, they are generally elongated and circular in cross-section. Bearded dragons, however, are horizontally compressed while arboreal lizards such as the chameleon are vertically compressed. Some species, like iguanas and chameleons, have dramatic sexual dimorphic characteristics: crests, spines, heavy jowls and pronounced femoral pores. The tail is usually long and can be prehensile, as in chameleons, or as a site of fat storage, as in the leopard gecko. Autotomy means self-amputation and is a mechanism present in some species such as iguanas, bearded dragons, skinks and geckos, to escape predators. The tail drops off owing to vertical fracture planes and in many cases a new tail tip may regrow. Many geckos have adhesive lamella on their digits to allow then walk vertically on smooth surfaces while the chameleon has pincer-like zygodactyl feet adapted for climbing.

Snakes

The snake has evolved its body for crawling so has few external features (Figure 2.1). Elongation has also resulted in organ asymmetry with the right-side organs lying cranial to and being larger than the left. The cranial third contains the heart, trachea, oesophagus, thyroid and proximal lung. The middle third has the stomach. liver, lung, spleen and pancreas. The caudal third has the small and large intestines, kidneys and gonads. The belly is slightly flattened to aid locomotion with single scales called gastropeges.

Integument

Contrary to popular belief, reptiles do not have a 'slimy skin' but in fact very dry skin, because they have few skin glands. Water loss is prevented by a heavily keratinized epithelium with a lipid layer. There are scent-type glands under the thigh in some lizards and musk glands near the cloaca in some snakes and turtles. These tubular skin invaginations are better developed in males and producing a waxy secretion that has a pheromonal function.

The epidermis is both thick and thin to form scales. These scales provide protection but also play a role in permeability. Within the epidermis there are three layers. The inner layer is called the stratum germinatum and consists of cuboidal cells that produce the protein keratin and the dividing cells of the intermediate layer. The intermediate layer contains lipids that help to provide a water permeable barrier in the skin. The outer stratum corneum is heavily keratinized into the scales. This thick keratinized skin means that reptile have far less sensory innervation in their skin, which is why they are at risk of thermal burns.

The dermis consists of connective tissue, blood, lymphatic vessels and nerves. Pigment cells or chromatophores provide elaborate colouration, most notably seen in the chameleon. In some species of lizards, such as skinks, the dermis has bony plates, called osteoderms, and in chelonia this has fused with the vertebrae to form the shell.

(a)

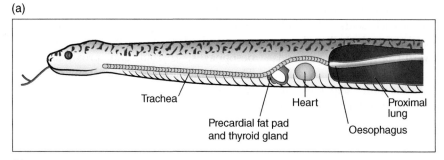

(b)

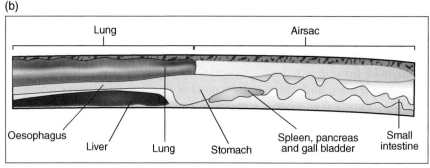

(c)

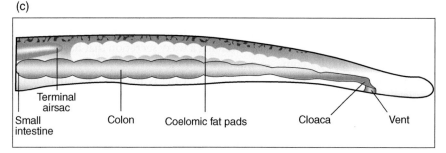

Figure 2.1 Internal anatomy of a snake: a) Cranial third: trachea, thyroid, heart, proximal lung and oesphagus; b) Middle third: liver, lung, stomach, spleen and pancreas; c) Caudal third: colon and coelomic fat pads.

Ecdysis

Ecdysis is the shedding of skin; it is controlled by the thyroid gland. Lizards and chelonians shed piecemeal. Snakes tend to shed the whole skin in one piece from snout to vent. It is colourless because the pigment cells are in the dermal layer. In a healthy snake the whole process can take up to abut 2 weeks. During ecdysis, the cells in the intermediate layer replicate to form a new three-layer epidermis. Once this is complete, lymph diffuses into the area between the two layers and enzymes are released to form the cleavage zone. The old skin is shed and the new epithelium hardens to form the new skin.

Dysecdysis or failure to shed occurs when there is low environmental humidity or when the reptile is ill. Malnutrition and debilitation leads to dehydration and hypoproteinaemia, rendering them unable to produce the enzymes needed to form the cleavage zone.

Skeletal System

Skull

Reptiles are divided into two subclasses based on the presence or absence of openings in the temporal region of the skull. These

Figure 2.2 Modified anapsid skull of chelonian, lateral and dorsoventral views.

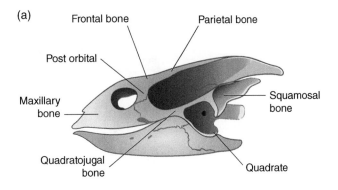

(a)

Frontal bone

Parietal bone

Post orbital

Maxillary bone

Squamosal bone

Quadratojugal bone

Quadrate

Lateral view

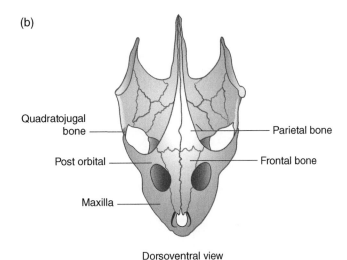

(b)

Quadratojugal bone

Parietal bone

Post orbital

Frontal bone

Maxilla

Dorsoventral view

'fenestrae' lie behind the eyes and provide better attachment for the jaw musculature (Figure 2.2).

Anapsid
Chelonia are anapsid (without arches) as they lack true temporal openings. The head is small so it can be retracted inside the shell but large adductor muscles, sturdy skull and short jaw still enables them to have a powerful bite.

Diapsid
The tuatara (Rhynchocephalia) and crocodile have two temporal openings on their skull so are truly diapsid while snakes and lizards are modified diapsid (Figure 2.3).

Lizards have only one dorsal opening while snakes have an even more modified diapsid skull, having lost the temporal arch between the two openings. This has enabled the quadrate bone to move backward and forwards with no firm connection in a condition known as streptostyly. This has given snakes and lizards a kinetic skull, which is thought to enable the upper and lower jaw to close over prey. Lizards have very strong adductor muscles which extend from the temporal region to the lower jaw enabling the jaw to snap close like a trapdoor over prey (and unwary fingers).

The snake has the most kinetic skull of all and the skull is designed to allow a reptile with a small mouth to eat large enough prey

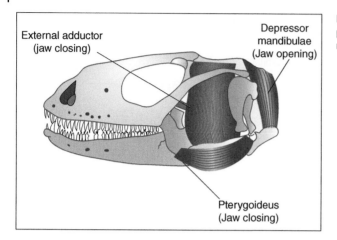

Figure 2.3 Lizard skull showing the powerful adductor (jaw closing) muscles.

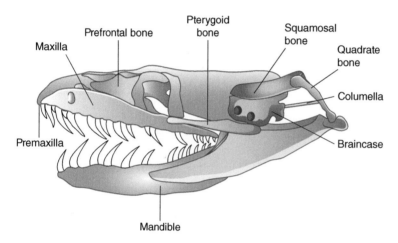

Figure 2.4 Skull of a simple snake.

to sustain its body size and length (Figure 2.4). It has no temporal arch, interorbital septum or middle ear cavity. The brain case is heavily ossified to protect it from struggling prey and all tooth bearing bones are able to move independently. Snakes lack a mandibular symphysis so the jaw bones can move apart and literally 'walk' its jaw along the prey. The quadrate bone, which articulates with the lower jaw and palatomaxillary arch, also has a very loose articulation. Snakes often yawn after a meal to allow their jawbones reposition themselves.

Vertebrae

Reptiles rest their belly along the ground so the backbone is not rigid but highly flexible. The spine is divided into presacral, sacral and caudal region. Chelonia have 18 presacral vertebrae – 8 free cervical and 10 trunk vertebrae fused into the dermal bone of the shell. The neck and tail are highly flexible with well developed epaxial and hypaxial muscles. Chelonia are classed into two suborders according to their mode of retracting their head into their shell. The pleurodira or side necks are more primitive, being unable to retract their head into their shell instead placing it sideways. The cryptodira have a neck that forms a vertical 'S' bend. This has enabled them to be more successful, as they are able to retract their head completely into their shell.

Lizards have a highly mobile and flexible backbone, well developed legs and a long tail for counterbalance. All the vertebrae except the cervical vertebrae bear ribs, leaving little

flank area. Primitive lizards and tortoises have short limbs directed sideways. Advanced lizards have their limbs rotated more towards their body so that the elbow faces caudally and the knee cranially, creating better shock absorption.

Snakes have up to 400 vertebrae pre-cloacally, each with its own pair of ribs and large axial skeletal muscles (Figure 2.5). Each vertebra has five separate articulations, creating an

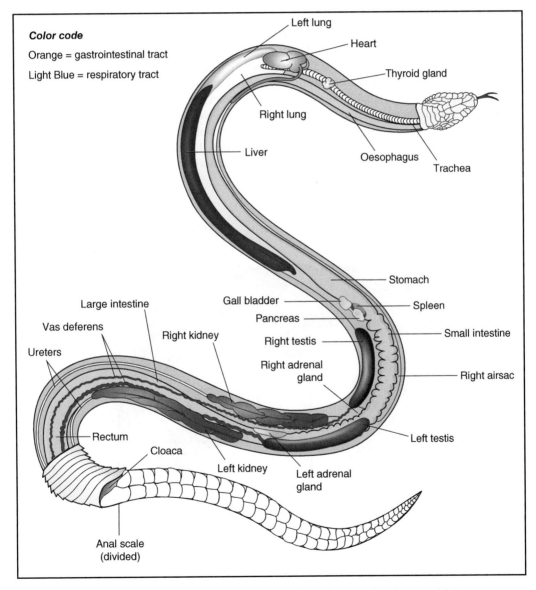

Figure 2.5 Internal anatomy of a snake (male) with coelomic fat pads removed to show caudal viscera.

extremely flexible backbone. The intercostal and hypaxial muscles not only help in locomotion but also in respiration and the passage of prey. In the process of elongation the snake has lost its pectoral and pelvic girdles. However, in some of the more primitive snakes such as boas and pythons, pelvic vestigial spurs can be seen on either side of the vent.

Cardiovascular System

In chelonians, the heart lies in the midline just caudal to the pectoral girdle (Figures 2.6 and 2.7). In most lizards (Figures 2.8 and 2.9), it lies at the level of the pectoral girdle but has descended caudally to the more mammalian location of mid-thoracoabdominal cavity in the more advanced monitor lizards. In snakes, the heart lies just cranioventral to the tracheal bifurcation, about one-quarter of the way down the body (Figure 2.1).

Chelonia, snakes and lizards have a three-chambered heart (two atria and one ventricle), whereas crocodiles have four chambers. The right atrium receives deoxygenated blood from the circulation via a large chamber the sinus venosus. There are two aortas: the left gives rise to the coeliac, cranial mesenteric and left gastric arteries before uniting with the right aorta caudal to the heart. A large ventral abdominal vein lies along the inner surface of the midline and must be avoided when making a coeliotomy incision. A renal portal system is also present (see urinary section).

The ventricle is divided into three sub chambers, the cavae venosum, arteriosum and pulmonale. Although there is no permanent division, oxygenated and deoxygenated blood never actually mixes, due to atrioventricular valves, a muscular ridge, pressure differential and the timing of ventricular contractions.

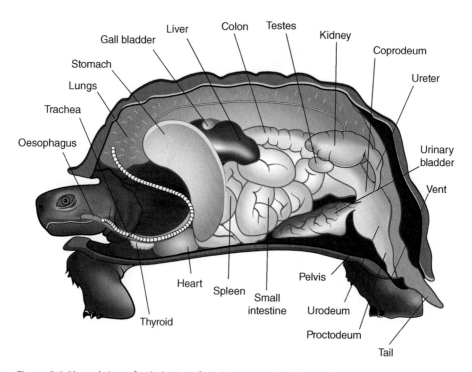

Figure 2.6 Ventral view of a chelonian after plastron and trunk muscles have been removed.

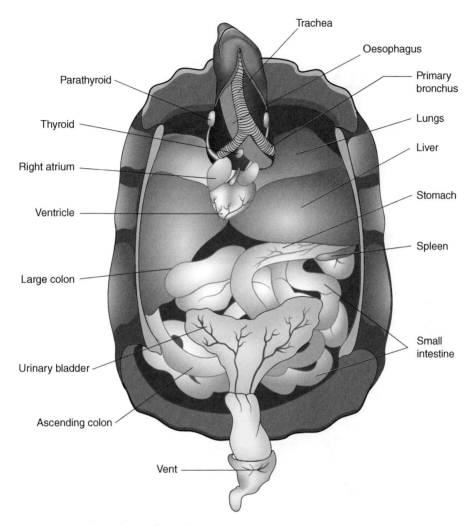

Figure 2.7 Midsagittal view of a chelonian.

Intracardiac Blood Shunting

The undivided ventricle also plays an important role in thermoregulation and the ability to breath hold because blood can be shunted towards or away from the lungs depending on pulmonary resistance. During peak respiration, pulmonary resistance is low so deoxygenated blood flows through the lungs. During periods of oxygen starvation (for example when snakes swallow prey or turtles dive) the pulmonary arteries vasoconstrict. This increases pulmonary resistance and shunts blood away from the lungs to the systemic circulation.

Clinical Significance of Blood Shunting

The ability of reptiles to shunt blood away from their lungs systemically and switch to anaerobic metabolism presents challenges for anaesthesia, especially with aquatic chelonians that can hold their breath for hours. It also explains why many reptiles with chronic pneumonia are slow to recover, as the increased lung resistance of the infection

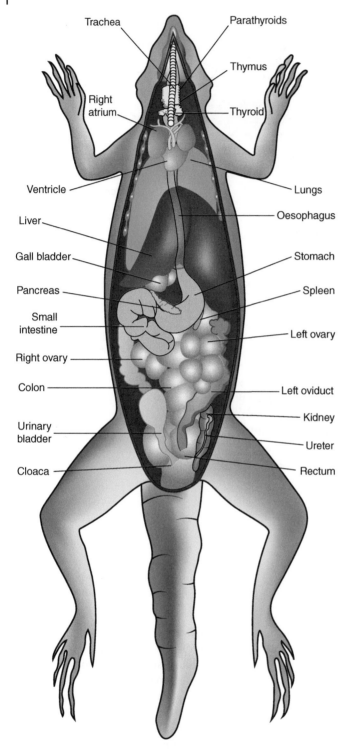

Figure 2.8 Ventral view of a female lizard.

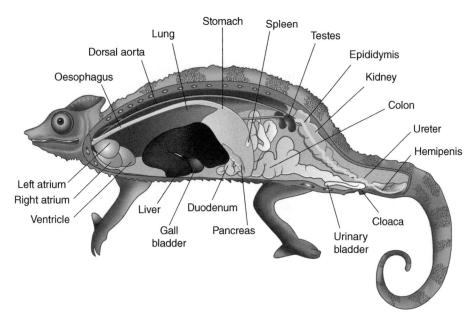

Figure 2.9 Lateral, mid-sagittal view of a male chameleon.

diverts the blood supply away from where it is most needed.

Blood Volume

Normal blood volume is approximately 5–8% body weight; 10% of this can be safely taken from a healthy reptile during blood sampling.

Blood Cells

Reptile erythrocytes are nucleated and have a longer lifespan than in mammals and birds. The haematocrit varies with temperature and season rather than high altitudes and hypoxia as in mammals. The white blood cells include heterophils, eosinophils, basophils, lymphocytes, monocytes and azurophils. Azurophils are unique to reptiles. They are like monocytes but are smaller in size and have a red-purple cytoplasm.

Immune System

Reptiles have a better developed lymphatic system than a venous system. They lack lymph nodes but have vast plexiform lymphatic networks and large reservoirs, called cisternae, at the site of mammalian lymph nodes. As the lymphatic system is so developed, dilution of blood samples with lymph during venepuncture is common.

Chelonia have a highly developed lymphatic system and this is why oedema is a common presenting symptom for many illnesses. Their skin has a network of lymphatic vessels that are widely meshed. These vessels become superficial as they near the attachment of the skin to the shell. The orbits have two lymphatic vessels that extend into both eyelids and some species, such as the red-eared terrapin, have a lymphatic ring around the base of the neck. In snakes, dilation of the lymph vessels (lymph hearts) is found on either side of the tail base where the vessels are protected by modified forked caudal vertebrae.

Respiratory System

Reptiles have large-volume lungs that function not only for gas exchange but are used for vocalization, display and buoyancy.

Upper Tract

Air enters through the external nares, the nasal sinus and internal nares. The glottis lies quite rostrally, usually just behind the tongue. It remains closed at rest, opening only for respiration via the glottis dilator muscles.

Lower Respiratory Tract

The trachea has incomplete tracheal rings, with the dorsal fourth being membranous. In contrast to mammals, the lung volume is large but only has 1% of the surface area of a mammal of equivalent size. The lung parenchyma is simple and sac like, with a honeycomb network of faveoli – the reptile unit of gaseous exchange. The mucociliary lining of the tract is primitive, making them poor at clearing exudates. There is no diaphragm and the combined pleuroperitoneal space is called the coelom. In more advanced species, such as monitor lizards, a membrane called the postpulmonary septum divides the pleural cavity from the peritoneal cavity.

There are three types of lung anatomy based on the degree of partition of the lungs. Snakes and some lizards have single-chambered, primitive unicameral lungs. Chameleons and iguanas have paucicameral (few-chambered) lungs with no intrapulmonary bronchus. Chelonians, monitor lizards and crocodiles have advanced multicameral (multichambered) lungs with an intrapulmonary bronchus.

Control of Respiration

Respiration in reptiles is controlled by rising temperature and not acid base balance and partial pressure of carbon dioxide as in mammals. A rise in temperature increases metabolic rate and hence oxygen demand, stimulating respiration and increasing tidal volume. Low oxygen levels also stimulates respiration – hence the need to be careful not to overventilate reptiles with oxygen during cardiopulmonary arrest.

Clinical Note

The lack of diaphragm and ability to cough and primitive bronchociliary transport system means that reptiles easily get respiratory disease. Reptiles suffering from pneumonia will tend to seek the cooler end of their vivarium to reduce the demand for oxygen.

Ventilation

Despite their lack of diaphragm, reptiles breathe via negative pressure breathing. Respiration is triphasic, with expiration, inspiration and relaxation (breath-holding). Air is inhaled and expired by the action of the intercostal and/or trunk muscles.

Chelonia

Chelonia have an easily visible glottis at the back of a short fleshy tongue. In cryptodira, the trachea is very short and bifurcates rapidly to allow for head retraction. The lungs are advanced, being multicameral, and occupy a large volume in the dorsal half of the body cavity. They are separated from the ventral cavity and the viscera by a thin nonmuscular postpulmonary septum. There is no expandable chest, as the ribs, sternum and backbone are modified into a hard shell, and there is no diaphragm (Figures 2.6 and 2.7). Instead, chelonians breathe by using their powerful trunk muscles to expand and contract the lungs by attachment to the postpulmonary septum.

Chelonians can hold their breath for very long periods (up to 33 hours in aquatic species) as they are very tolerant of hypoxia and are able to convert to anaerobic metabolism. They have the highest bicarbonate concentration of all vertebrates, which helps them to buffer lactic acid accumulation.

Lizards

Lizards breathe by expansion and contraction of the ribs. More primitive lizards have the heart at the level of the pectoral girdle and unicameral lungs. Intermediate species have paucicameral lungs, with some having air sacs (Figure 2.9). The more advanced species like the monitor lizards have multicameral lungs with a single intrapulmonary bronchus. As the lungs now extend cranioventrally, the heart lies more caudally in the mid-sternum.

Snakes

In snakes, the glottis is very mobile and can be extended laterally while feeding to allow breathing while ingesting prey. In the process of body elongation, more advanced species have evolved only one lung (Figures 2.1 and 2.5). The more primitive Boidae have two lungs, although the right lung is slightly longer. The lungs are simple and unicameral. Like some lizards, the caudal third is nonrespiratory and functions like an air sac. Respiration is via the dorsal and ventrolateral intercostal muscles and some species use the air sac like a bellows.

Digestive System

The digestive tract is shorter than that of mammals and can vary from the simple tract of carnivores to the larger colons and caecum of herbivores. All snakes are carnivorous. Most lizards are omnivorous or insectivorous, with only 3% being herbivorous. About 25% of the Chelonia are herbivorous.

Dentition

Reptile teeth are composed of enamel, dentine and cement but they lack a periodontal membrane. They are polyphyodontic, meaning that they are resorbed and replaced at a rapid rate during life. This enables simple teeth to be always sharp. There are three types of teeth, depending on the reptile's feeding habits. Acrodonts have teeth attached to the crest of the bone, as seen in chameleons and water dragons. Pleurodont teeth have an eroded labial side and are attached to a higher-sided labial wall (snakes and iguanas). Thecodonts have teeth embedded in a bony socket but with no periodontal membrane, as in crocodiles.

Chelonians have no teeth, so they are unable to chew but instead they have a short horny beak with sharp edges. Most snakes seen in veterinary practice have six rows of teeth – four upper and two lower. Their teeth are long, thin and backwards-pointing to prevent the escape of prey. Copious amounts of saliva are produced by the salivary glands during swallowing to moisten and lubricate the prey. In venomous species some maxillary teeth are modified into fangs.

Rear-Fanged Snakes

In about one-third of colubrids, the caudal labial salivary gland becomes modified into the Duvernoy's gland, which lies behind the eye (Figure 2.10). Venom passes from this

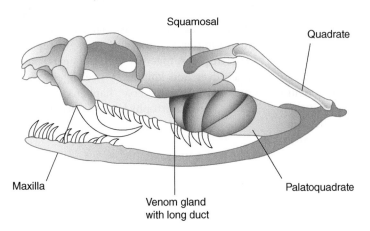

Squamosal

Quadrate

Maxilla

Venom gland
with long duct

Palatoquadrate

Figure 2.10 Skull of an advanced snake showing the location of the venom gland. The duct opens into the grooved front fangs.

gland into modified teeth at the caudal maxilla. These create rear fangs which incapacitate the prey so that it cannot damage the snake's mouth while it is being eaten.

Front-Fanged Snakes

In front-fanged snakes, the venom gland is large and separated from the labial gland and behind the eye with a large duct running rostrally into fangs at the rostral maxilla. In Elapidae, the fangs remain erect and cannot fold. Viperidae have highly modified fangs, which are so long that they have to be folded backwards in a sheath along the roof of the mouth when not raised for striking.

Gastrointestinal Tract

The stomach is small and gastroliths can often be seen on radiographs in Chelonia. In snakes, the stomach is fusiform with no well-developed cardiac sphincter, causing easy regurgitation of food. The liver is large in all reptiles and very elongated in snakes. A gall bladder is usually present and the main bile pigment is biliverdin. The pancreas is attached to the mesenteric border of the duodenal loop and in some snakes it is fused to create a splenopancreas. A caecum is prominent in herbivorous reptiles such as iguanas and tortoises. Reptiles do not have subcutaneous fat but instead store fat as 'fat bodies' in the caudal coelom or in the tail.

The rectum ends in a pouch called the cloaca (Latin for sewer.) The anterior chamber or coprodeum collects the faeces; a middle chamber called the urodeum is where the ureter and reproduction system enters and a posterior chamber called the proctodeum where all wastes collect prior to excretion. Cloacal scent glands are present in some snakes and serve as a warning mechanism, producing foul-smelling secretions.

Digestion

In snakes, digestion begins as soon as even part of the prey reaches the stomach and is a rapid process. Absorption, however, is very slow, as the whole prey is used, including the skeleton, it may take up to five days for large snake to digest a rat. The keratinous structures, such as fur, are finally excreted as an undigested pad called the felt. Herbivorous lizards are hind-gut fermenters (Figures 2.6–2.8). They have a short small intestine but the large intestine (caecum and colon) takes up 50% of the length. Gut transit time is much slower in herbivores, often taking several days to digest the cellulose food.

Clinical Note

Digestion is dependent on the ambient temperature, food composition and the physical health of the animal. The practice of force feeding solid food items to a sick or debilitated reptile leads to putrefaction, not digestion, so is not recommended.

Feeding Frequency

Reptiles, being ectoderms, can survive on a fraction of the food input of birds and mammals as they expend no energy on thermogenesis (Bennett and Nagy 1977). Their low metabolic rate and efficient food conversion allows them to eat less frequently. Large carnivorous snakes such as pythons can last months between each feed. To conserve energy, their gut and digestive enzymes become dormant during fasting and then experience a rapid increase in metabolic rate and enzymatic activity when they eat to help them digest their prey. They have also adapted their gastrointestinal tract so that when food enters, the quiescent gut rapidly hypertrophies, together with the heart, pancreas, liver and kidneys. Once digestion is completed, the reverse happens and all affected organs atrophy back to normal size.

Urinary System

The kidneys are lobed and are located in the dorsocaudal coelom. In chelonians and lizards they are symmetrical but the right kidney lies cranial to the left in snakes (Figures 2.1, 2.5–2.9). Chelonians and most lizards have a urinary bladder connected to the cloaca by a short urethra. In terrestrial chelonians that hibernate it is large and bilobed and serves as an organ for water storage. Snakes and lizards that lack a bladder reflux urine into the distal colon for water absorption. Reptile kidneys lack a loop of Henle, renal pelvis and pyramids. In male snakes and lizards, the terminal segment of the kidney has become a sexual segment, which is under androgen control.

Clinical Note

The dorsocaudal location of the kidneys means that nephromegaly commonly results in constipation – this is commonly seen in aged iguanas.

Osmoregulation

Tortoises and snakes drink by sucking up fluid while lizards can lap with their tongues. There is also some minor absorption through the skin and condensation of the nasal passages. As reptiles lack a loop of Henle, they are unable to concentrate urine beyond the osmotic values of blood plasma.

Aquatic and semi-aquatic reptiles have no need to conserve water so they excrete ammonia and urea. To help to conserve water, terrestrial species excrete uric acid, which precipitates out as pasty white urates, while aquatic species excrete urea. Although this helps to minimize water loss, one major disadvantage is that because uric acid is secreted via the kidney tubules it is still excreted even when the reptile is dehydrated. Consequently, dehydrated reptiles or those with renal problems can easily develop gout, a build-up of uric acid in the bloodstream which then precipitates into urate crystals deposited in joints (articular gout) and visceral organs (visceral gout).

Renal Portal System

The reptile kidney has a dual afferent blood supply consisting of the renal arteries and the renal portal vein. This vein bypasses the renal glomerulus and enters at the level of the kidney tubules, where it helps to secrete urates. It also plays a role in water conservation because when the glomerular filtration rate slows down during dehydration, the renal portal system will keep the renal tubules perfused to prevent necrosis. Control of the renal portal system in is unknown but it is thought that, like in birds, there is a valve system so that when the body is under stress these valves close and send blood directly to the heart.

Clinical Notes

As venous return from the hind limb goes straight to the kidney tubule, injecting drugs into the caudal half of the body could theoretically lower serum concentration and lead to renal toxicity from nephrotoxic drugs. However, this applies mainly to drugs excreted by tubular secretion so aminoglycosides such as gentamycin and amikacin, which are excreted via glomerular filtration, would not be affected. Although renal portal flow increases to the kidney when the animal is dehydrated, when the glomerulus is closed epithelial transport ceases. Thus, although more drug enters the kidney it will not necessarily be excreted.

Reproductive System

The Male

The right testis lie adjacent to the vena cava and is connected to it by tiny vessels. The left testis has its own blood supply but lies intimately with the left adrenal gland. Lizards and snakes have two extra cloacal hemipenes which lie just caudal to the cloaca. In many lizards they can be visualized externally as bulges in the proximal ventral tail base. They are blind-ended organs that become engorged by lymph and blood and evert during mating. Only one hemipene is used during copulation. The organ is erected by vascular engorgement and muscular action and is everted to protrude through the cloaca. Chelonia and crocodiles have developed the ventral proctodeum in a single intracloacal phallus which cannot be inverted. The hemipene and chelonian phallus is solely an organ of reproduction so can be amputated if damaged or necrotic.

The Female

The female has paired ovaries and oviducts which lie at the same level cranial to the kidneys in chelonians and lizards and lies asymmetrically in snakes. The ovaries function in the production of oestrogens and gametogenesis. They are saccular in shape and covered with follicles. The right ovary lies close to the vena cava while the left ovary lies close to the left adrenal gland. The oviducts not only provide egg transport but also albumin, protein and calcium for egg formation. In viviparous reptiles the uterine section is thickened and muscular to hold the developing embryo.

Endocrine System

Thyroid Glands

In chelonians and snakes, this gland is unpaired and spherical and lies just ventral to the trachea cranial the heart. It can be paired, bi-lobed (most common) or unpaired in lizards. It functions for metabolism (subject to temperature) and plays an important role in shedding and growth.

Parathyroid Gland

Unlike in mammals, the parathyroid glands are not found within the thyroid gland but are located near the thymus or ultimobranchial bodies. Chelonians and snakes have two pairs while lizards have one or two, depending on the species. The parathyroids control calcium and phosphorous levels. Lizards and chelonians on low calcium diets develop hypocalcaemia, which stimulates increase production of parathyroid hormone. This then acts to mobilize calcium from the

bones to increase serum calcium. Nutritional secondary hyperparathyroidism and osteopenia eventually results.

Adrenal Glands

These are yellow or red in colour and lie retroperitoneally in chelonians and closely adherent to the gonads in lizards and snakes.

Pancreas

This forms a C-shaped loop in chelonians. In lizards it has three parts and in snakes it is often pyramidal in shape and is often intimately linked to the spleen. As in mammals, it has both exocrine and endocrine functions.

Nervous System

Reptiles have 12 cranial nerves. The brain comprises 1% of the body mass and reptiles have well-developed optic lobes, reflecting their excellent vision. Unlike in mammals, the spinal cord extends to the tail tip and there is no cauda equina. The spinal cord has locomotor centres, giving it some local autonomy from the brain. This means that spinal cord injuries could have a better prognosis than in mammals.

Senses

Hearing

Only crocodiles have an external ear. In other reptile species the tympanic membrane is the outer limit of the middle ear and is covered by modified skin. The middle ear has only one bone, called the columella, which is attached to the tympanic membrane and the quadrate bone of the lower jaw. Vibrations pass from the air or ground to the tympanic membrane to the columella, which then moves the peri-lymphatic fluid to give rise to nerve impulses. A short broad auditory tube leads from the middle ear to the pharynx and, as in birds, is not closed. The inner ears contain the organs of balance, the three semicircular canals, the utricle and saccule and the organ of hearing, the cochlea.

Hearing in reptiles is poor. Lizards have the best hearing but they are sensitive only to a narrow range of low-frequency sounds. Snakes and burrowing lizards lack an external or middle ear and transmit sound instead by bone conduction.

Taste and Touch

Reptiles have taste buds on their tongue and oral epithelium. The tongue is an organ of taste, touch and smell.

Olfaction

All reptiles have an accessory olfactory organ called the Jacobson organ. These are paired domed cavities and lie over the vomer bones on the rostral roof of the oral cavity, innervated by a branch of the olfactory nerve. Olfaction is well developed in chelonians but most highly developed in snakes, which receive data by flickering their tongue in and out from a sheath beneath the glottis.

Sight

The principle receptors are the eyes, with the parietal gland and possibly the skin forming secondary receptors. In some lizards, such as the iguana, the parietal gland is well developed. It is located in the dorsal midline of the head and connects to the pineal gland. It consists of a lens and retina and although it does not form images it may function in thermoregulation, basking and reproduction.

Lizards and chelonians have scleral ossicles. As in birds, the iris is controlled by skeletal muscle so is nonresponsive to mydriatics like atropine. In chelonians, the lacrimal gland is modified into the salt gland. Chelonians have no nasolacrimal ducts so lose tears by evaporation – hence giving the impression they are weeping. Chelonians and most lizards have eyelids, with the upper eyelids being larger and less mobile than the lower. Snakes have fused their eyelids into a single protective scale over the cornea, called the spectacle or brille. Sight and colour vision is well developed in chelonians and insectivorous lizards, which need keen eyesight to catch prey. Most lizards have only a narrow binocular field, which is why they cock their head to get the best monocular vision. Chameleons have the best vision of all. Sight is poor in snakes.

Heat Sensing – The Sixth Sense

Some snakes possess specialized infrared reception or pits, which enable them to sense warm-blooded prey and strike to catch them, even in total darkness. These pits are richly innervated by the trigeminal nerve and are so sensitive that they can detect a temperature variation even $0.003\,°C$.

Reference

Bennett, A.F. and Nagy, K.A. (1977) Energy expenditure in free ranging lizards. *Ecology* 58 (3), 698–700.

Carmel, B. and Johnson, R. (2014) Husbandry, in *A Guide to Health and Disease in Reptiles and Amphibians*. Reptile Publications, Burleigh BC, Australia, pp. 39–91.

Rossi, J. V. (2006) General husbandry and management, in *Reptile Medicine and Surgery* 2nd ed. (D. Mader, ed.), Saunders Elsevier, St Louis, MO. pp. 25–41.

Further Reading

Bennett, A.F and Dawson, W.R. (1976) Metabolism, in *Biology of the Reptilia*, *Volume 5, Physiology A* (C. Gans and W.R. Dawson, eds). Academic Press, London, pp. 127–211.Bentley, P.J. (1976) Osmoregulation, in *Biology of the Reptilia, Volume 5, Physiology A* (C. Gans and W.R. Dawson, eds). Academic Press, London, pp. 356–408.

Dantzler, W.H. (1976) Renal Function, in *Biology of the Reptilia, Volume 5, Physiology A* (C. Gans and W.R. Dawson, eds). Academic Press, London, pp. 447–496.

Evans, H.E. (1986) Reptiles: introduction and anatomy, in *Zoo and Wildlife Medicine*, 2nd edn (M.E. Fowler, ed.). W.B. Saunders, Philadelphia, PA, pp. 108–132.

Fox, H. (1977) The urogenital system of reptiles, in *Biology of the Reptilia, Volume 6, Morphology E* (C. Gans and T.S. Parsons, eds). Academic Press, London, pp. 1–122.

Holz, P.H. (1999) The reptilian renal–portal system: influence on therapy, in *Zoo and Wild Animal Medicine, Current Therapy*, 4th edn (M.E. Fowler and R.E. Miller, eds). W.B Saunders, Philadelphia, PA, pp. 249–252.

Holz, P.H. Barker I.K., Burger J.P. et al (1997) The effect of the renal portal system on pharmokinetic parameters in the red eared slider (trachemys scripta elegans). *Journal of Zoo and Wildlife Medicine*, 28 (4), 386–393.

King, G.M. and Custance, D.R. (1982) The Lizard, in *Colour Atlas of Vertebrate Anatomy*. Blackwell Scientific, Oxford, pp. 4.1–4.10.

Minnich, J.E. (1982) The use of water, in *Biology of the Reptilia, Volume 12, Physiology C. Physiological Ecology* (C. Gans and F.H. Pough, eds). Academic Press, London, pp. 325–386.

Ottaviani, G. and Tazzi, A. (1977) The lymphatic system, in Biology of the Reptilia, Volume 6, Morphology E (C. Gans and T.S. Parsons, eds). Academic Press, London, pp. 315–458.

O'Malley, B. (2005) *Clinical Anatomy and Physiology of Exotic Species: Structure and Function of Mammals, Birds, Reptiles and Amphibians.* Elsevier Saunders, Philadelphia, PA.

Pincheira-Donoso, D., Bauer A.M., Meiri S. and Uetz P. (2013) Global taxonomic diversity of living reptile. *PLOS One*, 8 (3), e59741.

Pough, F.H., Andrew, R.M., Cadle, J.E. et al. (1998) *Herpetology*. Prentice Hall, Englewood cliffs, NJ.

Perry, S.F. and Duncker, H.R. (1978) Lung architecture, volume and static mechanics in five species of lizards. *Respiratory Physiology*, 34, 61–81.

Pough, F.H., Janis, C.M. and Heiser J.B. (2002) *Vertebrate Life*, 6th ed. Prentice Hall, Englewood Cliffs, NJ. pp. 270–341.

3

Behaviour in the Wild and in Captivity

Robert Johnson

Introduction

Little has been written on the behaviour of captive reptiles that is useful for the practising veterinarian. It is important that the clinician is able to distinguish between normally occurring behaviours and what is pathological. Owners and keepers may report behaviours as unusual when they are not. Animal behaviour, together with structure and function, are the three phenotypic manifestations shaped through natural selection and adaptation. It can be difficult to distinguish between pathophysiological responses and normal ethological components of reptilian behaviour. Often, disease will manifest as a direct result of behavioural factors. Observed behaviours in reptiles are often directly related to thermoregulatory and other physiological requirements. This chapter highlights some unique features of reptilian structure, function and behaviour pertinent to the exotic animal consultation.

Normal Needs and Behaviour of Captive Reptiles

The physical, social and behavioural requirements of captive reptiles have been described (Greenberg 1992):

Box 3.1 A hierarchy of reptilian needs.	
Homeostasis:	Thermoregulation, nutrition, water balance.
Safety	Predator evasion, hibernacula.
Sociality	Daily or seasonal social behaviour (predatory behaviour, social and reproductive behaviour, migration for food or reproductive sites, torpor).
Social dominance:	Does the animal manifest priority of access to valued resources (Figure 3.1)?
Reproductive success:	Fitness, fecundity.
(Greenberg 1992)	

Inextricably linked with this hierarchy of needs is the issue of animal welfare. General criteria for the welfare of captive animals have been previously described in the literature as the 'five freedoms of animal welfare' (freedom from hunger and thirst, discomfort, pain, injury and disease, fear and distress, and freedom to express normal behaviour). Trends in captive animal management are now moving beyond the five freedoms towards a life worth living. The absence of suffering is not necessarily good welfare. Animal care needs to be directed at more than mere survival, minimum standards or ability to reproduce. Keeping standards should include validated

Reptile Medicine and Surgery in Clinical Practice, First Edition. Edited by Bob Doneley, Deborah Monks, Robert Johnson and Brendan Carmel.

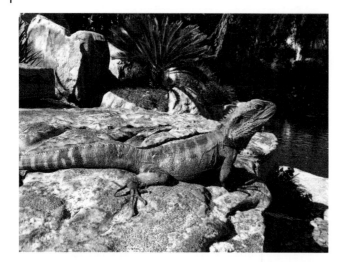

Figure 3.1 Male eastern water dragon assuming a dominant posture.

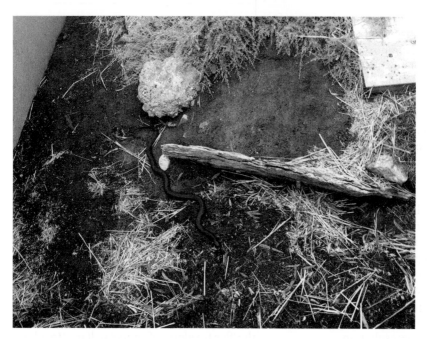

Figure 3.2 An outdoor enclosure provides a natural environment for a red-bellied black snake.

enrichments, replacing negative experiences with positive ones (Figure 3.2).

Physiological Responses

Health problems in captive reptiles can be related to an aspect of reptilian physiology or behaviour rather than to a primary disease process. Physiology and structure–function relationships have been shown to be important principles of normal species-specific behaviour. Physiological parameters to be considered when assessing normal behaviour in captive reptiles are thermoregulation, postprandial metabolism, olfaction, vision, chemosensation, water exchange, feeding response, digestion, respiration and circulatory factors (see Chapter 2 for more detailed information). Consequently, disease in captive reptiles is more often than not a manifestation of incorrect or inappropriate husbandry practices affecting these processes.

Body Temperature and Ectothermy

Reptiles are termed 'ectothermic' because they are dependent upon external heat sources rather than internal heat production. Unlike in endothermic animals such as mammals and birds, metabolic heat production in reptiles is usually insufficient to raise the body temperature significantly above that of the ambient surroundings. Two important consequences of ectothermy are highly relevant to husbandry.

First, energy use derived from food or fat stores is lower because metabolic heat is not required to maintain body temperature. The food requirement is further lowered by behaviours that entail relatively long periods of inactivity. The extent to which food requirements are connected with both body temperature and activity varies with species and the circumstances of captivity. Weight loss due to excessive energy expenditure related to 'escape' or exploratory activity can occur while in new or inadequate enclosures, with conspecific aggression or related stress and disease or parasitism. Collectively, these signs are termed maladaption.

Second, reptiles are not poikilothermic (cold-blooded) and most are capable of very precise thermoregulation by behaviour. Maintaining a prolonged constant body temperature is not required physiologically in most cases and can be harmful. Variability of body temperature has importance with respect to species variation, seasonal acclimatization, feeding and nutrition, activity reproduction and disease.

Thermoregulation can occur by:

- movement between a heat source (e.g. sunlight, warm substrate) and a heat sink (e.g. shade, water, burrow)
- postural adjustments (e.g. changes in body volume, shape orientation, posture; Figure 3.3)
- physiological responses (e.g. heat production in muscle tissues in some species,

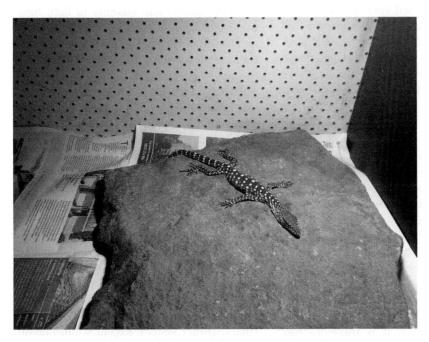

Figure 3.3 A juvenile perentie thermoregulating in a spread-eagled posture.

colour changes, circulatory changes and ventilatory adjustments to increase water evaporation from mucous membranes).

At high temperatures reptiles may pant or gape. Captive animals should not be kept in conditions where they are exposed to high temperatures without the opportunity of 'behavioural avoidance'. Conversely, at temperatures below the regulated range reptiles become torpid and sluggish and digestion ceases.

Preferred Body Temperature

Care of reptiles requires knowledge of the unique thermal requirements of a species. Preferred body temperature is species, and sometimes subspecies, dependent. In captivity, diurnal and/or arboreal species require a radiant heat source, whereas nocturnally active and/or predominately terrestrial species may avoid a photothermal (light and heat) source and may prefer a thermally variable substrate or subfloor heating. In most cases, however, a daily thermal cycle or behavioural access to thermal variation is desirable (Figure 3.4). Decreased environmental temperature plus a reduced photoperiod will stimulate oogenesis and spermatogenesis. Snakes and lizards become more aggressive with higher temperatures, especially above the preferred body temperature.

Body Temperature and Disease

Inappropriate thermal exposure can suppress the immune systems of reptiles and can operate in conjunction with other forms of stress imposed by captivity. The inability to cool below activity temperatures for prolonged periods can affect appetite and reproduction. Bacterial infections can induce reptiles to select a body temperature several degrees above 'normal' levels. Elevated body temperature enhances the survival of animals infected with a potentially lethal pathogen. It is therefore bad husbandry to cool sick reptiles.

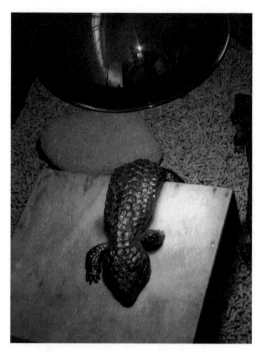

Figure 3.4 A shingleback skink is freely able to move to or away from a heat source.

Light and Photoreception

Both the quality and quantity of light have important consequences for the physiology and health of captive reptiles (see Chapter 6 for more detailed information). The eyes are the main receptors for light; however, the pineal gland (the third eye) and possibly the skin also have some role to play. Annual cycles of day length may affect appetite, metabolism and reproduction. However, environmental temperature rather than light appears to be the more influential factor affecting reproduction.

Unlike their mammalian counterparts, nocturnal snakes have small eyes compared with diurnal snakes. Geckos and most nocturnal mammals have large eyes, owing to their sole reliance on vision. Nocturnal hunters (snakes) rely upon a combination of scent, heat and vision (Figure 3.5). Most snakes and lizards have well-developed vision as well as a chemosensory system. Recent studies reveal that reptiles may perceive 'light-flicker', such

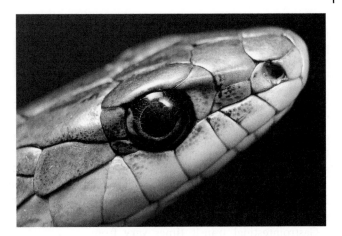

Figure 3.5 Common tree snakes are nocturnal hunters (courtesy of M. Wilson).

as that produced by ultraviolet lights connected to alternating current sources (Woo *et al.* 2009).

Chemoreception and Acoustic Sensation

Chemoreception in reptiles uses a combination of the olfactory system, taste buds (not in all squamates) and the vomeronasal system. Most squamates use visual and chemical signals for communication (geckos also use acoustic signs). Crocodiles also respond to acoustic stimuli. Chemoreception occurs in reptiles by tongue-flicking over the vomeronasal organ – paired sensory organs in the rostral aspect of the upper mouth (Figure 3.6). Tongue-flick rate is an accurate and proportional measure of a snake's level of interest in its environment, particularly while searching

for food. Tongue-flicking of captive elapids often indicates that they are about to defaecate. Flicking usually ceases once elimination is complete. Tongue-flicking may also be a sign of distress. Some keepers recommend not cleaning a hide box too scrupulously, leaving an odour for the snake to sense. Other keepers recommend the keeping of a small amount of faeces in a pot within the vivarium to satisfy the olfactory needs of the captive reptile.

Water Exchange and Humidity

Reptiles lose water by evaporation across the skin and respiratory membranes and by excretion (urine and faeces). Evaporation may account for more than half of the total water loss. As a result, exposure of captive reptiles to inappropriate levels of ambient humidity

Figure 3.6 A yellow-faced whip snake tongue flicking.

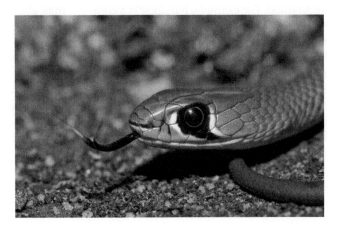

(if terrestrial) or salinity (if aquatic or amphibious) can alter hormone levels, cause weight loss and suppress reproduction.

Digestion and Nutrition

The rate of feeding varies with a multiplicity of factors, including species, animal size, age, temperature, activity, reproductive status, season, disease, parasite burden and stress. If a 'healthy' reptile habituated to captivity refuses food, the item should be removed until the next scheduled feeding.

Gastrointestinal transit times vary from species to species. While some reptiles, especially skinks, produce faeces within hours of feeding, others may retain faeces for months. Passage of faeces is facilitated by warmth and activity. Retention of gut contents can aid in water absorption. Recently fed reptiles need warmth and seclusion. Digestion ceases at low temperatures and food can putrefy in the gut of a cool animal.

Respiration and Circulation

Temperature change, excitement, activity and ecdysis can produce marked changes in respiration.

Pain and Stress

Pain perception and stress in reptiles and the resultant physiological responses are not well understood. For example, handling is a common stressor in captive reptiles. Improper handling, in addition to crowding and poor hygiene, can produce physiological deterioration leading to reduced growth, suppressed reproductive capacity and increased mortality from disease. Often, sick animals presented for veterinary examination have a history of over handling. Similar to birds and mammals, reptiles in pain will often exhibit aggressive behaviour. Snakes suffering from mite infestation will seek water for soaking to ease their discomfort.

Behaviour Patterns of Captive Reptiles

Behaviour patterns may be divided into maintenance and distance-reducing behaviours. Captive environments can easily create behavioural and spatial restrictions, leading to maladaptive reactions such as hyper- and hypoactivity, co-occupant aggression, variable environmental temperature preferences, interaction with transparent boundaries, aggression and adaptability.

Maintenance Behaviours

Maintenance behaviours include feeding and thermoregulatory responses.

Feeding

Prehension, chewing   The scleroglossa (geckos, snakes and monitor lizards) have prehensile jaws and actively seek out foods via sensory capabilities. Iguania (iguanas, chameleons) lack these characteristics and wait for the food to come to them. They capture food with their sticky tongues.

Heat sensing pits   Most pythons, except the reptile eaters (*Aspidites* spp., womas and black-headed pythons) possess heat sensing (labial) pits, small indentations in the upper and lower jaws. These infrared sensory organs work in conjunction with the visual system in seeking prey. It is also thought that infrared imaging systems may also be used for finding basking sites and shelter.

Constriction   Pythons, usually ambush hunters, strike violently when prehending their prey. The food item is then constricted and swallowed. Womas and black-headed pythons, being reptile-eating ground dwellers, will often push prey items up against a firm surface instead of constricting them, an adaptive behaviour useful in a burrow, where there is insufficient space for constriction.

Envenomation Elapids (most of the Australian venomous snakes) will strike and then release, following the prey for a few minutes after the attack to consume it. Some venomous snakes, such as brown snakes, constrict as well. It has been proposed that this is due to the short fangs in this species. Colubrid snakes will swallow prey items live in the wild.

Captive Feeding Routines

In order to train pythons to strike only at prey items, thereby reducing potential distress or injury to keepers, it is preferable to feed snakes in a container separate from their enclosure. The pythons should be accustomed to handling by gentle lifting with a probe or jigger every one to two days. The snake becomes used to being handled and lifted from its enclosure and will usually not strike. Despite being social reptiles, bearded dragons, especially juveniles, may need to be fed separately. Males tend to 'bully' females, dominating the food supply. Turtles often bite each other when feeding, particularly on the hind limbs and tail.

Hyperactivity and Hypoactivity

Reptiles will become hyperactive at ambient temperatures above their preferred body temperature. Signs of heat stress will become evident if the temperature increases above a tolerable level. These signs include panting and mouth gaping in lizards, hyperactivity, escape behaviour and seeking the point furthest from the heat source. Hypoactivity will occur when reptiles are kept below their preferred body temperature or preferred optimal temperature zone.

Distance-Reducing Behaviour

Distance-reducing behaviours include aggregation, courtship and mating, post-ovipositional, territorial, combat and anti-predator behaviour.

Social or Solitary?

It is important to know which species are naturally gregarious and which prefer to be solitary. Sometimes reptiles within one genus will display wide variations in social behaviour. Bearded dragons can be successfully kept in a harem situation with one male and several females; however, two males will often fight when placed in the same enclosure. Cannibalism is common in Antaresia species (children's pythons etc.), Aspidites species (womas and black-headed pythons) and most of the Elapidae.

Head Bobbing, Hand Waving, Digging, Tail Whipping

Bearded dragons of both sexes 'head bob' and wave their forelimbs. Males do it more vigorously. Females are more submissive and tend to mimic the behaviour of their male cage mate.

Courtship and Mating

After a period of cooling to stimulate spermatogenesis, males of most species of reptile will eat and enter a period of hyperactivity and mate-seeking behaviour. Males will also engage in mock combat. Snakes, monitors and skinks particularly show this behaviour. The beards of male bearded dragons turn black when they are sexually mature and active.

The Gravid State

A gravid python will typically expose its ventrum and shiver periodically. Pre-ovipositional anorexia is common. Dragons, chameleons, monitors and turtles will exhibit digging behaviour just prior to oviposition. Egg laying usually occurs within 24 hours. Often, pythons will become restless after oviposition and egg removal. Artificial eggs or egg shells from earlier clutches can be introduced to settle the snake.

Maternal Incubation

Morelia spp. are particularly good at maternal incubation of eggs. The snake will wrap around its eggs and shiver sporadically. The eggs may be left alone for extended periods as the female basks opportunistically and then returns to the eggs, maintaining them at a temperature of 29–30 °C and a humidity of approximately 65%. The female may not eat during the incubation period and will become protective and more aggressive.

Mock Combat

Male reptiles of many species engage in ritual or mock combat. This is particularly prevalent in lizards, monitors (Varanidae) and elapid snakes (Elapidae) and normally occurs in the mating season (Figure 3.7). Male pythons 'pace' the enclosure when they are ready to mate, appearing as if they are hungry. Defensive behaviours may be more prevalent during handling or attempts at handling, such as:

- catalepsy, tonic immobility
- tail flicking, tail autotomy
- eversion of hemipenis or phallus
- excretion of faeces, urine, urates, scent gland excretion (turtles)
- bluff and threat displays (Figure 3.8)
- colour change
- shedding skin

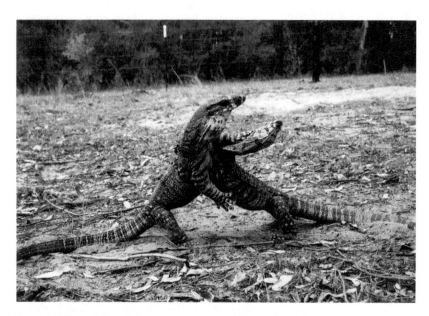

Figure 3.7 Two adult male lace monitors engaged in mock combat.

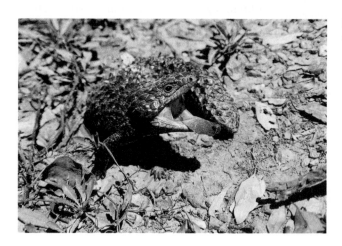

Figure 3.8 Shingleback skink in a bluff defensive posture.

Figure 3.9 Excessive constriction when handling is an indicator of stress.

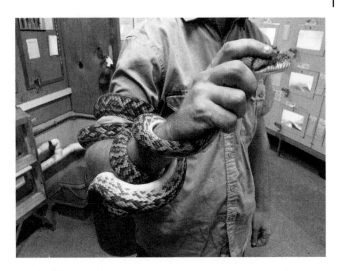

- constricting, balling (Figure 3.9)
- withdrawal of head, limbs and tail (chelonians)
- striking or attacking.

Fitness and Environmental Enhancement

Lack of fitness appears to have a negative effect on normal physiological responses in captive reptiles. Attention should be paid to the captive environment to maximize the opportunity for snakes to move around the exhibit and maintain muscle tone and strength.

Pythons

While most species of pythons spend a substantial part of the time on the ground, several species are also climbers, such as *Morelia spilota* (carpet and diamond pythons). In captivity, the opportunity to climb is not often provided. Captive pythons are predisposed to dystocia. Decreased muscle tone, reduced strength and lack of fitness may be mitigating factors in this process.

Green Pythons

In captivity, green pythons spend most of the time coiled on a perch (Figure 3.10). These snakes are much more active in the wild,

Figure 3.10 Captive green pythons spend much of their time perching.

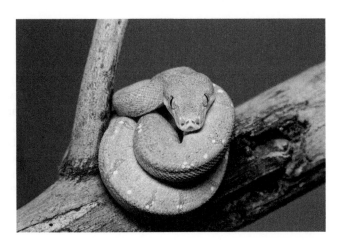

Table 3.1 Signs of comfort and discomfort in captive reptiles (adapted from Warwick 1995).

Comfort	Discomfort
Alertness	Hyper-alertness
Relaxed state	Escape attempts, repeated inflation/deflation cycles
Calmly smelling or tasting objects	Mock or actual attacks
Subtle changes in body posture	'Clutching' object or handler
Gradual body movements and locomotion	Feigning death
Moderate to relaxed grasp on handler	Hiding head
Normal to relaxed breathing	Inflation of the body
Sleeping	Rapid gular pulsation
Absence of signs of discomfort	Open-mouth defence posture
	Open-mouth breathing
	Defecation with handling
	Projection of penis or hemipenis
	Regurgitation
	Vocalization (crocodile, gecko)
	Pigmentation change

preferring to move or climb vertically as they hunt or seek a mate. Suggestions for improving captive conditions include the provision of more opportunities to climb. Enclosures tend to be very sterile and not enriching. Keepers of this species tend to be more focused on providing the perfect temperature and humidity and little else. Offering a thermal mosaic could stimulate snakes to move around the cage more.

Signs of Comfort and Discomfort

The comfort or discomfort of a captive reptile may be determined by assessing for the presence or absence of certain behavioural and physiological responses (Table 3.1).

References

Greenberg, N. (1992) The saurian psyche revisited: lizards in research, in *The Care and Use of Amphibians, Reptiles and Fish in Research* (D.O. Schaeffer, K.M. Kleinow and L. Krulisch, eds), Scientists Center for Animal Welfare, Bethesda, MD, pp. 75–91.

Warwick, C. (1995) Psychological and behavioural principles and problems, in *Health and Welfare of Captive Reptiles* (C. Warwick, F. Frye and J.B. Murphy, eds), Chapman and Hall, London, pp. 205–238.

Woo, K.L., Hunt, M., Harper, D. *et al.* (2009). Discrimination of flicker frequency rates in the reptile tuatara (Sphenodon). *Naturwissenschaften*, 96 (3), 415–419.

Further Reading

Bradley, T. (2002) Reptile behaviour basics for the veterinary clinician, in *Proceedings, Association of Reptilian and Amphibian Veterinarians Annual Conference, Reno, Nevada*. Association of Reptilian and Amphibian Veterinarians, Reno, NV, pp. 165–170.

Gillingham, J.C. (1995) Normal behaviour, in *Health and Welfare of Captive Reptiles*, (C. Warwick, F. Frye and J.B. Murphy, eds), Chapman and Hall, London, pp. 131–164.

Green, T.C. and Mellor, D.J. (2011) Extending ideas about animal welfare assessment to include 'quality of life' and related concepts. *New Zealand Veterinary Journal*, 59 (6), 263–271.

Greer, A. (1997) Pythonidae – Pythons, in *The Biology and Evolution of Australian Snakes*, Surrey, Beatty and Sons, Chipping Norton, NSW, pp. 24–83.

Hernandez-Divers, S.J. (2000) Reptile behaviour, in *Proceedings, Association of Reptilian and Amphibian Veterinarians Annual Conference, Reno, Nevada*, Association of Reptilian and Amphibian Veterinarians, Reno, NV, p. 183.

Lillywhite, H.B. and Gatten, R.E. (1995) Physiology and functional anatomy, in *Health and Welfare of Captive Reptiles* (C.Warwick, F. Frye and J.B. Murphy, eds), Chapman and Hall, London, pp. 5–31.

Lock, B.A. Behavioural and morphologic adaptations, in *Reptile Medicine and Surgery*, 2nd ed. (D.R. Mader ed.). Elsevier, St Louis, MO, 2006, pp. 163–179.

Luz, S, Keil, R., Meyer, W. and Martelli, P. (2002) Diagnosis of some common diseases in snakes, with respect to the understanding of disease-induced behavioural changes. Proceedings, European Association of Zoo and Wildlife Veterinarians (EAZVW) 4th Scientific Meeting, joint with the annual meeting of the European Wildlife Disease Association (EWDA) May 8–12, 2002, Heidelberg, Germany.

Pough, F.H. (2003) Communication, in *Herpetology*, 4th ed. (F.H. Pough, R.M. Andrews, J.E. Cadle, et al.). Prentice Hall, UpperSaddle River, NJ.

Warwick, C. (1990) Reptilian ethology in captivity: observations of some problems and an evaluation of their aetiology. *Applied Animal Behaviour Science*, 26, 1–13.

Warwick, C., Frye, F.L. and Murphy, J.B. (1995) Introduction: Health and welfare of captive reptiles, in *Health and Welfare of Captive Reptiles* (C. Warwick, F. Frye and J.B. Murphy, eds), Chapman and Hall, London, pp. 1–4.

4

Husbandry and Nutrition

Michelle Kischinovsky, Aidan Raftery and Shivananden Sawmy

Introduction

A large percentage of disease in reptiles can be referred back to inadequate husbandry and/or nutrition. A fundamental understanding of the requirements, habits and behaviours of the presented species is essential to provide optimal veterinary care and to improve chances of recovery.

Ectothermy

Ectothermy is the ability of an animal to regulate its body temperature by moving between the different temperature zones in its environment. This is in contrast to endotherms, which rely mainly on the heat from internal metabolic processes to control body temperature. All reptiles are classed as ectotherms but some are able to generate enough metabolic heat to raise their body temperature above that of the surrounding environment; for example, the incubation behaviour of some python species. Female pythons coil around the clutch of eggs and if the ambient temperature drops they shiver, producing heat and maintaining the eggs at an even temperature.

Behaviour and Environmental Enrichment

Historically, captive reptile environments were only enriched to provide more interesting viewing but, increasingly, the welfare value of enrichment is being recognized (see Chapter 3 for more details). Reptiles provided with environmental enrichment are more active and develop increased physical skills. The enrichment needs to be appropriate to the species to increase choices available to stimulate normal behaviour, at the same time allowing the reptile some control over their environment.

Basic Concepts

Housing

The captive environment should mimic the natural habitat. The shape and interior design of the enclosure will depend on whether the animal is arboreal, terrestrial, semi-aquatic or aquatic, so knowledge of the natural history of the species is essential. As a general rule, arboreal species should have a more vertical enclosure with furniture and foliage facilitating climbing and shelter, whereas terrestrial species require more horizontal space, with objects and substrate allowing for hiding and digging or burrowing. The size of the enclosure will be dependent on:

- the species; for example, some very active snakes such as racers (*Coluber* spp.), garter snakes (*Thamnophis* spp.)and corn snakes (*Pantherophis guttatus*), may need a larger space than less active snakes, such as boas and pythons, of similar body length
- the size of the animal (at time of acquiring and as it grows)
- the number of animals housed together
- whether it is a breeding pair (potential off-spring and breeding facilities)
- whether the same sex conspecifics are present (a larger enclosure will be required for territories; see conspecifics section).

Enclosure heat and humidity should be controlled to mimic the natural preferences of the species. The enclosure should also be large enough to accommodate a temperature gradient (horizontally or vertically), basking lights or spots, furniture and feeding bowls, a retreat box and appropriate environmental enrichment objects (see Chapter 3 for behaviour and Chapter 5 for enclosure design). For aquatic and semi-aquatic species, the enclosure should be large enough to house a land and a water area, as well as a water filtering system. Some aquatic species may require a submersible water heater.

The opening of the enclosure should be situated to allow easy and stress free retrieval of the reptile from the vivarium, as well as easy access for feeding and cleaning without risk of the animal escaping. Non-climbing species, such as turtles and tortoises, are often housed in enclosures without tops. An effective and secure closing mechanism is important as some reptiles, especially snakes, have a remarkable tendency to squeeze through seemingly impossibly small gaps. Venomous and dangerous species should be kept in a locked enclosure.

The positioning of the enclosure should be considered. Some reptiles thrive in habitats exposed to sunlight and high humidity, while others prefer shadier environments and good ventilation, such as many chameleon species. Species such as the African spurred tortoise (*Centrochelys sulcata*) and many lizards, aquatic and semi-aquatic turtles can, where the climate is appropriate, be kept in outdoor enclosures or ponds.

Environmental Enrichment

A stimulating habitat will, in most cases, enable the reptile to be more active and encourage natural species-specific behaviours such as foraging, hunting, hiding and burrowing (see also Chapter 3). This encourages exploration of the environment. Any objects potentially harmful if ingested should be securely placed or fastened. Knowledge of the species natural habitat and routines are invaluable. The environment should be safe; there should be no harmful materials or toxic plants and any large objects such as rocks should be fixed.

Mentally stimulating activities for all reptiles include foraging and the stalking of prey. Natural scent trails can be made by burrowing or dragging a prey item through the enclosures of snakes and carnivorous lizards. Insectivores can be fed a variety of different live insects, some winged, jumping and burrowing, for stimulation. Live fish and worms can be released for aquatic species and other partially aquatic reptiles such as garter snakes (*Thamnophis* spp.) and Chinese water dragons (*Physignathus cocincinus*). Omnivores and herbivores can be offered whole leaves and greens, still on their stalks or suspended high up to allow mimicking tearing food from bushes or trees.

The habitat should aim to stimulate the senses by varying temperatures, light and humidity to mimic natural conditions throughout a day. Social reptiles benefit from being housed with conspecifics, although knowledge of their social structure is imperative to avoid aggression or stress. Some may benefit from enclosures co-inhabited with other compatible species, such as arboreal lizards with terrestrial tortoises, choosing species that have similar climate requirements and no risk of transmissible pathogens.

Hygiene

Good hygiene is good husbandry. Faecal material, urates and any uneaten food should be removed on a daily basis. The importance is greater when dealing with decaying plant or animal feed. Removing leftover or uneaten live insects from the enclosure also allows for the monitoring of appetite and the task functions as part of a daily survey of the animals overall wellbeing. Additionally, some insect species will bite the reptile if not removed from the enclosure.

Some enclosure materials are easier to maintain and disinfect than others. Artificial plants are ideal in a hospital setting but may lack visual appeal and enrichment. Some natural materials commonly used, such as plywood, are difficult to disinfect if not correctly sealed with a waterproofing agent. An easily cleaned and inexpensive substrate such as newspaper or paper towelling should be used for sick animals.

If the humidity, temperature gradient or ventilation are incorrect, growth of unwanted pathogens (bacteria or fungus) may occur – even if the substrate or foliage is not harmful to the animal.

Good hand hygiene is indispensable, both before and after animal handling, not only to limit the risk of zoonotic infections but also to prevent cross-infection of other animals. Healthy animals should be handled or treated first and the sick or immunocompromised last. Excessive cleaning may remove naturally occurring healthy environmental organisms, may disturb the animals unnecessarily, causing a stress response which may lead to immunosuppression.

While adequate caging and environmental enrichment are imperative for the maintenance of a healthy and thriving animal in a private, zoo or school collection, the facilities provided in a hospital setting have different goals. Short-term patients will tolerate a stark environment, although humidity and heat should be provided and carefully controlled, especially given that sick reptiles often do not thermoregulate properly. The entire enclosure, furniture and its substrate should be easily cleaned out and disinfected.

Water Quality

Water must be available to all species at all times. Snakes will often drink out of a bowl, in which they often also submerge themselves (to aid shedding). Lizards and tortoises often rehydrate themselves when soaked in water baths but will readily learn to drink out of a shallow bowl in their enclosure. Some lizards, such as the crested geckos (*Correlophus ciliatus*) and anoles (*Anolis* spp.) tend to lick condensing water droplets off the sides of the enclosure after misting, whereas water drippers with catch systems are ideal for chameleons.

Good water quality is fundamental for the heath of aquatic species. Semi-aquatic and aquatic reptiles must be able to submerge themselves fully. Many reptiles defecate in the water. Turtles and some lizards and snakes will forage in or use water to facilitate swallowing and, in doing so, will leave food debris, which can act as a nidus for pathogens. Constant insults to the water can cause rapid changes in the salinity and pH levels and can increase nitrogen levels, which can promote unfavourable algae and bacterial blooms. Contaminated water or poor water quality may lead to disease.

As aquatic reptiles tend to produce more waste than fish, a high-quality water filtering system is advised. This can be chemical, biological or mechanical, and often a combination of the latter two is used. The water must be dechlorinated where there is biological filtration.

The frequency of cleaning of water dishes and pools will largely depend on the stocking density, temperatures, quality of the filtration system and the frequency and type of feed. A subjective visual assessment of the water can be made but even though it may look clean, it can still house excessive amounts of nitrogenous and bacterial waste. Readily available commercial water testing kits are recommended. Feeding the reptile in a separate container outside the enclosure can limit the frequency of water changes required.

Conspecifics

The majority of reptiles are solitary by nature and interact only with conspecifics during the breeding season. They will often form hierarchies, with the high-ranking animals sometimes competing for the best basking spots, feed or retreat sites, which may cause a chronic state of stress in lower-ranking animals or may even causing physical injuries. Males are usually more territorial, and more so in the presence of another male; this is especially true during breeding season. Sexually mature male green iguanas (*Iguana iguana*) have been known to exhibit very offensive aggression during breeding season (December to March in the northern hemisphere) and have even been known to attack human owners during this period. Extra care should be taken when handling large lizard or snake species. It is not uncommon for lizards to tolerate living together for a number of years and then to exhibit aggressive behaviour when reaching sexually maturity.

For the species tolerating social housing, one male should generally be kept with several females to avoid sexual dominance aggression (for more information, see Chapter 3).

Transport

Transport requirements will depend on the journey distance, species, size and number of individuals and, importantly, the ambient temperature. Reptiles must be provided with adequate ventilation during transport and kept warm (24–30 °C) while avoiding overheating. A thermometer should be used to monitor temperature. Improvised containers such as a jar or cardboard box with air holes punched in the lid or commercial rodent carriers can be used. Insulated containers are best, such as a commercial purpose- or homemade polystyrene or cooler box, to help to prevent the temperature from rising above 30 °C. All reptiles should be placed in an escape-proof container; for example a cloth bag tied with a knot placed within a secure box for snakes. A hot-water bottle wrapped in a towel (to ensure that there is no direct contact between the animal and the heat source) should be placed inside the container. Each animal should have some form of identification, such as a tag or microchip and, when transporting multiple reptiles, several boxes can be placed inside one larger insulated container. The containers should be secure in the transport vehicle to reduce the risk of trauma and movement. Note that venomous species should be transported in clearly labelled, locked, containers, together with the necessary documentation, anti-venom and envenomation emergency protocol (also see Chapter 10).

Handling and Restraint for Feeding and Husbandry Purposes

Please refer to the reptile consultation (Chapter 10) and clinical techniques (Chapter 13) chapters for a detailed description of handling and restraint techniques for veterinary examination purposes. Please note that only the chelonians and squamates are covered in this textbook.

Sex Identification

Sex identification of reptiles can be challenging, especially with juveniles. Some species exhibit varying degrees of sexual dimorphism. Please refer to Chapter 7 for further information.

Preventative Health Care

Key considerations for maintaining captive reptiles in good health include the following:

- Research the desired species prior to acquisition.
- Source new animals from a reputable and ethical source. Avoid purchasing wild-caught animals (illegal in some countries) as they are more likely to carry parasites and will be less capable of adapting into captivity.
- Maintain good husbandry and nutritional practices that mimic those in the wild where possible.
- Keep good records.
- Maintain effective biosecurity and quarantine protocols.
- Have an experienced reptilian veterinarian examine the animals on a regular basis.

Quarantine

A quarantine protocol should be in place for any reptile collection. All new acquisitions should be quarantined for a minimum of six months. Quarantine periods need to be constantly reviewed according to the most recent information available. See Chapter 16 (Infectious Diseases and Immunology) for further details.

New arrivals should be kept in a separate room with dedicated equipment and cage furniture. Owners or keepers should adhere to strict biosecurity measures such as foot baths, wearing disposable gloves and effective hand sanitization. Shower and change clothes between units and manage the newly acquired animals last during the daily routine.

Quarantined reptiles should be kept under optimum husbandry conditions and regularly monitored for their appetite, behaviour and defecation. Prior to acquisition, each individual reptile should ideally have had an examination and ancillary diagnostic tests, as determined by a veterinarian experienced with reptiles. This may not be performed in practice, so each specimen should undergo a full clinical examination, husbandry review and diagnostic tests while in quarantine. Faecal screening for pathogenic protozoa and helminths should be performed (see Chapter 31). Haematology, biochemistry and infectious disease screening should be considered where applicable for, for example, herpesvirus, inclusion body disease, sunshine virus, ferlavirus, adenovirus (see Chapter 16).

Record Keeping

Good record keeping allows the owner, keeper or veterinarian to recognize signs of ill health at an early stage, to address suboptimal husbandry and environmental parameters and may allow retrospective identification of a problem. It is essential to keep a detailed record of environmental parameters such as temperature, humidity and ultraviolet light emission (and the frequency that the light bulb needs changing).

Animals should be weighed regularly using accurate digital scales. Weight checks prior to, during and post-hibernation in tortoises are essential, for example.

Behavioural changes, clinical signs, appetite and frequency of defecation (including anomalies in consistency and colour) should be noted. Frequency of cleaning and disinfection or alterations to cage furniture should be logged. Measurements such as total length and snout-to-vent length in squamates and carapace length in chelonians can be useful for monitoring growth and body condition.

Nutrition

Reptiles have evolved to fill many ecological niches, resulting in large variations in dietary requirements. As a general rule, reptiles can be divided into herbivores, omnivores and carnivores.

Herbivory

There are no herbivorous snakes. The green iguana is the most common herbivorous lizard species seen in many parts of the world.

A large pitfall of herbivorous diets in captive reptiles is the inability of many keepers to provide the correct calcium to phosphorus ratio, which should be greater than two to one, and the appropriate level of calcium in the diet. Table 4.1 lists the greens that are commonly fed. Romaine and red lettuce varieties are often recommended but these plants have inadequate calcium to phosphorus ratios and a relatively low calcium content. The herbs listed in the table have a very high calcium to phosphorus ratio and a very high calcium content.

Oxalates are often stated as having an effect on the availability of the calcium in the diet. There are no studies looking at the impact of the oxalate content in the diet of herbivorous reptiles. Oxalates are broken down by bacteria in the gut of herbivorous mammals, releasing the calcium for absorption. Levels of oxalates found in the commonly fed plants listed here should not cause any problems.

Brassicas (plants in the cabbage family) contain varying amounts of thiocyanate which can interfere with iodine uptake. Hypothyroidism is, however, very rarely diagnosed in reptiles.

The reptile diet should be a mixture of different plant types. Care should be taken to ensure that a variety is actually eaten and that the animal does not selectively feed. Dietary imbalances will show up quickly in rapidly growing juveniles and reproductively active females. Other adult individuals may take months or years for some deficiencies to cause obvious clinical signs.

Omnivory

Many lizard and chelonian species are omnivorous. There are no omnivorous snakes. The main challenges of an omnivorous diet are the calcium content, the calcium to phosphorus ratio and the vitamin A content. Most of the omnivores commonly presented for treatment are eating a mixture of plant material and invertebrates. From Table 4.2 it can be seen that the calcium content of the commonly fed invertebrates is very low and there is a negative calcium to phosphorus ratio. The one exception in the chart are phoenix worms, the larvae of the black soldier fly, although there are concerns about the digestibility of their calcium content.

Good care of the invertebrates before feeding will help convert them into a more balanced food item. The feeder invertebrates are best fed a formulated diet that is fortified with calcium and vitamin A. Much of the calcium in the insect diet is not absorbed from the gastrointestinal tract so, with a short gut transit time, they need to be eaten within an hour of feeding.

Most plants contain high levels of vitamin A so hypovitaminosis A is only seen in reptiles that are predominantly insectivorous.

Carnivory

Some chelonians, some lizards and all snakes are carnivores. Carnivorous reptiles can be divided up into those feeding predominantly on vertebrates and those feeding on invertebrates. The limitations of a largely invertebrate diet are covered in the section on omnivory. Nutritional imbalances involving calcium and phosphorus are unlikely to occur when the diet is largely vertebrate species. Thiamine deficiency and obesity are the most commonly seen nutritional disorders with a diet of vertebrates (see Chapter 15).

Hypovitaminosis A is relatively common in insectivorous reptiles. Obesity is also a common problem in carnivorous reptiles, largely a result of overfeeding, although reduced activity will also play a part.

Snake Nutrition

Nutritional disorders are rarely reported in snakes as they are generally fed a whole prey item, which is usually a nutritionally

Table 4.1 Commonly fed greens.

Vegetable/herb	Calcium (mg/100 g)	Phosphorus (mg/100 g)	Ca : P ratio	Vitamin A (iu/100 g)	Fibre (g/100 g)	Carbohydrate (g/100 g)	Protein (g/100 g)	Water (g/100 g)
Parsley	138	58	2.4 : 1	8424	3.3	6.33	2.97	87.71
Lettuce:								
Cos/Romaine	33	30	1 : 1	8710	2.1	3.29	1.23	94.61
Red	33	28	1 : 1	7492	0.9	2.26	1.33	95.64
Iceberg	18	20	1 : 1	502	1.2	2.97	0.9	95.64
Cabbage	40	26	2 : 1	98	2.5	5.8	1.28	92.18
Kale	150	92	1.5 : 1	9990		8.8	4.3	
Cress	81	76	1 : 1	6917	1.1	5.5	2.6	89.4
Dandelion	187	66	3 : 1	10161	3.5	9.2	2.7	85.6
Pak choi	105	74	1 : 0.7	4468	1	2.1	1.5	95.32
Broccoli	47	66	1 : 1.5	623	2.6	6.64	2.82	89.3
Spinach	99	49	2 : 1	9377	2.2	3.63	2.86	91.4
Turnip greens	190	42	4.5 : 1	11587	3.2	7.13	1.5	89.67
Marjoram (dry)	1990	306	6 : 1	8068	40.3	60.56	12.66	7.64
Thyme	405	106	4 : 1	4651	14	24.45	5.56	65.11
Tarragon (dry)	1139	313	3.5 : 1	4200	7.4	50.22	22.77	7.74
Spearmint	199	60	3 : 1	4054	6.8	8.41	3.29	85.55

Source: US Department of Agriculture Food Composition Database.
Ca, calcium; P, phosphorus.

Table 4.2 Commonly fed invertebrates.

Species (cricket house)	Calcium (mg/100 g)	Phosphorus (mg/100 g)	Ca : P ratio	Vitamin A (iu/100 g)	Crude fat (g/100 g)	Crude protein (g/100 g)	Water (g/100 g)
Acheta domesticus	40.7	295	1 : 7.25	< 100	6.8	20.5	69.2
Mealworm larvae	16.9	285	1 : 16.86	< 100	5.4	23.7	61.9
Superworm larvae (*Zophobas morio*)	17.7	237	1 : 13.39	< 100	17.7	19.7	57.9
Waxworm (*Galleria mellonella*)	24.3	195	1 : 8.02	< 100	24.9	4.13	31.4
Phoenix worm (*Hermetia illucens*)	934	356	2.62 : 1		14	17.5	61.2

Source: modified from Latney and Clayton 2014.

complete package. Mammalian prey items (usually thawed rabbits, rats and mice) are fed, even though some of the more commonly kept reptile species feed on reptiles in the wild. They will usually readily accept mammals, especially if this is the only food provided from hatching. Some species of snakes eat mainly invertebrates in the wild but these species are very rarely maintained in captivity. Only humanely killed prey should be fed.

Overfeeding leading to obesity is a common problem in snakes. The prey item fed should be approximately equal to or slightly greater than the diameter of the snake at the level of its stomach. Feeding frequency will depend on the species of snake, its age and reproductive status. Some species are more active and feed more frequently; for example, the colubrids, whereas, in general, boas and pythons feed less frequently as they are less active. Juvenile animals need to feed more frequently because of their increased growth requirements. Larger snakes will eat much larger prey and, depending on size, may only feed every one to three months. Garter snakes mainly eat amphibians and fish in the wild. In captivity, they are commonly fed fish and thiamine deficiency may result (see Chapter 15).

Anorexia is a common presenting sign in snakes. Investigation of an anorexic snake should start with a thorough clinical examination together with an evaluation of the husbandry.

Clean water should always be available. The water bowl should be large enough to allow the snake to soak. This is especially important for some species, such as the short-tailed pythons.

Lizard Nutrition

Whether terrestrial or arboreal, lizards can be classed as herbivorous, omnivorous or carnivorous, with the vast majority being insectivorous (Table 4.3). Research is still lacking on the natural diets of some captive species. Some reptiles with a preferential food source in the wild may thrive well in captivity on an alternate or commercially manufactured diet. There may be seasonal variation of dietary choices, which should aim to be replicated in captivity. Knowledge of the lizard's natural diet is essential.

Herbivores

The commonly kept green iguana (*Iguana iguana*), chuckwallas (*Sauromalus* spp.), spiny-tailed lizards (*Uromastyx* spp.) and less so the prehensile-tailed skinks (*Corucia zebrata*) are considered primary herbivores. They thrive on a plant-based diet throughout life and rely on hind-gut fermentation to digest these high-fibre diets. Some other lizards generally considered herbivorous have undergone an ontogenetic shift from a carnivorous diet as juveniles towards herbivory as adults. There may also be variation in the type of foliage consumed as a juvenile compared with the adult stage.

A variety of fresh chopped greens dark green and leafy vegetables can be fed and some may benefit from high-protein foods such as beans, peas or lentils (Table 4.2). Many species tolerate fruit in their diets, as well and flowers and nectar, is preferential for some. Although still considered truly herbivorous, some have been known in the wild to occasionally supplement their diet with eggs or insects and in captivity these are often provided.

Some commercially available diets are sufficient for certain commonly kept species. Additional supplements (calcium, minerals and vitamins) can be added to the diet where indicated. Some herbivorous species have a very specialized diet, eating only one kind of plant or fruit; for example, many anoles only eat nectar. Some plants, flowers or vegetables may be toxic to lizards. Avocado, rhubarb, eggplant, tulips, daffodils and azaleas have all been suggested as toxic but little is known of these effects; so if uncertain, then it is best to omit from the diet.

Table 4.3 Commonly presented lizard species based on preferred food categories (food list not extensive).

Diet type	Species	Suggested diet
Herbivorous[a]	Green iguana (*Iguana iguana*)	Leafy greens, mixed vegetables and fruits, squash, peas, beans and alfalfa hay
	Prehensile-tailed skink (*Corucia zebrata*)	Generally as above
	Chuckwalla (*Sauromalus* spp.): Common chuckwalla (*S. ater*)	Mixed vegetables and fruits, squash, peas, flowers; occasional insects or egg
	Spiny-tailed lizard (*Uromastyx* spp.) Mali uromastyx (*Uromastyx (dispar) maliensis*)	Mixed leafy greens, flowers, seeds, carrots, sweet potato and squash; occasional insect
Omnivorous	Bearded dragon (*Pogona* spp.): Inland bearded dragon (*Pogona vitticeps*) Rankin's bearded dragon (*Pogona henrylawsoni*)	Approx. 60% invertebrates, 40% vegetable matter; juveniles more carnivorous than adults
	Argentine tegu (*Salvator merianae*)	Approx. 50% fruits and 50% whole vertebrates, invertebrates, egg; juveniles require more protein
	Veiled chameleon (*Chamaeleo calyptratus*)	40–70% invertebrates and 30–60% vegetable matter (more so adults)
	Water dragon: Chinese water dragon (*Physignathus cocincinus*) Eastern water dragon (*Intellagama lesueurii lesueurii*)	80–95% invertebrates and 10–15% vegetable matter; occasional small fish, snails and rodents
	Crested gecko (*Correlophus ciliatus*)	Mainly invertebrate insects; soft and pureed fruit baby food or custom blends
	Giant day gecko (*Phelsuma grandis*)	Generally as above
	Blue-tongued skink (*Tiliqua* spp.)	Approx. 50% vegetables, 25% fruits and 25% invertebrates (mainly snails)
Carnivorous: Vertebrates[b]	Bosc's (or savannah) monitor (*Varanus exanthematicus*)	Rodents (mice, rats), large insects, snails, fish
Invertebrates[c]	Green anole (*Anolis carolinensis*)	Primarily invertebrates; rarely will eat small amount of fruit and vegetables
	Leopard gecko (*Eublepharis macularius*)	Mixed invertebrates
	Fat-tailed gecko, African fat-tailed gecko (*Hemitheconyx caudicinctus*)	Mixed invertebrates
	Jackson's chameleon (*Trioceros jacksonii*)	Mixed invertebrates
	Panther chameleon (*Furcifer pardalis*)	Mixed invertebrates

[a] For example, vegetables, leafy greens, fruits, flowers, beans, lentils, seeds, nectar.
[b] For example, mice, rats, gerbils, day-old chicks.
[c] For example, beetles, hoppers, roaches, worms, flies, snails, crustaceans.

Omnivores

Most lizards are omnivorous, with some having a more herbivorous diet and others a more carnivorous. The majority of the carnivorous portion of the diet comprises invertebrates (insects), although some of the larger lizards will occasionally eat small rodents, chicks or other prepared meat. Often, owners will feed a few select insect species, so advice should be given to promote feeding of a highly varied diet. Feeding a uniform or unsuitable diet may lead to nutritional disorders (see Chapter 15 for more details).

Most lizards that feed on invertebrates will readily eat a wide variety of insect species. A general invertebrate diet typically includes a selection of cockroaches, crickets, grasshoppers, locusts, larvae, flies and worms (mealworms, silkworms, phoenix worms, giant mealworms, waxworms; Table 4.3). Some will eat earthworms, snails, spiders, beetles, moths and other wild caught insects. Most lizards respond to movement, so feeding live and well-nourished invertebrates (as discussed in the omnivory section) is good practice. Generally, the size of the prey item should be no larger than the distance between the lizard's eyes. Insects not consumed in one sitting should be removed as some are known to inflict bites.

Juvenile bearded dragons and tegu species rely on a more carnivorous diet and will shift towards a less protein-rich diet as they mature. Some skinks and geckos, such as the day gecko (*Phelsuma* spp.) and the crested gecko (*Correlophus ciliatus*), have unique nutritional requirements and commonly include fruit and nectar in their diet. In captivity, this is commonly substituted with sweet fruit puree and fruit-flavoured baby food, although proprietary fruit and nectar foods are available.

Carnivores

Lizards that feed purely on other vertebrates (mammals, birds or other reptiles) are not commonly kept as pets. The Bosc's monitor (*Varanus exanthematicus*), also known as the savannah monitor, is a lizard commonly encountered as a pet, which almost exclusively feeds on vertebrate prey. The Tokay gecko (*Gekko gecko*), with its opportunistic feeding habits, will readily eat small rodents and lizards as well as invertebrates. Most monitors, chameleons, collared lizards, anoles, basilisks, skinks and geckos have a predominantly invertebrate diet, described in more detail in the 'omnivore' section.

All vertebrate feed should be dead and served fresh or rapidly thawed. All feed, including uneaten invertebrates, should be removed if not consumed within a sitting, as they will decay or may bite and inflict injury on the lizard.

Chelonian Nutrition

Chelonians can be herbivorous, carnivorous or omnivorous (Table 4.4). Terrestrial chelonians are typically entirely herbivorous or omnivorous, while aquatic species tend be mostly omnivorous or carnivorous. Certain herbivorous species may also have opportunistic omnivorous habits. Herbivorous chelonians are hind-gut fermenters, with microbial fermentation of ingesta occurring in the large intestines. The gut flora also produces digestible energy from fibre, additional microbial-derived protein and volatile fatty acids by modifying plant material.

The ideal diet for captive chelonians should mimic that of the species in the wild. The key to nutritional management of captive chelonians is to avoid dependence on one or two food items. Nutritional disorders arise from poorly balanced or unsuitable diets, as well as from poor husbandry. In theory, a balanced diet and appropriate husbandry should preclude the use of dietary supplements. However, it is often recommended that all captive chelonians should be supplemented with calcium and appropriate vitamins to counteract the (likely) limitations of their diet and husbandry. All chelonians should also be offered regular access to fresh water for drinking and bathing.

Table 4.4 A classification of commonly presented chelonians based on diet and habitat.

Habitat	Herbivores	Omnivores	Carnivores
Terrestrial	Horsfield's tortoise (*Testudo horsfieldi*)	Red-footed tortoise (*Chelonoidis carbonaria*)	None
	Hermann's tortoise (*T. hermanni*)	Yellow-footed tortoise (*C. denticulata*)	
	Spur-thighed tortoises (e.g. *T. graeca*)	African hingeback tortoises (*Kinixys* spp.)	
	Marginated tortoise (*T. marginata*)	Elongated tortoises (*Indotestudo* spp.)	
	African spurred tortoise (*Geochelone [Centrochelys] sulcata*)		
	Leopard tortoise (*G. pardalis*)		
	Indian star tortoise (*G. elegans*)		
	Aldabra Giant tortoise (*Aldabrachelys gigantea*)		
	Radiated tortoise (*G.* or *Astrochelys radiata*)		
	North American gopher tortoises (*Gopherus* spp.)		
	Green sea turtle (*Chelonia mydas*)		
Semi-aquatic and Aquatic (marine) species	None	Red-eared slider (Trachemys scripta elegans)	Long-necked turtles (*Chelodina longicollis*)
		Map turtles (*Graptemys* spp.)	Snapping turtles (*Chelydra* spp.)
		Asian leaf turtle (*Cyclemys dentata*)	Matamata (*Chelus fimbriatus*)
		American side-necked turtles (*Platemys* spp.)	Soft-shelled turtles (*Trionyx* spp.)
		Short-necked turtles (*Emydura* spp.)	

Terrestrial Chelonians

Herbivores

To avoid selective feeding and to meet their nutritional requirements, herbivorous tortoises should be fed a wide variety of plants rich in fibre, minerals such as calcium, and vitamins (e.g. A and D3). The calcium to phosphorus ratio of the diet should be 1.5–2 to 1. Additionally, the diet should be low in protein (Table 4.5).

Herbivorous tortoises should ideally be fed daily with a variety of mixed vegetation supplemented with a multivitamin and mineral supplement. All food items should be thoroughly washed prior to feeding to remove any potential toxic residues. The use of commercial pelleted diets is currently not recommended as a complete diet because of their high protein content, which can cause an abnormally rapid growth and selective feeding in some species of tortoises.

Omnivores

Captive omnivorous chelonians (terrestrial and aquatic species) do well when fed plant

Table 4.5 A rough guide to feeding common terrestrial herbivorous chelonians.

Category	Examples	Comments
Greens	Grass	Grass can be used as a food source only by some species
	Kale	*Rhubarb should never be offered due to its toxic oxalate content*
	Rocket	
	Watercress	
	Dandelion leaves and flowers	
	Spring greens	
	Cabbage	
	Spinach	
Forage and wild plants	Clover	Ensure that no poisonous plants are present
	Nasturtium	
	Rose	
	Bramble	
	Plantain	
	Nettles	
	Lilac	

and animal matter in proportions ranging from 50 : 50 to 90 : 10, depending on species, age and habitat variations. Just like herbivorous tortoises, terrestrial omnivorous chelonians should be fed a wide variety of food items and it is essential to avoid items too high in animal protein (and hence phosphorus) as they can cause abnormal carapacial and bone growth. Supplementation with a high calcium and vitamin powder is recommended to maintain a good calcium to phosphorus ratio, since some food items, such as insect pupae and larvae, are high in phosphorus but low in calcium. They may also be dusted with calcium immediately prior to feeding but dusting on its own is not sufficient.

Semi-Aquatic Chelonians

The majority of semi-aquatic chelonians are omnivorous and exploit a wide variety of food sources in their natural habitats. Feeding recommendations for terrestrial and semi-aquatic chelonians are provided in Box 4.1. Most juveniles tend to be carnivorous but consume a higher proportion of plant material as they mature; for example, adult red-eared sliders (*Trachemys scripta elegans*) become increasingly more herbivorous. Nutritional imbalance and disease can result if semi-aquatic chelonians are fed meat, fish pieces or prawn-only diets and thus multivitamin and calcium supplementation must be provided if they are offered these food items. Adult semi-and aquatic chelonians should only be fed two to four times a week, depending on species and life stage, as obesity is common. Many semi-aquatic species will not eat unless they are fed in water. It is recommended to use a separate feeding tank to avoid soiling the main tank with uneaten food. Some species prefer to consume partly decomposed vegetation instead of fresh food items.

Aquatic Chelonians

Aquatic chelonians are initially carnivorous as hatchlings but become omnivores once they reach adult life (Box 4.2). Obligate carnivores include certain marine species, such as loggerhead turtles (*Caretta caretta*) and

Box 4.1 A general guide to feeding terrestrial and semi-aquatic omnivorous chelonians.

Vegetation (greens; 50–90% of diet)

- Collard greens
- Mustard greens
- Dandelion
- Chard
- Kale
- Parsley
- Squash
- Carrots
- Broccoli
- Spinach

Animal protein (10–50% of diet)

- Invertebrates (e.g. earthworms, crickets, waxworms, woodlice, slugs, silkworms and snails)
- Raw whole fish (e.g. sardines)
- Whole mice
- Pinkies
- Trout pellets (soaked)

Comments

- Whole fish are nutritionally more complete compared with gutted fish and should be offered periodically to provide vitamin A.
- Adult mice are nutritionally superior to pinkies.
- Cat and dog foods can have particularly high fat and vitamin D3 contents and should be avoided or only fed occasionally, as they can cause soft tissue mineralization.
- Commercial turtle flakes (rich in dried shrimp) may lack vitamins and minerals.

Box 4.2 Selected food preferences for carnivorous aquatic chelonians kept in captive environments.

Freshwater species:
- Long-necked turtles (*Chelodina longicollis*)
- Snapping turtles (*Chelydra* spp.)
- Matamata (*Chelus fimbriatus*)
- Softshell turtles (*Apalone* spp.)

Preferred foods:
- Mice
- Earthworms
- Shrimp (with shells)
- Trout
- Slugs
- Snails
- Wild-caught invertebrates
- Day-old chicks
- Trout chow
- Turtle flakes
- Tubifex worms
- Waxworms
- Mealworms
- Grasshoppers

Comments:
- Ideally feed whole vertebrate prey items.
- Insects should only be a minor part of the diet.
- Occasionally, a variety of greens and aquatic plants can also be offered.
- Commercial turtle and fish diets are poor nutritional substitutes, so should only be fed in minimal amounts.

Marine species:
- Green sea turtle (*Chelonia mydas*; the only herbivorous sea turtle)
- Hawksbill turtle (*Eretmochelys imbricata*)
- Loggerhead turtle (*Caretta caretta*)

Preferred foods:
- Crustaceans
- Molluscs
- Sea grasses
- Algae
- Trout pellets

Comments:
- Captive sea turtles will eat fish, crustaceans, and molluscs and may be acclimated to balanced diets in pellet or gelatin form.
- A fish-based multivitamin containing thiamine (25 mg/kg of fish) and vitamin E (100 iu/kg of fish) should be provided daily.
- In the wild:
  - Green sea turtles feed on sea grasses and algae.
  - Loggerhead, Kemp's ridley and Olive ridley turtles prey on molluscs and crustaceans.
  - Hawksbills prefer sponges.
  - Leatherback turtles specialize on jellyfish.

freshwater chelonians, such as soft-shell turtles (*Apalone* spp.), with the latter species also consuming a small amount of vegeta-tion. Obesity is common in captive adult aquatic chelonians, so they should only be fed three to four times a week.

Reference

Latney, L. and Clayton, L. (2014) Updates on amphibian nutrition and nutritive value of common feeder insects. *Veterinary Clinics of North America: Exotic Animal Practice*, 17 (3), 347–367.

Further Reading

Almli, L.M. and Burghardt, G.M. (2006) Environmental enrichment alters the behavioral profile of ratsnakes (Elaphe). *Journal of Applied Animal Welfare Science*, 9 (2): 85–109.

Barten, S.L. (2006) Lizards, in *Reptile Medicine and Surgery*, 2nd ed. (D.R. Mader, ed.). Elsevier, St Louis, MO, pp. 59–77.

Berger, S., Martin II, L.B., Wikelski, M. et al. (2005) Corticosterone suppresses immune activity in territorial Galápagos marine iguanas during reproduction. *Hormones and Behavior*, 47 (4), 419–429.

Boyer, T.H. and Boyer, D.M. (2006) Turtles, tortoises, and terrapins, in *Reptile Medicine and Surgery*, 2nd ed., (D.R. Mader, ed.). Elsevier, St Louis, MO, pp. 78–99.

Burghardt, G.M. (2013) Environmental enrichment and cognitive complexity in reptiles and amphibians: concepts, review, and implications for captive populations. *Applied Animal Behaviour Science*, 147 (3–4), 286–298.

Calvert, I. (2004) Nutrition, in *BSAVA Manual of Reptiles*, 2nd ed. (S.J. Girling and P. Raiti, eds). British Small Animal Veterinary Association, Gloucester, pp. 18–39.

Calvert, I. (2004) Nutritional problems, in *BSAVA Manual of Reptiles*, 2nd ed. (S.J. Girling and P. Raiti, eds). British Small Animal Veterinary Association, Gloucester, pp. 289–308.

Chapple, D.G. (2003) Ecology, life-history, and behavior in the Australian Scincid genus *Egernia*, with comments on the evolution of complex sociality in lizards. *Herpetological Monographs* 17: 145–180.

Cooper, J.E. (2010) Terrestrial reptiles: lizards, snakes and tortoises, in *The UFAW Handbook on the Care and Management of Laboratory and other Research Animals*, 8th ed. (R. Hubrecht and J. Kirkwood, eds). Wiley-Blackwell, Oxford, pp. 707–730.

Dierenfeld, E. and King, J (2008) Digestibility and mineral availability of Phoenix worms, *Hermetia illucens*, ingested by mountain chicken frogs, *Leptodactylus fallax*. *Journal of Herpetological Medicine and Surgery*, 18: 100–105.

Donoghue S. (2006) Nutrition, in *Reptile Medicine and Surgery*, 2nd ed. (D.R. Mader, ed.). Elsevier, St Louis, MO, pp. 251–298.

Eatwell, K. (2010) Lizards, in *BSAVA Manual of Exotic Pets: A Foundation Manual*, 5th ed. (A. Meredith and C. Johnson-Delaney, eds). British Small Animal Veterinary Association, Gloucester, pp. 273–293.

Ernst, C. and Barbour, R. (1989) *Turtles of the World*. Smithsonian Institution Press, Washington, D.C.

Flanagan, J.P. (2015) Chelonians (Turtles, Tortoises), in *Fowler's Zoo and Wild Animal Medicine, Volume* 8. (R.E. Miller and M.E. Fowler, eds). Elsevier Saunders, St Louis, MO, pp. 27–37.

Ganesh, C.B. and Yajurved, H.N. (2002) Stress inhibits seasonal and FSH-induced ovarian recrudescence in the lizard, *Mabuya carinata*. *Journal of Experimental Zoology*, 292 (7), 640–648.

Gardner, M.G., Pearson, S.K., Johnston, G.R. and Schwarz, M.P. (2016) Group living in squamate reptiles: a review of evidence for stable aggregations. *Biological reviews of the Cambridge Philosophical Society*, 91(4), 925–936.

Gramanzini, M., Di Girolamo, N., Gargiulo S. *et al.* (2013) Assessment of dual-energy x-ray absorptiometry for use in evaluating the effects of dietary and environmental management on Hermann's tortoises (*Testudo hermanni*). *American Journal of Veterinary Research*, 74 (6), 918–224.

Greenberg, N., and Crews, D. (1990) Endocrine and behavioral responses to aggression and social dominance in the green anole lizard, *Anolis carolinesis*. *General and Comparative Endocrinology*, 77, 246–255.

Jessop, M. and Bennett, T.D. (2010) Tortoises and Turtles, in *BSAVA Manual of Exotic Pets: A Foundation Manual*, 5th ed. (A. Meredith and C. Johnson-Delaney, eds). British Small Animal Veterinary Association, Glocester, pp. 249–272.

Johnson, J.H. (2004) Husbandry and medicine of aquatic reptiles. *Seminars in Avian and Exotic Pet Medicine*, 13 (4), 223–228.

Klaphake, E. (2010) A fresh look at metabolic bone diseases in reptiles and amphibians. *Veterinary Clinics of North America Exotic Animal Practice*, 13, 375–392.

McArthur, S., Wilkinson, R., Meyer, J., *et al.* (2004) *Medicine and Surgery of Tortoises and Turtles*. Blackwell Publishing, Oxford.

Mans, C. and Braun, J. (2014) Update on common nutritional disorders of captive reptiles. *Veterinary Clinics of North America Exotic Animal Practice*, 17, 369–395.

Molina, F.d.B. and Lightfoot, T.L. (2001) Class Reptilia, order Squamata, (lizards): iguanas,

tegus, in *Biology, Medicine, and Surgery of South American Wild Animals* (M.E. Fowler and Z.S. Cubas, eds), Iowa State University Press, Ames, IA, pp. 31–39.

Norton, T.M. and Walsh, M.T. (2012) *Sea turtle rehabilitation in Fowler's Zoo and Wild Animal Medicine: Current Therapy, Volume 7* (R.E. Miller and M.E. Fowler, eds), Elsevier-Saunders, St Louis, MO, pp. 239–246.

O'Malley, B. (2005) *Clinical Anatomy and Physiology of Exotic Species*. Saunders-Elsevier, St. Louis, MO.

Polis, G.A. and Myers, C.A. (1985) A Survey of intraspecific predation among reptiles and amphibians. *Journal of Herpetology*, 19 (1), 99–107.

Raftery, A. (2004) Clinical examination, in *BSAVA Manual of Reptiles*, 2nd ed. (S.J. Girling and P. Raiti, eds), British Small Animal Veterinary Association, Gloucester, pp. 51–70.

Raiti, P. (2010) Snakes, in *BSAVA Manual of Exotic Pets: A Foundation Manual*, 5th ed. (A. Meredith and C. Johnson-Delaney, eds), British Small Animal Veterinary Association, Gloucester, pp. 294–315.

Rossi, J.V. (2006) General husbandry and management, in *Reptile Medicine and Surgery* (D. R. Mader, ed.), St Louis, MO, Saunders, pp. 25–41.

Silvestre, A.M. (2014) How to assess stress in reptiles. *Journal of Exotic Pet Medicine*, 23 (3), 240–243.

Varga, M. (2004) Captive maintenance and welfare, in *BSAVA Manual of Reptiles*, 2nd ed. (S.J. Girling and P. Raiti, eds), British Small Animal Veterinary Association, Gloucester, pp. 6–17.

Wilkinson, S.L. (2015) Reptile wellness management. *Veterinary Clinics of North America Exotic Animal Practice*, 18, 281–304.

5

Enclosure Design

Michael McFadden, Deborah Monks, Bob Doneley and Robert Johnson

Introduction

Before acquiring any reptile species, careful consideration must be given to exactly how the species will be housed. This must take into account the species behaviour, size and thermoregulatory requirements. Reptile housing not only provides safety and security, it also allows specific physiological needs to be met. Being ectothermic, the provision of heat and ultraviolet light, with appropriate gradients for each, is crucial for reptilian health. With these facts in mind, possibly the first decision to make is whether the species will be housed indoors or outdoors.

Indoor or Outdoor Enclosures

There are many advantages to housing reptiles in indoor enclosures. They allow the keeper better control of the reptile's environment, as there is no exposure to natural elements such as rainfall or extreme fluctuations in temperature. Electrical devices such as heaters and lights can be safely employed without contact with water, and the temperature within the facility can be carefully controlled to suit the species. Housing reptiles inside also minimizes the risk of contact with wild reptiles or potential predators and reduces the risk posed by parasites (if managed appropriately). There are disadvantages, however. There is a need to replicate natural environmental cues, with the associated cost of purchasing and maintaining heating and lighting devices and the limitations of available space.

Conversely, there is a range of benefits to housing a species in an outside enclosure. Heating and lighting are free and readily available, assuming that the outdoor enclosure has been positioned in a location where the reptiles have access to sunlight for at least eight hours a day and the species being kept is from a climatically similar natural environment. By accessing natural sunlight, it provides the reptiles with a much better source of ultraviolet B than that provided by artificial light sources. Outdoor enclosures permit the species to be exposed to numerous cues (e.g. natural photoperiod and seasonal variations in temperature) that can stimulate normal behaviours, including feeding and reproduction. They are less restricted on space than indoor enclosures. Possibly the primary disadvantage is that outdoor enclosure use is

Reptile Medicine and Surgery in Clinical Practice, First Edition. Edited by Bob Doneley, Deborah Monks, Robert Johnson and Brendan Carmel.

largely limited to those species found in a similar climatic zone, otherwise artificial heating may need to be provided.

Almost any species of reptile can be maintained in an indoor enclosure assuming that all vital needs, such as spatial requirements, adequate basking sites and the provision of ultraviolet B light, are met. Smaller species can be much easier to maintain indoors, owing to their smaller spatial needs and the relative ease of providing temperature gradients. Larger species, such as large monitors and crocodilians, require much larger enclosures. However, this can be achieved successfully, as demonstrated by many zoos.

Species most suitable for outdoor enclosures are those that have evolved in a climate similar to that where the enclosure is located. Care must be taken to consider humidity, rather than just temperature, as housing arid species in humid coastal environments may result in respiratory infection during the cooler months. Other species may be kept outdoors as long as careful attention has been paid to ensure their requirements are met. For example, a tropical or sub-tropical species may be kept outdoors in a temperate environment assuming that additional basking sites and night heating have been provided.

General Housing Considerations

When designing enclosures, both indoors and out, there are some basic points to consider: location, design, construction materials, access, furniture, heating and lighting.

Location

Indoor
It is best to locate enclosures within a well-insulated room that does not fluctuate greatly in temperature. To make heating more cost effective, some larger hobbyists will heat a room to a minimum optimum body temperature for the species being housed and then

provide basking areas within each enclosure. Enclosures should generally be raised off the floor, to prevent the cold being absorbed from below, especially if facility flooring is concrete.

Direct sunlight directed on a glass enclosure can quickly raise the temperature to potentially lethal levels. This mistake is sometimes made by those erroneously believing that sunlight through a window will provide for the ultraviolet needs of the reptile, unaware that the ultraviolet light is filtered out by glass or plastic.

Outdoor
Outdoor enclosures are best positioned where they will receive direct sunlight for at least eight hours per day, allowing thermoregulation and providing access to natural ultraviolet light. Both basking areas and shade must be provided to allow the animal to thermoregulate. In those species in which breeding is anticipated, appropriate nesting sites (with appropriate substrate) should be provided (Figure 5.1).

Turtles, crocodilians, some agamids and some snakes are aquatic or require regular access to water. Stagnant water will cause numerous hygiene issues, so most outdoor enclosures have a pond and a filtration system both to remove particulate waste and to aerate the water. Regular water testing is still required, as is pond cleaning. Water loss due to evaporation needs to be carefully monitored, as this will concentrate soluble waste products within the water.

Design

Indoor
The ultimate design of any reptile enclosure will be largely dependent on the natural history and behaviour of the species being kept. Before designing an enclosure, it is important to research the key life history attributes of the species. This includes whether it is terrestrial or arboreal, to help to determine whether a horizontal or vertical enclosure is required. Determine whether it is nocturnal

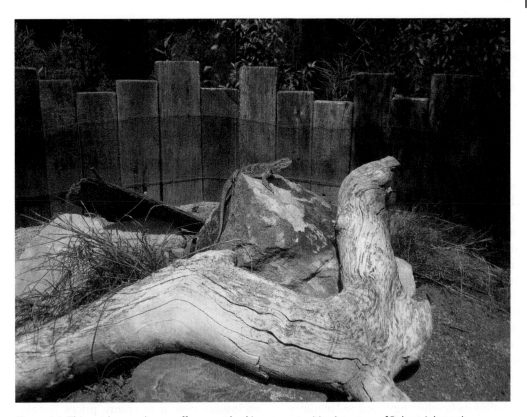

Figure 5.1 This outdoor enclosure offers great basking opportunities (courtesy of Robert Johnson).

or diurnal, which greatly affects how to optimize the heating of the enclosure. Other attributes, such as whether the species is partially aquatic or fossorial, is assessed as this will influence whether a focus should be made on providing a sizable water body or a suitable deep substrate.

The size of a reptile enclosure can be quite variable, depending on the species. There are no distinct rules that determine the size of an enclosure and the it can vary greatly, even within a genus or between species of the same size. However, there do exist minimum enclosure requirements in some jurisdictions. An ideal enclosure is large enough to allow the reptiles within it to exhibit natural behaviours, including basking, hiding, movement (whether terrestrial or arboreal) and the ability to use a temperature gradient.

Care should be taken not to provide an enclosure that is too large. Unfortunately, many well-meaning new keepers often provide their juvenile pythons with a large, open enclosure with a basking light for heat. These juvenile snakes inevitably occupy a shelter at a suboptimal temperature and refuse to feed. A smaller enclosure, particularly with several hides, will usually make a younger snake feel more secure, thus allowing it to feel safe while feeding and thermoregulating.

Outdoor

Housing a reptile outdoors usually allows for a larger, better ventilated enclosure. These enclosures need to be predator and pest proof, secure against both reptile escape and unauthorized human entry, provide adequate access to heat and light and sufficient protection from extremes of temperature, especially heat. The presence of aerial predators such as crows or hawks may necessitate roofing.

If the enclosure is well positioned, electricity costs can be reduced by permitting the reptiles to bask in natural sunlight, rather than supplying artificial ultraviolet light and heating. It should be noted that animals housed outdoors may still require some heated areas.

Construction Materials

Indoor

The selection of materials for indoor enclosures depends on the species, the desired enclosure design and the climatic conditions within the room in which it will be located. Factors that can often guide a decision on choice of materials include the weight of the materials, cost, insulation properties and how easy it is to clean and disinfect. Three of the most commonly chosen materials to construct enclosures are glass, plastic and timber. Although commonly used, caution should be applied when employing materials that may swell when exposed to moisture, including melamine, chipboard and medium-density fibreboard (MDF).

Glass Glass is one of the most commonly used construction materials for reptile enclosures. It can be aesthetically pleasing and is commercially available in a wide range of sizes, largely due to the aquarium trade. Traditionally, glass reptile terraria were purchased as fish tanks. If using a fish tank for a lizard or snake, great care must be taken to ensure that the lid will adequately contain the reptile, as most fish tanks are not sold with tight-fitting, well-ventilated lids. Currently, there is a range of glass terraria available specifically designed for reptiles. These include a number of attractive, front-opening enclosures with ventilation panels on the sides and/or roof. Aquatic turtles are usually maintained indoors in fish tanks with dry docking platforms. It is important that these are stable, as unstable platforms may not be used by the animal (Figures 5.2 and 5.3).

Disadvantages of glass include its cost, weight and insulation properties. Glass enclosures can be quite expensive, although the greater range of commercially available enclosures now may ensure prices remain competitive. Glass is a poor insulator, so heat

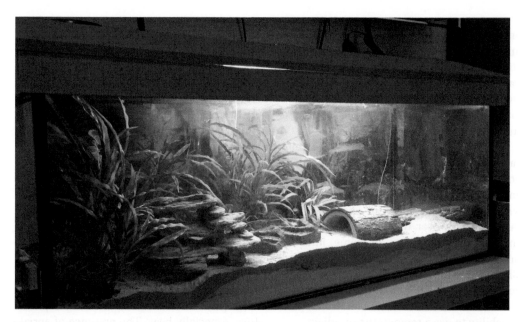

Figure 5.2 This converted aquarium tank houses *Nephrurus asper* geckos. The easily accessible lid prevents access of other animals into the enclosure. In this case, heating is by way of heat cord under the substrate (courtesy of Deborah Monks).

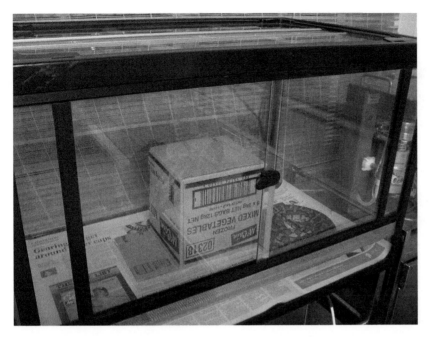

Figure 5.3 This glass reptile enclosure has inbuilt vents but can require insulation during colder seasons as glass does not tend to retain heat (courtesy of Bob Doneley).

can be rapidly lost from an enclosure if there is a significant difference between the temperature within and outside of the enclosure. Additionally, for nervous specimens, it is possible that they may feel less secure in an enclosure that is transparent on all sides. Certain animals may not perceive glass as a barrier and may cause severe rostral rub injuries through repeated abrasion while pacing.

Plastic There are a range of plastic enclosures widely used for housing reptiles. These include smaller plastic-lidded containers, plastic tubs positioned in a rack system and commercially available moulded plastic enclosures. They are generally light in weight, easy to disinfectant and are waterproof. However, plastic also has a number of disadvantages, including having poor insulation properties, becoming easily scratched and turning brittle or warping when exposed to heat or ultraviolet light.

The smaller plastic enclosures have been successfully used for juveniles or small species, such as geckos or young pythons.

However, they are generally only available in smaller sizes, restricting their use to only small specimens. For larger specimens, there is now a range of larger, aesthetically pleasing moulded plastic enclosures available from a number of suppliers. However, apart from cost, these enclosures also have some disadvantages. They may warp over time, affecting the ability of the glass doors to close tightly. In some brands, the raised front below the sliding doors can quite easily conceal a snake, making it difficult to see a specimen before opening the enclosure. Additionally, although the enclosures are designed to conveniently stack on top of each other to use the space efficiently, replacing a light globe may require removal of all of the enclosures (Figure 5.4).

Timber Timber is the most commonly used material for building reptile enclosures. It is sturdy, affordable and has good insulation properties. Timber enclosures can be built to any desired size or specification and the materials are readily available. However, care must be taken to ensure the timber and the

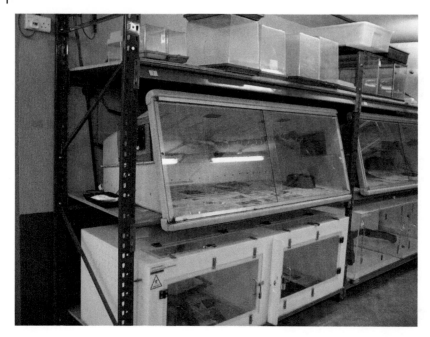

Figure 5.4 These plastic moulded enclosures are easy to disinfect (courtesy of Bob Doneley).

joins have been properly sealed to prevent moisture directly contacting the exposed timber, leading to the timber rotting. Marine grade timber is often used as it is more resistant to moisture and humidity as well as being very sturdy. Exposed hardware can sometimes cause lacerations or abrasions (Figure 5.5).

Outdoor

Although outdoor enclosures may be made of similar materials to indoor enclosures, simply using 'indoor' enclosures outside diminishes many of the benefits of housing reptiles outdoors.

- Pits: some species are amenable to being kept in dug-out, secured pits (Figures 5.1 and 5.6). The sides should offer limited purchase for escape, although top covers are often recommended to protect the animals from predators.
- Wire and wood/metal: some species, such as arboreal snakes, do well in aviary style enclosures made from wire mesh on wooden or metal frame. If using wood, it is important that it is sealed to prevent contamination. It should be non-toxic.

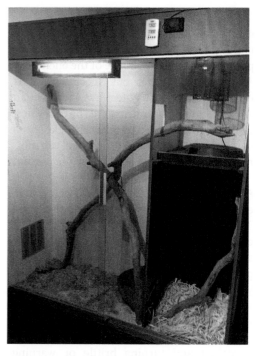

Figure 5.5 Timber enclosure suitable for a python. There is a range of thermal options for this snake, as well as different substrates to increase environmental stimulation (courtesy of Deborah Monks).

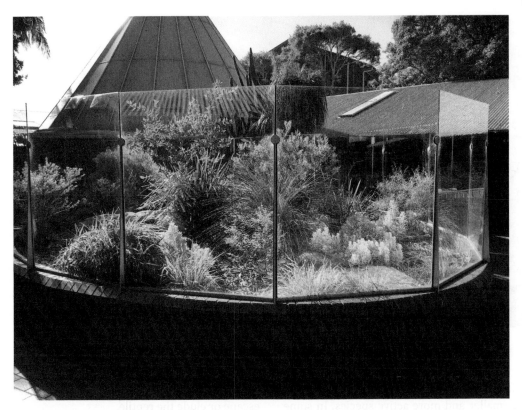

Figure 5.6 A secure outdoor enclosure, suitable for red-bellied black snakes (courtesy of Michael McFadden).

- Glass/Perspex: institutions displaying animals to the public often use half-length Perspex or glass to prevent contact but allow sight of the animals. Terrestrial animals can be housed this way, although arboreal animals may escape. It is important that there are no protuberances near the enclosure perimeter which could be used to assist escape.
- Ponds: aquatic animals such as turtles and crocodilians will require an outdoor water source as well as land. Filtration and water quality are discussed later in this chapter. It is important that the water source is accessible, with a non-slip substrate to facilitate entry and exit. Additionally, cleaning must be easy to accomplish and usually there needs to be some sort of filtration.

Whatever construction materials are used, it is important that there are no sharp points or areas in which the animals may be injured or trapped.

Access for Feeding, Cleaning when Dealing with Venomous Reptiles

Venomous reptiles should be housed in lockable enclosures within a locked room. Hide boxes fitted with sliding and secure doors can serve as transport containers or as temporary housing during cage cleaning (Figure 5.7). The appearance of the enclosure should strike a happy medium between providing a 'natural' enclosure and one that is easily maintained, and that access to the snake is not hindered by a proliferation of cage furniture. Front-opening enclosures are preferable; however, a barrier at ground level

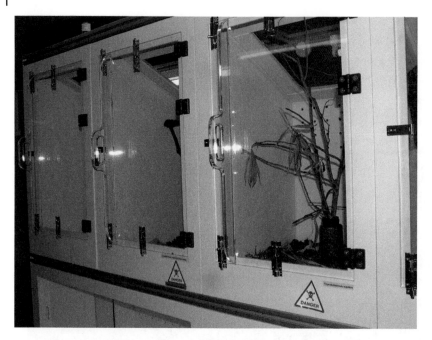

Figure 5.7 Venomous reptiles kept in locked enclosure (courtesy of Bob Doneley).

may need to be in place to prevent the escape of smaller and more active species. In some regions, venomous snakes can be kept outdoors in pits or in well-fenced enclosures (Figures 5.1 and 5.6). Access to these areas should be strictly controlled.

Furniture

Food and Water Dishes

Almost all species require a water dish, pond or other source of fresh water. The exceptions are species that will only accept water from rain or dew, including arboreal exotic species such as chameleons, which may need a daily spray or mist to rehydrate. Even so, water sources will add to enclosure humidity which is important for some tropical species.

Food dishes are used for species being fed non-live food items. After feeding is complete, they should be removed and cleaned. Additionally, food dishes may be used for live invertebrate feeding in situations where impaction from substrate may be a problem or where the species cannot be tong fed and there is a potential for the crickets to either escape or elude the reptile.

Privacy Shelters

Most reptiles require shelters that permit them to hide. Exceptions to this include large or arboreal reptiles that would sleep on a branch or in the open under natural conditions. A shelter will provide a sense of security in the reptile, reducing stress levels and permit the reptile to thrive. Some reptiles, such as hatchling pythons, may not commence feeding if a shelter site is not provided. Shelters can take many forms, including rock caves, disposable cardboard boxes or commercially sold plastic reptile hides. Shelters must not be excessively large or animals will not feel secure within. Entry points should be sufficiently wide to permit twice the animal's width. Outdoor enclosures can also use hollow logs, grass and shrubbery as a more naturalistic hide area.

Branches

Natural branches and vines or commercially available artificial alternatives can assist the aesthetics of an enclosure and support natural behaviours in an arboreal reptile. Care must be taken to secure these furnishings when installing them, so that they do not fall, potentially causing injury. Similarly for rock-dwelling reptiles, natural or artificial rocks can be placed in an enclosure to facilitate basking platforms and rock crevices in which to shelter. However, these must be situated carefully so as not to collapse upon the reptile.

Plants are often difficult to maintain inside without appropriate plant lighting, plants do improve the aesthetics of a cage. Often placed in aquaria, plants also fulfil a nutritional function for some species of turtles. Plants will often grow better in outdoor enclosures.

Other Furniture

Other pieces of cage furniture may be visually pleasing for the owner but not fulfil any useful function for the animal. Furniture must be sufficiently secured to avoid injury or entrapment.

Heat Source

See Chapters 4 and 6 for a detailed discussion on various heating options. It is worth noting that reptiles appear to be relatively insensitive to thermal pain, so direct contact with heating elements must be avoided. Heating elements should be enclosed to prevent reptiles coming into contact with them (Figure 5.8) and heat pads and heat rocks should have a secondary thermostat system to prevent overheating. Insufficient heating leads to immunosuppression, among other physiological issues. It is equally important to avoid overheating, as reptiles can perish in high temperatures. Even if the animals within an outdoor enclosure are acclimatized to the local conditions, there should be a back-up plan for heat provision in the case of poor or cold weather persisting for more than 24 hours.

Aquatic animals may need the water sources heated, which is done most commonly using a fish tank heater. As with any heating element, a secondary thermometer should be used to check the accuracy of the heat provision

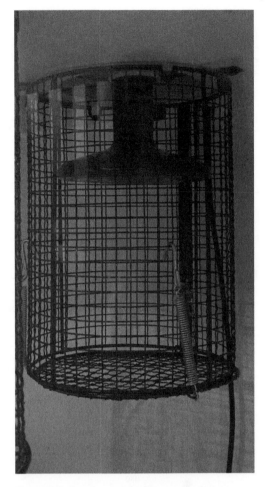

Figure 5.8 Cage to prevent direct animal access to heat lamp. This is an essential part of adequate husbandry (courtesy of Deborah Monks).

(Figure 5.9). With some large or aggressive animals, the heater should be caged to avoid damage and possible electrocution.

Lighting

Ultraviolet lighting is extremely important for calcium metabolism in many species (see Chapter 6 for more detail). Please note that lights can also cause burns from heat production, so should be caged if there is a chance that an animal may come into direct contact with them.

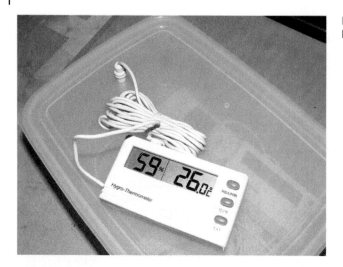

Figure 5.9 Thermometer and hygrometer (courtesy of Bob Doneley).

Table 5.1 Advantages and disadvantages of various substrate options.

Substrate	Cost	Ease of replacement and cleaning	Visualisation of droppings	Naturalistic	Risk of ingestion
Newspaper	£	☺☺☺	Easy	No	No
Recycled newspaper pellets (e.g. cat litter)	£	☺☺	Easy	No	Yes
Pine chips	££	☺☺	Moderate	No	Yes
Coconut fibre	£££	☺☺	Difficult	Yes	Yes
Synthetic turf	£££ but multiple use	☺☺☺	Easy	No	No
Sand	££	☺	Easy	Yes	Yes

Substrate

There are many different substrate options for reptiles and the appropriate substrate may vary according to time of year and clinical need (Table 5.1). Animals kept without substrate not uncommonly have difficulty with mobility, due to lack of traction. The glare from overhead lighting reflected from the flooring can cause stress, especially in glass-bottomed enclosures.

Pest Control

It is important that all outdoor enclosures are securely pest-proofed to ensure the safety of the reptiles and to prevent potential escape. Rats and mice are capable climbers and can also dig under a wall. For this reason, all enclosures should either have a solid or mesh base or the walls must be dug at least 50 cm into the ground. Enclosures for smaller species should be fully enclosed to prevent access from other predators, such as birds or cats. Depending on the local invertebrate population and the species kept, measures may need to be taken to protect insectivorous animals from ingesting poisonous or excessively hard bodied insects.

Breeding Racks

Breeding racks are a popular style of housing employed by larger breeders or keepers with large reptile collections. They are typically designed as a portable rack on wheels with many shelves containing plastic tubs (Figure 5.10). There are a number of instances where breeding racks can be useful. They allow for the efficient holding of a large number of reptiles in a relatively small space. Examples of where this may be beneficial include research programmes or for the rearing of large numbers of juvenile snakes. Other advantages of using a rack include the low electricity cost (as the enclosures are typically heated via energy efficient heat tape or cords) and ease of disinfection (as the tubs are typically plastic and easy to wash).

There are, however, disadvantages associated with breeding racks. It is usually not possible to provide effective lighting to the enclosures within a rack as, in most rack designs, lighting cannot be suspended above the tubs, leaving room lighting as the sole source of light. For this reason, these

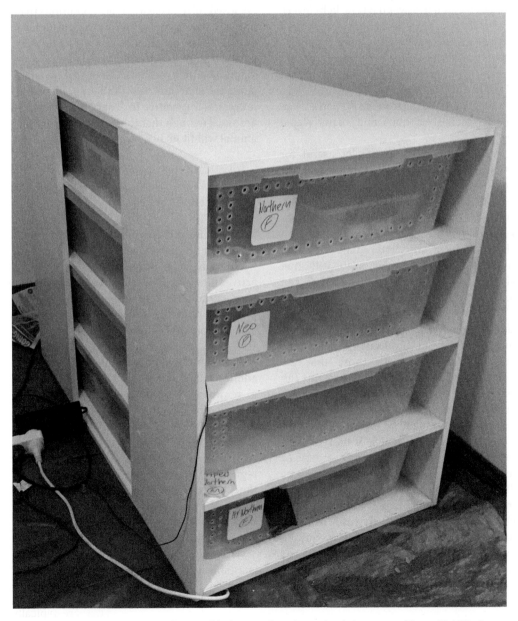

Figure 5.10 A small rack system, often used for housing breeding animals (courtesy of Emma McMillan).

enclosures have only limited use in diurnal basking species and should not be used for species requiring ultraviolet B. There are extremely limited opportunities to provide environmental enrichment to animals in breeding racks, which may cause welfare concerns. In the advent of a contagious disease, quarantine and infection control are very difficult to establish in a rack system.

Species most suitable for breeding racks are typically nocturnal species. These species are better suited to lower daytime light levels, have lower requirements of ultraviolet B light and naturally regulate their body temperature through the ambient temperature and by resting on warm surfaces, similar to that accessible on the heated base of a tub in a breeding rack. Such groups of reptiles can include geckos, pythons and many elapid snakes.

Breeding racks are especially useful for juvenile snakes. Juvenile snakes typically require a relatively small enclosure, with suitable hides, a water bowl and a heat gradient, with a warm spot provided by under-floor heating. They are also best housed individually to minimize stress and reduce the risk of cannibalism. These needs are easily met within a typical breeding rack, which can house hatchlings in an efficient manner.

The size of breeding racks is extremely variable. Commercial racks are available in a range of sizes from those suitable for geckos and hatchling snakes to those that are designed for large pythons. Rack systems can also be easily custom designed and constructed around a particular size of tub that best suits the reptile to be kept.

Breeding racks are typically heated using under-floor techniques, such as heat tape or heat cord. These heating products are quite efficient, as they have low wattage and can provide a suitable temperature gradient within a tub. They are usually easily installed but in all instances where wiring is required, always use a qualified electrician. Heat cords may need to be recessed within the base of the shelf of the rack to ensure that the tubs can be easily slid into and out of the rack

without catching. It may also be necessary to have more than one row of heat cord per shelf, especially for medium to larger tubs, to ensure that there is a suitably large heated area with an even heat distribution. To avoid malfunction, a thermometer should be used to confirm adequate heat provision, thus preventing both under- and over-heating.

It is important to ensure that the tubs within a rack system receive adequate ventilation. A lack of ventilation within an enclosed tub can easily create conditions that are excessively moist and humid, especially after a snake urinates or if a water bowl is partially spilled. Typically, ventilation is provided by either mesh panels or drilled holes along the sides and rear of the tub. If drilling holes, it is imperative to ensure that the holes are small enough that there is no risk that the animal will fit its head through them.

Aquatic Enclosure and Water Quality

Whether indoors or outdoors, aquatic and semi-aquatic species need to have access to healthy, hygienic water, preferably with an active nitrogen cycle. Faeces and urinary waste products, leftover food and decomposing plant material release toxic ammonia. The conversion of this ammonia to progressively less toxic chemicals is called the nitrogen cycle. Denitrifying bacteria convert ammonia into nitrite and then nitrate, which is removed via regular water changes or absorbed by aquatic plants. After first adding water, it takes about six weeks for a nitrogen cycle to completely establish. Plants and small amounts of organic material should be regularly but gradually added during this time. Filtration should be installed and active. Water quality should be tested regularly to track the establishment of the nitrogen cycle.

With indoor tanks, once the nitrogen cycle is established, between 10% and 20% of the water should be removed and replaced once a week. This is in addition to replacing any water loss from evaporation. Gravel or siphon vacuums are useful, as they clean the substrate at the same time as removing water. It is important to only clean between 10% and 20% of the substrate at any one time, avoiding disturbing large pockets of anaerobic bacteria and overloading the denitrifying bacteria or reducing total levels of denitrifying bacteria. Leftover food and floating faeces should be removed from the tank daily.

Filtration is very important, both to remove waste and to oxygenate the water. For indoor aquaria, at least one large, external canister filter is required, which will circulate three to four water volumes per hour. Tank volume can be calculated using the formula:

length multiplied by width by height of the water column (all in metres) = volume (litres)

For outdoor ponds, a similar water flow rate is recommended. Measure the height of the water level, not the height of the entire tank. External filters often have three types of filtration: chemical (activated charcoal), physical (sponge) and biological (ceramic or plastic 'biospheres' coated in denitrifying bacteria). The return of filtered water to the tank is usually via a spray bar that breaks the surface tension of the water and oxygenates it.

The internal components of the filter should be cleaned in a bucket of tank or pond water, *never* with tap water. This is to preserve all the good bacteria in the filter that assist with the nitrogen cycle. Water quality should be tested regularly, even after the nitrogen cycle is well established, as there may be differences throughout the year.

Summary

Ultimately, the choice of enclosure and the design is the owner's choice. Species requirements, individual behavioural needs, owner preference for naturalistic versus utilitarian, cost and ease of maintenance all factor into the choice. From a veterinary perspective, better-designed enclosures will tend to lead to healthier animals, as they supply a better microclimate and secure options for the animals.

Further Reading

More information on reptile enclosures can be found in herpetocutural literature, including the Australian Birdkeeper Publications series A Guide to ... books covering different reptile species (lizards, pythons, elapid snakes, varanids, etc.).

6

Lighting
Frances M. Baines

Introduction

Lighting is surely one of the most neglected and misunderstood aspects of reptile husbandry. The provision of species appropriate levels of full spectrum lighting is vital. Evolutionary processes determine that optimal levels of heat, light and ultraviolet (UV) are likely to be the 'natural' levels that the reptile experiences in its microhabitat with favourable environmental conditions. Reptiles self-regulate their exposure to solar radiation. Deviations from the optimal range are likely to act as stressors, with negative repercussions on health. Much attention has been paid in the past to thermoregulation and the need for thermal gradients in the vivarium; the importance of similar, superimposed visible light and UV gradients is now becoming more widely recognized.

The Solar Spectrum

The part of the electromagnetic spectrum that is found in sunlight (Figure 6.1) includes short-wavelength infrared (IR-A: 750–1500 nm), so-called visible light (visible to humans; 400–780 nm) and ultraviolet (UV). Ultraviolet light is subdivided into UVA (320–400 nm) and UVB, only part of which (290–295 nm, depending upon solar altitude, to 320 nm) is present in sunlight, since earth's atmosphere blocks hazardous shorter wavelengths (UVB below 290 nm and all UVC) from reaching the surface.

Infrared

Short-wavelength infrared (IR-A) is responsible for the warming effect of sunlight. During its passage through the atmosphere, water vapour absorbs certain wavelengths strongly, so that when it reaches earth's surface it is 'water filtered'. This naturally filtered IR-A penetrates deeply through the skin without excessive heating of water molecules in the tissues. Basking reptiles absorb water-filtered IR-A extremely effectively; solar radiation may pass right through the dorsal skin to the internal organs of small-bodied specimens. IR-A also warms the surface of the earth, which re-radiates in far longer wavelengths (IR-B and IR-C; 1400–1,000,000 nm). Long-wavelength infrared does not penetrate the epidermis. Its heat energy is absorbed entirely by the upper layers of the skin, from which it must be conducted or carried by convection in bodily fluids to deeper tissues. This type of radiation is absorbed from warm surroundings by the ventral skin of the reptile; where the skin is in contact with substrate, heat transfer by conduction also takes place. Infrared is invisible to humans and

Reptile Medicine and Surgery in Clinical Practice, First Edition. Edited by Bob Doneley, Deborah Monks, Robert Johnson and Brendan Carmel.
© 2018 John Wiley & Sons Ltd. Published 2018 by John Wiley & Sons Ltd.

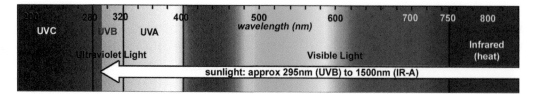

Figure 6.1 The solar spectrum is part of the electromagnetic spectrum which extends from around 290–295 nm (depending upon solar altitude) in the UVB range, to 1500 nm in the short-wavelength infrared.

most reptiles, although some snakes can perceive the longer wavelengths (above 3000 nm) through their facial pit organs.

Visible Light and Ultraviolet A

Retinal cone cells are responsible for colour vision. Humans have three types of cone cell, responding only to what we call 'visible light'. Most reptiles have a fourth cone type, which responds to UVA, enabling vision in the ultraviolet (Figure 6.2). This extra dimension to colour perception is vital to many reptile species for intraspecific recognition and detection of food items, since UVA-reflective markings are found on many animals and plants. Some nocturnal geckos lack the red-sensitive cone but their green-sensitive cone also responds to red light. Some have full colour vision in dim moonlight that humans can barely see.

Sunlight has powerful effects unrelated to conscious vision. Non-visual photoreceptors are found in the retina, the pineal body and the parietal eye (where present). Reptiles possess deep brain photoreceptors that respond to sunlight's glow through the skull. These transmit information as to the length of day and night, the sun's position in the sky and the intensity and proportion of short-wavelength light to the suprachiasmatic nuclei within the hypothalamus, which sets circadian and circannual rhythms. Pineal melatonin secretion, governed by the photoperiod and body temperature, is also part of this neuroendocrine network, which controls much daily and seasonal behaviour including activity levels, thermoregulation and the reproductive cycle. Non-visual perception can be very sensitive to small changes

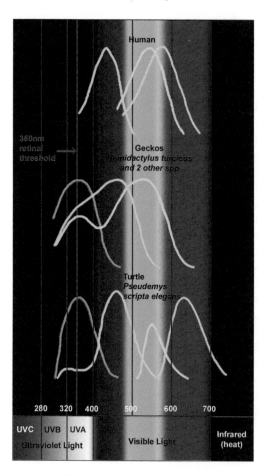

Figure 6.2 The spectral sensitivities of light-sensitive retinal cone cells in human (modified from Vorobyev 2004), geckos (modified from Roth and Kelber 2004) and turtle (modified from Loew and Govardovskii 2001). Humans have cone cells most responsive to blue, green and orange-red wavelengths, and the lens blocks wavelengths below 400 nm from reaching the retina. The reptile lens permits wavelengths from around 350 nm to reach the retina and cone cells maximally responsive to UVA expand their range of vision. Note also the differences in peak sensitivities and wavelength ranges between species. The turtle 'red' cone, for example, enables it to perceive longer wavelengths than either man or gecko.

in light levels; for example, nocturnal species monitor aspects of daylight from their hiding places.

Ultraviolet B

UVB in sunlight is an effective disinfectant. It has direct effects upon the immune system in the skin, upregulates melanin synthesis, stimulates production of beta endorphins (giving sunlight its feel-good factor), improves skin barrier functions and induces nitric oxide production, which has localized protective effects. UVB is best known for its role in enabling the skin synthesis of vitamin D3, the primary source of this essential pro-hormone in most vertebrates. For synthesis to occur, sunlight must contain UVB in wavelengths between 290 and 315 nanometres. Since short-wavelength UV is strongly scattered by the atmosphere, the amount of UV-B in sunlight depends upon the solar altitude. When the sun is low in the sky, near dawn and dusk or at higher latitudes in winter, there is very little UVB in the spectrum. As the sun rises, the rays have a shorter path through the atmosphere, so less scattering occurs and UV levels rise.

By midday in the tropics, the UV in direct sunlight may be extreme. The damaging effects of excessive exposure to ultraviolet radiation include DNA damage and oxidative stress. However, reptiles have evolved both behavioural traits and skin physiology to optimize their vitamin D3 production while maintaining adequate protection from the UV levels they encounter in their natural environment. Thermoregulatory behaviour is a major determinant of UV exposure. Many diurnal species, for example, bask primarily in the morning before UV levels are high. Some species also behaviourally regulate their UV exposure according to their vitamin D3 status. Nocturnal lizards have skin which permits much greater UV transmission than diurnal desert lizards exposed to strong sunlight. They may also synthesize vitamin D at a much faster rate, presumably enabling adequate synthesis despite reduced

opportunity for exposure. Some diurnal species have skin with a much higher resistance than mammals to UV damage from sunlight.

Vitamin D3

Vitamin D3 synthesis in reptiles requires ultraviolet light and warmth. UVB converts 7-dehydro-cholesterol, bound to the plasma membrane of cells in the epidermis, to previtamin-D3. A temperature-sensitive isomerization then transforms this into vitamin D3; when a reptile is within its preferred optimum temperature range, conversion will be much faster than at low temperatures. Overproduction does not occur; if exposure to sunlight is prolonged, excess previtamin-D3 and vitamin D3 in the epidermis are converted into apparently inert photoproducts.

Vitamin D3 is then transported in the bloodstream to the liver, where it is enzymatically converted into 25-hydroxy-vitamin D3 (25(OH)D3). This is the main storage form of the vitamin, measured to estimate vitamin D status. Circulating 25(OH)D3 is the substrate for the hormone, 1,25 di-hydroxy-vitamin D3 (1,25(OH)2D3), or calcitriol, synthesized within renal cells. Vitamin D receptors in kidney, intestine and bone cells respond to calcitriol to maintain calcium and phosphorus homeostasis. Serum calcitriol levels are normally extremely low, increasing in response to raised parathyroid hormone levels and low serum calcium or phosphorus.

Vitamin D receptors are also found in almost every organ in the vertebrate body. The cells of many organs, including the brain, vascular smooth muscle and macrophages, also possess enzymatic ability to produce intracellular calcitriol with a purely autocrine and paracrine function, in mammals, regulating genes controlling responses to seasonal changes, cell division and both innate and adaptive immune systems. Whether this occurs in reptiles is not yet known but its cutaneous synthesis in reptiles is well

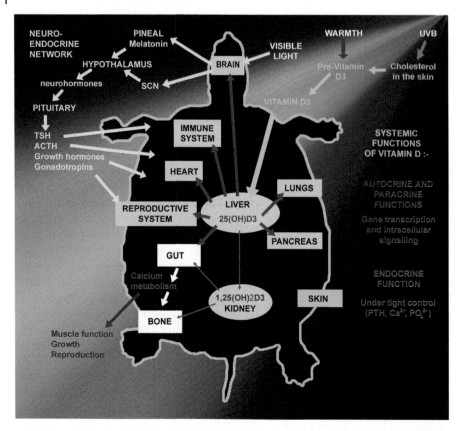

Figure 6.3 The effects of visible light (including UVA) upon the neuro-endocrine network, and UVB plus infrared upon the vitamin D3 pathway. Sunlight has significant effects upon the whole body, via these two systems.

established. Figure 6.3 is a graphical representation of some of the effects of sunlight upon the reptile body.

Natural Sunlight

No artificial lighting system can provide the full spectrum and intensity of natural sunlight, its subtle changes in colour as a day progresses, or approximate the sun's movement across the sky. Many reptiles benefit from outdoor enclosures whenever ambient temperatures are suitable. Direct sunlight requirement depends upon the species but all require access to full shade and shelter. Outdoor shelters within these enclosures can

now be covered with special horticultural, UV-transmitting plastic sheeting, which enables vitamin D3 synthesis 'under cover' and which may even prolong the season that can be spent outdoors.

Ordinary glass and most plastics block all UVB and some UVA. However, windows and skylights can be glazed with special UV-transmitting acrylics or low-iron glass. UV-transmitting acrylics allow up to 80% transmission of UVB; low iron glass may allow 50% through. Supplementary UVB may be required if natural sunlight levels outside are low. Heat build-up caused by direct sunlight through glass and plastics must never be ignored. Vivaria should never be positioned in front of sunlit windows.

Artificial Sunlight

Many reptiles in captivity must rely upon artificial lighting but it is virtually impossible to simulate sunlight using just one type of lamp. Varying degrees of success can be achieved by combining so-called 'basking lamps' with specialist reptile lamps emitting UVA and UVB. Providing a species-appropriate basking zone with a gradient into shade will allow the reptile to decide how much heat, visible light and UV radiation it experiences each day. Both the spectrum and the intensity of the infrared, light and UV must be considered when constructing the necessary gradients across the vivarium (Figure 6.4).

Basking Lamps

Incandescent (tungsten or halogen) lamps provide infrared and visible light for creating basking zones but this is deficient in blue and UVA, contains no UVB and is of low intensity. To simulate sunlight, additional high-intensity lighting is required. Incandescent lamps connected to timers can produce a simple 'sunrise and sunset' effect. Timers can switch them on just before, and off just after, other lamps in the vivarium.

Thermal burns are a hazard when using incandescent lamps. These emit primarily IR-A but this includes the wavelengths removed from natural sunlight by atmospheric moisture. They also emit longer-wavelength IR-B and some IR-C. Prolonged exposure may dangerously overheat the skin surface and water molecules in the epidermis before deeper structures reach optimum temperatures. If the beam is narrow and only warms a small portion of the body, the reptile may remain under the lamp long enough for serious burns to occur. It is therefore essential that any basking zone covers an area at least as large as the whole body of the animal and that the radiation is evenly distributed with no focal 'hot spots'. Thermal imaging (Figure 6.5)

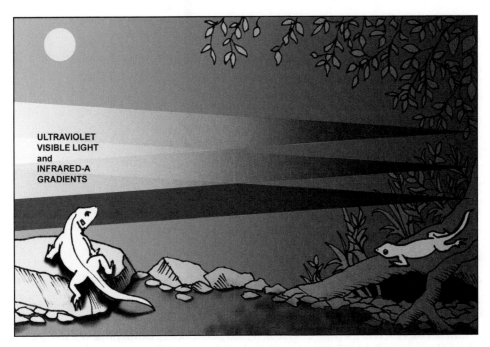

Figure 6.4 A simplified representation of a photo-microhabitat: ultraviolet, visible light and heat gradients are superimposed and all fall from a maximum in direct sunlight to a minimum in deep shade. When creating photo-microhabitats in captivity, this principle must apply, with species-appropriate maximum and minimum levels for each component of the 'artificial sunlight'.

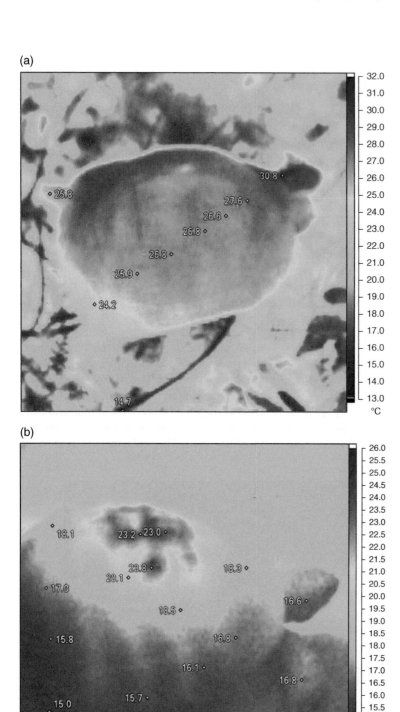

Figure 6.5 Thermal images. A: Wild specimen of an adult *Testudo graeca*, located basking in natural sunlight in its microhabitat, Murcia, Spain. B: Adult *T. graeca* in captivity, basking under a 100-watt mercury vapour 'spot' lamp. Note the contrast between the almost uniform body temperature of the sun-warmed animal and the extremely localized heating provided by the basking lamp. The head and limbs of animal B remain at ambient (air) temperature. The areas of greatest heating are along the sutures between the bones of the carapace, suggesting that there may be excessive heat transfer to water molecules in the tissues and blood vessels concentrated in these areas (images courtesy of A.C. Highfield).

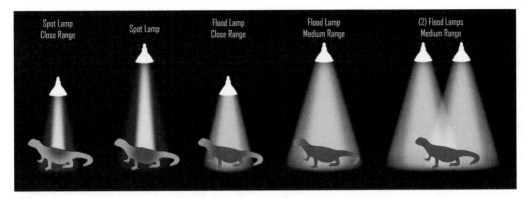

| Spot Lamp Close Range | Spot Lamp | Flood Lamp Close Range | Flood Lamp Medium Range | (2) Flood Lamps Medium Range |

Figure 6.6 A graphical representation of the infrared distribution from 'spot' and 'flood' type bulbs used at varying distances above a basking zone. The goal must be to achieve uniform basking zone temperatures across an area as wide as the entire body of the animal. Smaller 'spots' increase the risk of thermal burns as they cannot warm the whole animal evenly (courtesy of M. Versweyveld).

reveals the contrast between the uniform body temperature of a reptile basking in natural sunlight and one under a 'basking lamp' with a narrow beam. The abnormal heating of just the top of a tortoise carapace from 'spot' lamps may contribute to localized dehydration and development of pyramiding deformities often seen in captive tortoises.

Figure 6.6 is a graphic representation of the infrared distribution from 'spot' and 'flood' type bulbs used at varying distances above a basking zone. To create a large enough zone to accommodate the entire body of a reptile flood bulbs (with beam angles of 30 degrees or more) are essential. These must be positioned well above the animal and more than one bulb may be necessary.

Incandescent lamps should be controlled using dimming thermostats. Surface temperatures underneath basking lamps must be measured directly as they are very different from ambient (air) temperatures. Non-contact infrared thermometers (popularly known as 'temperature guns') are best for this purpose.

Ceramic heaters and heat mats are excellent background or night-time heaters but they emit no UV, visible light or IR-A, only IR-B and IR-C. These wavelengths are not found in sunlight so these products are not ideal for creating basking zones.

Coloured Lamps

Coloured lamps should be avoided. Reptiles need full-spectrum white light during the day. Most so-called 'infra-red' heat lamps are simply incandescent bulbs made with red glass. Their red light distorts colour vision and only weakly stimulates the non-visual pathways governing circadian rhythms.

The use of red or blue 'moonlight' lamps at night is not recommended. Reptiles can see both colours. Moonlight is not blue, being reflected sunlight – white light too dim for human colour vision. Reptiles should not be illuminated at night, as their circadian rhythms require regular periods of darkness and daylight, easily achieved by keeping the lamps on timers.

Visible Light

Metal halides are the only readily available products that can reproduce the full brilliance of sunlight. These are discharge lamps requiring external ballasts, which cannot be used with a thermostat. High-quality bulbs used for household and industrial floodlighting, in appropriate fixtures, produce good visible light including UVA but no UVB. 'Daylight' versions (colour temperature 5500–6500 K) are suitable choices for a large vivarium, when combined with a UVB lamp.

Positioning of the lamp is crucial. At close range, the visible light is extremely intense and could damage the eyes if placed in an animal's direct line of sight instead of directly above the vivarium. These lamps also emit significant infrared so similar cautions to those described above apply regarding the possibility of thermal injury.

'Daylight' fluorescent tubes and compact lamps are sometimes called 'full-spectrum' lights but most brands emit no UVB and very little UVA. They can be useful for improving general light levels in cooler areas of a vivarium. New 'high-output' slim fluorescent tubes (T5-HO; diameter 16 mm) produce much more intense illumination than traditional, wider tubes (T8; diameter 25 mm).

Light-emitting diode (LED) lighting is a recent innovation. There are two types of LED:

1) 'White' LEDs, which use a blue LED and a phosphor to simulate white light. The spectrum of these contains no UVA or UVB at all and is deficient in cyan (turquoise) and red.

2) LEDs that emit just one colour, in a very narrow band of wavelengths. 'White' is created using a combination of red, blue and green LEDs in a single bulb. This light will not appear white to any animal with retinal cones having different sensitivities to that of a human. In theory, multiple LEDs covering a wide range of wavelengths could be blended to create a more sun-like spectrum but, at present, suitable UVA and UVB LEDs are not available.

Neither type of LED should be the primary light source in a vivarium. They may be suitable for supplementary lighting or for enhancing plant growth.

Ultraviolet Lamps

Numerous manufacturers now make UVB-emitting bulbs for reptiles. There are four main types of UVB lamp (Figure 6.7). Although brands vary, certain characteristics such as beam shape, heat and light output are common to most lamps within each category. Both the UV and infrared output must be considered when positioning lamps over a basking zone. Narrow beams creating 'hot spots' of either type of radiation must be avoided. Some mercury vapour lamps and metal halides produce sufficient heat to contribute to basking zones and previously discussed cautions regarding infrared radiation apply.

High-quality products from well-known brands should be chosen. Cheap, inferior products may not have suitable spectra, output or longevity. Independent test results for a range of products are available (e.g. www.uvguide.co.uk) but these provide rough guides only. UV irradiance at reptile level will be affected by the size and wattage of the lamp, how long it has been in use, the fixture used and the presence of mesh or reflectors, as well as shade from branches, rocks and so on. Even the ambient temperature and fluctuations in the line voltage can affect irradiance. Solarization of the glass causes a slow loss of UVB transparency, and hence UVB output, over time. Ideally, lamps should be tested with a UV meter in place at the closest lamp-to-reptile distance, with tests repeated monthly to monitor decay.

The most suitable meter currently available is the Solarmeter® 6.5 model UV Index Meter (Solartech Inc; ZooMed Digital UV Index Radiometer, ZooMed Laboratories Inc). The UV Index is a measure of the solar UV intensity at the Earth's surface relevant to its effect on human skin but this meter's sensitivity response also follows the action spectrum for vitamin D3 synthesis fairly closely, making this meter suitable for measuring UV from both sunlight and lamps. It is a scientific instrument. Cheap 'sun-smart' UV Index meters are not an alternative. Many have sensors that do not register short wavelength UVB and so cannot give accurate readings with reptile lamps.

Concerns are sometimes expressed regarding the 100–120 Hz 'flicker' characteristic of self-ballasted mercury vapour lamps and fluorescent tubes run on magnetic ballasts. The flicker is too rapid for the human eye, which has a flicker fusion frequency of up to 60 Hz. Reptile flicker fusion frequency is similar to that of humans so lamp flicker should not be a problem for reptiles. If

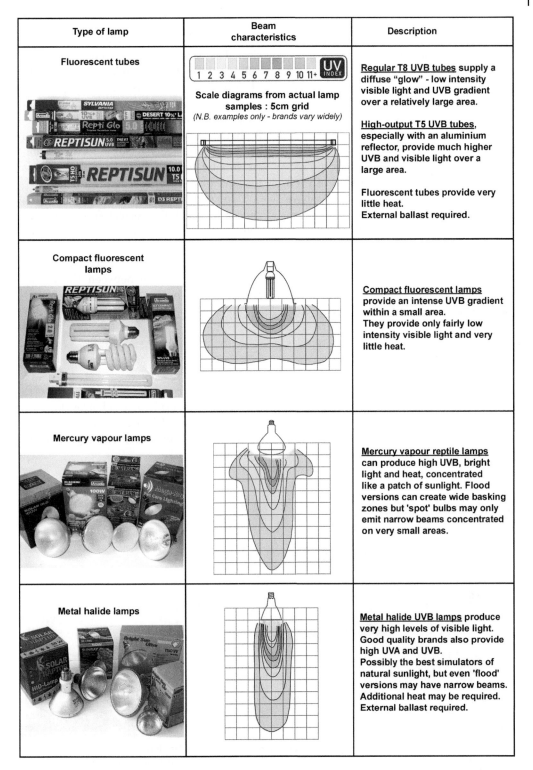

Type of lamp	Beam characteristics	Description
Fluorescent tubes	**Scale diagrams from actual lamp samples : 5cm grid** *(N.B. examples only - brands vary widely)*	**Regular T8 UVB tubes** supply a diffuse "glow" - low intensity visible light and UVB gradient over a relatively large area. **High-output T5 UVB tubes**, especially with an aluminium reflector, provide much higher UVB and visible light over a large area. Fluorescent tubes provide very little heat. External ballast required.
Compact fluorescent lamps		**Compact fluorescent lamps** provide an intense UVB gradient within a small area. They provide only fairly low intensity visible light and very little heat.
Mercury vapour lamps		**Mercury vapour reptile lamps** can produce high UVB, bright light and heat, concentrated like a patch of sunlight. Flood versions can create wide basking zones but 'spot' bulbs may only emit narrow beams concentrated on very small areas.
Metal halide lamps		**Metal halide UVB lamps** produce very high levels of visible light. Good quality brands also provide high UVA and UVB. Possibly the best simulators of natural sunlight, but even 'flood' versions may have narrow beams. Additional heat may be required. External ballast required.

Figure 6.7 The main types of UVB lamp used in reptile husbandry. In the middle column are graphical representations of the UV gradients which form beneath each lamp type when in use. The shapes of these gradients vary between brands, and are modified by reflectors, mesh, etc.

electronic ballasts are used, no species will see flicker, since these operate at 40,000–120,000 flicker fusion frequency Hz.

Estimating the Ultraviolet Requirement: The Ferguson Zone Concept

There are few scientific data to back the recommendation of any particular level of UVB for any species. Very few field studies have been made of the UV exposure of wild reptiles. Measurements must be taken in their microhabitat, where exposure varies widely, from diurnal species basking in full sun to nocturnal animals receiving low level UV while sleeping (Figure 6.8). Suitable UV levels for any species may be estimated using a concept described by Ferguson *et al.* (2010). The daytime UV exposure of 15 species of reptiles in the field was recorded. Species were assigned into four sun exposure ranges or 'zones' according to their basking and/or daylight exposure habits, which have since been designated 'UVB zones' or 'Ferguson zones' (Table 6.1). The average of all the readings

taken for each species might be seen as a suitable 'mid-background' level of UV for the species. The 'Maximum UV Index recorded' refers to the highest UV Index in which a reptile from this species was found. This provides a rough guide as to the upper acceptable limit for the UV gradient to be provided in captivity. In theory, any species may be assigned to a zone based on its behaviour in its microhabitat. Box 6.1 lists Ferguson zone designations for some popular reptile species.

A suitable UV gradient in the vivarium, chosen to match the correct Ferguson zone, will enable the animal to self-regulate its exposure. A full range of UV levels is vital, from zero (full shade) to a maximum at the closest point possible between the reptile and the UVB lamp.

Providing the Ultraviolet Gradient

UVB can be provided for indoor enclosures in two ways. The 'shade method' provides low-level 'background' UV over a large proportion of the animal's enclosure, with a gradient to

(a)

(b)

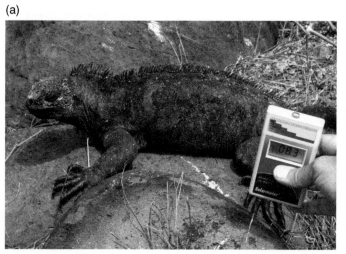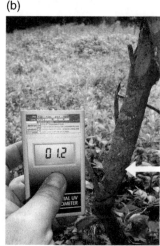

Figure 6.8 Measurement of the daytime UV Index exposure of two tropical lizards occupying very different microhabitats. (a) Basking marine iguana, *Amblyrhynchus cristatus venustissimus*, Galapagos, in direct sunlight; UV Index 8.3 (photo by the author). (b) Nocturnal animals may receive significant UV exposure during daylight hours. Sleeping leaf-tailed gecko, *Uroplatus* sp., Madagascar, on tree trunk in light shade; Madagascar UV Index 1.2. The arrow indicates the position of the eyes of this cryptic lizard, lying head down against the bark of the tree (courtesy of L. Warren).

Table 6.1 The Ferguson zones. The mean Ultraviolet Index (UVI) exposure levels of lizards and snakes spot-checked in the field during their activity period in the spring–early summer breeding season have determined their grouping into one of four photo-microhabitat 'zones', with increasing average exposure levels from zone 1 to zone 4. Fifteen species were studied. The average number of sightings per species was 14 (range 3–30); summarized from Ferguson *et al.* (2010).

Zone	Characteristics	Zone range UVI	Species	Common name	Maximum UVI recorded
1	Crepuscular or shade dweller, thermal conformer	0–0.7	*Agkistrodon piscivorus*	Cottonmouth water moccasin	0.6
			Elaphe obsoleta	Texas rat snake	0.8
			Anolis lineotopus	Jamaican brown anole	1.4
			Nerodia fasciata	Broad-banded water snake	1.1
2	Partial sun/ occasional basker, thermoregulator	0.7–1.0	*Thamnophis proximus*	Western ribbon snake	1.1
			Anolis grahami	Jamaican blue-pants anole	1.1
			Anolis carolinensis	Green anole	3.0
			Nerodia erythrogaster	Yellow-bellied water snake	2.7
3	Open or partial sun basker, thermoregulator	1.0–2.6	*Uta stansburiana stejnegeri*	Desert Side-blotched Lizard	2.9
			Sceloporus undulatus hyacinthinus	Eastern Fence Lizard	4.9
			Anolis sagrei	Cuban brown Anole	4.1
			Sceloporus olivaceous	Texas Spiny Lizard	7.4
4	Mid-day sun basker, thermoregulator	2.6–3.5	*Holbrookia maculata*	Lesser Earless Lizard	4.5
			Sceloporus graciosus	Sagebrush Lizard	9.5

Box 6.1 Ferguson zone designations for 55 reptile species commonly kept in captivity.

As assigned by the British and Irish Association of Zoos and Aquariums' Reptile & Amphibian Working Group (Baines *et al.* 2016).

Lizards (zone)
Crested gecko (1)
Crocodile skink (1)
Leopard gecko (1)
Tokay gecko (1)
Australian water dragon (2)
Emerald tree monitor (2)
Fire skink (2)
Green anole (2)
Monkey-tailed skink (2)
Pygmy chameleon (2)
Scheltopusik (2)
Wonder gecko (2)
Blue-tongued skink (2–3)
Chinese water dragon (2–3)
Electric blue day gecko (2–3)

Panther chameleon (2–3)
Black-and-white tegu (3)
Frilled lizard (3)
Standing's day gecko (3)
Sudan plated lizard (3)
Yemen chameleon (3)
Bearded dragon (3–4)
Bosc or savannah monitor (3–4)
Collared lizard (3–4)
Green iguana (3–4)
Chuckwalla (4)
Uromastyx (4)

Tortoises and turtles (zone)
Ornate box turtle (2)
Red Foot tortoise (2)

Yellow-footed tortoise (2)	Emerald tree boa (1)
Common musk turtle (2–3)	Green tree python (1)
European pond turtle (3)	Milksnake (1)
Indian star tortoise (3)	Reticulated python (1)
Leopard tortoise (3)	Amethystine python (1–2)
Spotted turtle (3)	Corn snake (1–2)
Cooter (3–4)	Rough green snake (1–2)
Painted turtle (3–4)	Boa constrictor (2)
Red-eared slider (3–4)	Red-tailed rat snake (2)
Sulcata or African spurred tortoise (3–4)	Rough green snake (1–2)
Yellow-bellied slider (3–4)	San Francisco garter snake (2)
	Western hognose snake (2)
Snakes (zone)	Diamond python (3)
Burmese python (1)	
Burmese python (1)	

zero in shade. This would be suitable for shade-dwelling reptiles and occasional baskers (i.e. those in Ferguson zones 1 and 2, such as the leopard gecko and many snakes; Table 6.2). A UV Index up to approximately 1.0 at the closest access point would seem appropriate. Fluorescent T8 (1-inch diameter) UVB tubes may be used if the animals will be close to the lamps; T5-HO UVB tubes would be suitable if positioned at much greater distances.

The 'sunbeam method' provides a higher level of UV for species known to bask in direct sunlight. The aim is to provide UV similar to that experienced during a typical early to mid-morning basking period, which is when most reptiles bask extensively. This higher level needs to be restricted to the basking zone (like a sunbeam) with a gradient to zero in shade. It can be provided for the full photoperiod. This method would seem appropriate for reptiles in Ferguson zones 3 and 4; for example, the bearded dragon (Table 6.2). T5-HO UVB tubes are suitable if used with an aluminium reflector; UVB metal halide and mercury vapour lamps may also be successful. Although some zone 4 reptiles will bask above UVI 7.0, even these bask mainly in the early morning and late afternoon, when levels are around UVI 3.0–5.0. For safety, a UV Index of 7.0–8.0 should be considered the absolute maximum UV Index at reptile level for both zone 3 and zone 4 reptiles, since the UV spectrum from artificial lighting is not the same as from natural sunlight. Figure 6.9 is a graphical representation of a basking zone created for a zone 3 reptile, showing superimposed heat, light and UV gradients produced by multiple lamps.

Zone 2 (occasional baskers) in larger enclosures providing plentiful shelter would probably use this type of UV gradient as well, with the lamps supplying a maximum UV Index of around 3.0.

UVI meter readings from a selection of new UVB lamps, on sale at the time of writing, are shown in Table 6.2. Readings were taken from directly beneath the lamps, with no mesh between lamp and reptile. Vivarium mesh screens typically block 30–40% of the light and UVB.

Excessive Ultraviolet Exposure/Non-Terrestrial UVB and UVC

All guidelines to date are still experimental. It is vital to watch the animals' responses and to adjust the UV levels immediately if problems

Table 6.2 UV Index readings from individual samples of 21 UVB emitting lamps sold for use with reptiles, available in the UK at the time of writing. The lamps were all 'seasoned' for approximately 100 hours before testing and measurements taken after 30 minutes warm-up time. Readings were taken with a Solarmeter® 6.5 UV Index Meter from directly beneath each lamp at the stated distances. Except where stated, tests were conducted on lamps in simple, open fixtures with no reflectors or shades. No mesh, glass or plastic was placed between the lamp and the meter. (Numbers in brackets: UV Index too high – lamp is unsuitable at this distance).

		Distance from lamp (cm)			
Brand name and type	Wattage	20	30	40	50
T8 fluorescent tubes (all 610 mm length):					
ExoTerra Repti-Glo 2.0	20 W	0			
Arcadia Natural Sunlight 2% UVB T8	18 W	0.3	0.2	0.1	0.1
Arcadia D3 Reptile 6% UVB T8	18 W	0.7	0.4	0.2	0.2
ExoTerra Repti-Glo 5.0	20 W	1.5	0.9	0.6	0.4
ZooMed Reptisun 10.0 T8	18 W	1.5	0.9	0.6	0.4
Arcadia D3+ 12% Reptile UVB T8	18 W	1.5	0.9	0.6	0.4
Arcadia D3+ Reptile 12% UVB T8 with reflector	18 W	3.2	2.0	1.3	0.9
T5 High Output fluorescent tubes (550 mm length):					
ZooMed Reptisun T5-HO 5.0	24 W	0.7	0.5	0.3	0.2
Arcadia D3 Reptile 6% UVB T5	24 W	2.0	1.2	0.7	0.5
ZooMed Reptisun T5-HO10.0	24 W	1.2	0.8	0.5	0.4
Arcadia D3+ Reptile 12% UVB T5	24 W	2.9	1.8	1.2	0.8
Arcadia D3+ Reptile 12% UVB T5 with reflector	24 W	6.3	3.6	2.3	1.6
Compact fluorescent lamps:					
ExoTerra Reptile UVB 100	25 W	1.6	0.8	0.4	0.3
ExoTerra Reptile UVB 200	25 W	1.8	0.9	0.5	0.3
Arcadia Natural Sunlight Compact Lamp	20 W	0.5	0.2	0.1	0.1
Arcadia D3+ 10%UVB Compact Reptile Lamp	23 W	2.7	1.3	0.8	0.5
ZooMed ReptiSun 5.0 Compact Lamp	26 W	0.5	0.3	0.1	0.1
ZooMed ReptiSun 10.0 Compact Lamp	26 W	1.8	0.9	0.4	0.3
Metal halides:					
Lucky Reptile Bright Sun UV Desert 35 W PAR30	35 W	(27.9)	(15.1)	(9.6)	6.5
Lucky Reptile Bright Sun UV Desert 70 W PAR30	70 W	3.9	1.7	0.8	0.5
Lucky Reptile Bright Sun Flood Jungle 150 W PAR38	150 W	(14.1)	6.3	3.5	2.1
ExoTerra SunRay 35 W PAR30	35 W	(26.2)	(10.3)	5.4	3.3
ExoTerra SunRay 50 W PAR30	50 W	(11.0)	5.0	2.8	1.7
ExoTerra SunRay 70 W PAR30	70 W	(17.3)	7.4	4.0	2.4
Mercury vapour lamps:					
ExoTerra Solar Glo 160 W	160 W	1.7	1.0	0.5	0.4
Arcadia D3 Basking Lamp 100 W	100 W	4.3	2.3	1.3	0.9
Arcadia D3 Basking Lamp 160 W	160 W	5.1	2.7	1.6	1.1

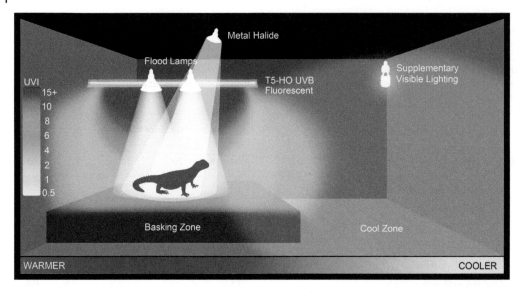

Figure 6.9 A graphical representation of a basking zone created for a reptile in Ferguson zone 3 or 4, using a combination of incandescent basking lamps for infrared and visible light, a metal halide lamp (non-UVB-emitting) for visible light and UVA, and a T5-HO UVB fluorescent tube. The UV Index gradient from an Arcadia T5 D3+ 12% UVB fluorescent tube fitted with a reflector is shown approximately to scale (courtesy of M. Versweyveld).

are seen. Albino and hypomelanistic animals, which lack protective melanin, may be at increased risk of UV-induced skin damage and cancer. They are likely to need much lower UV levels than normally pigmented conspecifics.

A few brands of lamp sold for use with reptiles were previously found to emit hazardous, very-short-wavelength UVB and UVC never found in natural sunlight. These have caused photo-kerato-conjunctivitis in many reptiles, with severe photo-dermatitis, burns and death in a significant number of cases (Figure 6.10). Once the problem was identified, the manufacturers withdrew these lamps from sale but there is the possibility that similar products may be available.

Excessive exposure to UV must also be avoided as high doses of 'solar' UVB and UVA can result in eye and skin damage and, in mammals, can lead to the formation of skin cancers. Squamous cell carcinomas have been reported in captive reptiles but the relevance of their association with use of artificial UV lighting is as yet undetermined.

General Recommendations for Reptile Keepers

- Captive reptiles need a sufficiently large, species-appropriate microhabitat with suitable heat, light and UV gradients, shelters and basking areas, so they can select their preferences at all times as they would in the wild. Provision of adequate shade is vital for all species.
- The sources of UV, visible light and infrared radiation must be positioned close together, simulating sunlight and creating a basking zone at least as large as the whole body of the animal. Multiple lamps may be required in some cases. The effects are additive for all wavelengths so overlapping beams must be used with caution.
- Suitable levels of UV for any species may be estimated from knowledge of their basking habits and micro-habitat in the wild. The Ferguson zones offer a range of suitable irradiances, using the UV Index, for four different categories of basking behaviour (Ferguson *et al*. 2010). The

(a)

(b)

(c)

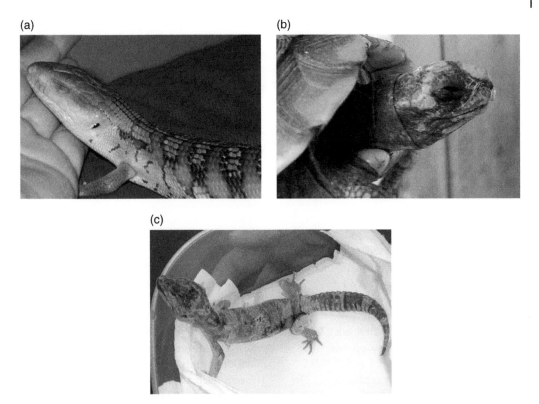

Figure 6.10 Three lizards exposed to hazardous, abnormally short-wavelength UVB from 'problem' compact fluorescent lamps marketed in 2006–07 (see text). A: Juvenile blue-tongue skink (*Tiliqua scincoides*) with photo-kerato-conjunctivitis, after 24 hours' exposure (courtesy of A. Murphree). B: Yellow-footed tortoise (*Geochelone denticulata*) with photo-kerato-conjunctivitis, after 3 days' exposure (courtesy of M. Buono). C: Albino leopard gecko hatchling (*Eublepharis macularius*) with extensive, very severe UV 'burns' after 2 days of exposure; the animal died two days later (courtesy of M. Buono).

Solarmeter model 6.5 UV Index Meter is a suitable tool to measure lamp irradiance in the vivarium.

- Basking temperatures and ambient temperatures must be suitable to ensure basking behaviours – and therefore UV exposure times – are natural, neither abnormally short nor prolonged. It is vital to check the temperatures reached under a lamp. Take into account the height of the animal.
- Lamps should always be positioned above the animals so the shape of the head and upper eyelids, and eyebrow ridges when present, shade the eyes from the direct light. Lights shining sideways may cause stress, and intense visible light, as well as UV, can cause eye damage.

- All lamps present an electrical risk. Many can also cause thermal and/or UV burns at close range. All bulbs should be inaccessible to the animals; wire guards may be necessary. Wide wire mesh should be chosen where possible, to maximize light and UV transmission.
- Ordinary glass or plastics must not be placed anywhere between the lamp and the animal as these typically block transmission of all UVB.
- Reptiles rely upon a distinct day and night to set their circadian rhythms. Timers should be used to provide the correct photoperiod for the species. If background heat is required at night, ceramic heaters or heat mats mounted on a rear wall are appropriate, as they emit no visible light.

References

Ferguson, G.W., Brinker, A. M., Gehrmann, W. H. *et al.* (2010) Voluntary exposure of some western-hemisphere snake and lizard species to ultraviolet-B radiation in the field: how much ultraviolet-B should a lizard or snake receive in captivity? *Zoo Biology*, 29 (3), 317–334.

Loew, E.R. and Govardovskii, V.I. (2001) Photoreceptors and visual pigments in the red-eared turtle, *Trachemys scripta elegans. Visual Neuroscience*, 18 (5), 753–757.

Roth, L.S.V. and Kelber, A. (2004) Nocturnal colour vision in geckos. *Proceedings of the Royal Society of London Biological Sciences*, 271 (Suppl 6), S485–S487.

Vorobyev, M. (2004) Ecology and evolution of primate colour vision. *Clinical and Experimental Optometry*, 87 (4/5), 230–238.

Further Reading

Baines, F.M. (2010) Photo-kerato-conjunctivitis in reptiles, in Proceedings ARAV 1st International Conference on Reptile and Amphibian Medicine, Munich, 4–7 March 2010. (S. Öfner and F. Weinzierl, eds), Verlag Dr. Hut, München, Germany, pp. 141–145.

Baines, F.M., Chattell, J., Dale, J. *et al.* (2016) How much UV-B does my reptile need? The UV-Tool, a guide to the selection of UV lighting for reptiles and amphibians in captivity. *Journal of Zoo and Aquarium Research*, 4 (1), 42–63.

Highfield, A.C. (2015) The Effect of Basking Lamps on the Health of Captive Tortoises and other Reptiles. Tortoise Trust, http://www.tortoisetrust.org/articles/baskinghealth.html (accessed 2 June 2017).

Hossein-nezhad, A. and Holick, M.F. (2013) Vitamin D for health: a global perspective. *Mayo Clinic Proceedings*, 88 (7), 720–755.

7

Reproduction
Timothy J. Portas

Reproductive Strategies in Reptiles

Considerable variation exists in the reproductive strategies both between and within the various reptilian taxa, including reproductive activity, frequency of reproduction in seasonal breeders, clutch size, degree of parental care and age at sexual maturity. Reptiles are either oviparous (egg laying) or viviparous (live bearing), with most species being oviparous. Viviparity does not occur in crocodilians or chelonians but occurs in approximately 20% of squamate species, including blue-tongued skinks and shingle-back lizards (*Tiliqua* spp.), various chameleon species, most vipers and rattle snakes (*Crotalus* spp.), most boas and some colubrids. Reproduction in temperate species tends to be seasonal, reflecting the thermal requirements for embryogenesis, while in tropical species reproduction may be continuous or influenced by other environmental factors such as rainfall or seasonal variations in resource availability. Seasonally breeding reptiles may produce a single or multiple clutches in a given season.

Anatomy and Physiology

The reader is referred to Chapter 2 for a brief discussion of reproductive anatomy. Pertinent aspects of reproductive physiology and egg anatomy are discussed in this chapter.

Reptile Reproductive Physiology

The reproductive physiology of many reptile species is poorly understood, although two broad patterns of reproductive behaviour are evident in reptiles – associated and dissociated. In the associated pattern, sexual behaviour is correlated with gonadal steroid concentrations and, in the case of females, is associated with ovulation. In the dissociated pattern, sexual behaviour is not mediated by gonadal steroid concentration and is related to environmental factors such as temperature. For males that exhibit a dissociated pattern, mating occurs at a time when gonadal activity is low and hence stored gametes produced in the previous breeding season are used. For females that exhibit a dissociated pattern, mating occurs early in the breeding season and sperm are stored for fertilization

Reptile Medicine and Surgery in Clinical Practice, First Edition. Edited by Bob Doneley, Deborah Monks, Robert Johnson and Brendan Carmel.
© 2018 John Wiley & Sons Ltd. Published 2018 by John Wiley & Sons Ltd.

of ova that subsequently develop. Sperm storage has been demonstrated in a number of reptile species and in some species sperm may be stored for up to several years. In some species, females frequently mate with multiple males and multiple paternity is possible in the resulting clutches.

Egg Anatomy

Reptile egg shell morphology varies both between and within the various taxonomic groups largely as a result of the degree of egg shell calcification. The eggs of crocodilians, some chelonians and some gekkonids have rigid shells, while other chelonians, most squamates and the tuatara (*Sphenodon punctatus*) produce eggs with a parchment-like, soft and pliable shell. Reptile eggs lack a chalaza, the fibrous ligament that suspends the yolk centrally within the albumen. Consequently, the yolk, which has a higher specific gravity than albumen, settles to the bottom of the egg while the embryo floats and subsequently attaches to the top of the egg. As a result, rotation of the egg during incubation may result in embryonic mortality. Except in the immediate post-oviposition period, care should be taken to ensure that eggs are not rotated during incubation.

Parthenogenesis

Parthenogenesis refers to asexual reproduction in which an egg develops without fertilization by spermatozoa. Parthenogenesis is uncommon in reptiles but has been reported most frequently in lizards (various species of Gekkonidae, Agamidae, Chamaelonidae, Xantusiidae, Lacertidae and Teiidae) and rarely in snakes.

Gender Assessment in Reptiles

Accurate determination of the sex of individual captive reptiles is imperative for successful breeding. Given the immense variation in anatomical form between and even within taxonomic groups, accurate gender assessment can be challenging. Additionally, some species of reptile, particularly snakes, are monomorphic and sex cannot be accurately determined on the basis of external morphology.

Chelonians

Adult chelonians generally exhibit sexual dimorphism. Males tend to have longer tails and a greater distance between the caudal margin of the carapace and the cloacal opening than females (Figure 7.1). Additionally, males frequently have a concave plastron to facilitate mounting the female during copulation. Other secondary sexual characteristics that provide clues to the gender of chelonians include elongated toenails on the forelimbs of male terrapins, eye colouration in terrapins, carapace shape and a generally larger body size in females compared with males. While sexually mature chelonians exhibit dimorphism, sexual maturity may not be reached until 10 years of age or later in some species. Sub-adult and juvenile (including hatchlings) chelonians may be sexed by coelioscopic examination of the gonads.

Crocodilians

Gender assessment in crocodilians is typically achieved by digital examination of the cranioventral cloaca; males have a larger penis while females have a smaller clitoris. The penis may be exteriorized for visual examination if there is doubt on palpation (Figure 7.2). Adult male crocodilians typically grow to a larger size than females.

Lizards

A number of techniques may be employed for gender assessment in lizards. Males possess paired hemipenes, which are inverted in the ventral tail base. In some species, a prominent hemipenal bulge is apparent, which can be used for gender assessment. A hemipenal

(a)

(b)

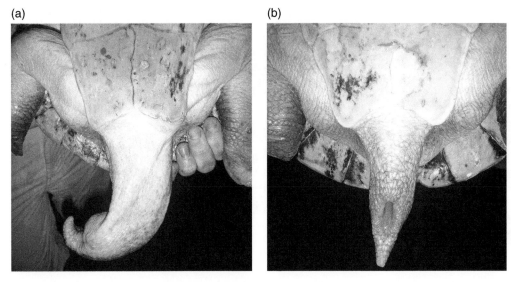

Figure 7.1 Comparison of the tails of male (a) and female (b) broad-shelled turtles (*Chelodina expansa*).

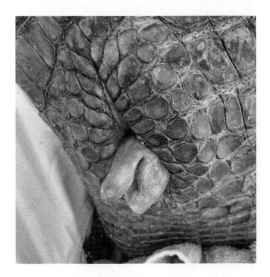

Figure 7.2 Phallus extruded through the cloacal opening of an American alligator (*Alligator mississipiensis*).

bulge is present in some iguanids and varanids and in most gekkonids. Some male gekkonids have prominent paracloacal spurs (Figure 7.3). The hemipenes of some varanids contain mineralized, radiodense hemibacula and radiography of the tail base can be used to determine the sex of those species where these occur (Figure 7.4). Hemipenal transillumination, using a suitably bright light applied to the tail base, can be used to identify the presence of absence of hemipenes in small species of agamids, gekkonids, varanids and scincids. Repeatable sex identification was demonstrated in free living eastern blue-tongued lizards (*Tiliqua scincoides*) using ratios of head width to snout vent length and head width to trunk length. The technique showed significant predictability with respect to sex identification in both adult and sub-adult lizards.

'Probing' or the introduction of a sterile, lubricated, blunt-tipped, sexing probe into the invaginated or inverted hemipenal pocket, can be used for gender assessment. A probe inserted into the hemipenal pocket will penetrate further in a male than in a conspecific female. Manual eversion of the hemipenes, as described below for snakes, may also be used. Ultrasonographic visualization of the hemipenes and gonads has been described in bearded dragons (Pogona vitticeps). Contrast radiography and contrast computed tomography have been effectively used to identify the hemipenes of a range of lizard species. Some gekkonids, iguanids and agamids have femoral pores on the ventral aspects of the thigh which are noticeably larger in adult males than adult females but

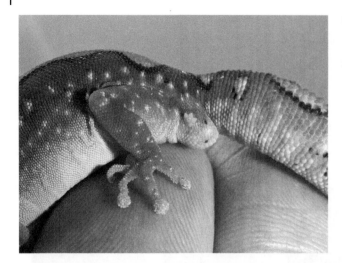

Figure 7.3 Hemipenal bulge and paracloacal spurs evident in a male helmeted gecko (*Diplodactylus galeatus*).

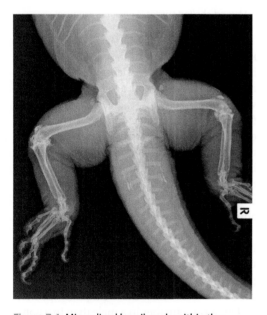

Figure 7.4 Mineralized hemibacula within the hemipenes are clearly evident in this radiograph of an adult male perentie (*Varanus giganteus*).

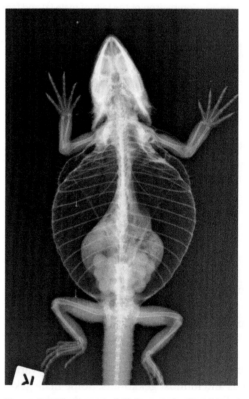

Figure 7.5 Vitellogenic follicles are clearly evident in this radiograph of an eastern bearded dragon (*Pogona barbarta*). The homogenous nature of coelomic cavity contents can make radiographic visualization of follicles challenging but, in this case, contrast provided by the lizard inflating itself with air in a threat display, enables the follicles to be clearly visualized.

are of a similar size in juvenile lizards (Funk 2002). Ultrasonography and radiography may be used to identify ovaries, follicles or eggs in females (Figure 7.5). Coelioscopy may also be used to visualize the gonads for gender assessment. Molecular sex assessment has also been described for some lizard species (Phillips *et al.* 2016).

(a)

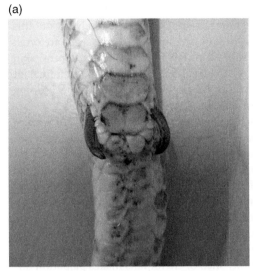

(b)

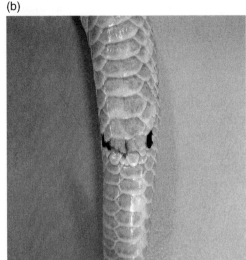

Figure 7.6 Comparison of cloacal spurs in the green tree python (*Morelia viridis*). The male is on the left (a) and the female on the right (b).

Snakes

'Probing', as described for lizards, is the most common method for assessing the sex of snakes. In female snakes, the sexing probe can be inserted to a depth of between 0–5 subcaudal scales, depending on the species. In male snakes, the sexing probe can be inserted to a depth of between 7–19 subcaudal scales depending on the species. For neonatal and juvenile snakes, in which probing carries a higher risk of trauma, manual eversion of the hemipenes is used. The hemipenes are most commonly everted using digital pressure. Saline, injected caudal to the hemipenes, may also be used to evert the hemipenes but carries a risk of infection, prolapse and hemipenal trauma, and is not recommended. Ultrasonography and contrast radiography for identification of the hemipenes have both been employed for gender assessment in snakes with ultrasonography more consistently accurate. Various secondary sexual characteristics may be used for assessing the gender of snakes, including a broader more slowly tapering tail in males compared with females and the presence of spurs lateral to the cloaca in pythons and boas that are generally larger in males than females

(Figure 7.6). Owing to variation between and within species, secondary sexual characteristics should not be relied on alone for gender assessment in snakes.

Breeding Management

Prior to breeding, female reptiles must be in appropriate body condition to support the metabolic demands of egg or fetus production and free from underlying disease to maximize the chances of successful reproduction. To ensure that adequate resources are available to support reproduction, captive reptiles should be in excellent body condition prior to cooling and the subsequent breeding season.

Appropriate environmental cues are necessary for the induction of reproductive behaviour in reptiles. Cooling or brumation is frequently used in temperate species to initiate breeding behaviour. Feeding of temperate species should cease before cooling or brumation commences: at least two weeks for snakes and several days for chelonians and lizards. Ensuring that animals are in good health and free from disease prior to cooling or brumation is important as these temperature changes may be associated with reduced immune function. In tropical species, photoperiod adjustment and dietary manipulation may be sufficient with excessive or inappropriate cooling being potentially detrimental to the reptile's health. If cooling is used in tropical species, temperature drops should be smaller and of shorter duration; typically, a reduction in the overnight temperature while still providing a limited period of heating during the day.

Mating

Males and females may be left together year round or separated outside of the breeding season and introduced for breeding purposes. The presence of a male prior to the breeding season has been shown to be necessary for folliculogenesis, vitellogenesis, ovulation and oviposition in some snake and chelonian species. The sequential introduction of multiple males may be necessary to stimulate breeding behaviour in some squamate and chelonian species and ensure fertilization. The decision to permanently house together or introduce only for breeding purposes will depend upon the species in question, the propensity for aggression both during and after the breeding season and the experience and preference of the herpetoculturalist. Mating in many species is preceded by a period of courtship behaviour.

Determination of Gravidity

The ability to determine whether a female reptile is gravid or pregnant is clinically important to allow for optimal management and monitoring through to oviposition or birth and for the diagnosis of dystocia. In many squamate species, the mid or caudal body becomes distended due to the presence of eggs or fetuses. The presence of large intracoelomic fat pads in some females will complicate diagnosis when relying on this technique. In many gekkonids, eggs are often visible through the translucent ventral skin and can be differentiated from abdominal fat pads by the slightly asymmetrical positioning of the eggs. Transillumination of the coelomic cavity may aid in diagnosis of species with less translucent skin. In many agamids, the outline of eggs are readily visible against the body wall. Behavioural changes in gravid females, including increased basking behaviour, inappetance and positional changes, may also provide some indication of reproductive status. Palpation is most applicable in snakes but can also be used in lizards. The bony shell of chelonians makes palpation difficult in this group but, with practice, eggs may be detected via palpation and ballotment through the inguinal fossa. During vitellogenesis, females reptiles can be expected to have elevations in total calcium, phosphorus, total protein, albumin, globulin, cholesterol (often marked) and triglycerides.

For definitive diagnosis of gravidity, radiography and/or ultrasonography are often employed. Radiography is particularly useful in chelonians as the calcified shells of their eggs are readily apparent. While eggs can be detected ultrasonographically via the inguinal fossa, the number of eggs cannot be determined by this method. In contrast, the poorly mineralized shells of many squamate species, particularly in the immediate post-ovulatory period, can be difficult to differentiate radiographically from preovulatory follicles (Figure 7.7). Ultrasound examination is therefore useful for determining gravidity in many squamate species in the immediate post-ovulatory period (Figure 7.8). The relatively homogenous radiographic appearance of coelomic cavity structures in many species limits the usefulness of radiography for assessing reproductive status in the preovulatory period. For viviparous species, ultrasonography is also appropriate, although in the later stages of gestation fetuses are also readily apparent with radiography.

(a) (b)

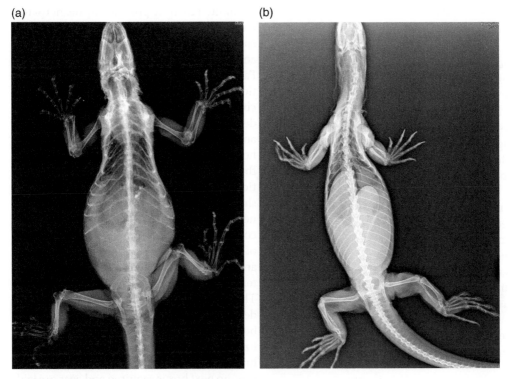

Figure 7.7 (a) In the immediate post-ovulatory period, the poorly mineralized shells and large number of eggs produced by some squamate species such as this green iguana (*Iguana iguana*) may be difficult to differentiate from preovulatory follicles radiographically. (b) In this lace monitor (*Varanus varius*), the large egg size and more mineralized shells immediately prior to oviposition are readily distinguishable radiographically.

Figure 7.8 Ultrasonographic appearance of an egg in a reticulated python (*Python reticulatus*). Note the hyperechoic shell and relatively homogenous echogenicity of the egg contents.

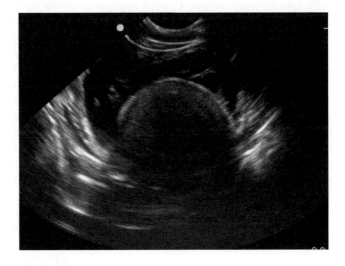

Determination of Length of Gestation

Determining the length of gestation in reptiles can be challenging, as it is influenced not only by species specific factors but also various environmental and physiological factors. Environmental factors can influence the length of gestation, with higher temperatures reducing gestation length. In some species, copulation and ovulation may be separated by significant periods of time and sperm storage has been documented in numerous species. Impending oviposition or parturition can be preceded by various species-specific behavioural changes such as the excavation of nest chambers in chelonians, some oviparous lizards and some crocodilians, the construction of nesting mounds in some crocodilians, and ecdysis at a variable interval before oviposition (termed a pre-lay shed) in many snakes and gekkonids.

Managing Gravid Females

Reproduction requires increased metabolic expenditure on the part of breeding females. Females producing multiple clutches over the course of a breeding season have a high metabolic cost of reproduction. Careful management of nutrition is required and, given that many species cease to eat and lose weight prior to oviposition, optimal nutrition in the immediate postpartum period is required. These animals also have a high demand for various vitamin and minerals, in particular calcium. Inappropriate nutritional management of breeding females poses a risk not only to the health of the female but also to the viability of any offspring produced. The reader is referred to Chapter 15 for a more complete discussion of metabolic and nutritional diseases.

Egg Laying

Wild gravid females are able to choose appropriate oviposition sites within their environment. In captivity, oviposition sites are limited to those provided by the herpetoculturalist. A sound knowledge of species-specific requirements is necessary to ensure an appropriate oviposition site is provided. Failure to provide an appropriate oviposition site may result in dystocia (common in chelonians and some iguanids) or the rapid desiccation of deposited eggs. Most chelonians and many lizards will excavate a nest hole for oviposition. A substrate that meets the species specific requirements for excavation, moisture content and temperature should be provided. Potentially suitable nesting substrates include sand, peat moss, coir peat, sphagnum moss or a combination of these, depending upon the species. In lizards, this nesting material is generally moistened and provided in a secure nesting box. The nesting substrate should be of sufficient depth for excavation of an adequate chamber; at least twice the snout-vent length of lizards and deeper than the length of the hind limbs in chelonians. In some lizard species, no next box is required and eggs are laid under bark (or cage furniture) or, in the case of some gekkonids, glued to cage furniture. For snakes, a secure nesting hide with moistened substrate is provided, although no nest chamber is excavated. Mound nesting crocodilians will need to be provided with sufficient vegetation to build a mound of decomposing material in which the eggs can be laid.

Egg brooding, in which the female coils tightly around the egg mass, occurs in most python species. In addition to providing protection for the egg mass from predators, some python species are facultatively endothermic, providing a stable thermal environment for the eggs. Egg brooding behaviour has also been shown to ensure stable environmental humidity for the egg mass.

Clutch size varies enormously between taxonomic groups. Some examples are: terrestrial chelonians and anoles (*Anolis* spp.), which lay a single egg per clutch; scincids and gekkonids, which lay two eggs; through to some marine turtles, which lay up to 200 eggs in a single clutch. Similar variation occurs in viviparous species. Knowing the number of eggs likely to be produced is important in helping to establish cases of dystocia. The number of clutches produced each season varies, with some species producing multiple clutches, through to the tuatara, which only produces eggs once every four years. Those species producing a smaller number of eggs per clutch tend to lay multiple clutches per seasons. In the captive setting, environmental manipulation can be employed to obtain multiple clutches from animals that would typically only produce one clutch per season in the wild. Viviparous species typically produce a maximum of one clutch per year. Cessation of feeding in the later stages of pregnancy is common in viviparous species and females tend to be in poor body condition postpartum.

Excavation of multiple nesting chambers without oviposition, straining, inappetance, dehydration and coelomic cavity distension, and lethargy are all potential clinical signs of dystocia. The reader is referred to Chapter 22 for a detailed discussion of the diagnosis and management of dystocia. Potential causes of egg mortality include inappropriate humidity, hyper- and hypothermia and microbial infections.

Multiple Clutches

Snakes tend to produce larger clutches of eggs than do lizards of a similar body mass but they typically only produce one clutch per season. In captivity, many herpetoculturalists seek to maximize the reproductive output of their animals. Some snakes, in particular some colubrids and pythons, can be 'pushed' to reproduce at a much earlier age than in the wild by feeding more regularly than required for maintenance (Stahl 2001). Reproductive maturity is associated with body size rather than age in many reptiles. This 'hypernutritional' approach can also be used to obtain two to three clutches from a female in a season. A reduced reproductive life span and health problems are more likely with this approach. In some species of lizard in which multiple clutches of eggs are produced in one season, overbreeding can result in marked loss of body condition in the female and metabolic imbalances, such as hypocalcaemia, as the female's body reserves are depleted through excessive egg production. Strategies for halting reproduction in these animals include removal of the male, although additional clutches may still be produced due to sperm storage, cessation of feeding and lowering environmental temperature. Manipulating food intake and environmental temperatures may be detrimental in females in poor body condition and should be undertaken with caution.

Egg Incubation

In the captive setting, most eggs are removed from the oviposition site and artificially incubated. Suitable substrates in which to incubate reptile eggs include vermiculite, perlite, sphagnum moss, peat moss, coir peat moss and sand (Figure 7.9). Species-specific requirements will dictate the suitability of these various incubation media and also the amount of water required to ensure appropriate hydration during incubation. Key physiological factors influencing artificially incubated eggs include temperature, humidity and gas exchange.

Temperature variably influences incubation duration, gender determination (in species with temperature-dependent sex determination), pigmentation, hatchling size, post-embryonic growth, locomotor performance and behaviour, and the incidence of developmental anomalies. Most reptile eggs are incubated at between 28 °C and 32 °C, although considerable species specific variation in optimum incubation temperature exists (Table 7.1). Lower incubation temperatures generally result in larger hatchlings with smaller yolk reserves. Higher incubation temperatures typically result in a shorter duration of incubation as embryonic metabolic processes are temperature dependent. However, this relationship is not linear and is also determined by genetic factors. Higher incubation temperatures generally result in

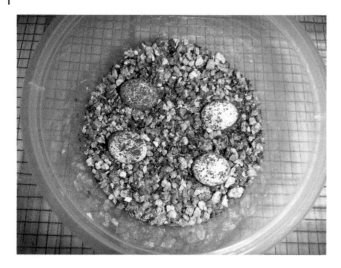

Figure 7.9 Two clutches of eggs from Cooktown ring-tailed geckos (*Cytrodactylus tuberculatus*) being incubated in moistened vermiculate. The adherence of substrate to the shell is common in gekkonids.

Table 7.1 Average clutch size, recommended egg incubation temperatures and incubation length for selected reptile species.

Species	Average clutch (*n*)	Incubation Temperature (°C)	Incubation Length (days)
Green iguana (*Iguana iguana*)	10–35	28–32	64–113
Bearded dragon (*Pogona vitticeps*)	4–35	27–31	55–86
Veiled chameleon (*Chamaeleo calyptratus*)	30–80	27–31	120–209
Leopard gecko (*Eublepharis macularius*)	2	26–31	45–65
Savannah monitor (*Varanus exanthematicus*)	12–20	27–30	138–194
Reticulated python (*Python reticulatus*)	40–45	29–31	70–105
Ball python (*Python regius*)	2–15	29–32	53–60
Burmese python (*Python bivittatus*)	30–40	30–32	55–70
Green tree python (*Morelia viridis*)	10–20	30–31.5	52–53
Carpet python (*Morelia spilota*)	9–54	31–32	57–78
Corn snake (*Pantherophis guttatus*)	20–25	25–29	60–65
Black rat snake (*Pantherophis obsoletus*)	6–16	25–29	50–76
Spectacled cobra (*Naja naja*)	10–45	26–28	54–80
Red–eared slider (*Trachemys scripta elegans*)	1–22	28–30	60–90
Eastern long–necked turtle (*Chelodina longicollis*)	4–24	27–31	60–85
Eastern box turtle (*Terrapene carolina carolina*)	2–7	28–30	50–75
Leopard tortoise (*Stigmochelys pardalis*)	3–19	28–30	120–200
Hermann's tortoise (*Testudo hermanni*)	4–5	28–31	60–66
African spurred tortoise (*Centrochelys sulcata*)	1–17	27–31	81–170
American alligator (*Alligator mississippiensis*)	2–28	28–33	55–76
Fresh water crocodile (*Crocodylus johnstoni*)	4–20	29–34	75–85
Tuatara (*Sphenodon punctatus*)	6–18	18–22	330–450

faster growth after hatching. Excessively high incubation temperatures may result in embryonic mortality and an increased incidence of embryonic abnormalities.

Temperature-dependent sex determination occurs in all crocodilians, some chelonians and lizards and the tuatara but has not been documented in snakes. Higher or lower temperature in reptiles exhibiting temperature-dependent sex determination variably produces more or less individuals of a given sex, depending upon the species. There is typically a transitional temperature range of 2–3 °C in which equal numbers of males and females are produced. Four broad classes of temperature-dependent sex determination are recognized:

- type 1 – in which higher incubation temperatures produce more females and lower temperatures more males (many chelonians)
- type 2 – in which higher incubation temperatures produce more males and lower temperatures more females (some crocodilians and lizards)
- type 3 – in which both higher and lower incubation temperatures produce more females while more males are produced at midrange temperatures (some crocodilians, lizards and chelonians)
- type 4 – in which lower incubation temperatures produce more males, intermediate temperatures produce more females and higher incubation temperatures produce equal numbers of both sexes (one gekkonid species).

Incubation humidity is influenced by environmental humidity, the moisture content of the substrate and the water potential of the substrate. Water is absorbed by the egg principally in its gaseous phase, although absorption of liquid water is also possible. Water absorption and loss is greatest in soft-shelled eggs and the egg volume and weight change in response to water absorption or loss. Water exchange in eggs is influenced by temperature and contact with the substrate. The water potential of the substrate (the amount of water available to the egg from the substrate) and resulting gas exchange can have profound influences on hatchling size and yolk metabolism. Monitoring and active management of both temperature and humidity is therefore vitally important during incubation. This information is critical to the veterinarian investigating egg mortality during incubation and morbidity and mortality in the immediate post-hatching period.

Determination of Egg Viability

Determining whether or not eggs are fertile and monitoring of fertile eggs is usually achieved by transillumination of the egg using a bright light source in a darkened room. This technique, known as candling, allows for visualization of the internal structures of the egg, including the air cell and developing blood vessels. Nonviable eggs may also exhibit abnormal colouration, excessive adherence of substrate, obvious microbial contamination and, for soft-shelled eggs, changes to the normal turgidity of the egg.

Hatching

Impending hatching may be evidenced by various changes to the egg up to several days before hatching, including the loss of calcareous shards from hard-shelled eggs, and fluid formation or dimpling of the surface of soft-shelled eggs. At hatching, a tooth or tooth-like structure on the tip of the upper jaw or beak, which is shed post-hatching, is used to rupture the embryonic membranes and egg shell, allowing the neonatal reptile to escape the confines of the egg. In crocodilians, chelonians and the tuatara, the egg tooth or

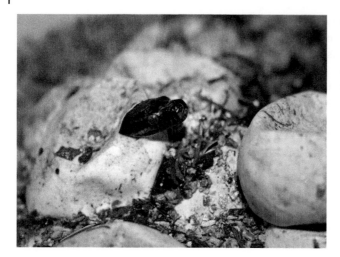

Figure 7.10 A neonatal carpet python (*Morelia spilota*) emerging from the recently pipped egg. Note the presence of depressions in the shells of the other eggs. This is a normal change seen immediately before hatching in many species with soft-shelled eggs.

caruncle is a horny outgrowth of the upper jaw. In squamates, the egg tooth is a true dentinal tooth attached to the premaxilla. Following opening of the egg shell or 'pipping', the neonatal reptile may remain in the egg from several hours to several days (Figure 7.10). The duration of time the neonate remains in the egg varies considerably among taxonomic groups and during this transitional phase, various physiological and anatomical changes may occur, including resorption of the remnant yolk sack, the transition to pulmonary respiration and unfolding of the carapace and plastron in chelonians. Knowledge of species-specific times spent in the egg shell following pipping is important when deciding whether to assist in the hatching process, as early removal from the shell may be deleterious to the hatchling.

Embryonic Mortality

Late embryonic death is a relatively common problem that may affect entire or partial clutches of oviparous species from all reptile taxa. Affected embryos are typically full term or near term at the time of death and are discovered when fertile eggs fail to hatch at the expected time. Potential causes may be related to maternal nutrition and body condition; incubation parameters such as temperature, humidity and gaseous exchange; infection; inbreeding; and egg rotation during incubation. Determining the cause of embryonic mortality requires a thorough review of the husbandry regime under which the adult reptiles are managed, a review of incubation parameters and necropsy and microbiological examination of dead embryos.

References

Funk, R.S. (2002) Lizard reproductive medicine and surgery. *Veterinary Clinics of North America Exotic Animal Practice*, 5, 579–613.

Phillips, C.A. Roffey, J.B. Hall, E. and Johnson R. (2016) Sex identification in the eastern blue-tongued lizard (Tiliqua scincoides White, ex Shaw, 1790) using morphometrics. *Australian Veterinary Journal*, 94 (7), 256–259.

Stahl, S.J. (2001) Reptile production medicine. *Seminars in Avian and Exotic Pet Medicine*, 10, 140–150.

Further Reading

Brown, D. (2014) *A Guide to Australian Lizards in Captivity*. Reptile Publications, Burleigh.

Bucy, D.S., Guzman, D.S. and Zwingenburger, A.L. (2015) Ultrasonographic anatomy of bearded dragons (*Pogona vitticeps*). *Journal of the American Veterinary Medical Association*, 246, 868–876.

DeNardo, D. (2006) Reproductive biology, in *Reptile Medicine and Surgery* 2nd ed. (D.R. Mader, ed.), Elsevier, St. Louis, MO, pp. 376–390.

Di Ianni, F., Volta, A., Pelizzone, I. *et al.* (2015) Diagnostic sensitivity of ultrasound, radiography and computed tomography for gender determination in four species of lizard. *Veterinary Radiology and Ultrasound*, 56, 40–45.

Divers, S.J. (2014) Diagnostic endoscopy, in *Current Therapy in Reptile and Medicine and Surgery*, (D.R. Mader and S.J. Divers, eds). Elsevier, St. Louis, MO, pp. 154–178.

Gnudi, G., Volta, A., Di Ianni, F. *et al.* (2009) Use of ultrasonography and contrast radiography for snake gender determination. *Veterinary Radiology and Ultrasound*, 50, 309–311.

Hochleithner, C. and Holland, M. (2014) Ultrasonography, in *Current Therapy in Reptile and Medicine and Surgery*

(D.R. Mader and S J. Divers, eds), Elsevier, St. Louis, MO, pp. 107–127.

Köhler, G. (2005) *Incubation of Reptile Eggs*. Krieger Publishing Company, Melbourne, Australia.

Lourdais, O., Hoffman, T.C.M. and DeNardo, D.F. (2007) Maternal brooding in the Children's python (*Antaresia childreni*) promotes egg water balance. *Journal of Comparative Physiology B*, 177, 569–577.

McArthur, S. (2004) Reproductive system, in *Medicine and Surgery of Tortoises and Turtles* (S. McArthur, R. Wilkinson and J. Meyer, eds), Blackwell Publishing, Oxford, pp. 57–63.

Rivera, S. (2008) Health assessment of the reptile reproductive tract. *Journal of Exotic Pet Medicine*, 17, 259–256.

Shine, R. (2003) Reproductive strategies in snakes. *Proceedings of the Royal Society of London B*, 270, 995–1004.

Sykes, J.M. (2010) Updates and practical approaches to reproductive disorders in reptiles. *Veterinary Clinics of North America Exotic Animal Practice*, 13, 349–373.

Wright, K.M. (2004) Breeding and neonatal care, in *BSAVA Manual of Reptiles*, 2nd ed. (S.J. Girling and P. Raiti, eds). British Small Animal Veterinary Association, Gloucester, pp. 40–50.

8

Reptile Paediatrics

Deborah Monks and Bob Doneley

Introduction

Paediatrics is the medicine and surgery of neonatal, juvenile and sub-adult animals. As with other groups, reptile paediatrics has considerable overlap with other disciplines of medicine and surgery. Reptiles have a variety of reproductive strategies (see Chapter 7), which means that development of foetuses can occur either externally (oviparous) or internally (as either viviparous or ovovivaparous young).

Hatching/Birth

Oviparous neonates

Assuming that the egg is successfully fertilized and that oviposition has occurred without incident, foetal development of oviparous species is entirely dependent on external conditions. Hygiene is, of course, critical, as is the provision of species appropriate temperature and humidity (see Chapter 7). Veterinary intervention during the incubation process is usually limited to egg necropsies. An egg necropsy is performed when neonates fail to hatch or are diagnosed as dead in shell after development has started. Although there are documented species-specific incubation times, temperature and humidity may alter those times (within a small window), which can obscure the expected date of hatch. In general terms, assisted hatching is performed when:

- the remainder of the clutch has hatched and a small number of eggs have exhibited minimal activity suggestive of imminent hatch
- the hatching process is initiated by a neonate but stalls
- candling reveals a live hatchling past the longest expected duration of incubation
- the egg was damaged at some point and required repair; the hatchling may have difficulty exiting the egg unassisted because of the means or amount of repair required.

The process of hatching heralds a massive physiological change for the neonate, especially of the respiratory system (Figures 8.1 and 8.2). Given these complexities, it is ironic that hatch interventions are usually limited to simple incisions of the shell (to allow the change to air from egg respiration while the foetus rests) and assisted fluids and hydration to foetuses that have become weakened during the hatching process. It is important to avoid forceful removal of the foetus from the egg, as the yolk sac must be internalized before hatching commences. If this does not occur, the yolk sac is prone to trauma and infection, both of which carry a poor prognosis.

Reptile Medicine and Surgery in Clinical Practice, First Edition. Edited by Bob Doneley, Deborah Monks, Robert Johnson and Brendan Carmel.

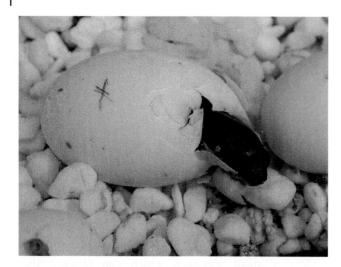

Figure 8.1 Australian broad-shelled turtle hatching (courtesy of Bob Doneley).

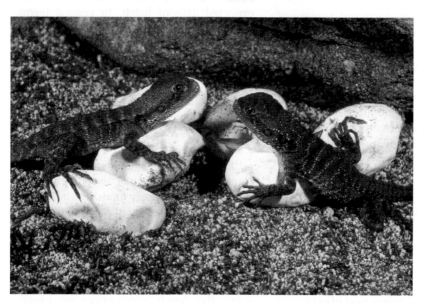

Figure 8.2 Eastern water dragons immediately post-hatching (courtesy of Bob Doneley).

Should a neonate hatch with a small volume of non-resorbed or still externalized yolk sac, dilute povidone iodine solution may be dabbed on to the umbilicus and a protective wrapping placed around it (even clear plastic wrap may suffice in the very short term). In cases involving more significantly externalized yolk sacs, the extraneous portion may be ligated close to the umbilicus and excised. The affected neonate will need to be fed much sooner than the conspecifics, as the nutrition provided by the yolk sac will be reduced. The more externalized the yolk sac, the poorer the prognosis (Figures 8.3 and 8.4). In these cases, the decision to use antibiotics should be made on an individual basis. While the internal aspect of the egg is sterile, the external environment is not, and yolk sac infections can be terminal. On the other hand, antibiotics given at such an early age may compromise the ability of the neonate to develop normal flora. Herbivorous species that rely on bacterial assistance for digestion are particularly at risk. Attention to

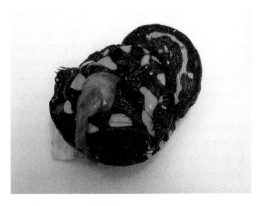

Figure 8.3 Externalized yolk sac in Australian broad-shelled turtle hatchling (courtesy of Bob Doneley).

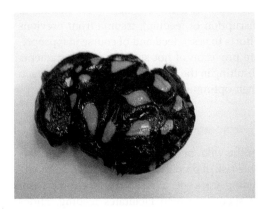

Figure 8.4 Normal umbilicus in Australian broad-shelled turtle hatchling (courtesy of Bob Doneley).

husbandry and hygiene is critical and arguably frontline management. There is a high mortality in hatchlings with larger exteriorized yolk sacs, regardless of intervention.

Ovoviviparous/Viviparous Neonates

Generally, dystocia is rare in species which give birth to live young. In the unusual event of obstructive dystocia, the involved foetus is usually dead. While obstructive dystocia may be a result of deformed or oversize foetuses, previous trauma resulting in maternal pelvic deformity can occur. Young born with congenital anatomical defects may be more prone to causing dystocia and less viable, even if successfully delivered (Figure 8.5).

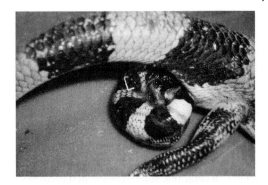

Figure 8.5 Blue-tongued lizard giving birth (courtesy of Annette Bird).

When surgical intervention (caesarean section) is required to alleviate dystocia, resuscitation of any delivered young is done according to standard mammalian processes – first clearing the oral cavity of mucus and debris, stimulating the body using gentle stroking pressure laterally around the thorax, and using resuscitative drugs if needed. A Doppler probe will be required to detect the presence of a heartbeat in reptiles, as auscultation is problematic.

Neonatal Care

Maternal Factors

Although little scientific research has been conducted in this area, it stands to reason that well-nourished females are much more likely to produce robust offspring. The shell provides the initial calcium for the neonatal skeleton, so the offspring of a calcium-depleted female are likely to have low body levels of calcium from the outset. While this can be addressed if identified, the practice of selling young reptiles as early as possible can lead to exacerbation of these underlying nutritional issues.

Post-Hatch/Birth Inappetence

Most reptiles do not need to eat immediately after birth, surviving on the nutrition provided by their yolk sacs for a variable period of time. The exact duration will vary according to species and should be previously researched.

The appropriate species-specific food must be offered but care must be taken to source size-appropriate items. Tiny maggots, crickets and other insects are often used for species that are insectivorous as young animals. Hand feeding may be required initially as neonates may need time to develop hunting skills.

Occasionally, developmentally delayed neonates refuse to eat for substantial periods of time. Once the yolk sac is absorbed, they progress to a catabolic state, from which recovery is unlikely unless eating commences. It is advisable for all anorexic neonates to have a complete physical examination, including disease testing if at all possible. The causes can be varied. Breeders use a number of techniques to encourage self-feeding, including:

- changing the species of food item offered
- offering a more 'natural' prey item
- scenting 'abnormal' food, such as rodents, with the scent of more 'natural' prey items
- hand feeding with normal foods, including moving or wriggling dead prey items to simulate life
- assist feeding with baby foods or commercial veterinary convalescence foods
- force feeding.

It is important to remember that some species are ambush predators rather than active hunters. Those species will commonly refuse to feed if they are feeling insecure, so an environmental audit ensuring sufficient hiding areas is important. If force feeding is required, it must be done extremely carefully, as damage can occur during the process. This is a particular concern with snakes. Animals that are not thermoregulating can suffer from maldigestion, meaning that the ingested food can decompose before it is digested. It is crucial to ensure that the animal is kept at the optimal body temperature in the postprandial phase of digestion.

In recently purchased young animals, common iatrogenic causes of inappetence include excessively large enclosures (leading to insufficient thermoregulation and feelings of insecurity); excessive interaction or handling of the new animal; inappropriate positioning of the enclosure in a thoroughfare (also leading to disruption of feeding); trauma from previous efforts to assist feed and of course inappropriate provision of hot spots and heat gradients resulting in the animals not being able to reach their optimum body temperature.

Thermoregulation

In the wild, neonatal reptiles are at considerable risk of predation. Sufficient and adequate hiding areas within an enclosure allow a sense of security, which facilitates feeding. Hides must be provided in multiple areas of the enclosure, including hot, warm and cool thermal zones, or the animals may refuse to thermoregulate in preference to staying hidden (Figure 8.6). Specific hot spots can be draped

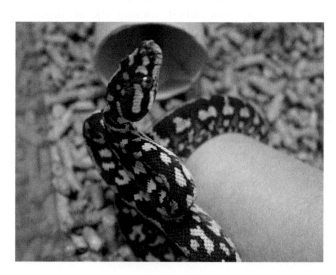

Figure 8.6 This juvenile jungle carpet python has toilet rolls as hides to allow for a sense of security in the enclosure (courtesy of Bob Doneley).

in artificial vines or other cover to improve the sense of security of neonates and encourage basking. While the maximum enclosure size possible is usually recommended for adult animals, young reptiles housed in excessively large enclosures will often thermoregulate poorly, presumably due to insecurity.

As well as the obvious improvement to immune function, adequate thermoregulation also facilitates the absorption of nutrients (including calcium) from the gastrointestinal tract.

Conspecific Aggression

It is common practice to house multiple neonates together but this often results in aggression and trauma. Some species (e.g. bearded dragons and blue-tongued skinks) are notorious for this. Not only can aggression result in damage to other babies but low level 'bullying' and 'intimidation' can also lead to delayed feeding and stunted growth for subordinate animals. Reduced access to resources, including prime basking areas, can compromise immunity. In many cases, paediatric reptiles do better kept individually, although this does vary according to species. In any case, previously traumatized young animals should be removed from group housing and any wounds treated according to first principles. It is not uncommon for bite wounds to crush the vascular supply of the skin, leading to progressive distal limb necrosis over several days. Treatment of such wounds involves aggressive, early diagnosis and treatment. Hot and cold poultices may stimulate blood supply to the extremity. Antibiotics are usually indicated. Traumatic amputation may occur from bites to limbs or tails or may be subsequently required at a later date due to tissue necrosis.

Examination and Diagnostic Testing

Paediatric reptiles are usually small, which confers particular difficulties with physical examination and diagnostic testing. Palpation of the body and limbs should be performed but diagnostic sensitivity is often poor. Specialized equipment can be used in specific instances (for instance paediatric and neonatal stethoscopes have much smaller heads). Ingenuity and creativity is often useful, as is inspiration acquired from other practitioners at conferences and presentations.

Oral and cytological smears can be made from samples taken with tiny cotton tips. Often, viral swabs provided by pathology companies have particularly small tips. Vascular access can be challenging, both due to the mechanical difficulties of drawing blood and the restriction in available volume if venepuncture is successful (see Chapter 13 for venepuncture sites). Using the smallest insulin syringe available (e.g. a 0.3 ml with a 29 g needle), it is often possible to get a small sample. Haemodilution with lymph is not uncommon and results must be interpreted in light of this. In the author's opinion, a blood smear for haematological analysis is the most useful test to prioritize, with a packed cell volume/total solids being the next most beneficial parameter. Even though venepuncture may be challenging, it is still not recommended to take blood via toe nail clipping.

Faecal analysis (floatation and direct smear) can be performed on freely passed specimens, thus avoiding issues of size on collection.

Given these challenges, comparatively more reliance needs to be placed on anamnesis to identify the likely aetiology of illness. A careful history may elicit information more consistent with congenital deformity, for instance, or indicate an animal that initially appeared healthy and then deteriorated, which may make infection more likely. If confirmatory testing cannot be done, the clinician must be prepared to prepare a treatment plan based on the most likely or most serious possibilities.

Treatment

If there is a high index of suspicion for a particular condition or a disease has been confirmed, then treatment specific to that problem must be instituted. In most cases, the drugs used will be the same regardless of age, although paediatric cases often require drug dilution to be accurate. Some drugs do not distribute or may be unstable in dilution and the practitioner must be aware of this. Compounded drugs may be the solution to this problem. Regardless of the underlying pathology, paediatric animals are prone to several serious secondary conditions.

Hypothermia

A small total body size and a high surface area to volume ratio leaves paediatric patients at risk of hypothermia. Additionally, unwell young animals may not properly thermoregulate. A lack of secure hides will make this more likely. When treating paediatric patients, it is advisable to provide a relatively small enclosure with a tightly controlled thermal gradient. Water should be provided, as insufficient humidity can worsen dehydration. Care must be taken to prevent total body immersion in the water dish, as evaporative cooling of the patient can occur. Paediatric patients presenting with hypothermia must be gently rewarmed, using stages to reach preferred optimum body temperature. Aggressive rewarming can lead to rebound hyperthermia. As immunocompromise is often associated with an episode of hypothermia, prophylactic antibiotics are often indicated.

Hypoglycaemia

After the yolk sac is exhausted, paediatric animals need to eat regularly to maintain euglycaemia. The frequency of feeding is mainly dictated by species, with snakes needing the least frequent feeding. Hyporexia and anorexia are common in unhealthy paediatric patients and secondary hypoglycaemia is not uncommon. Clinical signs can range from lethargy to an obtunded demeanour. Tremors can be present, and animals can even be seizuring on presentation. Hypoglycaemia can be difficult to differentiate from viral infection, septicaemia or structural neurological disease.

A blood glucose test to confirm the diagnosis is ideal, although it is not uncommon to treat on the presumption of hypoglycaemia rather than wait for confirmation, given the low risk of administration of glucose and the high consequence of incorrectly withholding treatment. In many situations, the blood taken for testing can be better used for other parameters, such as haematological examination. The accuracy of some patient-side testing kits has been called into question. Depending on the degree of hypoglycaemia, treatment may include the administration of oral glucose supplements, the use of stomach tubes to administer glucose and/or electrolyte solutions, or even subcutaneous injections or intravenous injections of glucose or dextrose solutions, providing intravenous access is possible. For oral and subcutaneous measures to be effective, the animal must be in the preferred optimal temperature zone. Once initially stabilized, normal assist feeding should begin, remembering that many paediatric animals have higher dietary protein requirements than adults. Caution needs to be exercised during assist feeding, as iatrogenic mandibular fractures can occur. The use of metal or other hard, narrow feeding tubes is contraindicated.

Hypocalcaemia

Young animals are generally undergoing great skeletal growth. This rapid growth commonly highlights husbandry deficiencies, meaning that hypocalcaemia is a common paediatric problem (see Chapters 4, 6, 15 and 25 for further information). True hypocalcaemia is a medical emergency, as acute cardiac failure, seizures and death can occur. Other common clinical signs include depression, lethargy, generalized muscle weakness and twitching. Patient-side testing can be done and is useful to gauge the severity of the deficiency and can determine the aggressiveness of treatment, with more severe cases receiving increased treatment frequency. Treatment options range from oral calcium/vitamin D to parenterally administered calcium (either subcutaneously, intravenously or intracoelomically).

Prevention of hypocalcaemia can be achieved with excellent husbandry, including appropriate provision of hot spots and thermal gradient, appropriate calcium and vitamin D supplementation of food, appropriate provision of ultraviolet lighting. An underappreciated cause of metabolic bone disease is insecurity of the reptile leading to constant hiding and lack of exposure to both ultraviolet light and basking areas. In some cases, curtains over the front of the enclosure can restore a feeling of security (see Chapters 4, 6 and 25).

Dehydration

Dehydration can occur rapidly, as much from a dry environment as insufficient drinking. Regardless of the patient's condition, in most cases it is crucial to have a shallow bowl of water in the enclosure of a sick paediatric to maintain humidity. The amount of humidity varies according to species, with chondropythons requiring a high humidity, while species such as shingleback lizards need a much drier environment. Gauze swabs can be used within the water dish to prevent animals from drowning or immersing themselves in water. Positioning water dishes close to heat sources will increase enclosure humidity. Dehydration is rectified using oral or parenteral means. Fluid requirements must be carefully calculated, as it is easy to cause iatrogenic overhydration.

Anaesthesia

Most injectable and gaseous anaesthetic agents used for adult reptiles may be used in paediatric patients, although the delivery of the drugs may be more complex. Dilution of injectable drugs to ensure an accurate dose is common. Insulin syringes are also useful for delivery and measurement of these amounts.

The relative amount of damage (and therefore pain) caused by intramuscular injection into small muscle volumes is greater in paediatric patients.

Vascular access is difficult in paediatric patients. Intraosseous catheterization is extremely useful; however, anaesthesia must be induced before an intraosseous catheter can be placed. Not all drugs are appropriate for intramedullary injection and the clinician is advised to check before administration. See Chapter 13 for placement of intraosseous catheters.

Intubation can also be challenging and many practitioners fashion 'home-made' endotracheal tubes from various items including intravenous catheters to allow intubation of small patients (Figure 8.7). Mucous blockage of small tubes can occur, so intermittent positive pressure ventilation is important. Additionally, the percentage decrease of the airway diameter is much greater in smaller animals.

Specific Conditions

Genetic Defects

The popularity of morphological mutations within the reptile trade means that congenital deformities and developmental issues are becoming more common. Unfortunately, in many cases, the economics of producing 'designer' traits supersedes the poor welfare outcomes experienced by these animals. This ethical tension needs to be resolved by the hobby. Examples include neurological deficits in jaguar carpet pythons ('jags') and lethal genes associated with some homozygous dominant colour traits like leucism. A good history of the affected individual and family tree, as well as knowledge of the industry will help differentiate random congenital deformity and intrinsic genetic deficits.

Infectious Diseases

Paediatric reptiles are initially reliant on maternal factors for protection against specific diseases (via maternal antibody transfer

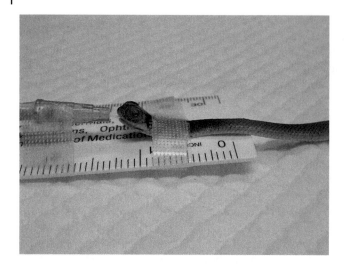

Figure 8.7 Eastern brown snake juvenile with endotracheal tube made from a 26-guage catheter (courtesy of Bob Doneley).

into the egg). Subsequently, appropriate husbandry should allow good general immunity. While young reptiles can be afflicted by any of the infectious diseases of older animals, the course of the disease is often more acute and more severe. An example is adenovirus in bearded dragons, which is often unapparent in adults; however, young dragons demonstrate a range of particular signs, including:

- chronic ill thrift
- stunting
- secondary infections due to immune suppression
- neurologic changes (tremors, star gazing, seizuring)
- diarrhoea and other gastrointestinal abnormalities.

See Chapter 16 for specific diseases. Given the emerging nature of reptile viral diseases, adequate quarantine is essential for any reptile keeper, more so those with paediatric animals. See Chapter 5 for a more detailed discussion of quarantine.

Substrate Ingestion

As young animals are acquiring the skills of hunting and prehension, it is more likely that they will accidentally ingest substrate. For this reason, saw shavings and wood chips are inadvisable as substrates. Rarely, indigestible food items may also cause gastrointestinal obstructions.

Endoscopic gastric retrieval under anaesthesia is possible. Sand can sometimes move through to the colon and cause constipation, which may be relieved using enemas.

Failure to Thrive

Some animals fail to thrive after hatching or birth. In the wild, this is an expected occurrence and not every animal survives to adulthood. In captivity, there are emotional and financial reasons to have a more individualized focus. At the outset, stunted patients should have a full examination including physical examination, faecal examination and preferably haematological examination (if possible). Consideration must be given to viral testing where appropriate (e.g. adenovirus in neonatal bearded dragons).

It is likely that, in some cases, the diagnostic sensitivity of the available testing is too poor to identify the underlying problem. It is also likely that some of these animals are suffering from emerging pathogens that have not yet been elucidated. Nonetheless, it is likely that paediatric patients failing to meet normal developmental milestones may not thrive long-term unless excellent support and husbandry is maintained, including attention to hygiene, assist feeding and appropriate lighting and heating for species (Annette Bird, personal communication).

Further Reading

Johnson, J.D. (2012) Reptile and amphibian pediatric medicine and surgery. *Veterinary Clinics North America, Exotic Animal Practice*, 15 (2), 251–264.

9

Setting Up and Equipping a Reptile Practice

Bob Doneley, Shane Simpson, Angela M. Lennox and John Chitty

Marketing A Reptile Practice

Introduction

The decision to start a reptile practice or incorporate reptiles into an existing practice should, like all business decisions, be based on research and planning detailed in a business plan. While a reptile practice is a niche concept it can and should be promoted like any mainstream business entity, with both internal and external marketing focusing on how you intend to advertise your interest and willingness to see and treat reptiles and amphibians.

Internal Marketing

Internal marketing is the process of promoting your services to both your staff and existing clients. It is vital that staff appreciate the services you are able to provide and actively discuss them with current and potential clients of the practice. It may be of no surprise to discover that many of the practice's current clients are reptile owners; by simply marketing to current clients the practice may already have a reptile client base.

Providing the staff with tools to allow them to promote the practice's services is vital, as is developing a brand that reflects the practice's interest in reptiles. Logos, client handouts, brochures, reminders, an informative website and social media outlets such as Facebook are all key components. In addition, reception and nursing staff need to be trained not only in handling reptile patients but also in how to handle and answer questions from clients. Employing staff who own reptiles or having one or two pet reptiles in the practice waiting room can go a long way to creating an air of confidence with the sometimes sceptical reptile owner.

External Marketing

Attracting new clients is essential should a reptile practice wish to succeed. Avenues for obtaining new clients include:

- Actively encouraging current clients to refer friends and family members who own reptiles. This can be achieved by offering discounts and other incentives to both the current and potential client.
- Advertising: an advertising budget can form part of a marketing plan to allow for promotion in locations such as business directories, Google AdWords, online forum banners and reptile-related magazines. Writing articles for magazines is also a great way of promoting your practice.

Reptile Medicine and Surgery in Clinical Practice, First Edition. Edited by Bob Doneley, Deborah Monks, Robert Johnson and Brendan Carmel.
© 2018 John Wiley & Sons Ltd. Published 2018 by John Wiley & Sons Ltd.

- Involvement with local herpetological groups. Becoming an active member by attending meetings, expos and speaking at events will quickly result in new clients. Reptile keepers know how hard it is to find a vet able to treat their animals and will appreciate your participation.
- Referrals: develop relationships with local pet stores and other veterinary clinics. These businesses will often readily forward clients to veterinarians who exhibit an interest in reptiles. Ensure you update these contacts with the progress of referred cases to keep the lines of communication open.

Fee Setting for the Reptile Practice

In principle, fees for services for reptiles should be similar to those for other pet species. In well-managed practices, veterinarians determine prices based on one of several strategies: competitive, cost-based, variable or value-based pricing. The competitive pricing strategy recommends setting fees somewhere in between the middle and the high end of local competition. Cost-based pricing uses a standard mark up over the purchase prices of goods. For variable pricing, prices change depending on demand or include strategies such as loyalty programmes or wellness programmes. Value-based pricing aligns the price of all services with the examination fee, which can be determined by what the economy in the area is expected to bear.

Regardless of strategy, most management consultants recommend there should be no difference between fees for reptiles and fees for more traditional pets, as veterinarians in general spend the same amount of time (and often more) during consultations and, in many cases, have invested significant resources into continuing education or other specialized equipment necessary to treat reptiles. Regardless, many practitioners

feel obligated to reduce fees for species seen less frequently. Reasons that have been given include feelings of inadequacy in terms of veterinary competency and sympathy for owners whom the practitioner perceives may not have funds for veterinary services.

Veterinarians who truly feel they have nothing to offer reptile owners should refrain from accepting them as clients. For the rest, the veterinary visit often consists of significant amounts of time discussing husbandry, the actual physical examination, consultation with books, journal or proceedings to support a diagnostic plan, diagnostic testing, which usually takes more time than for more familiar traditional pet species, and a return to the literature to interpret diagnostic testing and to formulate and put in place a treatment plan. In most cases, this takes much more time that the typical traditional pet consultation. Many exotic pet practitioners and practice consultants actually recommend that exotic services should be priced higher than a traditional pet examination. Some charge more for the physical examination only; others charge more for individual items such as specialized hospitalization or diagnostic testing.

Measuring the Financial Health of the Reptile Practice

Using traditional strategies to measure practice growth and health can be applied to the reptile practice. Key performance indicators (KPIs) are standardized calculations of quantifiable and measurable data reflecting performance or trends occurring within a business that impact on achievement of business goals and objectives. They can be measured across a number of areas of a business (including business performance, human resources, marketing and the operations of the business) and can be used for comparison of performance within a business (e.g. from year to year) or to similar businesses. A successful

Table 9.1 Suggested key performance indicators (KPIs) for a reptile practice.

Category	KPI	Explanation
Financial ratio	Rates of return	Investment income or loss for a specified time period, calculated as a percentage gain or loss on initial cost of investment
	Solvency	Ability of a business to meet financial obligations
	Debt	Ratio of debt to assets
	Inventory turnover	Frequency of sale and replacement of inventory
	Receivables turnover and debtor days	Ability of the business to collect monies owed
Sales	Income area sales	Measurement of income area (professional fees and inventory) sales as a percentage of total income
	Veterinarian productivity	Sales income, annual number of transactions, active clients, new clients, and lapsed clients, expressed as a ratio to full time equivalent veterinarians
	Transaction sales	Average transaction charge, professional fee average transaction charge, and number of transactions per active client
Cost control[a]	Total costs	Generally measure the relationship between total costs and total income and can help identify where a practice can trim costs to improve profitability
	Cost centres: • Drugs and medical supplies • Veterinary staff costs • Support staff costs • Pathology costs	Can be related to total income to help monitor the effectiveness or degree of influence expenditure in these areas has on profitability

[a] As a percentage of total income.

veterinary practice monitors a range of KPIs to seek ways of improving service provision and profitability. Improvements to veterinary practice performance can only be made when data are collected and interpreted using KPIs.

Veterinary business KPIs can be grouped into three broad categories (Table 9.1). These KPIs can be obtained, in many cases, from veterinary practice software, bank statements and the practice accountant. The practice owner or manager should measure these indicators each month and compare to previous months and years to monitor the practice performance.

KPIs often include items such as client turnover. Unlike in dog and cat practice, reptile owners are much less likely to use wellness care and do not present for routine vaccinations. Most consultations are for sick reptiles; if the reptile recovers, the owner is often unlikely to return until the next illness. Thus, certain KPIs may be less useful than for traditional pet practice.

The Consultation Room

The consultation room is a key element in any veterinary practice and is no less important in the reptile practice. It serves as the main interface between the veterinarian and the client. As such, it is important that it sends the right messages to clients – professionalism, hygiene, competence, and confidence. The room should be escape-proof for the eventuality of a reptile responding unexpectedly to handling and suddenly finding itself unrestrained. Possible escape routes include doors, windows and drains; likely hiding places include behind cupboards, refrigerators, chairs and bins. All of these features should be taken into consideration when designing or altering a room to serve as a consultation room.

The room and its fittings should be constructed of impervious material that not only looks professional but is also easy to clean and disinfect between patients. Handwashing facilities and an alcohol hand rinse add to the level of hygiene (and the client's perception of cleanliness).

Doors should be lockable and staff should be advised to always knock before entering. This is particularly important when dealing with dangerous reptiles such as venomous snakes and large monitors. When dealing with such animals, the display of warning signs on the doors is an appropriate safety measure.

The walls of the room can be used to display awards and certificates that attest to the veterinarian's knowledge and skills, and pictures or paintings that demonstrate an interest in reptiles.

Equipment

Most of the equipment needed to practice reptile medicine can be found in nearly all veterinary practices. There are some additional pieces that will make the consultation process smoother and easier. Digital scales, capable of weighing to 1 gram, are essential when examining a reptile. Larger scales will be required for large patients such as large monitors or tortoises. Easily cleaned (or disposable) containers are useful when weighing small patients, such as hatchling pythons or small lizards; plastic containers and cardboard boxes with lids are ideal, as are washable cloth bags (e.g. pillow slips).

Magnification and illumination are useful when examining small patients or lesions. Binocular loupes or ophthalmic equipment can fill this role.

Examination of a reptile's mouth and the administration of oral medications are always a challenge for the reptile veterinarian. Mouth gags, either stainless steel or acrylic, are useful items to have in the consultation room (Figures 9.1 and 9.2). Wooden tongue depressors or the plunger of a syringe can make useful substitutes. Care must be taken to minimize or prevent damage to the patient's gingiva and teeth.

Reptile sexing probes can be purchased as a set in different sizes (Figure 9.3). These are useful for identifying the sex of many snakes, look professional and are easy to clean. They must be used carefully, with adequate lubrication, and must be disinfected after use.

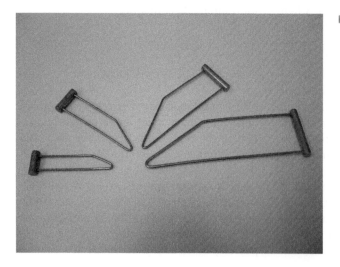

Figure 9.1 Metal oral specula.

Figure 9.2 Acrylic oral specula.

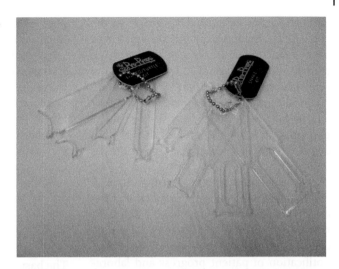

Figure 9.3 Reptile sexing probes.

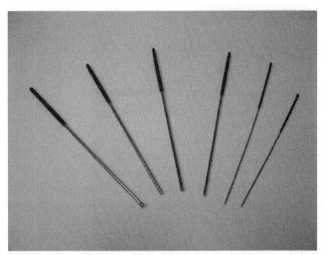

A tape measure is useful for recording details such as carapace length and measuring snakes for determination of organ location and the investigation of lumps.

If diagnostic sampling is performed in the consultation room a supply of sampling equipment should be kept on hand. This includes syringes, needles, cotton buds, sterile culture swabs, microscope slides, coverslips and paediatric blood collection tubes (lithium heparin and sodium EDTA).

Medical Records

Medical records are maintained for three reasons: to preserve a database of previous clinical findings for future reference and comparison; to prompt the clinician's memory on details when a patient has not been seen for weeks, months or years; and to demonstrate a clear (and defensible) thought process when the records are reviewed by another party, whether they be another clinician or a court of law. They also are invaluable for marketing and management purposes, such as reminders and billing. Records should be generated at the time of clinical examination or shortly afterwards, and in such a manner that the record is regarded as accurate and trustworthy.

Whether the record is handwritten or computerized, the use of a template encourages a methodical and organized approach to the clinical examination, assisting the clinician in both organizing their thoughts and ensuring that nothing is overlooked. After an initial record is created on the first visit, a separate record should be created for each subsequent day in hospital, revisit or visits for other problems. The record should also contain copies of laboratory and radiology reports or indicate where these records are held.

It is also important that records contain communications between the client and the clinic, including recommended treatments that were declined by the client, telephone calls made by either party, cost estimates and notification of patient progress and laboratory results to the client.

Hospitalization of Reptiles

Reptiles frequently require prolonged hospitalization. They have a much lower metabolic rate than birds or mammals, so their response to both illness and treatment will be accordingly slower. They are often a lot sicker than they initially appear and so extensive supportive care is often necessary to stabilize them. They may be as difficult to medicate, especially at home. Suboptimal husbandry practices are the primary cause of many reptile diseases. It is therefore imperative to hospitalize these patients in optimal conditions as an essential part of their therapy.

Hospitalization facilities must be planned with the anticipation that patients will be kept for much longer periods than a sick bird or mammal (in the case of an anorexic tortoise, for example, it is not unusual to hospitalize patients for over a month). To provide optimal therapy, the veterinarian must provide optimal husbandry. Hospitalization in suboptimal conditions will result in poor success rates.

Facilities

The basic facilities required are:

- the enclosure itself
- a heat source
- humidity
- light
- hiding places
- handling aids.

The Enclosure

Reptile enclosures (Figure 9.4) must be escape proof with tight-fitting, lockable doors (especially for small lizards and snakes) and strong hinges and locks (for large lizards and snakes). Access to the enclosure must be sufficient for easy capture of the patient.

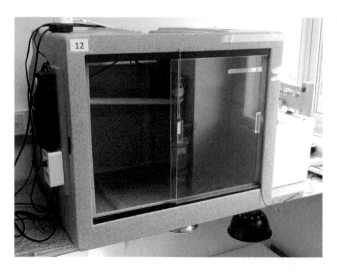

Figure 9.4 Reptile hospital cage.

Dimensions are dependent on species need; for example, arboreal species need some capacity to climb and hang, as this can aid passively clearance of respiratory discharges (Figure 9.5). Non-climbing tortoises can be maintained in an open 'tray' with a thermal gradient (Figure 9.6). Ambient heating is likely to be required to ensure lower temperatures are sufficient. Using old pet cages is not recommended, as disinfection is usually problematic. Aquatic species are difficult to hospitalize. They may be maintained in an aquarium or plastic tub, which can be part-filled with water and tilted to give a varying depth of water, with the shallowest end allowing the animal to leave the water. Water quality should be monitored and, preferably, changed daily. Semi-aquatic species, such as

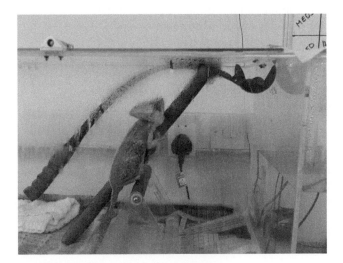

Figure 9.5 Climbing perches allow arboreal species to display normal behaviour.

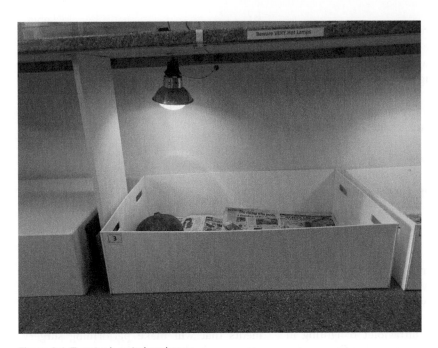

Figure 9.6 Tortoise hospital enclosure.

red-eared sliders, may be 'dry docked' and kept in the same way as tortoises. In these cases, bathing in deep water (e.g. in a plastic tub) should be provided as required. Post-surgery patients should only be provided with shallow bathing each day.

For practices that do not see many reptiles, it may seem logical to use the owner's vivarium. However, it must be remembered that many of the disease syndromes are due to a failure in husbandry; using an inappropriate vivarium may not be helpful to the patient.

Heat Source

All reptiles require keeping in the 'preferred optimum temperature zone'. This will vary according to species and may be altered by disease (see Chapter 5 for more detail). Temperatures should be monitored by a minimum–maximum thermometer. Hyper-thermia can be rapidly fatal, so vivaria should never be placed in direct sunlight and the entire room should be adequately ventilated in hot weather.

Humidity

Different species require different humidity and gradients (see Chapter 1). Even desert species require a humidity chamber to mimic the trapping of water under rocks: a wet towel in a box can be used and is easily changed each day. Humidity could also be provided by misting regularly or allowing evaporation from open dishes of water. Misting is vital when hospitalizing some species, such as chameleons, as they will only drink by taking droplets from the vivarium walls.

Light

Full-spectrum ultraviolet light should be provided. This may be incorporated into the heat source or may be separate. A 12-hour: 12-hour light–dark cycle is generally appropriate. The use of ultraviolet B lighting in reptile enclosures is discussed in Chapter 6.

Hiding Places

Many reptiles are shy and benefit from a place to hide. This may be a small box or humidity chamber, paper or substrate. This must be easily accessible for regular monitoring through the day. Covering the front of the vivarium may also help for some nervous individuals.

Handling Aids

While most species can be easily restrained using a towel, some handling aids may be required for more aggressive species, especially snakes. These should always be kept close to the vivarium whenever the animal is handled. All practices seeing reptiles should have the following aids:

- gloves – both thick gauntlets and thinner anti-needle stick gloves
- snake hook
- snake grabs or tongs
- snake tubes, if venomous species are being hospitalized.

Biosecurity

Many reptile pathogens are spread by direct contact or fomite. Biosecurity is therefore paramount and all patients must be barrier nursed (see Chapter 32). Enclosures should be thoroughly cleaned and disinfected between patients. All equipment used should be cleaned and disinfected between uses. Separate equipment (e.g. bath trays, bowls) should be labelled and only used for an individual patient.

The Surgical Suite

The surgical suite of most small animal practices can be easily modified to cater for reptilian patients. There are specific requirements that will make performing surgery safer for both the patient and operating staff, allow for a more efficient use of space, staff and time, resulting in an improved standard of care.

Instrumentation

Most veterinary practices already have surgical instruments that could be used satisfactorily in reptilian patients. In addition to these, ophthalmic instruments are useful when operating on small patients. A basic kit for reptile surgery may include:

- small scalpel handle and blade
- fine needle holders such as Olsen-Hegar or Castroviejo
- straight and curved Halsted mosquito forceps and Allis tissue forceps for tissue handling and haemostasis
- a selection of fine forceps such as Bishop Harmon or Debakey, as well as atraumatic forceps, e.g. Adson Brown tissue forceps
- at least one pair of good quality fine scissors, such as Iris (both straight and curved), Castroviejo or strabismus scissors.

In addition to these basic surgical instruments, the surgeon may have need for:

- eye speculums, such as Barraquer or Castroviejo, which are very effective retractors for coelomic surgery on small reptiles

- bulldog clamps; these small atraumatic clamps are useful in gastrointestinal surgery.

Other Equipment

In addition to the surgical instruments, some ancillary equipment is useful, including:

- vascular clips: haemostasis in small patients can problematic. The use of stainless steel or titanium vascular clips (e.g. Hemoclips® and Ligaclips®) can help greatly to reduce blood loss and surgery time (Figure 9.7).
- laser or radiosurgical unit: reduced swelling and pain at the surgery site, accurate haemostasis and a further reduction in anaesthetic time are some of the benefits of these modalities.
- reuseable retractor rings (e.g. Lone Star Retractor®): adequate surgical exposure can be a challenge in reptiles, particularly when performing a coeliotomy. The use of a Lone Star Retractor will greatly improve exposure and again reduce surgery time (Figure 9.8).
- magnification loupes: being able to actually see what you are performing surgery on is obviously vital, especially with very small patients.
- heating: keeping the patient warm throughout surgery and recovery is imperative for a good outcome. This can be achieved

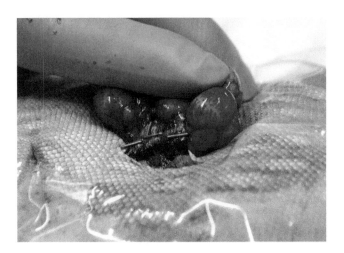

Figure 9.7 Haemoclips are used to ligate blood vessels, such as the ovarian vasculature in this bearded dragon.

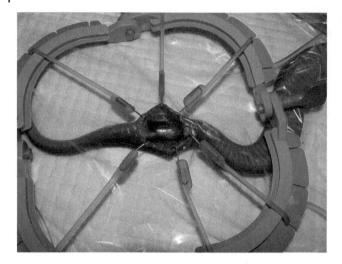

Figure 9.8 Lone Star retractor in use.

through the use of heating mats, forced warm air blankets and heat lamps.

- consumables: using clear patient drapes, swaged on suture needles, and sterilized cotton buds can improve patient care and increase the chances of a positive outcome of surgery.

Anaesthetic Equipment

Having the correct surgical equipment is useless if the animal cannot be safely and adequately anaesthetized for surgery. See Chapter 27 for more information on anaesthesia in reptiles.

10

The Reptile Consultation
Bob Doneley and Brendan Carmel

The Appointment

Before an examination can be performed, an appointment has to be made. This requires an interaction between your reception staff and a potential client, either in person or on the telephone. Some pointers that have proven to be successful include:

- Allow up to 1 hour for a new reptile client and 30 minutes for a regular client. Your receptionist must be bright, friendly and comfortable with reptiles and, above all, must exude confidence that your practice can competently examine and treat a reptile.
- Give the client clear instructions on what to bring:
  - a fresh faecal sample (not urates)
  - a water sample from the tank of aquatic reptiles (the client should bring at least 100 ml in a sealed bottle, without the reptile in it
  - digital photographs of the enclosure
  - the reptile in a suitable container, not draped over the client's neck or down their shirt front. The enclosure should be escape and leak proof and should have supplemental heat; for example, a hot water bottle or heat pack, to keep the reptile warm.

- Ensure that the receptionist obtains exact details of what is coming in – species, age, sex and problem. Having these details before the client arrives allows the veterinarian to do some quick research on the husbandry requirements and biological characteristics of any unfamiliar species. There is nothing worse than seeing an appointment in the scheduler that simply says 'Mr Jones, sick snake'.
- Ask the client to arrive at least 10 minutes before their appointment. If possible, e-mail them a new client questionnaire and ask them to bring it with them already filled in. Alternatively, have a link to a downloadable history form on your website.

More information on making an appointment is contained Chapter 32. On the arrival of the client and patient, details can be confirmed and entered into the computer database. Faecal and water samples provided by the client can be passed to a staff member for testing: water quality (pH, ammonia, nitrates, and nitrites), a faecal smear and a faecal flotation. These tests can be running while a history is taken and the reptile is being examined and the results available to the veterinarian before the completion of the consultation.

Reptile Medicine and Surgery in Clinical Practice, First Edition. Edited by Bob Doneley, Deborah Monks, Robert Johnson and Brendan Carmel.
© 2018 John Wiley & Sons Ltd. Published 2018 by John Wiley & Sons Ltd.

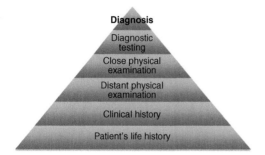

Figure 10.1 The diagnostic pyramid.

The Diagnostic Pyramid

The process of arriving at a diagnosis can be likened to building a pyramid (Figure 10.1). A solid base – the patient's history – is necessary for a good start and strong support. Layers can then be added (the physical examination and diagnostic testing) before arriving at the apex, the diagnosis. Bypassing any of these steps leads to a shaky and unstable diagnosis. But by working on them steadily and adding them in the right order, a solid diagnosis can be achieved.

Taking a History

A patient's history can be divided into two areas: what happened to the reptile before it became ill, and 'why are you here today?'. Most health problems in reptiles are due to incorrect or poor husbandry and, without an idea of how the reptile has been cared for, it can be difficult to determine what has gone wrong.

By using a computerized template, the first part of the history can be collected by the reception or nursing staff and then reviewed by the veterinarian at the beginning of the consultation. As mentioned above, a history form can be provided to the client before the consultation for completion. A list of suggested headings for such a template are shown in Box 10.1.

The second part of the history (Why are you here today?) can be started by the receptionist or nurse but will need to be explored in greater depth by the veterinarian after reviewing the first part of the history. An indication of the problem, when it was first noticed, whether is it progressing and what effect it is having on the animal (appetite, thirst, urination, defecation, shedding and activity levels) needs to be ascertained. It is important to know if any other animals have been affected and, if so, what happened to them.

Having the right tools in the consultation room to examine a reptile is essential. Much of the required equipment is already present in the general small animal practice, although some equipment specific for dealing with reptiles is required (see Chapter 9 for more details).

The Physical Examination

This is the part of the consultation the owner is keenest to get to, and a mistake made by many veterinarians is to go straight to a physical examination without first obtaining a good history. The clinician must resist the temptation to open that bag or container too soon!

All animals should be weighed and the weight recorded. A set of digital scales is an essential piece of consulting room equipment. Weighing the reptile in the bag or container before taking it out and then weighing the bag or container after removing the reptile is the simplest means of weighing fidgety reptiles. Recording the weight allows the clinician to calculate drug doses accurately, to monitor response to treatment and to compare the weight against previously recorded weights and against expected weights for that species. (It is also useful to encourage clients to weigh their reptiles regularly at home as weight loss may be the only subtle indicator of ill health in some reptiles.)

Successful reptile practice is based on a sound knowledge of the biology of the commonly presented species; perhaps more so than when dealing with other animal classes. In clinical reptile practice, a problem-based

---

Box 10.1 Suggested headings for a history form.

- The origin of the animal: where did the client obtain this animal and how long ago?
- The animal's age, sex, weight and reproductive history.
- Are there any other reptiles in the collection? If so, where are they housed in relation to the animal that has been presented?
- Have there been any new arrivals? If so, where did they come from? What quarantine procedures were followed and were any prophylactic treatments given?
- Details of the enclosure:
  - indoor/outdoor
  - orientation (horizontal or vertical)
  - size
  - construction materials
  - cage furniture (substrate, hides; climbing branches, water and feed dishes)
  - ventilation
  - frequency and method of cleaning.
- Heating:
  - At what temperature is the enclosure kept?
  - Is there a temperature gradient?
  - How is the heat provided?
  - How is it monitored (thermometer)?
  - How is it controlled (thermostat)?
  - Is the enclosure cooled during winter?
- Humidity:
  - What is the humidity in the cage?
  - How is it provided?
  - How is it monitored and controlled?
- Ultraviolet B (UVB) lighting: how is it provided? Is there access to unfiltered sunlight? How old are any artificial UVB sources and how often are they changed?
- Water (for aquatic reptiles):
  - Quality (temperature; pH; ammonia; nitrates; nitrites; hardness).
  - How is it filtered?
  - Water changes (how often, how much).
  - How is water quality monitored and how often?
- Feeding:
  - What with?
  - How often?
  - Any supplements?
  - When was the animal last fed?
- When did the reptile last defecate?
- When did the reptile last shed? Were there any difficulties with any shedding? Was any assistance required?
- Routine prophylactic treatments against external and internal parasites:
  - Has anything been done?
  - What with and how frequently?
  - When was the last treatment?
- Previous medical history:
  - Has this animal been unwell before?
  - What was the problem, how was it treated, and who treated it?
  - How did the animal respond to this treatment?

---

approach to diagnosis and treatment, outlining the commonly occurring clinical conditions, can be used (see Chapter 17). As with any species, examining normal or well animals to learn the normal is essential to detect the abnormal. Consider inspecting reptiles at pet shops, local herpetological societies or local zoos or wildlife parks to gain experience and to learn what is normal.

Although the history will have somewhat narrowed the clinician's list of differential diagnoses, care must be taken not to 'jump to the obvious'. A thorough physical examination, followed by a detailed examination of the problem area, may reveal other problems of which the owner was not aware; for example, necrotic stomatitis in a snake with skin lesions.

The physical examination should also include sex identification. Many owners, especially of pet reptiles (as distinct from breeding animals) are unaware or uncertain of their reptile's sex and seek veterinary advice on how to identify whether their pet is male or female. Knowing the animal's sex is a key element of establishing a list of differential diagnoses.

As with the examination of any species, a systematic approach is recommended: a methodical approach to examination of the reptile will lessen the chance of a missed diagnosis. Most reptiles resent oral examination so preferably examine the mouth last. Disposable gloves should be worn when examining reptiles, both for personal hygiene and also to help to minimize the potential transmission of disease between reptiles (e.g. sunshinevirus in snakes).

The first step of the examination is to observe: assess the demeanour, general alertness, posture and conformation of the reptile. This is done before picking the animal up; for example, observing a snake for any unusual coiling, twisting motions or weakness (Figure 10.2). If the reptile appears particularly lethargic, distressed or unwell, stop the physical examination and concentrate on stabilizing the patient (Figure 10.3). An outline of the approach to the physical examination is provided in Box 10.2.

The physical examination of a reptile is often unrewarding with respect to the development of a differential diagnosis list. There is then a resultant need for collection of diagnostic samples (see Chapter 11).

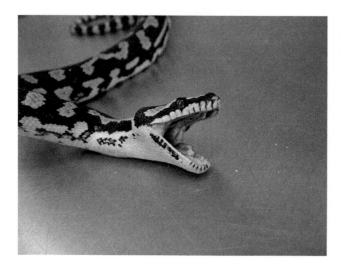

Figure 10.2 Abnormal posture and mouth breathing in a jungle carpet python with sunshinevirus.

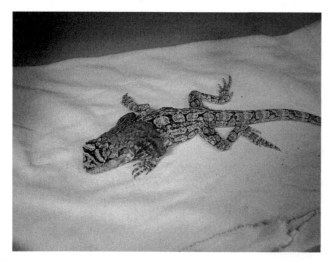

Figure 10.3 This juvenile frilled lizard may benefit from supportive care before conducting a detailed physical examination.

Box 10.2 Some general notes regarding the physical examination of reptiles.

- Begin with the external examination (Figure 10.4). Examine the skin, looking for abnormalities such as dysecdysis (abnormal shedding), lumps or bumps, discolouration, ulceration, wounds or parasites. Visually compare the symmetry of body parts. The nares, eyes, mouth, cloaca and ear openings (where present) should be free from discharge, swelling or discolouration.
- Performing a neurological examination on a reptile can be challenging. Reptiles do not have a consensual light response but do have a pupillary light response, although this is often sluggish compared with other species. Basic proprioceptive testing can be performed in some species.
- The reptilian eye is extremely variable in appearance. Familiarize yourself with the normal appearance of the species being examined. In snakes, the cornea is covered by the eye scale, or spectacle. (Figure 10.5) Some lizards have fused eyelids that form a spectacle

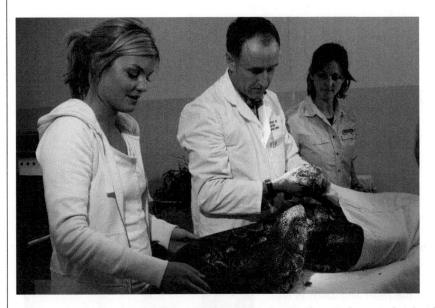

Figure 10.4 The clinical examination of this large reticulated python (*Python reticulatus*) with dysecdysis is aided by keeping most of the snake in a bag, with the help of assistants.

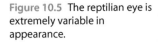

Figure 10.5 The reptilian eye is extremely variable in appearance.

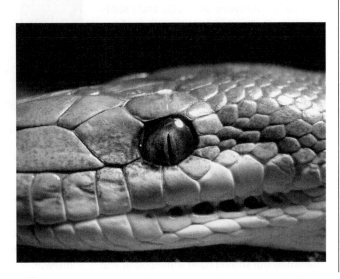

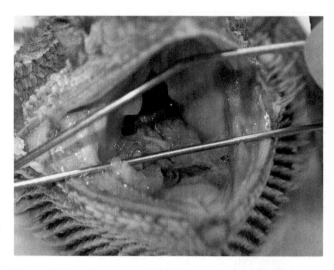

Figure 10.6 Oral examination of the pharynx of this bearded dragon revealed impaction with fibrous plant material.

as in snakes. See Chapter 2 for more details on the anatomy of the reptilian eye.

- The reptile mite (*Ophionyssus natricis*) is often found in grooves or crevices, such as inside the edge of the orbit, or in the gular groove (ventral chin region) of snakes.
- The cloacal region should be closely inspected. Does it appear enlarged or swollen or tender to the touch? Is there sufficient cloacal tone (akin to anal tone in mammals)? There should not be any accumulation of faecal or other matter around the cloaca.
- Auscultation of the heart and lungs in reptiles can be problematic. Some clinicians find the use of a wet swab or small towel as an interface between the reptile and a stethoscope will allow some assessment of respiratory or cardiac noises. Using a Doppler is highly recommended as a method to assess heart rate and rhythm in the consultation. Cardiac disease is increasingly being diagnosed in reptiles. See Chapter 20 for more information on cardiovascular diseases.
- Palpation of the coelomic region is possible in some reptiles.
- The mouth should be examined last, as most reptiles resent examination of the oral cavity, as mentioned previously (Figure 10.6). Pigmentation of the oral cavity varies widely between reptile species. Mucous membranes in reptiles are typically paler than in mammals but should have some colour and

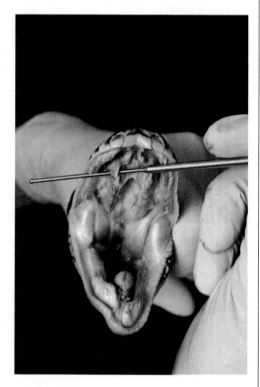

Figure 10.7 The mucous membrane colour of reptiles can be variable, from pale pink to darkly pigmented, such as in this snake.

should not appear dry (Figure 10.7). Pay attention to the choanae on the dorsal surface of the oral cavity; any discharge or swelling may point towards respiratory disease.

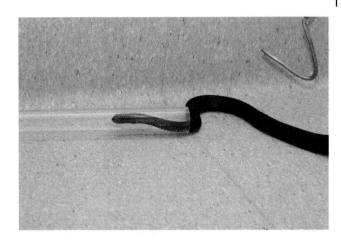

Figure 10.8 This venomous snake is 'tubed' to allow it to be examined safely. Only experienced veterinarians should examine and treat venomous or dangerous reptiles.

Venomous Reptiles

Warning: It is recommended that only experienced reptile veterinarians examine and treat venomous species. Safety is the prime consideration. Strict handling protocols must be in place and implemented (Figure 10.8).

Examination of the Lizard

A useful method of restraining many lizards for examination is to place the animal in a pillowcase or bag and extract the part of the lizard that you wish to examine (for example, a leg), leaving the rest of the lizard covered. This allows the head to be covered, keeping the lizard in the dark, which has a calming effect.

The internal organs of some small lizards such as geckos can be visualized via transillumination, using a focal light such as an otoscope light source. Palpation of the coelomic region in many lizards can be rewarding. Bearded dragons, for example, can be palpated to assess the size of the caudal abdominal fat pads and females can be palpated to feel for follicular stasis, a common concern in these species.

Sex Identification
Some lizards, such as the eastern water dragon (*Intellagama lesueurii lesueurii*) display obvious sexual dimorphism, with the male larger and with brighter, more prominent markings than the female. Others may be more subtle; for example, hemipenal bulges and the presence of femoral pores in the bearded dragon (*Pogona vitticeps*) and the iguana (*Iguana iguana*). Even more subtle dimorphism can be seen in species such as the blue-tongued skink (*Tiliqua scincoides*) where careful measurement of certain physical characteristics (head length, tail base width, etc.) can be used to identify the sex of this species.

Techniques used in sexually monomorphic species include eversion of the hemipenis ('popping', Figure 10.9), radiology of the hemipenis with or without contrast media,

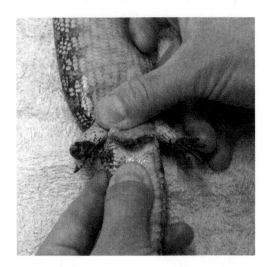

Figure 10.9 Manual eversion of a hemipenis in a blue-tongued lizard.

transillumination of the tail base, ultrasound, and endoscopy (see Chapter 7 for further detail).

Examination of the Snake

Initially, the snake should be weighed and its movements closely observed, watching for any unusual coiling, twisting motions or weakness of the distal body and decreased constriction. This can be done as a distant or hands-off examination for non-venomous or non-fractious species, allowing the snake to move over the consulting room table. It will usually try to find a secure point to which to anchor its tail, such as the table leg or underside of the table top. An alert snake will intermittently flick its tongue.

Palpate the entire length of the snake ventrally to feel between the ribs, assessing for masses and organ location. The snake is a conveniently linear animal and the position of the organs can be ascertained by using linear charts according to species. For example, the heart is located approximately 25% of the snout–vent length and can be palpated or monitored via a Doppler probe.

Sex Identification

Many snakes can be sexed by gently probing one or both hemipenes sulci to determine its length or by everting the hemipenes. Many pythons have a vestigial spur – the remnants of the pelvic girdle – on either side of the vent. In males, this spur is often (but not always) noticeably larger than that of the female. Ultrasonic detection of ovarian follicles is relatively simple in mature female snakes and requires less restraint than many other techniques (see Chapter 7 for further detail).

Examination of the Chelonian

On initial examination, place the chelonian on a flat surface, taking care to ensure that it cannot fall. Check muscle tone and strength as the turtle moves. Limbs should be strong and easily retract back under the carapace. Head and neck should also retract to resist handling.

Chelonians should be weighed and measured (straight carapace length). Carapace and plastron injuries and lesions are common and skin lesions may be an indication of more serious disease, such as a systemic illness. Oral examination may be revealing in an otherwise healthy animal, although opening the mouth can be a challenge in healthy species. Consider the use of a credit card or guitar plectrum as a lever to open the mouth. Abscesses occur frequently, especially around the eyes and ears. Oedema of the neck and limbs, with accompanying petechial haemorrhages, may indicate septicaemia (Figure 10.10). Palpation or ballottement of the inguinal and axillary fossae can be rewarding, for example to detect gravidity. Placing a turtle into lukewarm water can be a useful method to detect abnormal flotation.

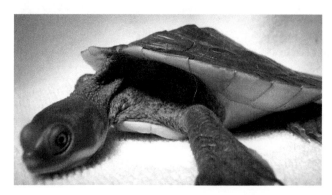

Figure 10.10 Petechial haemorrhages, often an indicator of septicaemia, in a moribund eastern long-necked turtle (*Chelodina longicollis*).

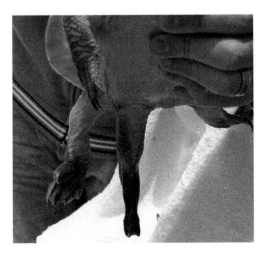

Figure 10.11 A chelonian may evert its phallus during the physical examination.

Sex Identification

Turtles and tortoises are often sexed by the shape of the shell (especially the plastron), the shape of the caudal plastron notch or by the length of the tail. The red-eared slider (*Trachemys scripta elegans*) shows a pronounced difference between the male and female front claws, with the claws on the males' front legs being longer than the claws of female turtles.

Young male tortoises may 'flash' their phallus (i.e. allow it to protrude from the cloaca) when immersed in a warm bath (Figure 10.11).

Ultrasonic examination via the pre-femoral fossa can be used in some larger tortoises to identify ovarian follicles, as can endoscopic cystoscopy (the ovaries can be visualized through the thin bladder wall). See Chapter 7 for further detail.

Summary

Other than to point out lesions during the examination, the clinician should resist the temptation to discuss findings and conclusions with the client until the physical examination has been concluded. Once the examination has been completed, the reptile can be returned to its carrier and then a summary of findings can be discussed with the client. This avoids distractions and allows the client to focus on the veterinarian. The discussion could include:

- problems identified with the husbandry and nutrition of the reptile
- problems identified during the examination
- how these problems could be linked
- a short list of possible diagnoses
- where to go to from here: radiology, haematology, biochemistry, etc.
- likely costs of these further tests and why the tests are needed
- the likely prognosis.

If the client declines further testing, this should be noted in the clinical record (and the client made aware that their decision is been recorded) and a treatment plan outlined.

Diagnosis

The apex of the diagnostic pyramid (Figure 10.1) is the diagnosis. In an ideal world, this would be a single, confirmed disease or problem. In the real world, however, such a diagnosis is often only obtained by necropsy and histopathology. In the live patient, we are often left with a short list (two to three items) of tentative diagnoses. In this situation, after explaining this outcome to the owner, a final diagnosis may be achieved by observing the patient's response to treatment.

Keep in mind that disease is usually the result of a combination of many factors: environment, husbandry, nutrition and exposure to a potential pathogen. Correcting many of these contributing factors often results in a clinical improvement and 'cure', and a final diagnosis may be obscured by this improvement.

11

Diagnostic Testing

Rachel E. Marschang, Frank Pasmans, Tim Hyndman, Mark Mitchell and An Martel

Introduction

Reptiles have evolved to mask their illnesses. This method of preservation is useful to animals in the wild but can make it challenging for veterinarians attempting to assess the health status of these patients. In addition, many disease processes found in reptiles are multifactorial and may involve husbandry issues and multiple infectious agents. Many infectious agents found in reptiles may only be pathogenic in conjunction with other issues or immune suppression. Diagnostic testing should therefore always be interpreted together with other findings, including history, clinical signs and adjunct testing methods. The methods used for laboratory testing for reptiles differ from testing in mammals. Contact your laboratory before submitting samples in order to optimize the samples submitted and the results obtained.

Haematology

Haematology can be used to provide physiological information regarding the health of reptile patients. Limitations with current analytical equipment require veterinarians to use manual methods of measuring blood cells. In mammals, it is common to evaluate erythrocytes as part of a complete blood count but, in reptiles, clinicians are typically limited to analyzing a packed cell volume. References for packed cell volume in reptiles are highly variable (20–40%) and should be interpreted based on the general condition and health of the patient. In cases where there are concerns that erythrocyte numbers are low (e.g., anaemia), erythrocytes can be counted (using the Unopette® system) manually or a review of the blood smear can be performed. Typically, a subjective, ordinal scale (1–4+) is used to assess the presence of anisocytosis and anisokaryosis from the blood smear. Immature erythrocytes have a higher nuclear to cytoplasmic ratio than mature cells and, using Romanowsky-type stains, have a more basophilic cytoplasm than mature cells. Review of the blood smear can provide additional information regarding potential anomalies of erythrocytes (e.g., viral inclusions and blood parasites; Figures 11.1 and 11.2).

Slide preparation for blood smears can affect the differential count. Direct blood smears made using glass microscope slides are found to be associated with significantly higher 'smudgeocytes' (cells that could not be differentiated) than other techniques such as

Reptile Medicine and Surgery in Clinical Practice, First Edition. Edited by Bob Doneley, Deborah Monks, Robert Johnson and Brendan Carmel.
© 2018 John Wiley & Sons Ltd. Published 2018 by John Wiley & Sons Ltd.

blood smear preparation using coverslips. Significant loss of blood cells due to incorrect slide preparation can affect the estimated leucocyte or differential counts.

Manual leucocyte counts for reptiles are typically performed using semi-quantitative methods. The first and simpler method is using a stained blood smear (e.g. Diff-Quik or Wright–Giemsa stain; Wright– Giemsa staining is less likely to be associated with leucocyte degranulation). Review the slide near the edge of the smear where the cells are evenly distributed in a monolayer. Using the high dry objective (400–450×), ten fields are scanned. The total number of white cells can be divided by 10 to obtain an average, which is multiplied by 2000 to calculate an estimated total leucocyte count (cells/µl). A differential count is then performed. A 100 or 250 cell count differential is recommended. A second method of estimation is done using phloxine B stain. A blood sample is mixed with the stain and the cells are then loaded on to a haemocytometer. The stain is used to identify heterophils and eosinophils. Once a differential is found, the following formula is used to estimate the leucocyte blood count:

Total leucocyte count

$$= \frac{\left[(\text{total haemocytometer count}) \times (32) \times 100 \right]}{(\% \text{ heterophils and eosinophils}) \times 100}$$

Reptiles have similar types of white blood cells to other non-mammalian vertebrates, with some species specific morphological differences. Table 11.1 gives examples of the blood cells and their function.

Biochemical Analyses

Biochemical analyses can also provide physiological information about a reptile patient's health status. Many of the same biochemical measures in mammals are also evaluated in reptiles; however, unlike

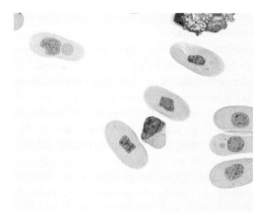

Figure 11.1 Inclusion bodies in blood cells of a boa constrictor with inclusion body disease (courtesy of Kim Heckers, Laboklin).

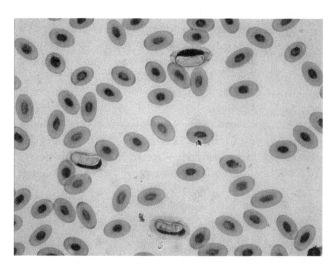

Figure 11.2 Haemogregarines (*Karyolysis* sp.) in a blood smear (stained with Hemacolor®) of the lizard *Podarcis melisellensis*. The parasites are visible inside the erythrocytes.

Table 11.1 Leucocytes commonly found in reptiles.

Cell type	Appearance	Function
Heterophil	Eosinophilic granules, round to lobed nucleus	Elevated with acute inflammation (e.g., infection, trauma, neoplasia)
Lymphocyte	Agranulocyte (high nuclear : cytoplasmic ratio)	Cell-mediated immunity Antibody production
Monocyte	Agranulocyte (low nuclear : cytoplasmic ratio)	Chronic inflammation
Azurophil	Same as monocyte, azure staining cytoplasm	Chronic inflammation
Eosinophil	Eosinophilic or basophilic granules	Hypersensitivity, parasitaemia
Basophils	Basophilic granules	Histamine release

mammals, interpretation can be difficult (while there is only one species of dog, there are over 9000 different species of reptile). Many of the biochemistry references available for reptiles are based on study populations of limited size or unknown health status. Because of these limitations, it is best to develop individual patient biochemistry references using known disease-free intervals for the patient (e.g. on annual health checks). These data can then be used in combination with published references to better assess a reptile's health status.

Sample collection and processing are important considerations when evaluating biochemistries in reptiles. Haemolysis and lymph dilution can have deleterious effects on the results. Lymph vessels are closely associated with blood vessels and may be accidentally sampled, diluting the blood sample. Either serum or plasma can be used to analyse biochemistries in reptiles; in either case, the normal appearance of the sample will be clear. The serum and plasma should be removed from the cells immediately to minimize artefacts.

Glucose concentrations in reptiles are highly variable but generally range between 2 mmol/l and 10 mmol/l (40–180 mg/dl). Lower concentrations are more commonly noted in large snakes, while higher concentrations are common in animals under stress. Diabetes mellitus is rare in reptiles.

Total protein, albumin and globulins can provide insight into the hydration, immunological and reproductive status of a reptile. Concentrations for total protein may range from 35 g/l to 75 g/l (3.5–7.5 mg/dl) and there should be a positive albumin to globulin ratio. Elevated total protein and albumin are common in dehydrated reptiles, while elevated globulins are common in reptiles with inflammatory disease. Protein electrophoresis is recommended to better ascertain which proteins are elevated in these cases. Elevated albumin concentrations in female reptiles during the breeding season are indicative of impending egg-laying; concurrent elevations in calcium and phosphorus are common in these individuals. Albumin may be artificially lower in some species (e.g., tortoises) because of a weakened affinity for bromocresol dye binding.

The end-products of protein catabolism in vertebrates include ammonia, uric acid and urea nitrogen. In reptiles, uric acid is generally considered the most common catabolite to be excreted; however, in some species (e.g. some tortoises) urea nitrogen is more common. This is important to consider, as it may result in misclassifying a reptile's health status. Hyperuricaemia is commonly associated with high-protein diets, a recent meal, dehydration and gout. Hyperuricaemia is not commonly observed in reptiles with renal disease. This is because urea is excreted in the proximal tubules; thus, it is usually widespread renal disease that affects blood concentrations. Uric acid concentrations are generally less than 595 µmol/l (less than 10 mg/dl) in healthy reptiles, although concentrations up to 1487 µmol/l (25 mg/dl) may be observed in carnivorous reptiles post-prandially. Urea nitrogen concentrations are typically less than 12.5 mmol/l (less than 35 mg/dl) in chelonians. Elevations in urea nitrogen may be associated with pre-renal, renal or post-renal disease.

Sodium (125–155 mmol/l), potassium (2.5–6.0 mmol/l) and chloride (90–120 mmol/l) are the electrolytes most commonly measured in reptiles. Elevations in sodium and chloride concentrations most commonly occur with dehydration; evaluating these electrolytes with total protein, albumin and packed cell volume can better define hydration status. Elevations in potassium are common with haemolysis and renal disease.

Calcium and phosphorus circulate in both bound and unbound forms. Most analysers measure total calcium (2–3.5 mmol/l; 8–14 mg/dl) and total phosphorus (0.97–2.26 mmol/l; 3–7 mg/dl), although some also measure unbound (ionized) calcium (1.0–1.5 mmol/l; 4–6 mg/dl). Hypocalcaemia and hyperphosphataemia are common in reptiles with renal disease; biopsy and histopathology are recommended for these cases to confirm a diagnosis. Hypercalcaemia and hyperphosphataemia are common with folliculogenesis and may be used to confirm a reptile's sex as female in non-dimorphic species. Normal calcium and phosphorous levels do not confirm that the reptile is male.

There are a number of enzymes commonly measured in biochemistry analyses, including creatine kinase, aspartate aminotransferase, alkaline phosphatase, lactate dehydrogenase and lactate. Few studies have assessed tissue specificity for these enzymes; however, only creatine kinase appears to be tissue specific, with the highest concentrations found in skeletal, cardiac and smooth muscles. The lack of site specificity for these enzymes suggests that clinicians should use caution when interpreting results. Best results will be achieved using biopsy and histopathology in association with enzyme concentrations.

Bile acids are considered an important liver function test in mammals and birds. Reptiles can produce different types of bile acids, limiting the value of some analysers if they only measure one type. Research in green iguanas (*Iguana iguana*) suggests that elevated bile acids (greater than 70 µmol/l) are indicative of hepatic disease.

Cytology

Cytological examination of samples can be used to make a diagnosis or to guide a clinician to additional diagnostic tests. The primary benefits of cytology are that it is rapid and inexpensive, if done in-house. Unfortunately, this diagnostic method only has a fair sensitivity (i.e. it is subject to false negatives). In cases where cytology proves limiting, biopsy and histopathology should be considered.

Fine-needle aspirates are commonly used to evaluate masses, joints, fluid-filled spaces (e.g., ascites), bone marrow or internal masses in reptiles. Needle and syringe sizes used for collecting the samples may vary based on patient size but a 25-gauge needle and 3–6 ml syringe are commonly used for sample collection. The surface of any site being sampled should be disinfected using standard aseptic techniques. For external masses, two different fine-needle aspiration techniques can be used. The first technique requires the needle to be attached to the syringe; the needle is inserted into the mass and negative pressure is applied by pulling back on the syringe plunger. Negative pressure should be released before removing the needle from the mass to prevent aspiration of the sample into the syringe and the loss of any cells. The second technique requires that the needle be inserted directly into the mass (with no syringe attached). This technique attempts to collect 'cores' of cells for evaluation. In both cases, the needle needs to be redirected through the sample multiple times to maximize the collection of cells. Once obtained, the samples should be placed on slides for staining. Ultrasound is recommended for collecting samples from within the coelomic cavity to ensure that the appropriate site is sampled.

Stain selection should be based on the presumed differentials. The most common findings from fine-needle aspiration and cytology are inflammation, infection, foreign material and cancer. Romanowsky-type stains, such as Diff-Quik stains, are commonly used because they are inexpensive, easy to prepare and can identify many of the common findings noted above. Gram stains are also useful for screening samples for bacteria. Direct smears prepared with saline are recommended for assessing protozoal populations.

Because reptiles are stoic in nature and mask illness, they typically present with varying stages of inflammation. Acute inflammation is often characterized by a significant number of heterophils (greater than 75%) on the smear. The presence of toxic heterophils (e.g., degranulation and vacuolation) is suggestive of a more aggressive response from the host. These slides should be screened closely for pathogens (e.g., bacteria, fungi). If pathogens are suspected, additional samples should be collected and submitted for culture or polymerase chain reaction testing. Chronic inflammation is a more common presentation and is characterized by a mixed population of lymphocytes, macrophages and heterophils. These slides should also be screened for pathogens, although other inflammatory diseases, such as neoplasia, should be considered. Diagnosing neoplasia from cytological samples can be challenging. Cells should be evaluated for the presence of multiple nuclei or nucleoli, the nuclear to cytoplasmic ratio and the types and densities of cells.

Serology

Serological testing is used in reptile medicine to determine whether an animal has been exposed to certain infectious agents. It is important to realize that the reptile immune system is dependent on environmental factors to function optimally. Antibody responses to infection will depend on temperature and time of year, stress, animal age and other infections. Serology is only capable of detecting a portion of the humoral immune response. In many cases, the cellular immune response may be more important for removal of pathogens from the system. While a positive serological test will provide information if an animal has been exposed to an infectious agent (or a similar antigen), it will not generally provide information on the current infection status of that animal. In these cases, paired testing may prove more valuable. Serological testing in reptiles is not standardized and results from different laboratories may not be comparable. Contact the laboratory to determine test methods used, antigens used, antibodies being measured (immunoglobulin M or Y, or both), cut-off points and any standardization of methods. Most methods used for the detection of antibodies against specific agents in reptiles require reagents with somewhat limited availability, including isolates or other source of antigen, specific antibodies or cell lines. This limits these tests to laboratories in which all of the necessary reagents are available and increases the costs. Here, we provide an overview of tests commonly described in reptile medicine and their interpretation.

Virus or Serum Neutralization Tests

Neutralization tests measure the ability of antibodies in serum or plasma to prevent a given pathogen from infecting susceptible cells. In reptiles, this method has been used for multiple viruses including herpesviruses, adenoviruses, reoviruses and picornaviruses. It is most commonly used to detect antibodies against testudinid herpesvirus in tortoises. Since herpesviruses cause persistent infections, any animal with detectable antibodies against these viruses must be considered infected, regardless of clinical status.

Haemagglutination Inhibition Tests

Haemagglutination inhibition is used to detect antibodies against pathogens that bind to and haemagglutinate red blood cells. In reptiles, this method is used to detect antibodies against ferlaviruses (also known as ophidian paramyxoviruses). Ferlaviruses have been shown to be serologically diverse and the use of different isolates and different cut-off values can lead to extreme differences in results obtained from different laboratories. It is not known whether ferlaviruses cause persistent infections in reptiles and so the presence of ferlavirus antibodies should not be automatically interpreted to mean that the animal is infected. The detection of antibodies against viruses in healthy reptiles should always be interpreted carefully.

Enzyme-linked Immunosorbent Assay

A number of enzyme-linked immunosorbent assays (ELISAs) for the detection of antibodies against specific pathogens have been described for reptiles. In general, antibodies in the sample bind to antigen. The reptile antibodies are then detected using secondary antibodies that target the reptile antibodies. ELISAs are most commonly used for the detection of antibodies against *Mycoplasma agassizii* in tortoises. Since this pathogen causes persistent infections, the detection of antibodies is an indication of infection, regardless of clinical status.

Molecular Diagnostics

In reptile practice, molecular diagnostics are usually used to detect the nucleic acids (DNA and RNA) of infectious agents. In the early 21st century, the technology and availability of molecular diagnostics has advanced at a staggering rate. Molecular diagnostics offer a number of advantages over traditional tests. For example, the viability of the infectious organism does not need to be maintained because the agent will not be required to replicate in the laboratory. This has the added advantage that molecular testing can detect agents that have fastidious in vitro growth requirements (e.g. arenavirus) or grow very slowly (e.g. *Mycobacteria*). Finally, the detection limits of molecular testing nearly always outperform those of more traditional tests such as culturing. A more detailed overview of these methods can be found in the excellent review by Johnson *et al.* (2007).

Polymerase Chain Reaction

In the polymerase chain reaction (PCR), nucleic acid (DNA or RNA) specific to the infectious agent of interest is amplified into large amounts of DNA. If a detectable amount of agent-specific DNA is found, the sample is considered to be positive for the presence of that agent. If not, the sample is considered negative. The interpretations of positive and negative PCR results, together with recommended courses of action, are listed in Table 11.2. Some PCR tests used to screen reptile samples are broadly reactive and so false positives are possible. For example, if a PCR for adenovirus was used that can detect all known adenoviruses, it is important that the test result is validated (by sequencing) to make sure that a reptilian adenovirus was identified and not a contaminating human adenovirus.

Traditionally, PCR has been a test that only provides a positive or negative result. Some more modern PCRs are able to quantify the amount of infectious agent in a sample, referred to as real-time or quantitative PCRs. From the clinician's perspective, many of these quantitative PCRs have limits of detection that are superior to traditional PCRs and thus represent a better test.

Culture

Bacterial and fungal cultivation is a standard procedure in reptile diagnostics but seldom used for viruses and parasites. Advantages of culture compared over

Table 11.2 Interpretation of polymerase chain reaction results.

| | PCR result | |
	Positive	Negative
Interpretation	Animal is infected. **or** Animal is uninfected but sample was contaminated with infectious agent.	Animal is uninfected. **or** Animal is infected but: • sample contained infectious agent in quantities below the detection limit of the PCR • wrong type of sample was collected (e.g. swab vs. blood) • sample was degraded (e.g. exposure to high temperature) • did not have agent in that sampling space (swab, blood) at the time of sampling e.g. intermittent shedding of infectious agent.
Recommended course of action	If comfortable sample contamination did not occur, then assume animal is infected. If there are doubts about inter-sample contamination, repeat testing.	Repeat testing ensuring the correct sample is taken and that it is stored and transported to the laboratory correctly. Multiple negative results will increase the confidence that the animal is truly uninfected.

molecular diagnostics are a less biased estimate of pathogen presence and diversity, the possibility of obtaining antimicrobial susceptibility profiles to redirect treatment (see Chapter 14) and, in the case of novel pathogens, detection of novel disease entities. Interpretation of mixed cultures can be hampered by the bias towards organisms that grow well on routine culture media and the currently poor understanding of bacterial and mycotic pathogens in reptile disease (Figures 11.3 and 11.4). Important pathogens that require specific growth conditions will be missed (e.g. intracellular bacteria that need cell cultures for growth such as Chlamydiales, many mycobacteria and most *Mycoplasma* spp.).

Standard techniques for bacteriology and mycology can be applied to reptile samples, with some modifications. Although many

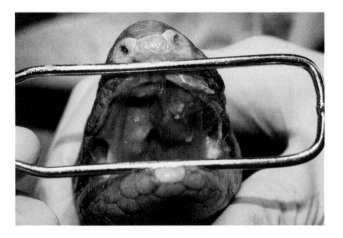

Figure 11.3 Open intra-oral abscesses (here in the skink *Corucia zebrata*) often yield abundant growth of a large variety of bacteria, which seriously hampers interpretation of bacterial cultures.

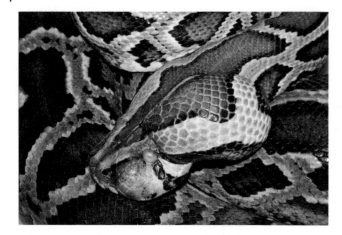

Figure 11.4 Bacterial cultures obtained from closed abscesses, such as this large abscess in a *Python molurus* are generally far easier to interpret, often yielding abundant growth of a limited number of bacterial and/or fungal taxa.

reptile-derived bacteria and fungi will grow well at typical clinical laboratory incubator temperatures (35–37 °C), incubation of samples should ideally reflect the preferred body temperature of the species or temperature of the reptile's environment (e.g., cooler temperatures with fungi). Generally, an incubation temperature of 30 °C supports the growth of bacterial and mycotic reptile pathogens. Both aerobic and anaerobic culture conditions should be used. Fungal cultures should be incubated for at least 10 days to decrease the likelihood of false negatives. Cultures can be identified using culture growth characteristics and morphology, biochemical typing, DNA sequencing (typically 16S rDNA for bacteria and internal transcribed spacer sequencing for fungi) or protein and peptide profiling (matrix-assisted laser desorption/ionization–time-of-flight mass spectrometry). A detailed laboratory report should include the bacteria and fungi that were identified and (semi-)quantitative data regarding the organisms to allow meaningful interpretation. The following guidelines are suggested:

- In cases where pure and abundant cultures are obtained from lesions, the bacteria or fungi identified can be expected to play a role in the disease process.
- In cases with mixed cultures (e.g. gastrointestinal, respiratory and skin samples), interpretation may be difficult. Isolation of a

known bacterial or fungal reptile pathogen from a lesion or site should only be considered as a presumptive diagnosis; histopathology is required to confirm the association. Despite the publication of reptile pathogens and their pathogenic relevance, epidemiological knowledge of bacterial (and mycotic) pathogens in reptiles is very limited. Few bacteria and fungi have been shown to be primary reptile pathogens (e.g. several *Mycoplasma* sp., *Devriesea agamarum* (Figure 11.5), fungi belonging to the family Onygenaceae; Figure 11.6). Identification of these pathogens in a sample from a patient with lesions consistent with the disease syndrome should be considered highly suspicious. Many potentially pathogenic taxa (e.g. *Salmonella* sp., *Aeromonas* sp., *Pseudomonas* sp.) are commonly found in the digestive and/or respiratory tract of healthy reptiles. In these cases, high relative abundance of a potentially pathogenic bacterium or fungus in a clinical sample is suggestive that it may play a role in the disease process.

- It is hard, if not impossible, to interpret the significance of bacteriological and mycological results from intestinal and faecal reptile samples. Intestinal bacterial and mycotic pathogens, let alone microbiota imbalances, in reptiles have been very poorly characterized. Since the majority of reptiles carry potential pathogens in the gut (e.g. *Salmonella*), the mere presence of

Figure 11.5 Although the cheilitis in this collared lizard (*Crotaphytus collaris*) is suggestive of an infection with *Devriesea agamarum*, bacterial cultures are necessary to confirm the diagnosis.

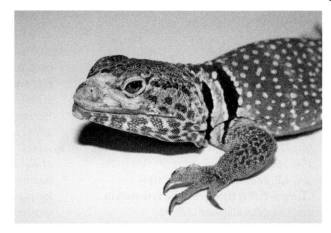

Figure 11.6 Growth of *Nannizziopsis guarroi*, isolated from a bearded dragon (*Pogona vitticeps*) on Sabouraud dextrose agar. Fungal cultures should be incubated for at least 10 days.

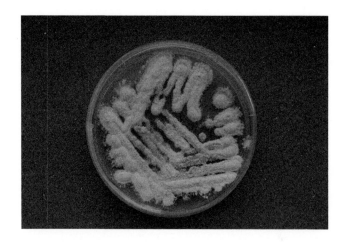

these pathogens is insufficient to draw any sound conclusions with regard to their role in the disease.

Overall, except for a few cases, bacterial and fungal infections in reptiles should generally be considered to be secondary to any cause that compromises reptile defences, such as other infections (e.g. viruses, parasites), stress or inadequate husbandry. Although parasitological examination should form part of any clinical or post-mortem examination of a reptile, parasite cultivation is not routinely done.

Viral cultures are rarely used in reptile diagnostics and generally require highly specialized laboratories. Viral cultures are sometimes considered when there is clear indication on histopathology that there is a viral aetiology but routine tests (PCR, serology) do not return any positive results.

Reference

Johnson, A.J., Origgi, F.C. and Wellehan, J.F.X. (2007) *Molecular Diagnostics in Infectious* *Disease and Pathology of Reptiles*. CRC Press, Boca Raton, FL.

Further Reading

Allender, M.C., Mitchell, M.A., Dreslik, M.J. *et al.* (2008) Measuring agreement and discord among hemagglutination inhibition assays against different ophidian paramyxovirus strains in the Eastern massasauga (*Sistrurus catenatus catenatus*). *Journal of Zoo and Wildlife Medicine*, 39 (3), 358–361.

Bogan, J.E. and Mitchell, M.A. (2014) Characterizing tissue enzyme activities in the American alligator (*Alligator mississipiensis*). *Journal of Herpetological Medicine and Surgery*, 24 (3–4), 77–81.

McBride, M., Hernandez-Divers, S.J., Koch, T. *et al.* 2006. Preliminary evaluation of pre- and post-prandial 3α hydroxyl bile acids in green iguanas. *Journal of Herpetological Medicine and Surgery*, 16 (4), 129–134.

Myers, D.A., Mitchell, M.A., Fleming, G. *et al.* (2008) Determining the value of bovine albumin as a blood cell stabilizer for pancake tortoise, *Malacochersus tornieri*, blood smears. *Journal of Herpetological Medicine and Surgery*, 3 (4), 95–99.

12

Diagnostic Imaging

Zdeněk Knotek, Shane Simpson and Paolo Martelli

Radiography

Radiography is part of the comprehensive clinical examination of reptiles and can be used to evaluate bone structures, confirm or rule out the presence of mineralized eggs, identify areas of differing soft-tissue density, including penetrating bite wounds, pulmonary granulomas and gastrointestinal foreign bodies.

Sedation and Anaesthesia

Sedation or short-acting anaesthesia is recommended for box turtles, shy tortoises that refuse to protrude from the shell, dangerous animals, very stressed or delicate individuals or when precise positioning is required.

Positioning

For correct radiographical interpretation, proper positioning and restraint are mandatory. Practitioners are encouraged to invest in equipment that allows the use of a horizontal beam. Not only is lateral recumbency difficult (or impossible) to maintain, it is likely to be resisted by the reptile. It also allows internal organs to move within the

coelom, complicating interpretation of radiographs (Pees 2011, Raiti 2004, Silverman *et al.* 2006, Wilkinson *et al.* 2004).

Chelonians

Three projections (dorsoventral, laterallateral, and craniocaudal) can be used in chelonians. When taking these views, patients should be in their natural ventral position lying on their plastron (Pees 2011, Raiti 2004, Silverman *et al.* 2006, Wilkinson *et al.* 2004). The patient's head and limbs should be extended out of the shell, which can be achieved by placing the patient on an elevated stand that touches the plastron only (Figure 12.1). The lungs are superimposed over other coelom organs and difficult to assess on a dorsoventral view, although collapsed or over-expanded lungs may be diagnosed. Better images of the lung fields can be obtained with laterolateral and craniocaudal projections using a horizontal beam. The cassette is placed vertically with the edge of the shell touching the cassette. The centre of the beam should be aimed at the lateral scutes in the middle of the animal (laterolateral view) or the centre of the body (craniocaudal view). The craniocaudal view is used as a complementary projection to

Reptile Medicine and Surgery in Clinical Practice, First Edition. Edited by Bob Doneley, Deborah Monks, Robert Johnson and Brendan Carmel.
© 2018 John Wiley & Sons Ltd. Published 2018 by John Wiley & Sons Ltd.

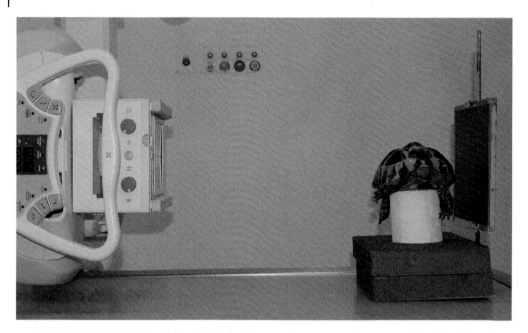

Figure 12.1 Positioning of a tortoise for a laterolateral view x-ray.

compare the inflation and densities of the left and right lung. Positioning of the chelonian is as symmetrical as possible so that both sides of the lungs can be compared (Pees 2011, Raiti 2004, Silverman *et al*. 2006, Wilkinson *et al*. 2004).

Snakes

In snakes, dorsoventral and laterolateral projections are used. Individual segments of the body should be properly identified using radio-opaque markers so that the same area can be compared in an orthogonal view. Dorsoventral projections of a coiled snake placed on the cassette are of limited value because of the possible movement of coelom organs and asymmetry of spine and ribs (Pees 2011, Raiti 2004, Silverman *et al*. 2006, Wilkinson *et al*. 2004). When dorsoventral projection is used, the patient is positioned in ventral recumbency using sedation and/or translucent plastic tubes to keep the spine as straight as possible. Better results are obtained if the laterolateral projection is performed using a horizontal beam (Pees 2011, Raiti 2004, Silverman *et al*. 2006, Wilkinson *et al*. 2004).

Lizards

In lizards, the appendicular skeleton is evaluated using dorsoventral and laterolateral projections, with the patient's limbs being as close as possible to the cassette (Pees 2011, Raiti 2004, Silverman *et al*. 2006, Wilkinson *et al*. 2004). For the laterolateral projection, the pectoral limbs are extended cranially and the pelvic limbs extended caudally. A translucent box or tube may assist in keeping the spine straight.

Crocodilians

Crocodilians are challenging to image on account of their large size and the presence of osteoderms, which mask underlying structures (Figure 12.2).

Exposure

Reptilian skeletal structures are less radiopaque compared with mammalian, therefore higher milliangstrom (mA) and lower kilovolt (kV) values are generally recommended (Pees 2011, Raiti 2004, Silverman *et al*. 2006, Wilkinson *et al*. 2004). While specific exposure settings depend primarily on the x-ray

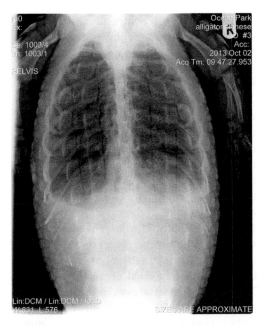

Figure 12.2 The presence of osteoderms in crocodilians may mask underlying structures or pathology.

system being used they generally range from 40 kV to 100 kV for 1.25–20 mA depending on the size of the animal and whether grids are used.

Plain Radiographs

Standard examination of the patient begins with taking plain radiographs. Data obtained from the clinical examination and plain radiographs will determine whether other special imaging procedures are warranted. Because organ densities may be very similar because of the absence of peritoneal fat, coelom insufflation with a small volume of surgical grade carbon dioxide is useful in differentiating organs.

Contrast Radiology

Contrast radiology is performed primarily to illustrate individual segments of the gastrointestinal tract, to identify radiolucent foreign bodies and to distinguish between intra- and extraluminal masses. Contrast

media may also be used to assess the size and position of other organs and masses (kidneys, urinary bladder or tumours; Pees 2011, Raiti 2004, Silverman *et al.* 2006, Wilkinson *et al.* 2004). In reptiles, gastrointestinal passage is very slow and variable, depending on the ambient temperature, the season and the reptile species. It has been reported that bowel transit time in a healthy chelonian is more than three weeks.

Barium Sulphate

The recommended maximum dose of barium sulphate is 20 ml/kg (Raiti 2004); however, a dose of 5–10 ml/kg is generally adequate. Ideally, the solution is administered by oesophageal tube into the stomach or, in large snakes and marine turtles, as caudally as possible within the oesophagus (Figure 12.3). It can also be injected or mixed into the diet for transit time studies. The administration of barium is contraindicated when the integrity of the gastrointestinal tract wall is suspect.

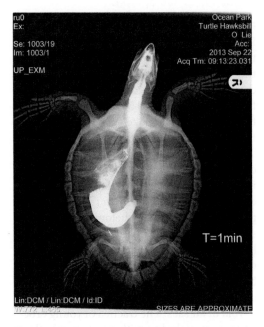

Figure 12.3 A contrast study of the gastrointestinal tract of a hawksbill turtle (*Eretmochelys imbricata*).

Iodine-Based Contrast Agents

Iodine compounds are the contrast media of choice in patients with intestinal wall perforation (Schumacher and Toal 2001). The recommended dose of iodine-based contrast agents is 10 ml/kg (250 mg iodine/ml). The advantage of these substances is a shorter transit time through the gastrointestinal tract. As iodine-based contrast media are gradually diluted by intestinal fluid in the intestine (they bind water), their contrast capacity decreases in caudal segments of the gastrointestinal tract. Retrograde application of a contrast medium via the cloaca is used to view caudal segments of the intestine, urinary bladder and cloaca. Iodine contrast agents are eliminated by means of glomerular filtration, so it is always critical to check the patient's hydration status and renal function.

Angiography, Excretory Nephrography

The principles of intravenous administration of contrast agents to reptiles are the same as in mammals; however, reliable intravenous access is more difficult in reptiles.

Evaluation of Radiographs

Respiratory Tract

In most reptiles, the lungs are located dorsal to the liver and extend to the dorsal wall of the coelom. Chelonian lungs are located directly beneath the carapace with the lung field representing 30–50% of the height of the coelom. Most snake species have only a right lung, terminating in a caudal air sac. The commonly kept Boidae have two lungs of similar size, with the right air sac extending more caudally. Detailed radiographic evaluation of the lung field in reptiles is hampered by the shell in chelonians and thick skin and skin derivatives in crocodiles and lizards. To properly evaluate the lung field of chelonians, the neck and limbs should be fully extended. Crocodiles have two well-developed, symmetrical and fleshy lungs devoid of air sacs. The trachea of young crocodiles is straight but with age a double flexure develops at the thoracic inlet. Unilaterally collapsed lung with contralateral overexpansion are not uncommonly seen after penetrating injuries.

Heart

The heart of most lizards is located between the pectoral girdle and it is therefore not easily viewed on radiographs. The heart of monitor lizards and crocodiles is located more caudally, halfway between the pelvic and pectoral girdles. Good visualization of the cardiac silhouette in chameleons is achieved only when their pectoral limbs are extended cranially. The heart of chelonians is masked by the superposition of the plastron and the carapace (dorsoventral view) and the liver and other internal organs in all views. The heart of most snakes is located within the cranial 15–25% of the snout–vent length (more cranial in arboreal snakes, more caudal in sea snakes).

With notable exceptions, such as in gout (when the pericardium is filled with uric acid crystals), radiography of the heart is of limited diagnostic significance; it is better evaluated with other imaging modalities.

Gastrointestinal Tract

Radiographic evaluation of the gastrointestinal tract is affected by the presence of gas or radio-opaque material (Figure 12.4). In many reptile species, a small amount of gas or small stones in the digestive tract is generally considered to be normal.

The chelonian stomach is tubular and is located in the left cranial third of the coelom. Accurate delineation of individual segments of the intestine is impossible unless they are filled with a radiopaque material or gas.

If the location of individual organs of snakes is expressed as a percentage of the snout–vent length, the stomach, small intestine and colon of Boidae are located at 50–70%, 60–80% and 80%, respectively.

Certain lizard species (iguanas) have a distinct caecum located in the right caudal coelom. The full stomach of bearded dragons is elongated and is located near the median axis. In chameleons, the stomach turns in a

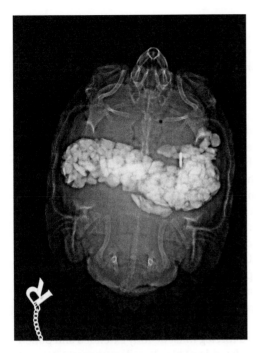

Figure 12.4 The stomach of a tortoise full of stones and pebbles due to lithophagia.

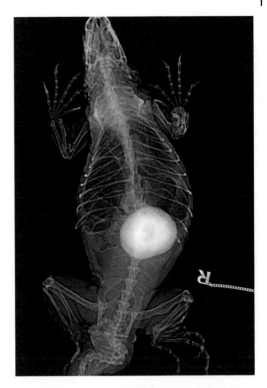

Figure 12.5 Urolith in the bladder of a green iguana (*Iguana iguana*).

cranioventral direction and the intestine is located in the caudal coelom.

In lizards and snakes, the triangular hepatic shadow is distinct, with the base located on the floor of the coelom cavity.

Urogenital Tract

Inactive ovaries and oviducts cannot be evaluated using radiography. However, in the reproductively active reptile, ovarian follicles and eggs occupy a considerable amount of the coelom, displacing other organs. Ovarian follicles cannot be evaluated in chelonians, although eggs are usually visible. Depending on the stage of gestation, the skeletons of foetuses can be radiographed in viviparous snakes and lizards. If the radiograph shows the spines as elongated linear formations, it is evidence of damage of fetal membranes and fetal death. The ability to evaluate the presence and shape of eggs in oviparous snakes is based on the degree of mineralization of eggshells. In lizards such as chameleons, iguanas and agamids, preovulatory follicles can be seen as nodular, soft-tissue formations located in the caudal coelom.

The major radiographical findings of the excretory system include radiopaque uroliths or sediment within the urinary bladder. Uroliths are most often found in chelonians and green iguanas (*Iguana iguana*; Figure 12.5). The kidneys of boid snakes are found 65–80% of the snout–vent length, with the right kidney cranial to the left. In chameleons, the kidneys are found cranial to the pelvis, near the vertebral column, especially when a laterolateral projection is used. The healthy kidneys of green iguanas, agamids and numerous other lizard species are intrapelvic and are only visible radiographically if they are enlarged. In monitor lizards, the kidneys are located cranial to the pelvis.

The hemipenes of rattlesnakes and hemibacula of monitor species are clearly visible on radiographs, offering a safe and accurate alternative for sexing these dangerous animals.

Skeleton

The density of bone in reptiles is evaluated by radiographic imaging of the ribs of snakes, the limbs of lizards and the shell and pectoral and pelvic girdles of chelonians. Some geckoes store calcium in specialized structures in the cervical area, the endolymphatic sacs. Congenital defects (lordosis, kyphosis and scoliosis) may be the consequences of problems during embryogenesis.

In young animals suffering from metabolic bone diseases, radiographs may show reduced radio-opacity of bones or shells and thickening of the long-bone cortices. In adult animals, these signs, as well as pathological fractures, may be present. Radiographic examination of chelonians may reveal shells with a 'moth-eaten' appearance.

Fractured ribs are common in free-living and captive reptiles and are seldom of clinical significance. Fractures of other bones take longer to heal in reptiles compared with mammals; follow-up radiographs should be taken at 6, 12 and 18 weeks.

Ultrasonography

Ultrasonography is a feasible non-invasive diagnostic imaging modality in reptiles. Anaesthesia is seldom necessary, although sedation is recommended in aggressive or dangerous (venomous) animals. Organs can be easily visualized and differentiated by their specific echogenicity. Ultrasonography is the major imaging tool for obstetrical work in reptiles, being useful in fertility assessment, sex identification, determination of the number of follicles and the timing of oviposition.

Chelonians

For chelonians, either a 7.5 MHz or 7–12 (14) MHz transducer with a small footprint is recommended (Hochleithner and Holland 2014, Schumacher and Toal 2001). For giant tortoises and sea turtles, frequencies of 2.5–5 MHz are recommended. The animal is held in ventral recumbency with the feet held away from the table to prevent movement, or on a pedestal, as previously described. For all but the largest species, one person can restrain the animal while another performs the ultrasound examination. The acoustic windows are in the pre-femoral fossa, the cervical region and the axilla (in soft-shelled chelonians, the coelom can be scanned through the plastron). An acoustic stand-off material such as a glove filled with acoustic coupling gel or water can be used to provide adequate contact with the skin (Hochleithner and Holland 2014, Schumacher and Toal 2001). Soaking the patient in warm water for approximately 20–30 minutes before investigation will also improve the contact of the transducer with the skin.

To access the cervical window, the head and foreleg must be fully extended and pulled to the side. This site allows examination of the cranial coelom. The heart is imaged on the midline in the dorsal third just caudal to the scapulae. The ventricular and atrial walls, atrioventricular valves and main coronary vessels can be imaged. Blood-flow patterns and velocities can be measured using the colour Doppler display and spectral analysis (Figure 12.6). The valves can be seen as highly reflective ribbons.

The pre-femoral window is the preferred site for examination of the liver, gastrointestinal and genitourinary tracts. In chelonians, the liver is bi-lobed, the right lobe is larger and the anechoic gallbladder is attached to it. The structure of the liver is homogenously hypoechoic with anechoic vessels. The portal vein, hepatic veins and the caudal vena cava can be individually assessed. Hyperechogenicity and enlargement of the liver is seen in cases of fatty liver deposition degeneration. A heterogeneous pattern of the liver parenchyma with anechoic areas is common with focal necrosis or inflammation (Hochleithner and Holland 2014, Schumacher and Toal 2001). Anechoic round or oval structures can be visualized in patients with cystic changes. The ovaries are

Figure 12.6 Ultrasound colour Doppler image of a chelonian kidney.

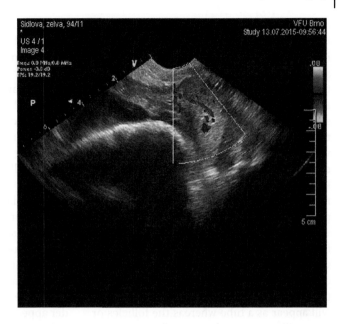

paired, hyperechoic elongated organs attached to the peritoneum on either side of the dorsal midline cranial to the pelvic girdle. Ultrasound can penetrate the thin-walled eggs of some species (e.g. red-eared sliders) to detect the inspissated contents within retained eggs. This technique has proved useful in determining the age of the egg and hence diagnosing dystocia. Eggs that are in the distal tract may be imaged through the post-femoral fossa (between the tail and legs). The testes are located cranial and ventral to the kidneys, appearing uniformly echogenic and slightly more hypoechoic than the adjacent kidneys.

The kidneys show higher echogenicity than the liver and the fat body. Large hyperechoic granules may be detected in enlarged kidneys in animals with renal disease. Anechoic spherical structures indicate cystic changes. The thin-walled urinary bladder is located ventrally in the caudal section of the coelom. The round or oval bladder is either anechoic or hyperechoic. Calculi can be distinguished by their solid structure and the distal shadowing of the ultrasound beam. Pathologically, there can be eggs within the urinary bladder. In herbivores, the stomach is small with a thin wall and the intestines are elongated and show mucosal folds.

Lizards

In small lizards, transducers with high frequency (10–18 MHz) are recommended. In larger lizards (iguanas, monitors), 7.5–12 MHz linear or convex transducers can be used; for animals heavier than 10 kg 3.5–7.5 MHz probes are suitable (Hochleithner and Holland 2014, Schumacher and Toal 2001). Acoustic coupling gel should be applied to the skin and the transducer. As with chelonians, the use of stand-offs and warm water baths is useful. The animal may be scanned in either lateral or dorsal recumbency. Lizards may also be restrained vertically with the head uppermost and the ventral surface facing the scanner operator. The limiting factors for ultrasonography in lizards are the presence of ossified scales (in *Tiliqua* and *Heloderma* spp.) and ecdysis, when the space between the layers of the cutis is filled with lymph. The atrioventricular valves and the hepatic vein extending from the liver to the sinus venosus is imaged on the longitudinal view of the heart. The liver is bi-lobed, with the gallbladder situated in the larger right lobe as an anechoic structure. The portal vein, hepatic veins and the caudal vena cava may be individually assessed. The twin fat bodies lie on either side, cranial to the pelvis. The echogenic pattern is hyperechoic compared with the liver with a granular structure and typical hyperechoic septa. The gonads are cranial to the kidneys. The ovaries, containing many small round, hypoechoic previtelline follicles, are positioned dorsally. An ovary containing vitelline follicles (large, up to 2.5 cm, round, hyperechoic structures) is easily detected. Care must be taken to differentiate poorly calcified eggs from bowel loops by rotating the transducer through 90 degrees: the bowel will appear as a tube whereas the follicles or eggs will remain spherical. The testes are small oval structures in the dorsal coelom, hyperechoic compared with the kidneys. The kidneys are located within the pelvis but, in cases of enlargement, the cranial pole may extend beyond the pelvic region. The urinary bladder, round to oval in shape, is identified by a thin wall and anechoic contents.

Snakes

Snakes can often be scanned using gentle restraint but very active or dangerous (venomous) snakes require anaesthesia. A 7.5 MHz sector transducer is generally used, although small snakes may require a 10 MHz transducer (Hochleithner and Holland 2014, Schumacher and Toal 2001). As with other reptiles, a stand-off is required, although, alternatively, the patient and transducer may be partially submerged in water to achieve an optimal image. In larger snakes, intercostal placement of the transducer may avoid the ribs interfering with the ultrasound picture but, in smaller snakes, acoustic shadows may be present.

The standard procedure should start cranially, beginning with the heart, and end with the cloaca (Hochleithner and Holland 2014, Schumacher and Toal 2001). The heart is located by visualizing the beating organ beneath the scales ventrally at 15–25% of the snout–vent length. In larger snakes, the atrial ventricles and atrioventricular valves may be seen. In larger individuals, the right and left aortic arches may be followed cranially to the common carotid artery. The liver in snakes is located immediately caudal to the heart extending to the middle of the body.

The gall bladder is extrahepatic, located caudal to the empty stomach. The stomach may be identified at the caudal edge of the liver, distinguished by its folded appearance or the presence of food particles or fluid. The triad of the spleen, pancreas and gall bladder (located at 50% snout–vent length) serves as a useful landmark, caudal to the liver yet cranial to the gonads and kidneys. The gall bladder appears as an anechoic focal area.

The pancreas may be seen as a less hyperechoic form in the group. In cases of anorexia, the gall bladder is often greatly enlarged and can fill one third of the diameter of the snake. The spleen can be visualised as a circular shaped organ with higher echogenicity than the liver.

The testes have uniform echotexture. In larger snakes, the deferent duct may be seen as hyperechoic parallel lines originating from the testis. The ovaries may be difficult to locate in non-cycling, young females but with progressive breeding seasons the follicles become more apparent, just caudal to the gall bladder. In mature females the ovaries may fill a large part of the coelom. Ovarian follicles appear as hypoechoic spherical structures. In snakes, the eggs seem to contain two layers with the upper layer consisting of the anechoic albumin and the inner layer is the highly echoic yolk. In viviparous snakes (boid snakes, anacondas, vipers) an embryo/foetus is seen. The kidneys are located caudal to the gonads (the right kidney is located cranial to the left kidney) and are cylindrical in shape with a stacked book appearance. On ultrasound, they show a homogenous texture with a higher echogenicity than the fat body and a granulated structure. Faecal pellets may be imaged within the large intestine. In males, the inverted hemipenes are located caudal to the vent and can be detected as a hyperechoic area.

Crocodilians

For diagnostic imaging, adult crocodilians need to be sedated (midazolam) or anaesthetised. In young specimens, manual restraint can be used. Crocodilians are kept in ventral recumbency. Ultrasonography is particularly useful in crocodilians and is strongly indicated for general examination and health assessment. The heart is located centrally in the body, below the lungs and between the two liver lobes. Crocodilian cardiac anatomy is unique and probably the most complex of vertebrate hearts. The liver is bi-lobed and together with the heart separates the cranial coelom from the caudal part. The right liver lobe is slightly larger than the left and both can be scanned in their entirety.

The gallbladder is centrally situated caudal to the liver. The spleen is located almost directly caudal to the gall bladder. Another important abdominal organ is the single fat body. The kidneys can be very hard to identify as they are intrapelvic and consist of inverted renal tissue folded within a fatty stroma. The two ovaries are cranial and medial to the kidneys and consist of flat,

folded tissue in the hatchling, small bunched follicles in the immature female or, in the preovulatory stage, they may appear as numerous large follicles filling the caudal coelom. Testicles are elliptical in shape and similar in texture to those of other vertebrates. The diameter of the intestines increases and the thickness of the intestinal wall decreases from duodenum to rectum.

Computed Tomography

Computed tomography (CT) makes use of computer-processed x-rays to produce tomographic images ('slices') of the scanned object (Figure 12.7). The x-ray slice data is generated using an x-ray source that rotates around the object as the object passes through the beam; x-ray sensors are positioned on the opposite side of the circle from the x-ray source. Increasing the number of sensors increases the resolution; for example a 16-slice scanner has 16 sensors (Kiefer and Pees 2011, Wyneken 2014). The data are then processed by a computer to generate images in a number of planes (transverse, sagittal and coronal) and even three-dimensional reconstructions. Sedation or short-acting anaesthesia is recommended to prevent movement artefacts, although chelonians may be restrained within a sac or fixed on

Figure 12.7 Computed tomography of a green turtle (*Chelonia mydas*).

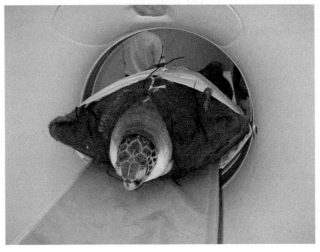

wooden blocks. Densitometry, the qualitative assessment of density of tissues, is expressed in Hounsfield units (HU; Kiefer and Pees 2011, Wyneken 2014). As an example, the normal densitometry of the chelonian shell measures 950–1300 HU but, in chelonians with metabolic bone disease, the densitometry may measure only 350–550 HU (Kiefer and Pees 2011, Wyneken 2014).

A stomach filled with gas is easy to find but the bowel loops are difficult to identify in the normal animal. Enlargement of the liver is easily detected. The densitometry of the liver decreases with fatty liver disease from 50–70 HU to −10 to −40 HU (Kiefer and Pees 2011). CT scans give detailed information about the number, size, shape, density and position of follicles and eggs. In most patients, the kidneys are easily located using plain sagittal views, especially when enlarged. Using plain CT, kidneys from the clinically healthy tortoises range in density from 33 HU to 42 HU. Gout often causes increased density of the kidneys. Urine retention or urate deposits in the reptile urinary bladder are easy to find. In tortoises, the normal kidney length is 1.7–2.7 cm and, when compared with the length of the endoplastron (equivalent to the breast bone), the ratio of endoplastron to kidney is 1.37 to 1. The slow respiratory rate permits high-quality scans of the typical reticular pattern of the chelonian lung. The value for density of lungs in python is about −744 HU (Kiefer and Pees 2011).

Iodinated contrast medium (370 mg I/ml) at a dose of 1 ml/kg, 2 ml/kg or 3 ml/kg is injected into the jugular vein and coelom organs are measured 1, 5, 10 and 15 minutes post-administration. After intravenous administration of the contrast medium, the kidney density varies with the dosage given (55–62 HU for 1 ml/kg contrast medium, 58–110 HU for 2 ml/kg contrast medium and 92–93 HU for 3 ml/kg contrast medium). In the majority of reptiles, maximum enhancement may be visible immediately, while in some animals maximum enhancement is evident after 5–10 minutes (Kiefer and Pees 2011, Wyneken 2014).

Magnetic Resonance Imaging

Magnetic resonance imaging (MRI) in reptiles is suitable for imaging of the respiratory tract, liver, gastrointestinal tract, urogenital tract and soft-tissue masses (tumours). As an MRI procedure takes longer than conventional radiography or CT examination, sedation or light anaesthesia is recommended (Ludewig and Pees 2011). For MRI examination, the reptile is positioned in ventral recumbency as symmetrically as possible (Figure 12.8). The three standard scanning planes are used – coronal, transverse and sagittal. The most important weightings are classified as T1 and T2. Fat tissue has a very high signal intensity (bright), while fluids have low signal intensity (dark) with T1-weighting. In contrast, in the T2-weighting, free fluid has high signal intensity and fat has low signal intensity (grey). T1-weighting is used for the assessment of structures that contain more fat, while T2-weighting is used for the assessment of ascites, inflammatory exudates and effusions. Further image enhancement can be achieved with the use of intravenous injectable paramagnetic compounds (via intravenous catheter). Within 20–30 minutes, it is possible to obtain sufficient images to build up a complete three-dimensional picture of the patient's internal structure (Ludewig and Pees 2011).

Diagnostic Endoscopy

Endoscopy is a minimally invasive diagnostic method for direct visual examination and antemortem biopsy. The standard equipment for diagnostic endoscopy in reptiles includes (Divers 2014):

- 2.7 mm diameter × 18 cm telescope, 30-degree forward-oblique with 4.8 mm operating sheath
- 1.9 mm diameter × 18 cm telescope, 30-degree forward-oblique with 4 mm operating sheath

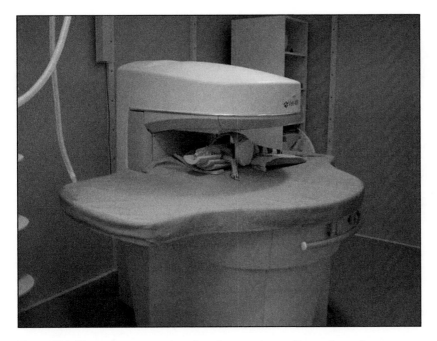

Figure 12.8 Magnetic resonance imaging of a green iguana (*Iguana iguana*).

- 1.7 mm flexible grasping forceps
- 1.7 mm flexible biopsy forceps with double-action jaws
- insufflator machine
- fluids (e.g. 0.9% sterile saline solution bag with infusion set)
- xenon cold light source and light cable
- endovideo camera and monitor.

Alternatively, the mobile endoscopic imaging systems (Tele Pack® system or AIDA-Vet® system) can replace the need for a light source, cable, camera and monitor).

In most cases, animals should be sedated or anaesthetised to achieve safe and good quality endoscopy. If necessary, sedation can be supplemented with local anaesthetic blocks (Divers 2014).

Oculoscopy, otoscopy

Oculoscopy in snakes and otoscopy in lizards are performed using similar approaches to other animals. These simple techniques require minimal training and allow good visualization and magnification of the ocular/ear structures. Sedation is required

for oculoscopy in snakes, while manual restraint is sufficient for otoscopy in small to medium sized lizards.

Tracheoscopy, Pulmonoscopy

In small to medium snake or lizard species, direct endoscopy of the trachea and proximal part of the lungs is easy to perform under sedation, while in larger animals pulmonoscopy (air sac endoscopy) is required to access the lungs and requires general anaesthesia. Pulmonoscopy in snakes can be performed via either a tracheal and transcutaneous approach. For transcutaneous pulmonoscopy, the snake is positioned in left lateral recumbency (for examination of right air sac and lung in all snake species) or right lateral recumbency (for examination of the smaller left lung in *Boidae*). After aseptic preparation, a short incision is made in the skin on the right side of the snake's body, at 35–45% along its length and parallel with the horizontal axis of the body. The incision is made between the second and third row of lateral skin scales. After incising the skin and blunt

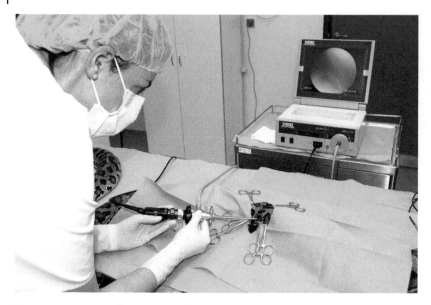

Figure 12.9 Air sac endoscopy in a python.

dissecting through the muscle and coelom membranes, the avascular transparent wall of the air sac can be visualized. Stay sutures are placed in the air sac wall and it is gently perforated; the telescope is introduced and directed cranially into the lung (Figure 12.9) and caudally into the air sac. Some of the visceral organs can be viewed through the transparent air sac. After selected parts of the air sac and lungs are observed, the air sac, muscle wall and skin are closed in separate layers (Knotek and Jekl 2015).

Oesophagoscopy and Gastroscopy

Oesophagoscopy can be performed on reptiles using 'twilight' anaesthesia (intravenous alfaxalone or propofol), while gastroscopy requires a surgical plane of anaesthesia. A bag of warm sterile saline fluid is connected via an infusion set to the port of the operating sheath. A second set, although rarely required, can be connected to a second port, with the other end placed into a collection bucket under the table (Divers 2014). A telescope (1.9 mm or 2.7 mm) with operating sheath is gently introduced into the proximal part of oesophagus. The saline irrigation

helps to gently dilate the oesophagus, allowing the telescope to be easily directed into the distal part of the oesophagus and the stomach. Flexible forceps (grasping or biopsy) are passed through the working channel of the operating sheath as required (Divers 2014).

Cloacoscopy–Cystoscopy, Colonoscopy

Cloacoscopy can be performed using sedation or short-acting anaesthesia but cystoscopy and colonoscopy require a surgical plane of anaesthesia. Cloacoscopy is useful for examining the cloacal mucosa and the chelonian phallus or clitoris. Cloacoscopy combined with cystoscopy is used in chelonians for direct visualization of the urinary bladder and indirect visualization of the coelom cavity (gonads, fat, liver and intestine; Divers 2014). The telescope with working sheath attached is inserted into the cloaca while placing a finger and thumb around the vent to act as a valve to control the infusion and outflow of fluid. Flushing of the cloaca with warm saline through the operating sheath allows a clear view of the accessory vesicles (Figure 12.10). The telescope is

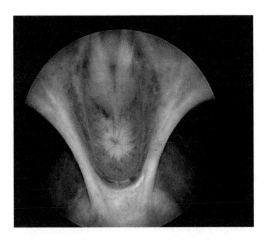

Figure 12.10 Cloacoscopic examination of a red-eared slider (*Trachemys scripta elegans*).

gently inserted into the urinary bladder, making sure that the volume of saline infused is controlled to prevent overfilling the bladder.

Coelioscopy

Coelioscopy is used for the examination of the reptilian coelom and biopsy collection (Divers 2014). General anaesthesia combined with effective analgesia is mandatory. Lizards, snakes and chelonians are placed in ventral, lateral or oblique (some chelonians) recumbency. Insufflation of the coelom with medical grade carbon dioxide (or irrigation of the coelom with warm saline fluid), allows a clearer view of the coelom. One finger and thumb are placed around the operating sheath and incision in the skin to form a seal, regulating the outflow of saline or carbon dioxide. After coelioscopy is finished, the carbon dioxide (or saline fluid) is released out of the coelom through the operating sheath, while the body wall is gently pushed.

Chelonians
Coelioscopy is performed through the pre-femoral approach (Divers 2014). After incising the skin and blunt dissecting the subcutaneous fat, the tendinous aponeurosis of the ventral and oblique abdominal muscles is opened, exposing the underlying coelom membrane. This is perforated and the

telescope introduced into the coelom and directed proximally. The telescope with the operating sheath is then introduced and directed into the proximal coelom.

Lizards

Coelioscopy is performed on lizards using a caudolateral approach. Following the skin incision, a haemostat is used for blunt perforation of the subcutaneous tissues, including the coelom membrane. The telescope with operating sheath is introduced and directed into the proximal coelom while the haemostat is withdrawn.

Snakes

Coelioscopy is performed on snakes using a left lateral approach in the caudal coelom. The skin incision is made between the second and third row of lateral skin scales and a haemostat is used for blunt perforation of the subcutaneous tissues including the coelom membrane (Divers 2014). The telescope with operating sheath is introduced and directed into the proximal coelom while the haemostat is withdrawn.

Training

Diagnostic endoscopy is not an innate skill and appropriate training (with the use of training models and cadavers) is required to obtain and maintain competency (Divers 2014).

References

Divers, S.J. (2014) Diagnostic endoscopy. in *Reptile Medicine and Surgery*, 2nd ed. (D.R. Madder, ed.). W.B. Saunders, Philadelphia, pp. 154–178.

Hochleithner, C. and Holland, M. (2014) Ultrasonography, in *Current Therapy in Reptile Medicine and Surgery* (D.R. Mader and S.J. Divers, eds). Elsevier, St. Louis, MO, pp. 107–127.

Kiefer, I. and Pees, M. (2011) Computed tomography, in *Diagnostic Imaging of Exotic Pets* (M.E. Kraurwald-Junghanns, M. Pees, S. Reese *et al.*, eds). Schlutersche, Hannover, pp. 358–367.

Knotek, Z. and Jekl, V. (2015) Pulmonoscopy of snakes. *Veterinary Clinics of North America Exotic Animal Practice*, 18, 493–506.

Ludewig, E. and Pees, M. (2011) Magnetic resonance imaging in *Diagnostic Imaging of Exotic Pets* (M.E. Kraurwald-Junghanns, M. Pees, S. Reese *et al.*, eds). Schlutersche, Hannover, pp. 368–377.

Pees, M. (2011) Reptiles, in *Diagnostic Imaging of Exotic Pets* M.E. Krautwald-Junghanns, M. Pees, S. Reese and T. Tully, eds). Schlütersche, Hannover, pp. 309–333.

Raiti, P. (2004) Non-invasive imaging in *BSAVA Manual of Reptiles*, 2nd ed. (S.J. Girling and P. Raiti, eds). British Small Animal Veterinary Association, Gloucester, pp. 87–93.

Schumacher, J. and Toal, R.L. (2001) Advanced radiography and ultrasonography in reptiles. *Seminars in Avian and Exotic Pet Medicine*, 10, 162–168.

Silvermann, S. (2006) Diagnostic imaging, in *Reptile Medicine and Surgery*, 2nd ed. (D.R. Madder, ed.). W.B. Saunders, Philadelphia, pp. 471–489.

Wilkinson, R. Hernandez-Divers, S., Lafortune, M. *et al.* (2004) Diagnostic imaging techniques, in *Medicine and Surgery of Tortoises and Turtles* (S. McArthur, R. Wilkinson and J. Meyer, eds). Blackwell, Oxford, pp. 187–238.

Wyneken, J. (2014) Computed tomography and magnetic resonance imaging, in *Current Therapy in Reptile Medicine and Surgery* (D.R. Mader and S.J. Divers, eds). Elsevier, St. Louis, MO, pp. 93–106.

13

Clinical Techniques and Supportive Care
Kimberly Vinette Herrin

General Handling

Patient knowledge and proper restraint are key to avoiding injury. Snakes that tend to bite may be restrained in plastic restraint tubes. Venomous snakes should be restrained by licensed handlers using snake hooks and tubes. Lizards may bite, scratch or flick their tails. Freshwater turtles may bite, particularly short-necked turtles. Long-necked turtles also have glands along the margin of the plastron that may discharge a strong odour when handled. Sea turtles may occasionally bite but more often flap their front flippers strongly when handled. This may cause trauma to the handler if they are holding the turtle from the sides of the carapace. There is also a spur on the leading edge of the front flippers that may cut and scratch.

In addition to injuries, reptiles may naturally carry strains of *Salmonella* sp. that could be shed in the faeces and be a source of zoonotic infection. Proper hygiene, especially hand washing and dedicated enclosure cleaning areas, is important when handling and keeping reptiles.

An initial visual or distant examination may reveal an immense amount of information about a reptile's condition, including activity, appetite, posture, excrement or any visible signs of illness or injury. A calico bag or pillowcase may be used to restrain reptiles safely for radiographs or to expose a specific part of the body through the opening.

Snakes

Snakes should be supported throughout the entire length of their body, to avoid excessive pressure on the spine, which can lead to fractures and subsequent arthritis (Figure 13.1). For very large snakes, multiple handlers may be required to support the snake's weight. Allow non-venomous snakes to move slowly. Nervous or aggressive snakes may be restrained in snake tubes and may require injectable sedation or anaesthesia for examination (e.g. alfaxalone intravenously). Oral examinations may necessitate gently holding the animal behind the base of the head to allow opening of the mouth by the clinician. To restrain the head, hold the lateral cranium behind the occiput with thumb and middle finger, with the index finger on top of the snake's head.

Lizards

Most lizards may be restrained by supporting the body. Small lizards often do not require much restraint (particularly bearded dragons, blue-tongued or shingle-backed lizards)

Reptile Medicine and Surgery in Clinical Practice, First Edition. Edited by Bob Doneley, Deborah Monks, Robert Johnson and Brendan Carmel.
© 2018 John Wiley & Sons Ltd. Published 2018 by John Wiley & Sons Ltd.

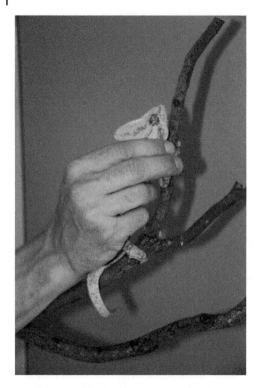

Figure 13.1 Veiled chameleon (*Chamaeleo calyptratus*) restraint. Chameleons are more comfortable when grasping something with their feet.

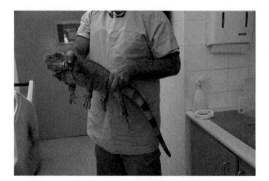

Figure 13.2 Restraint of a large green iguana (*Iguana iguana*).

while others that are more active (smaller skinks) may be held around the pectoral girdle with the forelimbs against the body. Remember that small skinks and geckos can drop their tails. In lizards exhibiting tail autotomy, take care not to grab them by the tail. In larger lizards (such as monitors), restraint may be best achieved by holding the front legs against the thorax with the hind legs extended alongside the tail. To avoid a flicking tail interfering with examination or diagnostics, secure the tail by restraining it under an arm. Alternatively, flicking may be avoided by holding the lizard away from the handler's body (Figure 13.2). If necessary, lizards may be wrapped in towels for restraint.

Turtles

Freshwater turtles may be restrained by holding the sides or the tail end of the carapace. Tortoises may also be restrained by holding the sides of the carapace or by supporting from the plastron. Smaller sea turtles (less than 15 kg) may be restrained by holding the cranial part of the carapace (behind the head) and caudal carapace (above tail). Larger sea turtles may require two or more handlers.

Crocodilians

Restraint varies on size and species. For crocodilians up to 0.8 m, manual restraint can be performed with one hand holding the neck (if examining mouth) or by holding the mouth closed and having the other hand holding the lower body. Always be mindful of the teeth, which are partially exposed even when the jaw is closed, and the tail that may lash around. When not being examined, the mouth can be taped closed. Crocodilians between 1 m and 3 m can be restrained with a catchpole to snare around the neck and by grabbing the tail to help stabilize and prevent rolling. They may also be strapped to a restraining board to help control movement. The head can then be pinned and the mouth taped closed. Larger crocodilians should be restrained by two or three experienced handlers and chemical restraint should be considered.

For some reptiles (e.g. iguanids, crocodilians), a calming effect may be achieved by simultaneously applying gentle pressure to both eyes to induce vasovagal response.

Diagnostic Techniques

Blood Collection

Blood collection in reptiles can be challenging to the uninitiated practitioner. When collecting blood, take care not to contaminate the sample with lymph fluid as this may alter the values of the complete blood cell count (dilution) as well as some chemical parameters (total phosphorus and potassium).

Snakes

In snakes, the primary site for blood collection is the caudal tail vein. This vein runs just below the vertebral processes. Short-tailed snakes are slightly more challenging. Access is via the ventral midline at a point approximately one-quarter to halfway along the tail (distal to the male hemipenes or female musk glands). Use an appropriately sized needle and syringe at a 45–60-degree angle, aiming craniodorsally while maintaining gentle negative pressure. Advance until the needle reaches the vertebral body and then slightly withdraw. If venepuncture via the tail vein is unsuccessful, cardiac puncture may be attempted. With the snake in dorsal recumbency, the heartbeat may be visualized on the ventral aspect of snake at approximately the cranial third of the body. This is often easier to perform in an anaesthetized snake. In a study of repeated cardiocentesis in ball pythons, there was no evidence of clinical complications and only minimal histological evidence of trauma from this technique; however, there is still a chance of causing some degree of haemopericardium. If the heartbeat is not readily visible, ultrasound is a quick and simple means of identifying the heart. The heart can be isolated by the forefinger (cranial aspect) and by the thumb (caudal aspect). The approach to cardiocentesis is to enter through the skin under the ventral scute (approximately 1 scute caudal to heart) at 45 degrees in a craniodorsal direction into the ventricle. Apply pressure for up to 60 seconds after cardiocentesis.

Lizards

In lizards, the tail vein is the most common venepuncture site. It is accessed through a ventral midline approach at either a 90 or 45-degree angle in the craniodorsal direction. Maintain negative pressure until the needle reaches the vertebral body and slightly withdraw to find the ventral tail vein; redirect slightly if needed. The approach may also be on lateral midline by angling 45–90 degrees craniomedially towards the lateral process of the vertebral body. Lymph contamination may occur from the lateral approach. Another option in lizards is venepuncture of the ventral abdominal or jugular vein (Figure 13.3a,b).

Turtles

Common venepuncture sites include the dorsal coccygeal (tail) vein, jugular vein, brachial vein and subcarapacial vein. Tortoises and freshwater turtles often have visible jugular veins on both sides and there is little risk of lymph contamination. The dorsal coccygeal vein can be accessed at the cranial aspect of the tail by aiming cranioventrally at a 45–90-degree approach from the dorsal midline of the tail, maintaining some negative pressure. The subcarapacial venous sinus can be accessed if the head is retracted by bending the needle and approaching midline behind the head where the carapace and skin meet. The needle is advanced in a caudodorsal direction toward the vertebra. Maintain slight negative pressure and redirect slightly if needed. In larger tortoises, the brachial vein may be accessed via the caudal aspect of the forelimb. In sea turtles, the supravertebral sinus is a common collection site and can be accessed by advancing the needle on either side of the nuchal crest approximately 2–4 cm behind the skull and directed toward the vertebra (Figure 13.3c). The external jugular vein is another site that can be accessed with the head extended. The needle is advanced at approximately 45 degrees (around one-third of the distance laterally from the spine and around one-third of the distance from the carapace to the skull). Ultrasound is useful in locating this site.

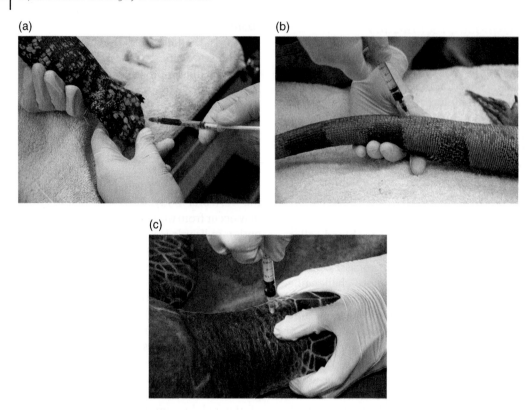

Figure 13.3 Blood collection from the ventral tail vein of (a) a shingleback lizard; (b) a green iguana; (c) Blood collection from the supravertebral sinus in a green turtle.

Crocodilians

The supravertebral venous sinus may be accessed in crocodilians through a 90-degree dorsal midline approach directly behind the occiput. Advance slowly with negative pressure to avoid deep penetration that could lead to spinal trauma. Alternatively, the ventral tail vein may be used (as described for lizards).

Blood Handling

Lithium heparin is the anticoagulant of choice for reptile blood. Fresh slides should be prepared before placing the sample in heparin, as there is less clumping of leucocytes and thrombocytes, leading to an improved differential count. Samples may be stored at 4 °C for up to 24 hours. If there is a delay in testing, packed cell volume and total protein should be run in-house and the blood smear fixed in methanol (estimated leucocyte count and differential). Blood for biochemical analysis should be separated.

As a general rule, the amount of blood volume that may be removed is between 0.5% and 0.8% of the body weight in lizards, snakes, chelonians and 0.3–0.5% in crocodilians.

Occasionally, because of the patient's size, the sample may be too small for routine biochemical analysis; however, in most cases, packed cell volume, total protein and blood smear (differential cell count, check for haemoparasites) can still be analyzed. Small plastic sample tubes (e.g. 0.8 ml tubes) are available commercially. In some laboratories a full blood count (manual method) and chemistry can be performed on as little as 0.2 ml of whole blood.

A typical chemistry panel for reptiles may include total protein, albumin, glucose, uric acid, aspartate aminotransferase, creatine kinase, calcium and phosphorous. Special tests may require serum for analysis and details may be obtained from reference laboratories. If excess plasma or serum has been collected, it may be frozen at −20 °C or preferably −80 °C freezer in cryovials and banked for later use.

Microbiology

Fungal and bacterial diseases are often diagnosed in reptiles. Sampling sites will vary depending on the condition. Microbiology, including both bacterial and fungal cultures, may be useful tools in diagnosing reptile conditions. Good sample technique and sterile collection of samples is important. Sampling of the skin by deep scrapings or biopsy is recommended to exclude the possibility of environmental contamination.

Fluid-filled structures may be aspirated and submitted in a sterile container for cytology and culture/sensitivity. In some cases, tissue biopsies may yield the greatest information. Tissue biopsies may be submitted directly in a sterile container with sterile saline. Biopsies may be split in half with one part frozen or submitted for culture and the other half placed in 10% buffered formalin for histopathology.

If viral testing is indicated, contact the reference laboratory for specific viral culture or molecular testing advice (e.g. sunshinevirus, adenovirus). Blood culture may be indicated in cases of sepsis. Skin should be sterilized and a blood sample taken using a sterile technique. Aerobic and anaerobic cultures may be carried out on as little as 0.5 ml of blood.

Cytology

Cytology may be very useful diagnostic tool in assessing lesion aetiology. Slides should be dried and fixed in methanol in preparation for Diff-Quik staining. Diff-Quik is the most commonly used stain, however some clinicians recommend a modified Giemsa technique (Pappenheim method: May-Grünwald plus Giemsa–Romanowsky staining). If bacterial or fungal pathology is suspected, slides should be heat fixed in preparation for Gram staining. A Ziehl–Neesen stain can be added to either type of preparation to assess the slide for acid-fast bacteria.

Parasitology

Faecal samples can be collected opportunistically and are often a valuable diagnostic tool in a sick reptile. Faecal samples may be infrequent or even absent, owing to feeding patterns or anorexia. Repeat faecal examinations may be helpful to monitor parasite burdens or catch eggs of species that shed intermittently. The practitioner should be familiar with gastrointestinal helminths and which protozoa and amoebae are parasitic and which are natural, beneficial fauna. Keep in mind that pseuodoparasites (parasites of prey items) may also pass through reptile faeces and should not be interpreted as pathogenic. Wet preparations are used to detect flagellates, ciliates, larvae and amoeba. If amoebae are detected, Lugol's iodine can help highlight their structure. For animals that have died, necropsy should reveal the actual parasite burden, which may not be reflected in the egg counts.

External parasites include ticks (usually readily visible), mites (often hidden under scales, use magnification to view) and leeches on aquatic species. A thorough external examination should be carried out. Myiasis (maggot infestation) may also be seen in debilitated reptiles. For sample identification, ectoparasites may be collected in 70% ethanol and submitted to laboratory if further identification is required.

Treatment Techniques

Heating

Reptiles are ectothermic, generally requiring an external heat source to maintain body temperature. The preferred optimum temperature range should be known for patients that are in care to allow for best healing and recovery (see Chapters 1 and 2). Effort should be made in hospital enclosures to provide reptiles with their complete temperature range, allowing the reptile to choose its preferred temperature. Refer to Chapter 6 for further details on heating.

Lighting

Most reptiles require some degree of ultraviolet B light (wavelength 290–320 nm) for vitamin D3 synthesis. Vitamin D3 is required to absorb dietary calcium and subsequent prevention of nutritional metabolic bone disease. An ultraviolet B gradient may allow reptiles to regulate their exposure and lamps may be set to a timer to provide the appropriate amount of ultraviolet light. In species that can absorb oral vitamin D3, short-term hospital stays may not require ultraviolet lighting if they are supplemented with oral vitamin D3 and calcium. Refer to Chapter 6 for further details on lighting.

Fluid Therapy

Assessment of dehydration and fluid deficit may be difficult in reptiles. Some indicators include skin turgor, sunken eyes and thick mucus in the mouth. Understanding how fluids are obtained is critical for each species, as many do not drink directly (e.g. chameleons lick water droplets off their face and require misting). Recommended daily fluid therapy doses range from 10 ml/kg/day to 40 ml/kg/day. Calculation of daily fluid therapy (Table 13.1) has also been estimated at 15 ml/kg for large reptiles and up to 25 ml/kg for small reptiles (author's preference).

Recommended routes and management of fluid therapy include oral, subcutaneous, intracoelomic, intravenous, intraosseous and cloacal. Fluids should be administered orally if the animal is less than 5% dehydrated and is capable of absorbing oral fluids (no vomiting, ileus or diarrhoea). Administer by syringe or stomach tube (red rubber catheter measured to distal oesophagus or stomach). When passing a stomach tube, use a soft spatula to open the mouth to avoid damaging the teeth or the beak (turtles). A bite block may be useful in chelonians as they tend to bite soft feeding tubes. Avoid the glottis, which is at the base of the tongue. Fluids should be pre-warmed and the volume delivered should be no more than 3% of the body weight at a time. During gavage, identify the glottis and stop if the stomach overfills and fluid starts to back up. Fluid therapy may need to be divided into several treatments if this occurs.

The subcutaneous space may also be used if dehydration is less than 5%. Administer at body temperature. The subcutaneous space is limited in reptiles and subcutaneous fluid administration may cause trauma in lizards with tight or fragile skin. In lizards, access areas include the lateral body wall or over the scapulae (Figure 13.4); in snakes, the paravertebral space; in chelonians, the axillary or inguinal regions; this route is rarely used in crocodilians.

The intracoelomic route is recommended for more dehydrated cases, as it offers rapid administration of larger volumes of fluid and the coelom has good fluid absorption. In chelonians, inject in the ventrocaudal coelomic cavity to avoid the lungs and other internal organs. In lizards and snakes, the injection may be given with the patient in dorsal recumbency to move the viscera and lungs away, injecting the fluids intracoelomically in the caudal third of the body. Alternatively, lizards may be tilted on their side, which may be less distressing. Aspirate before giving intracoelomic fluids to ensure that the needle has not entered the lungs or a viscus. This may also be performed via a catheter placed in the pre-femoral fossa to help to avoid needle trauma. The intracoelomic route allows large volumes of fluids to be administered at the one time. Beware of overhydration, as exceeding coelomic absorption levels will reduce the capacity of the lungs to expand due to iatrogenic ascites.

The intravenous route is the best route for rapid fluid administration, especially in reptiles that are more than 8% dehydrated. Intravenous fluid administration typically requires cut-down surgery for catheter placement.

Table 13.1 Fluid therapy.

Solution	Administration			Comments
	Dose	Frequency	Route	
Oral electrolyte	10–20 ml/kg	q24h prn	PO	Oral fluid therapy, anorexia
Crystalloids:	10–30 ml/kg	q24h prn		Dose depends on patient dehydration and ongoing losses
Non-lactate sodium chloride (0.45%)			PO, SC, IV, IC, EpiCe, IO prn	Hypertonic dehydration; can mix with other crystalloid solutions
Sodium chloride (0.9%)			SC, IV, IO, IC, EpiCe prn	Hyperkalaemia, hypercalcaemia, hypochloraemic metabolic alkalosis; can mix with other crystalloid solutions
Dextrose (2.5%, 5.0%)			PO, SC, IV, IC, EpiCe, IO	Fluid therapy, hyperkalaemia; can mix 5% dextrose with other crystalloid solutions in equal parts if patient is hypoglycaemic
Lactated Ringer's solution			SC, IV, IO, IC, EpiCe (chelonians)	Fluid replacement, prevention of aminoglycoside nephrotoxicity; can use EpiCe in chelonians; avoid using with hepatic insufficiency
Ringer's solution for reptiles			SC, IV, IO, IC, EpiCe (chelonians)	Hypertonic dehydration or prevention of aminoglycoside nephrotoxicity; can use epiCe in chelonians Formula: 1 part LRS, 2 parts 2.5% dextrose/0.45% saline 1 part LRS, 1 part 5% dextrose, 1 part 0.9% saline

EpiCe, epicoelemic; IC, intracoelomic; IO, intraosseous; IV, intravenous; PO, oral; prn, as needed; q24h, every 24 hours; SC, subcutaneously.
Sources: Carpenter et al. (2014), Carpenter (2013), Funk and Diethelm (2006), Mader and Rudloff (2006), Kirchgessner (2009), Gibbons (2009), Jarchow (1988).

Figure 13.4 Subcutaneous fluid administration to a double-crested basilisk (*Basiliscus plumifrons*).

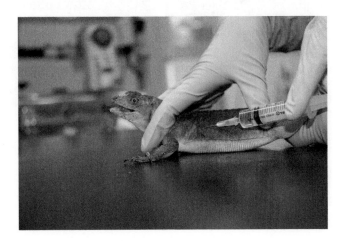

The intraosseous route is useful when rapid absorption is needed and intravenous access is limited or unavailable. Intraosseous catheters may be used in lizards and small crocodilians. They may also be placed in tortoises but with some difficulty. In lizards, placement is in the distal femur or tibial crest. Aseptic technique is imperative and local anaesthesia should be used over the tibial crest to numb the periosteum. With the leg in flexion, a spinal needle with stylet is advanced into the tibial plateau, anterior to the joint capsule and manipulated into the marrow cavity. Once placed, the stylet is removed and the needle secured. Placement must be confirmed by radiography as the needle may deviate out of the tibial medullary cavity. Catheter placement may also be carried out in the distal femur by entering the anterior surface of the metaphysis. Intraosseous catheters are useful for constant rate infusion since the marrow has limited space and is not suitable for bolus fluid administration (Figure 13.5a,b).

Cloacal absorption of fluids may be beneficial on a routine basis (daily bathing) and for mild dehydration but should not be considered a replacement for fluid therapy.

Nutritional Support

Nutritional support for the hospitalized reptile can be challenging. Attempts should be made to provide the species specific diet. Sick, hyporexic reptiles will often be reluctant to eat their normal diet. Many wild reptiles placed in captivity, particularly chelonians, are often reluctant to eat and may require supplemental feeding. Dehydration is common in sick reptiles and proper hydration should be established prior to supplemental feeding.

Standard metabolic rate (SMR) for reptiles is 32 ($BW^{0.75}$), measured in kilocalories (kcal) per day, where BW is body weight in kilograms (a 1-kg animal has an SMR of approximately 32 kcal/day). SMR in reptiles is only 25–35% of estimated values for mammals (personal communication, Michelle Shaw). In reptiles, daily intake is calculated as 1.1–4 times SMR, so a 1-kg animal requires 35–128 kcal/day. This amount may decrease during fasting and with less activity and/or lower ambient temperatures or may increase with more activity, reproduction, growth and protein synthesis required for healing. If the animal is in good condition, give approximately 75–100% of daily estimated calories

(a)　　　(b)

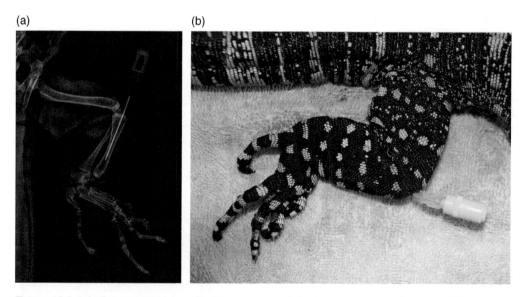

Figures 13.5 (a,b) Correct positioning of an intraosseous catheter in a lace monitor (*Varanus varius*).

Table 13.2 Percentage energy requirements for reptile dietary classifications.

Dietary type	Protein (%) (range)	Fat (%) (range)	Carbohydrate (%)
Carnivorous (snakes, crocodiles, some lizards, juvenile aquatic turtles)	50 (25–60)	45 (30–60)	5
Omnivorous (adult aquatic turtles, tortoises, some lizards)	25 (20–40)	25	50
Herbivorous (some tortoises, iguanas)	20	5	75

Source: Donoghue (2006).

to a hospitalized patient. If the reptile is in a debilitated condition, start with 40–75% and increase gradually so as to not cause gastrointestinal upsets (Donoghue 2006). For example, a 300-g bearded dragon would have an SMR of approximately 13 kcal/day and daily requirements would range from 14–52 kcal depending on the considerations listed here.

Carnivorous reptiles have a higher protein requirement than omnivorous reptiles. Some species alter their diet as they age, usually becoming less carnivorous (aquatic turtles and bearded dragons). Herbivores tend to have diets higher in carbohydrates (Donoghue 2006). Table 13.2 gives the energy requirements for reptile dietary classifications.

There are several commercial critical care diets available for gavage feeding in hospital, including a variety of commercial diets covering the nutritional range of carnivorous (including insectivorous), omnivorous and herbivorous reptiles. Some of the products used are human nutritional support products. When deciding when to feed the hospitalized reptile, it is important to understand the feeding frequency of the species in care.

Nutritional Delivery

Reptiles that are not eating on their own but are still alert may tolerate assist feeding by gently opening the mouth with a soft spatula and inserting food items that the reptile can easily swallow. If feeding whole prey, ensure that the prey is dead. If the reptile is difficult to assist feed, gavage feeding may be necessary.

Soft, flexible feeding tubes (e.g. red rubber catheter) or steel feeding needles can be used to deliver liquid or puréed diets. The tube should extend to the distal oesophagus or stomach. The practitioner can visually place the well-lubricated tube past the glottis to ensure that it enters the oesophagus. A bite block or speculum may be used to protect the reptile from biting on the feeding tube. When delivering soft food through the tube, identify the glottis during the process to ensure that food does not back up and become aspirated (Figure 13.6). Regurgitation could be a concern if the meal is too large. If it is tolerated by the patient, consider dividing the daily calorie requirement into two daily feeds.

Additional oil (e.g. olive oil) may be added to boost energy intake, particularly if the volume is restricted during assisted feeding (personal communication, Shaw).

Oesophagostomy Tube Support

Oesophagostomy tubes are useful for nutritional support in anorexic chelonians that cannot or will not eat. Chelonians are often difficult to assist feed due to their long necks and resistance to mouth opening relative to other reptiles. An oesophagostomy tube can be easily placed in chelonians in debilitated condition using local anaesthesia or they may require general anaesthesia if they are more active. See Chapter 28 for a description of the technique.

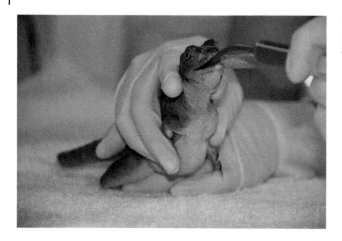

Figure 13.6 Gavage feeding a double-crested basilisk (*Basiliscus plumifrons*).

Liquid enteral nutrition is often required and can be made up from prepared sources or natural food items. Commercial critical care diets exist for herbivorous, omnivorous and carnivorous reptiles. In addition, human nutritional support products have also been useful for recovery from long-term anorexia, and may be mixed with vegetables or fruits for herbivores.

Respiratory Support

Assess respiratory rate and effort in the reptile patient. If the reptile is dyspnoeic, place it in an oxygen chamber for support. If it is sufficiently moribund and dyspneic, the reptile may need to be intubated and oxygen supplied through assisted ventilation, making sure the trachea is clear first. Once stabilized, diagnosis of the underlying respiratory condition may be assessed, including use of pulmonoscopy.

In instances of tracheal obstruction in snakes, saccular lung cannulation can be performed by transcutaneously accessing the air sacs to allow ventilation of the snake. Through a skin incision, the air sac may be accessed through blunt dissection of the intercostal muscles, allowing a tube to be placed through a small incision into the caudal aspect of the saccular lung (air sac). This has been performed successfully in ball and Burmese pythons with minimal damage to the surrounding tissue.

Administering Medications

The most common medication routes include: oral, subcutaneous, intramuscular, intravenous, intracoelomic and intraosseous.

Oral and Parenteral Dosing

Oral treatment may be given in the food and may be flavoured to avoid rejection. Gavage/tube feeding is another option for chelonians, snakes and lizards but care is needed to avoid damaging the mouth by repeated manipulation. Chelonians also tolerate oesophagostomy tubes. Crocodilians are typically treated in food. In some animals, such as bearded dragons, simply dripping measured amounts of liquid medication into the mouth is successful.

Parenteral dosing is often more effective than oral dosing in reptiles. Injection techniques may vary slightly in different species but should always be performed using sterile technique. With parenteral administration, there is evidence that some drugs removed by renal excretion or hepatic metabolism may be partially eliminated by the first-pass effect. When possible, subcutaneous or intramuscular injections may be given in the cranial half of the body, except in cases where a specific drug has been proven to be acceptable for caudal administration (e.g. carbenicillin, gentamicin).

Subcutaneous Dosing

Subcutaneous space is limited in reptiles and is poorly vascularized, therefore having variable absorption. In lizards, the lateral body wall or scapular area is often used; in chelonians, the axillary and inguinal areas are preferred; in snakes, the paravertebral space; in crocodilians, this route is rarely used.

Intramuscular Dosing

This is a common route of drug administration as it has rapid uptake and distribution. A common injection site is in the forelimbs. Some drugs are irritating when given intramuscularly and may cause pain and inflammation at the injection site. Enrofloxacin 50 mg/ml may cause muscle necrosis and sloughing when given in large volumes at full strength but may be diluted to 25 mg/ml with sterile water at a ratio of one to one to alleviate this problem. Avoid injecting into small muscle masses if possible, particularly in small animals, as this may impair mobility. Rotate injection sites if ongoing treatments are required.

Intravenous Dosing

The intravenous route has rapid uptake and distribution but may pose some difficulty with access in a debilitated patient. If a catheter is in place, intravenous drug administration is accessible and should be used. It is the best route for drug administration if a patient is dehydrated and hypothermic. Dehydration should be corrected prior to administration of any organotoxic drugs (e.g. gentamicin, nonsteroidal anti-inflammatory drugs).

Intraosseous Dosing

The intraosseous route is adequate for drug administration if access is available but only if the drugs have no known adverse marrow effects.

Intracoelomic Dosing

The intracoelomic route is a rare route for drug administration, although it is very good for fluid administration. For many drugs, the intracoelomic route is recommended only if all other routes are unavailable as absorption across coelomic membranes may be variable.

Maintaining Vascular Access

Once vascular access is achieved (which can be difficult), intravenous catheters can be secured in many reptilian species. Reptile skin is thick and tough and requires aseptic surgical cut-down technique for catheter placement. This is best performed in heavily sedated or anaesthetized animals but may be performed in emergency situations with moribund animals and local anaesthesia. Consider analgesia for pain relief.

Lizards

The typical site for intravenous catheter placement is the cephalic vein on the medial to lateral forelimb. A transverse cut-down can be performed with the incision running perpendicular to the vein. Dissect down to vein through subcutaneous tissue to place the catheter. Secure the catheter into the vein with tape or glue and bandage for protection. The jugular vein is also an option but is usually more difficult to access.

Chelonians

In tortoises and semi-aquatic turtles, the left and right jugular veins are used for intravenous catheters. *Note that the right jugular may be larger than the left.* The jugular vein may be visualized starting at the tympanic membrane and extending caudally. In some cases, a skin incision may not be necessary. With thicker skin, a small nick in the skin near the jugular vein will allow access to the vein. Catheter placement should be near the cranial third of the neck. The catheter should be flexible and its length should be one-third of the neck length to compensate for neck flexion and retraction. The catheter may be sutured or glued in place (no bandage is necessary).

In sea turtles, the external jugular vein is fairly accessible through cut-down and dissection technique.

Snakes

The left or right jugular vein is the intravenous catheter site for snakes. Placement is 9–10 ventral scales cranial to the heart. With the snake in dorsal recumbency, an incision is made between the first and second rows of dorsal scales (just above the ventral scales). The rectus abdominis muscle needs to be bluntly dissected to reveal the jugular vein (medial to ribs). Once the catheter (largest bore possible) is inserted, it may be sutured in place.

Blood Transfusion

The literature is scant regarding whole blood transfusions in reptiles but reptile practitioners do perform transfusions. Anaemia may be chronic or acute. Acute anaemia from acute blood loss is typically an indication for transfusion if the overall blood loss exceeds 20%. Packed cell volume and total protein of the recipient are critical in determining the need for a transfusion. Normal reptile packed cell volume ranges are typically between 20% and 40% and total protein levels of 3–8 g/dl. In an anaemic reptile, packed cell volume may drop quite low (less than 10%) and the patient should be monitored closely. Many reptiles may be able to cope with anaemia and will recover with supportive care. However, clinical signs such as weakness and lethargy are good indicators of when a transfusion is warranted.

Whole blood from a healthy conspecific (not to exceed 0.8% of the body weight of the donor) can be collected aseptically in anticoagulant. The anticoagulant commonly used is heparin at 5–10 units/ml of blood. If available, acid citrate dextrose solution can also be used at a ratio of one to nine with blood. Blood must be collected with strict aseptic technique and should be used within six hours of collection as red blood cells lose viability over time, especially in heparin, which lacks preservatives. Blood should be stored cooled and then warmed prior to administration.

Whole blood may be administered to the recipient via the intravenous or intraosseous route. Use a large gauge intravenous or butterfly catheter to prevent red blood cell haemolysis and platelet clumping. This may be difficult in snakes and the transfusion may instead be given via the intracoelomic route.

The blood should be warmed to 25–30 °C and may be given by syringe at a rate of 5–10 ml/kg/hour. In shocked patients, 20 ml/kg/hour is recommended. Monitor for signs of circulatory overload, particularly in small reptiles. A positive response to transfusion is often noted within two hours.

Note that a slide agglutination test can be performed on patients with a history of previous transfusions.

While filters (80 μm pore) have previously been recommended for clot and debris removal, one report recommended *not* using a standard Millipore filter as large reptilian erythrocytes would not pass through.

Bandaging and Wound Management

There are a variety of bandage materials available for use in reptiles. Small open wounds may be cleaned and dressed with topical antibiotic if infected (e.g. acute cadexomer iodine powder) covered in hydrocolloid paste to maintain moisture (e.g. DuoDERM®; Figure 13.7). The same principle may be applied to larger wounds with an additional secondary dressing. Change bandaging as needed; typically every two to three days as the wound is monitored. Some practitioners recommend suturing bandage material to the skin. Wound healing typically progresses similar to that of other animals but at a slower rate. Do note that in snakes, bandages are difficult to maintain because of their body shape.

Enemas

Impaction due to constipation or obstipation may be seen in some reptiles. Adequate hydration status should be maintained and fluid correction often resolves constipation. If not, warm water enemas given per cloaca may be performed. Red rubber catheters may be gently advanced and warm water instilled into the lower intestine. Alternatively, a mixture of 50% lubricant and 50% warm water at a rate of 1–3 ml/100 g body weight may be used.

Figure 13.7 The use of DuoDERM®/Iodosorb® in a shell fracture repair on an eastern long-necked turtle.

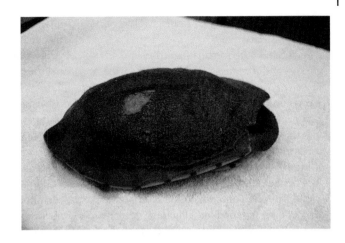

Acknowledgements

Taronga Zoo Wildlife Hospital: Michelle Shaw, nutritionist, Paul Thompson, laboratory manager, and the nurses and Reptile Division keepers for assistance with this chapter, and Robert Johnson.

Reference

Donoghue, S. (2006) Nutrition, in *Reptile Medicine and Surgery*, 2nd ed. (D. Mader, ed.), Saunders Elsevier, St Louis, MO, pp. 251–298.

Further Reading

Barten, S.L. (2006) Lizards, in *Reptile Medicine and Surgery*, 2nd ed. (D. Mader, ed.), Saunders Elsevier, St Louis, MO, pp. 59–77.

Barten, S.L. and Fleming, G.J. (2014) Current herpetologic husbandry and products, in *Current Therapy in Reptile Medicine and Surgery* (D.R. Mader and S.J. Divers, eds). Elsevier Saunders, St Louis, MO, pp. 2–12.

Boyer, T.H. and Boyer, D.M. (2006) Turtles, tortoises and terrapins, in *Reptile Medicine and Surgery*, 2nd ed. (D. Mader, ed.), Saunders Elsevier, St Louis, MO, pp. 78–99.

Campbell, T.W. (2006) Clinical pathology of reptiles, in *Reptile Medicine and Surgery*, 2nd ed. (D. Mader, ed.), Saunders Elsevier, St Louis, MO, pp. 453–470.

Campbell, T.W. (2014) Clinical pathology, in *Current Therapy in Reptile Medicine and Surgery* (D.R. Mader and S.J. Divers, eds). Elsevier Saunders, St Louis, MO, pp. 70–92.

Campbell, T.W. (2006) Hemoparasites, in *Reptile Medicine and Surgery*, 2nd ed. (D. Mader, ed.), Saunders Elsevier, St Louis, MO, pp. 801–805.

Carpenter, J.W. (2013) Reptiles, in *Exotic Animal Formulary*, 4th ed. (J.W. Carpenter and C.J. Marion, eds.), Elsevier Saunders, St Louis, MO, pp. 116–121.

Carpenter, J.W., Klaphake, E. and Gibbons, P.M. (2014) Reptiles, in *Current Therapy in Reptile Medicine and Surgery* (D.R. Mader and S.J. Divers, eds). Elsevier Saunders, St Louis, MO, pp. 70–92.

Cooper, J.E. (2006) Dermatology, in *Reptile Medicine and Surgery*, 2nd ed. (D. Mader, ed.), Saunders Elsevier, St Louis, MO, pp. 196–216.

DeVoe, R.S. (2015)Lacertilia (lizards, skinks, geckos) and *Amphisbaenids* (worm lizards), in *Zoo and Wild Animal Medicine* (M.E. Fowler and R.E. Miller, eds) Volume 8, Elsevier Saunders, St Louis, MO,pp. 52–60.

Flanagan, J.P. (2015) Chelonians (turtles, tortoises), in *Zoo and Wild Animal Medicine* (M.E. Fowler and R.E. Miller, eds) Volume 8, Elsevier Saunders, St Louis, MO, pp. 27–38.

Fleming, G.J. and Fontenot, D.K. (2015) Crocodilians (crocodiles, alligators, caiman, gharial), in *Zoo and Wild Animal Medicine* (M.E. Fowler and R.E. Miller, eds) Volume 8, Elsevier Saunders, St Louis, MO, pp. 38–49.

Funk R.S. and Diethelm, G. (2006) Reptile formulary, in *Reptile Medicine and Surgery*, 2nd ed. (D. Mader, ed.), Saunders Elsevier, St Louis, MO, pp. 1119–1139.

Gibbons, P.M. (2009) Critical care nutrition and fluid therapy in reptiles. Proceedings of the 15th Annual International Veterinary Emergency and Critical Care Symposium, September 9–13, Chicago, Illinois, pp. 91–94.

Gibbons, P.M. (2014) Therapeutics, in *Current Therapy in Reptile Medicine and Surgery* (D.R. Mader and S.J. Divers, eds). Elsevier Saunders, St Louis, MO, pp. 57–69.

Gibbons, P. M., Klaphake, E. and Carpenter, J. W. (2013) Reptiles, in *Exotic Animal Formulary*, 4th ed. (J.W. Carpenter and C.J. Marion), Elsevier Saunders, St Louis, MO, pp. 116–121.

Greiner, E.C. and Mader, D.R. (2006) Parasitology, in *Reptile Medicine and Surgery*, 2nd ed. (D. Mader, ed.), Saunders Elsevier, St Louis, MO, pp. 343–364.

Hernandez-Divers, S.J. (2006) Diagnostic techniques, in *Reptile Medicine and Surgery*, 2nd ed. (D. Mader, ed.), Saunders Elsevier, St Louis, MO, pp. 490–532.

Holz, P., Barker I.K., Burger, J.P. *et al.* (1997) The effect of the renal portal system on pharmacokinetic parameters in the red-eared slider (*Trachemys scripta elegans*). *Journal of Zoo and Wildlife Medicine*, 28 (4), 386–393.

Innis, C. (2008) Zoo Med 2008: Reptile Medicine. Tufts Open Courseware, Tufts University. http://ocw.tufts.edu/Content/60/lecturenotes/843397 (accessed 5 June 2017).

Innis, C., Papich, M., and Young, D. (2007) Pharmacokinetics of metronidazole in the red-eared slider turtle (Trachemys scripta elegans) after single intracoelomic injection. *Journal of Veterinary Pharmacology and Therapeutics*, 30, 168–171.

Isaza, R. and Jacobson, E.R. (2013) Antimicrobial drug use in reptiles, in *Antimicrobial Therapy in Veterinary Medicine*, 5th ed. (S. Giguère, J.F. Prescott and P.M. Dowling, eds), Wiley-Blackwell, Chichester, pp. 623–636.

Isaza, R., Andrews, G.A., Coke, R.L. and Hunter, R.P. (2004) Assessment of multiple cardiocentesis in ball pythons (*Python regius*). *Contemporary Topics in Laboratory Animal Science*, 43 (6), 35–38.

Jarchow, J.L. (1988) Hospital care of the reptile patient, in *Exotic Animals* (E.T. Jacobson and G.V. Killias Jr, eds). Churchill Livingstone, New York, New York, pp. 19–34.

Kirchgessner, M. and Mitchell, M.A. (2009) Chelonians, in *Manual of Exotic Pet Practice* (M.A. Mitchell and T.N. Tully Jr, eds). Elsevier Saunders, St Louis, MO, pp. 207–249.

Knotková, Z., Doubek, Z., Knotek, Z. and Hajková, P. (2002) Blood cell morphology and plasma biochemistry in Russian tortoises (*Agrionemys horsfieldi*). *Acta Veterinaria Brno*, 71, 191–198.

Lane, T. (2006) Crocodilians, in *Reptile Medicine and Surgery*, 2nd ed. (D. Mader, ed.), Saunders Elsevier, St Louis, MO, pp. 100–117.

Lock, B.A., and Wellehan, J. (2015) Ophidia (snakes), in *Zoo and Wild Animal Medicine* (M.E. Fowler and R.E. Miller, eds) Volume 8, Elsevier Saunders, St Louis, MO, pp. 60–74.

Mader, D.R. (2006) Medical care of seaturtles: medicine and surgery, in *Reptile Medicine and Surgery*, 2nd ed. (D. Mader, ed.), Saunders Elsevier, St Louis, MO, pp. 977–1000.

Mader, D.R. and Rudloff, E. (2006) Emergency and critical care, in *Reptile Medicine and Surgery*, 2nd ed. (D. Mader, ed.), Saunders Elsevier, St Louis, MO, pp. 533–548.

Mitchell, M.A. (2006) Therapeutics, in *Reptile Medicine and Surgery*, 2nd ed. (D. Mader, ed.), Saunders Elsevier, St Louis, MO, pp. 631–664.

Myers, D.A., Wellehan, J.F.X. and Isaza, R. (2009) Saccular lung cannulation in a ball python (*Python regius*) to treat a tracheal obstruction. *Journal of Zoo and Wildlife Medicine*, 40 (1), 214–216.

Pare, J A, Sigler, L., Rosenthal, K.L. and Mader, D.R. (2006) Microbiology: fungal and bacterial diseases of reptiles, in *Reptile Medicine and Surgery*, 2nd ed. (D. Mader, ed.), Saunders Elsevier, St Louis, MO, pp. 801–805.

Schumacher, J. (2015) Fluid therapy in reptiles, in *Zoo and Wild Animal Medicine* (M.E. Fowler and R.E. Miller, eds) Volume 8, Elsevier Saunders, St Louis, MO, pp. 160–164.

Schumacher, J. and Mans, C. (2014) Anesthesia, in *Current Therapy in Reptile Medicine and Surgery* (D.R. Mader and S.J. Divers, eds). Elsevier Saunders, St Louis, MO, pp. 134–153.

Schumacher, J. and Yelen, T. (2006) Anesthesia and analgesia, in *Reptile Medicine and Surgery*, 2nd ed. (D. Mader, ed.), Saunders Elsevier, St Louis, MO, pp. 442–452.

Stacy, N. I., Alleman, A.R. and Sayler, K.A. (2011) Diagnostic hematology of reptiles. *Clinics in Laboratory Medicine*, 31, 87–108.

Thompson, P. (2012) Practical Laboratory Skills Workshop, Wildlife Pathology Short Course. Taronga Conservation Society Australia, Mosman, NSW, pp. 4–18. http://arwh.org/sites/default/files/2017-01/WILDLIFE%20PATHOLOGY_Practical%20Laboratory%20Skills_2012_v2.pdf.

14

Reptile Pharmacology

Tim Hyndman

Introduction

*Primum non nocere (First, do no harm)
Post hoc ergo propter hoc (After this,
therefore, because of this; He was sick,
he is now well, and therefore the treatment cured him)*

These two Latin phrases eloquently summa-
rize the guiding principles of drug therapy in
all species. First, the goal of all veterinarians
when administering therapy to animals is not
to cause harm. Second, it is important that
the veterinarian understands that the resolution of a clinical disease was not necessarily
because of the therapy they administered. To
automatically assume that it was can result in
self-fulfilling prophecies, and not scientific
evidence, justifying therapeutic decisions.
These teachings are especially pertinent to
reptile drug therapy because the veterinarian
only has limited information to guide their
decisions as to how they employ their drug
armamentarium for an incredibly diverse
group of species. Despite these challenges,
the veterinarian is already well trained to
apply their knowledge of pharmacology to
these remarkable animals.

The reader is reminded that the drug formulary found in Appendix 1 of this book
provides information specific to individual
drugs (e.g. doses) and so serves as a

complement to the discussion presented in
this chapter. Box 14.1 outlines 10 rules to
remember when treating reptiles with drugs.

Administration of Drugs
for Reptiles

The clinician should know what species (or
at least what family) of reptile has been presented to them. This will then allow helpful
husbandry recommendations to be made.
The second fundamental piece of information that should be established before any
drug therapy starts is an accurate diagnosis.
It is accepted that delaying supportive therapy until all diagnostic tests have been completed can compromise the animal's welfare.
It is also accepted that treatment trials can
provide valuable information about underlying disease processes but, nevertheless,
determining a definitive diagnosis should
always remain the goal of the veterinarian,
as it will direct the clinician to the most
appropriate treatment modality.

All reptiles are ectothermic and each species has a natural preference for a specific
range of ambient temperatures they will seek
to regulate their body temperature. This is
referred to as the preferred optimal body temperature or the preferred optimal temperature
zone. The assumption is made that a reptile

Reptile Medicine and Surgery in Clinical Practice, First Edition. Edited by Bob Doneley, Deborah Monks,
Robert Johnson and Brendan Carmel.
© 2018 John Wiley & Sons Ltd. Published 2018 by John Wiley & Sons Ltd.

Box 14.1 Ten rules to remember when treating reptiles with drugs.

1) Ensure that the owner has provided informed consent for the therapy you would like to instigate. The vast majority of drugs administered to reptiles are not registered for them.

2) Do not use macrocyclic lactones in turtles and tortoises. Great care should also be exercised when considering these drugs for crocodilians, skinks and indigo snakes.

3) Be kind and compassionate to your reptilian patients. Our capacity to interpret pain and distress in reptiles is limited. Assume that reptiles require the same levels of analgesia afforded to companion mammals.

4) Husbandry can always be improved. Improved husbandry is unfailingly the best medicine.

5) Ensure that each reptilian patient is kept at their preferred optimal body temperature during drug therapy. This should mean that drug absorption, distribution, metabolism and elimination will be as reliable as possible.

6) Courses of medication will generally need to be longer in reptiles than mammals.

7) 'Baytril® (enrofloxacin) deficiency' is not a diagnosis. Reptile patients deserve our best efforts to reach a correct diagnosis.

8) Avoid serial injections of enrofloxacin into the muscle and subcutaneously. This practice is painful and is associated with tissue necrosis and abscess formation.

9) Intramuscular injections should be injected into the front half (e.g. forelimbs) of reptiles. This may avoid first pass renal clearance of some drugs.

10) There is very little justification to use corticosteroids in reptiles. Nonsteroidal anti-inflammatory drugs will nearly always represent a better option.

---

will function optimally at their preferred optimal body temperature. It is therefore also assumed that if a reptile is held at its preferred optimal body temperature, any drugs that are administered to it will be absorbed, distributed, metabolized and eliminated as reliably as possible (see also Chapter 2).

Once a drug has been selected for therapy and the animal has been provided with its preferred optimal temperature zone, a route of administration needs to be chosen. The most reliable ways to deliver a drug to the blood are by intravenous or intracardiac injection. For intravenous injections, the ventral tail vein is usually chosen for snakes and lizards but for turtles and tortoises the dorsal tail vein, jugular vein, occipital sinus, subcarapacial sinus and brachial vein can be tried (see Chapter 13). Intravenous injections can be very challenging in reptiles. Injections directly into the heart are typically reserved for the administration of euthanasia solutions in anaesthetized or heavily sedated patients.

Injections administered into the muscle and the subcutaneous tissue are two common routes of drug administration for reptiles. Larger boluses can be administered under the skin rather than into the muscle and especially large volumes should be injected into multiple sites (see Chapter 13). For snakes, back (epaxial) muscles are usually chosen for intramuscular injections but, for turtles, tortoises and lizards, the front limb is usually chosen. There is debate as to whether drugs should be preferentially injected into the cranial half of reptiles. Reptiles have a unique vascular system and part of it, the renal portal system, means that venous drainage from the caudal half of the animal may be delivered directly to the kidney before returning to the heart. For drugs that are primarily eliminated by the renal tubules (e.g. beta-lactam antibiotics), this may mean that some of the administered drug is extracted by the kidney before it can be distributed throughout the body. This may have clinical consequences if this results in blood drug concentrations becoming subtherapeutic. Obviously, the clinical consequences of injecting drugs into the caudal half of reptiles have not been quantified for every drug in every species. Considering that it is rarely more difficult to inject a reptile in the cranial half of the body compared with the caudal half of the body, injections into the cranial half of the body are encouraged. It should also be noted that intravenous injections into the tail vein may also result in drugs being delivered directly the kidney.

Injecting drugs into the body cavities of reptiles (the coelomic cavity) cannot be recommended because of the risk of lacerating the alimentary tract, highly vascular organs and the reproductive tract, especially in females during their breeding seasons. The inadvertent injection of drug into the lumen of the alimentary tract may decrease drug absorption.

Drugs can be administered directly into the alimentary tract of reptiles. This can be through instilling drug into the mouth, depositing it lower down into the oesophagus or stomach or even by inserting the drug into the reptile's food item. This last method is sometimes used for venomous or otherwise dangerous reptiles and, although it represents a safe method of drug administration, drug absorption will likely be unpredictable.

Some drugs are administered directly on to the skin of reptiles. As a generalization, it should be assumed that this route of administration is only suitable for those drugs being used for a topical effect; for example, for treating external parasite burdens such as mite infestations. Due care should still be exercised as systemic toxicity has been associated with topical drug administration in reptiles (e.g. pyrethroids).

Drug Compounding

Drug compounding is defined as the manipulation of a drug to form a medicine. It is typically performed by compounding pharmacists or veterinarians and is done extemporaneously (ad hoc) to meet the medical needs of an individual patient. Owing to the limited arsenal of drugs that are registered for use in reptiles, it can be tempting to

obtain medicines from compounding pharmacists. By this means, specific drug concentrations can be obtained, drugs can be combined into 'polypills', particular palatants (flavours) can be added to drugs and, often, this can be done at a cheaper price than if the clinician were to purchase registered drugs. These advantages may be partially or totally offset by a number of disadvantages, namely the unproven safety, efficacy, manufacturing standards and stability for the particular medication being sought. In one study on two concentrations of compounded oral doxycycline, 33 mg/ml and 167 mg/ml, the doxycycline was found to be stable for between 7 and 14 days, at both room temperature and when stored in a refrigerator (Papich *et al.* 2013). The compounding pharmacist had assigned an expiry date of 28 days to these two preparations.

It is prudent to be cautious about compounded drugs. This caution should extend especially to low-concentration medications (e.g. drugs presented in microgram amounts), those intended for injection and those associated with claims of systemic absorption following their application to the skin (transdermals).

Antibiotic Therapy

Antibiotic resistance is emerging and spreading more rapidly than ever. Compounding this resistance, new antibiotics are arriving to market at their slowest rates ever. This means that antibiotics should be used sparingly and appropriately. Once the decision has been made to administer an antibiotic (or antibiotics), the dose and dosing interval must be considered carefully. The duration of the antibiotic course should be decided during therapy.

Which Antibiotic(s) Should be Used?

A bacterial culture and sensitivity continues to be the gold standard for determining the bacteria present in a clinical sample and for predicting which antibiotic(s) will have in vivo efficacy against the cultured bacterium. If possible, culture and sensitivity should be ordered in parallel with cytology or histopathology. These pathology tests can provide further insights into the significance of the bacteria that has been cultured. For example, seeing Gram-negative rods within heterophils and monocytes would support that a culture result of *Escherichia coli* was significant. The added benefit of cytology and histopathology is that non-bacterial causes of disease can be investigated (e.g. neoplasia, fungal infections).

In the absence of culture and sensitivity, the clinician is forced to make a clinical judgement as to whether they consider there is a bacterial infection at all, and which bacteria are involved. As a starting guide, *Pseudomonas* and *Aeromonas* are commonly isolated from ulcerative stomatitis, pneumonia, cutaneous lesions and septicaemias. *Serratia* is commonly isolated from bite wounds and other cutaneous lesions. *Mycobacteria* can be isolated (and/or detected by special stains) in cutaneous lesions and in septic reptiles. *Providencia* can be an opportunistic pathogen of the mouth and *Klebsiella* can be associated with ocular infections and pneumonia. *Salmonella* and *Escherichia* are associated with gut infections. It is not surprising then that empirically selected antibiotics should have good efficacy against Gram-negative bacteria. Some empirical antibiotic choices for a selection of common reptile presentations are listed in Table 14.1.

A culture and sensitivity result predicts susceptibility but if the antibiotic does not reach the site of infection because of decreased blood flow to that area (e.g. the core of an abscess), antibiotic efficacy will be diminished. This is one of the reasons why the surgical treatment of reptilian abscesses is so important. Antibiotics such as fluoroquinolones and macrolides will concentrate in abscesses while sulphonamides are inactivated in purulent environments. For slow-growing bacteria, the beta-lactams are expected to have diminished activity because these antibiotics are dependent on bacterial replication to be effective. The aminoglycosides have no activity against anaerobic bacteria.

What Dose and Dose Interval Should be Used?

The dose of an antibiotic should not be a static number that is independent of the clinical case. Rather than 'What is the dose rate for antibiotic X?', the clinician is encouraged to tailor their dose to suit the clinical presentation. Therefore, the question of 'What dose should I choose for this case?' is far more relevant. It is naïve to assume that all bacterial infections will respond equally to the same dose of a particular antibiotic.

Broad generalizations can still be made about dose selection, and the recommendations are strongly linked to the particular class of antibiotic. For dose (concentration)-dependent antibiotics, such as the fluoroquinolones, aminoglycosides, metronidazole and azithromycin, higher doses result in improved efficacy. For time-dependent antibiotics such as the beta-lactams and the macrolides (except azithromycin), the efficacy of the antibiotic is enhanced by prolonging the length of time that the plasma concentration exceeds the susceptibility of the bacterium (e.g. the minimum inhibitory concentration). For these drugs, increasing the dose frequency is the best way of improving drug efficacy. The tetracyclines and the sulphonamides do not fit neatly into either of these categories. A practical example would be to consider increasing the dose rate of enrofloxacin from 10 mg/kg once daily to 20 mg/kg once daily if you were targeting a bacterium that was harder to kill (e.g. *Pseudomonas*). Similarly, administering the typical 20 mg/kg dose of ceftazidime at a higher dose frequency (e.g. every 48 hours compared with every 72 hours) should result in improved drug efficacy for this commonly used beta-lactam.

The sensitivity profile presented as part of a culture and sensitivity report is derived

Table 14.1 Treatment recommendations for specific conditions.

Disease process	Anti-infective options	Other drugs	Comments
Abscess: *subspectactular abscesses, internal abscesses*	**Bacterial:** ceftazidime, ceftiofur	NSAIDs	Surgery is nearly always more important than medical therapy. Topical ocular preparations are inappropriate for reptiles with undamaged spectacles; e.g. all snakes and most geckos.
Alimentary: *periodontal disease, diarrhoea, regurgitation*	**Bacterial:** ceftazidime, ceftiofur **Fungal:** nystatin, itraconazole **Coccidia:** toltrazuril, ponazuril, potentiated sulphonamides **Cryptosporidium:** paromomycin **Flagellates:** metronidazole **Nematodes:** fenbendazole, ivermectin[a]	NSAIDs Fluid therapy, especially if diarrhoea and stomatitis (not drinking)	Beware of zoonotic potential of salmonella.
Neurological	**Protozoal** (rare): metronidazole, potentiated sulphonamides	NSAIDs Calcium for hypocalcaemia Glucose for hypoglycaemia Fluid therapy to hasten elimination of toxins	Drug therapy may not help (e.g. viral infections) and so may need to consider euthanasia.
Reproductive: *egg binding (dystocia), prolapse*	**Bacterial/prophylactic:** ceftazidime, ceftiofur	NSAIDs Calcium and fluid therapy for many dystocias (see Chapter 22 for more medical options)	Some eggs can be manually passed and so drug therapy may not be needed. Many cases will be surgical.
Respiratory: *upper and lower respiratory disease*	**Bacterial:** ceftiofur, ceftazidime, piperacillin **Mycoplasma:** enrofloxacin, macrolides (e.g. azithromycin, tylosin) **Fungal:** itraconazole, voriconazole **Protozoal:** potentiated sulphonamides, toltrazuril **Herpesvirus:** acyclovir **Helminth:** ivermectin[a]	NSAIDs Vitamin A in turtles and tortoises with swollen eyelids	Ensure that humidity is correct.

(*Continued*)

Table 14.1 (Continued)

Disease process	Anti-infective options	Other drugs	Comments
Sepsis	**Bacterial**: amoxicillin/clavulanate and either ceftazidime or ceftiofur	NSAIDs Fluid therapy	Aggressively look for underlying cause
Skin/shell: *thermal burns, trauma (cage mate, dog attack, motor vehicle)*	**Mixed bacterial/fungal**: topical silver sulfadiazine, chlorhexidine, iodine or clotrimazole; systemic ceftiofur, ceftazidime **Fungal**: itraconazole, voriconazole **Tapeworm**: praziquantel **Ectoparasites**: topical ivermectin,[a] fipronil and pyrethroids	NSAIDs Fluid therapy, especially for burns	Neoplasias are not uncommon Adequate humidity is important for addressing shedding problems. Drug therapy rarely needed Regular substrate changes are very important for ectoparasite management Tapeworm cysts should be surgically resected

[a] Do not use the macrocyclic lactones in turtles, tortoises, indigo snakes, crocodilians or skinks. Toxicity is treated with fluid therapy.
NSAID, nonsteroidal anti-inflammatory drugs.

from interactions between the cultured bacterium and standardized concentrations of each antibiotic. The corollary to this is that if a sensitivity profile returns with a lot of 'resistants', a dose-dependent antibiotic, for example, may still be effective if a very high dose is chosen. Obviously, the adverse-effect profile of the drug must also be considered.

What Antibiotic Course Duration Should be Used?

There are numerous factors that should be considered when choosing the duration of an antibiotic course. The idea that an antibiotic course for a reptile should always extend for 14, 21 or 28 days is overly simplistic. For every antibiotic course that is started, the most common scenarios that the clinician will face are 'It's not working' and 'This is working really well, but how long do I go for?'. With 'It's not working', be prepared to change the plan. The definition of a fool is someone who does the same thing over and over expecting a different outcome. The clinician is strongly encouraged to revisit diagnostics. It is acceptable to change to a new antibiotic if the decision was directed by recent culture and sensitivity results. However, it is rare that changing from one empirically selected antibiotic to another one will provide a more favourable outcome.

When asked 'This is working really well, but how long do I go for?', try to have a checkpoint in mind that you see as an indicator that the patient has 'turned the corner'. At this checkpoint, consider administering an antibiotic for a short while longer (e.g. 4–5 days, but using common sense as you reflect on the progression of recovery). The 'turned the corner' checkpoint may be that the animal is now eating, walking, perching, supporting their own body weight, has defecated or passed urates for the first time since being hospitalized. An important exception to this generalization about stopping an antibiotic course involves the treatment of some chelonian shell infections. These infections typically require months of antibiotic therapy.

Antifungals

Fungal infections in reptiles occur most commonly on the skin. They are most often secondary to thermal burns or trauma and so specific treatment of the fungal infection should always occur in parallel to addressing the underlying problem, which will often be related to husbandry. Some fungal infections can be primary diseases (e.g. yellow fungus disease in dragons; see Chapter 16). These infections are usually treated topically with broad-spectrum antimicrobial creams such as silver sulfadiazine or with antifungal creams such as clotrimazole. Some fungal infections are treated systemically with terbinafine or antifungal azoles such as itraconazole or voriconazole. Antifungal courses vary in length from a couple of weeks to many weeks. Systemic fungal infections in reptiles are rare.

Antivirals

Our understanding of viral infections in reptiles is still very limited. Some infections can have no signs of disease (e.g. some adenovirus infections), while others can be highly infectious and pathogenic (e.g. some ferlavirus outbreaks). This creates a challenge for the clinician as to how these infections should be managed. These viruses can usually only be avoided through good biosecurity, as commercially available vaccines do not exist. The most extensively studied antivirals in reptiles are all purine analogues (acyclovir, ganciclovir and valacyclovir) and they have been associated with varying degrees of success in treating herpesvirus infections in tortoises. For some iridoviral infections, increasing the ambient temperature has been trialled. With this method, the animal is kept at an elevated temperature where viral replication is reduced. This can have animal welfare implications for the reptile and so this treatment should only be considered as a last resort, and only in heat-tolerant species. Sadly, for many reptiles clinically affected by viral infections, treatment is often palliative (e.g. nonsteroidal anti-inflammatory drugs) and sometimes euthanasia is the most suitable option.

Antiparasitics

Reptiles can be infested (often simultaneously) with a suite of parasites that cover a broad range of taxonomic groupings, most commonly nematodes, protozoa and a selection of external parasites (see Chapter 31). The majority of antiparasitics used in reptiles for internal helminths are administered orally and these include the benzimidazoles (e.g. fenbendazole) and the macrocyclic lactones (e.g. ivermectin, moxidectin). Both these drug classes are capable of causing toxicity under certain situations. The benzimidazoles have been associated with toxicity of the bone marrow (myelosuppression), intestinal epithelium, liver and fetuses, especially at higher doses given for longer periods (e.g. fenbendazole 100 mg/kg every 24 hours for 3 days with food or even 25 mg/kg as a single dose). It is important that only modern dose recommendations are followed for the benzimidazoles. Ivermectin has been associated with dose-dependent toxicity in a number of chelonian species (Teare and Bush 1983). It is suspected that the mechanism of toxicity is similar to that seen in susceptible dog breeds, where there is a deficiency in the P-glycoprotein pumps at the blood–brain barrier that would ordinarily prevent toxic concentrations in the brain. Toxic effects are predominantly neuromotor (e.g. paresis). The entire group of macrocyclic lactones should be avoided in turtles and tortoises.

Coccidiosis is a common infestation of reptiles, especially dragons, that can be very difficult to treat. Toltrazuril and its metabolite ponazuril are both coccidiocidal and have been shown to be effective in eliminating organism shedding. However, not all studies support these findings and longer-term studies that include post-mortem histological examinations are needed. The sulphonamides have also been used for this indication but similar reservations about drug efficacy need to be made. The owner should be informed about the difficulty in treating these infestations.

The drug paromomycin has been used for cryptosporidiosis but successful drug therapy is usually temporary. This parasite is notoriously difficult to treat.

Studies on topical imidacloprid–moxidectin and emodepside–praziquantel have revealed encouraging signs of efficacy against nematodes. Safety studies of these drugs in reptiles are lacking, so the use of these topical drugs should only occur following informed owner consent.

Topical antiparasitics are most commonly used for treating mite infestations in snakes. Ivermectin diluted in tap water, fipronil spray (not spot on) and the synthetic pyrethroids have all been used with success. Careful monitoring is required as neurological adverse effects have been observed with all three drugs.

Anti-Inflammatories and Analgesics

It can be very difficult to detect pain in reptiles but, despite this, it should be assumed that whatever causes pain in a mammal will cause similar levels of pain in reptiles. The corollary to this assumption is that inflammation in reptiles will be associated with pain and we assume that it can be attenuated by anti-inflammatory medications. Inflammatory pain can be caused by various noxious stimuli: thermal (e.g. thermal burns), mechanical (e.g. cage-mate trauma) and chemical (e.g. proinflammatory mediators secondary to infectious processes). It is typically treated with non-steroidal anti-inflammatory drugs (NSAIDs). Although controlled clinical trials are lacking that compare the efficacy and safety of the NSAIDs in reptiles, meloxicam is the NSAID that is preferred by a number of reptile practitioners. There have been recent pharmacokinetic studies that have assessed the plasma concentrations of meloxicam following the administration of standard doses, usually 0.1–0.2 mg/kg (Divers *et al.* 2010; Lai *et al.* 2015; Uney *et al.* 2016). Plasma concentrations associated with analgesia in mammals were found in green iguanas but not in loggerhead sea turtles or red-eared sliders.

The opioids represent a vitally important class of analgesics. Excepting euthanasia, they represent the most powerful method of pain relief available from a systemically administered drug. Furthermore, they generally have minimal effects on the cardiovascular system. Traditionally, their use in reptiles has been based on extrapolations from avian dosing. However, since the early 2000s, the results of a number of experiments on the efficacy of opioids in reptiles have been published. The opioids morphine (1–5 mg/kg subcutaneously or intramuscularly every 24 hours) and methadone (3–5 mg/kg subcutaneously or intramuscularly every 24 hours) and the opioid-like drug tramadol (5–10 mg/kg orally every 48–72 hours) have shown the best results in the few reptile species tested. The results of testing butorphanol and buprenorphine have been disappointing.

There are insufficient data to be able to recommend the use of corticosteroids as anti-inflammatories and analgesics, and similarly, the efficacy of other analgesics such amantadine, gabapentin, ketamine and alpha-2 agonists has not been properly substantiated. An excellent summary of clinical analgesia in reptiles is provided by Sladky and Mans (2012).

As mentioned earlier in this chapter, it can be difficult to assess pain (and therefore analgesia) in reptiles. This does not mean that the clinician should not attempt to do it. There are number of signs that reptiles can be display as manifestations of pain. Examples include aggression, decreased movement, guarding parts of their bodies and decreased intake of food and water. These signs are obviously non-specific to pain but improvement in these signs should be viewed favourably.

Learning More

The reader interested in learning more about reptile pharmacology and drug therapy is referred to the overview written by Mitchell (2006) and for a review of published literature on reptilian therapeutics, the work by Gibbons (2014) is recommended. Recommended reptile formularies can be found in Appendix 1 of this book and in the most recent edition of the *Exotic Animal Formulary* (Carpenter 2012). Information about drug stability and drug interactions can be found in product inserts (dossiers) and the veterinary drug formularies by Papich (2015) and Plumb (2015). For objective information about drug compounding produced by veterinary advocacy groups, the reader is referred to the guidelines produced by the American Veterinary Medical Association and the Australian Veterinary Association.

References

Carpenter, J.W. (2012) *Exotic Animal Formulary*, 4th ed. Elsevier Saunders, St Louis, MO.

Divers, S.J., Papich, M., McBride, M. *et al.* (2010). Pharmacokinetics of meloxicam following intravenous and oral administration in green iguanas (*Iguana iguana*). *American Journal of Veterinary Research,*. 71 (11), 1277–1283.

Gibbons P. (2014) Therapeutics, in *Current Therapy in Reptile Medicine and Surgery* (D. Mader and S. Divers, eds). Elsevier, St. Louis, MO, pp. 57–69.

Mitchell, M. (2006) Therapeutics, in *Reptile Medicine and Surgery*, 2nd ed. (D. Mader, ed.). Elsevier, St. Louis, MO, pp. 631–664.

Lai, R.O., Di Bello, A., Soloperto, S. *et al.* (2015). Pharmacokinetic behavior of meloxicam in loggerhead sea turtles (*Caretta caretta*) after intramuscular and Intravenous administration. *Journal of Wildlife Diseases*, 51 (2), 509–512.

Papich, M.G. (2015) *Saunders Handbook of Veterinary Drugs: Small and Large Animal*, 4th ed. Elsevier Saunders, St. Louis, MO.

Papich, M.G., Davidson, G.S. and Fortier, L.A. (2013) Doxycycline concentration over time after storage in a compounded veterinary preparation. *Journal of the American Veterinary Medical Association*, 242, 1674–1678.

Plumb, D. (2015) *Plumb's Veterinary Drug Handbook*, 8th ed. Wiley-Blackwell, Oxford, 2015.

Sladky, K.K. and Mans, C. (2012) Clinical analgesia in reptiles. *Journal of Exotic Pet Medicine*, 21, 158–167.

Teare, J. and Bush, M. (1983) Toxicity and efficacy of ivermectin in chelonians. *Journal of the American Veterinary Medical Association*, 183, 1195–1197.

Uney, K., Altan, F., Aboubakr, M. *et al.* (2016). Pharmacokinetics of meloxicam in red-eared slider turtles (*Trachemys scripta elegans*) after single intravenous and intramuscular injections. *American Journal of Veterinary Research*, 77 (5), 439–444.

Further Reading

American Veterinary Medical Association. Compounding. https://www.avma.org/KB/Resources/Reference/Pages/Compounding.aspx. 2016 (accessed 5 June 2017).

Australian Veterinary Association. Guidelines for the Preparation and Use of Compounded Pharmaceuticals. http://www.ava.com.au/newsarticle/guidelines-prescribing-and-using-compounded-medicines (accessed 5 June 2017).

Svendsen, O., Kok, L. and Lauritzenā, B. (2007) Nociception after intraperitoneal injection of a sodium pentobarbitone formulation with and without lidocaine in rats quantified by expression of neuronal c-fos in the spinal cord: a preliminary study. *Laboratory Animals*, 41, 197–203.

15

Nutritional and Metabolic Diseases

Brendan Carmel and Robert Johnson

Metabolic Bone Disease

The term 'metabolic bone disease' is not a single disease entity but rather a term used to describe a collection of medical disorders that affect the integrity and function of bones (see Chapter 25 for further discussion). Nonetheless, the term metabolic bone disease is used in this chapter as a broad phrase to cover the complex disease. Metabolic bone diseases likely comprise the most common disease conditions affecting captive reptiles.

Previously the forms of metabolic bone disease linked to improper diet, inadequate exposure to ultraviolet lighting or kidney dysfunction have been termed fibrous nutritional metabolic disease, osteodystrophy, nutritional secondary hyperparathyroidism (NSHP), osteodystrophia fibrosa, osteomalacia, renal osteodystrophy and rickets. There are other synonyms. For the purpose of this discussion, and for clarity, the general term metabolic bone disease will be used and will concentrate on the common forms of disease seen in captive reptiles.

The aetiology of metabolic bone disease is typically nutritional environmental or renal.

Causes

The predominant causes of metabolic bone disease in reptiles are prolonged deficiency of dietary calcium or vitamin D3, an imbalance of the calcium–phosphorus ratio in the diet (usually an excess of phosphorus), inadequate exposure to UVB radiation of appropriate wavelength or a lack of a suitable temperature zone (Figure 15.1).

Metabolic bone disease is most common in lizards and turtles. The condition is uncommon to rare in snakes as they usually eat whole food items and are more likely to receive and absorb adequate dietary levels of calcium and vitamin D3. Note than many reptiles that actively bask (heliothermic) may not have developed mechanisms to absorb or store dietary forms of vitamin D3, relying on the pathways described in this chapter to produce active vitamin D3 via UVB light.

Vitamin D Synthesis

In reptiles, UVB of the wavelength 290–315 nm reacts with the reptile skin and provitamin precursors are converted to previtamin D3. The previtamin D3 is then converted to vitamin D3 (cholecalciferol) via temperature-dependent isomerization (Hedley

Reptile Medicine and Surgery in Clinical Practice, First Edition. Edited by Bob Doneley, Deborah Monks, Robert Johnson and Brendan Carmel.
© 2018 John Wiley & Sons Ltd. Published 2018 by John Wiley & Sons Ltd.

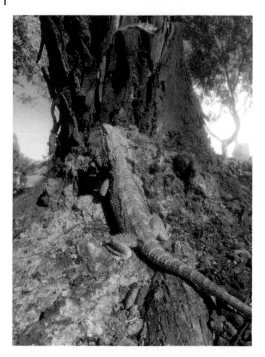

Figure 15.1 A free living central bearded dragon (*Pogona vitticeps*) basking. Metabolic bone disease only occurs in captive reptiles.

2012a). This is an important point: adequate temperature (via a basking zone in the reptile enclosure) is required for vitamin D3 synthesis to occur. Cholecalciferol is metabolized via renal and hepatic pathways to the active form of vitamin D3, calcitriol (1,25-DHCC). Calcitriol is required for absorption of calcium from the intestinal tract.

Captive animals may not have adequate exposure to UVB due to several factors, such as ultraviolet light not passing through Perspex or glass, inadequate ultraviolet lighting in the vivarium or infrequent replacement of ultraviolet globes: ultraviolet output diminishes with time (see Chapter 6 for more details).

To summarise: the most common causes of metabolic bone disease in captive reptiles are inadequate ultraviolet light, inadequate dietary calcium, an inappropriate calcium to phosphorous ratio and inadequate temperature zone (the reptile needs to be at an appropriate temperature to absorb ultraviolet light).

Pathogenesis

Homeostatic mechanisms work to maintain a constant blood calcium level, which is essential for normal function of cells. Any reduction in the blood calcium level from metabolic bone disease triggers production of parathyroid hormone. Parathyroid hormone stimulates an increase in blood calcium levels by increasing bone resorption, renal tubular reabsorption of calcium and phosphate excretion in the urine. Parathyroid hormone also stimulates the formation of calcitriol (1,25-DHCC), which in turn increases the absorption of intestinal calcium.

If insufficient calcium is available from the diet, calcium is resorbed from the bones to compensate. With a prolonged deficiency, the resultant osteopenia weakens the bones leading to rickets (young animals) or osteomalacia (adult animal). Susceptible reptile groups include most diurnal species: agamids (dragons), skinks, turtles, iguanas, varanids (monitors) and chameleons (Figure 15.2). Young, actively growing reptiles, mature, reproductively active females and herbivorous and insectivorous species are particularly prone to developing metabolic bone disease, (insectivorous species due to the difficulty of providing an appropriate captive diet with the right balance of calcium).

Clinical metabolic bone disease is uncommon in adult reptiles, which have a lesser demand for calcium, the exception being breeding females. Reptiles fed on a whole-animal diet, such as most snakes, are unlikely to exhibit clinical metabolic bone disease, as the diet likely provides adequate vitamin D and calcium. Subclinical disease may be present, although no studies have investigated this theory.

Clinical Signs

Common clinical signs include weakness, musculoskeletal deformities, anorexia, poor growth or weight loss, abnormal shell

Figure 15.2 Severe stunting, bone loss and rubber jaw in a juvenile lace monitor (*Varanus varius*).

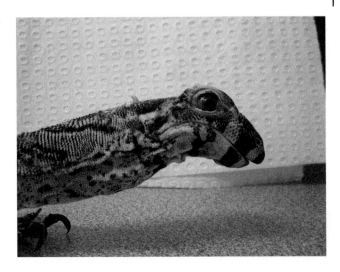

Figure 15.3 Kyphosis, lordosis in an eastern blue-tongued skink (*Tiliqua scincoides*).

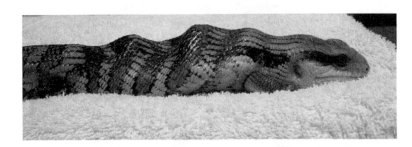

Figure 15.4 Spinal deformity in a central bearded dragon (*Pogona vitticeps*) with metabolic bone disease.

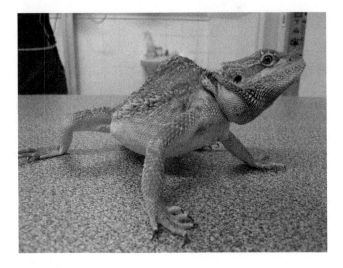

growth in chelonians, paresis/paralysis and tremors. Other more specific signs may include an inability to walk, hyperreflexia, hypermetria, tetany, seizures; lordosis, kyphosis, scoliosis, pathological fractures and stunted growth (rostral 'rounding', small head); prolapse of the cloaca, colon, hemipenis, oviduct or tongue (occurring in Old World chameleons; Figures 15.3 and 15.4). Fibrous osteodystrophy is common in green

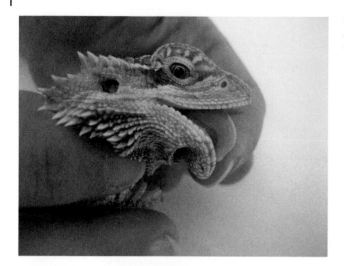

Figure 15.5 Rubber jaw in a juvenile central bearded dragon (*Pogona vitticeps*).

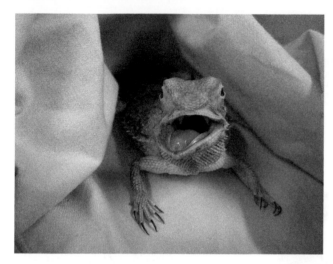

Figure 15.6 Rubber jaw in a juvenile pygmy bearded dragon (*Pogona henrylawsoni*).

iguanas, manifesting as a thickness and swelling of the long bones and mandible. Demineralization of bony tissue may lead to softer, more pliable bones, particularly the mandible (Figures 15.5 and 15.6). Bloating and decreased gastrointestinal motility may also occur. It has been suggested that metabolic bone disease may be a factor in spinal osteopathy (proliferative spinal osteoathropathy; see Chapter 25).

Differential Diagnosis

Other disease processes which may result in similar clinical signs include renal metabolic bone disease (RMBD), spinal osteopathy (proliferative spinal osteoathropathy), osteomyelitis, trauma, sepsis, neoplasia, toxins/poisons, other vitamin/mineral deficiency or excess, and osteomalacia.

Diagnosis

Metabolic bone disease is strongly suspected in many cases based on clinical history (diet and husbandry in particular) and physical examination. Whole-body radiographs often confirm suspicions, with characteristic changes of decreased bone density, pathological fractures (often 'folding' fractures; Figure 15.7 and 15.8), bending and distortion of bones and increased

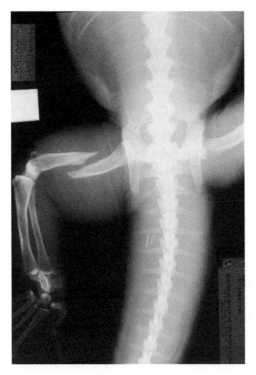

Figure 15.7 Pathological fracture of the femur in an adult perentie (*Varanus giganteus*).

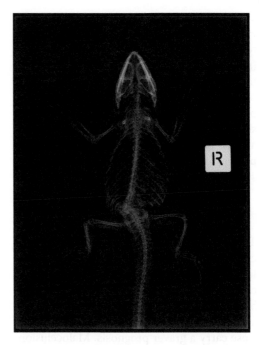

Figure 15.8 Spinal deformity of the caudal lumbar spine and tibia and fibula fracture in a central bearded dragon (*Pogona vitticeps*) with metabolic bone disease.

and uneven cortical widening due to fibrous osteodystrophy.

Clinical pathology results may be normal, as the reptile will try to keep calcium levels within normal range. Reptiles with renal metabolic bone disease are typically hypocalcaemic and have high phosphorus levels. Ionized calcium is a more accurate representation of physiologically active calcium, although normal ranges are available for very few species.

Treatment

Stabilize the patient and treat life-threatening signs first. Long-term treatment is usually required for many weeks to months, during which time husbandry deficiencies can be addressed. An early assessment of the client and their commitment is required. Euthanasia may be recommended for patients where there is little chance of success or when dealing with a client who is not dedicated.

Initial Treatment

Warm the patient and provide the preferred optimal temperature zone for the species to allow the patient to thermoregulate and achieve its preferred body temperature. Commence nutritional support and give fluid therapy if required. Analgesia is indicated in most cases as metabolic bone disease is thought to be a painful condition. If signs of hypocalcaemia, such as tremors, seizures or tetany, are present, give calcium gluconate intramuscularly until the signs have abated. Provide appropriate lighting (see Chapter 6). Once stabilized, oral calcium supplementation (calcium glubionate) and Vitamin D3 should be provided. See Appendix 1 for dose rates.

Long-term Treatment

Husbandry improvements should be made to ensure adequate exposure to UVB light (see Chapter 6) and the opportunity to thermoregulate within the species' preferred optimal temperature zone. A diet with suitable levels of vitamins D2, D3 and calcium should be provided. Specific attention should also be paid to the management of chronic pain associated with secondary conditions such as degenerative joint disease.

Prognosis

The prognosis will vary according to the chronicity and severity of clinical signs. Ideally early identification and treatment of clinical signs will prevent or at least lessen bony changes, such as fibrous osteodystrophy and pathological fractures, paralysis or prolapse carry a graver prognosis. Malocclusion secondary to fibrous dystrophy may also occur, leading to dysphagia and weakness.

Renal Secondary Hyperparathyroidism

Causes

Causes of renal secondary hyperparathyroidism (RSHP) include dehydration, a high-protein diet, hypervitaminosis D, toxins and primary renal disease.

Pathogenesis

In cases of chronic renal insufficiency, decreased filtration of phosphate occurs, leading to hyperphosphataemia. In the healthy animal, parathyroid hormone promotes renal hydroxylation of 25-hydroxycholecalciferol to form calcitriol, the most active form of vitamin D. However, hyperphosphataemia has a negative effect on hydroxylation in renal tubular cells and decreases calcitriol production, leading to RSHP and osteodystrophy.

Diagnosis

A blood calcium to phosphorus ratio of less than one is a reliable diagnostic indicator of renal disease in reptiles. Hypoproteinaemia is also a common finding in lizards with metabolic bone disease, particularly green iguanas. Hyperuricaemia is not commonly observed in reptiles with renal disease (discussed in Chapter 11). Differential diagnoses of RSHP include NSHP, hypertrophic osteopathy and osteomyelitis.

Treatment

Treatment of RSHP is mostly supportive, as the prognosis is poor in most cases. Supportive care is instituted as for metabolic bone disease. See Chapter 13 for information on fluid therapy. Phosphate binders such as aluminium hydroxide or calcium carbonate and chitosan may be of some use in helping to control hyperphosphataemia.

Reptiles with renal disease may present with concurrent illness such as gut impaction, preovulatory follicular stasis or gout (see Chapter 23 for more detail). The underlying renal disease may not be apparent initially and the practitioner is advised to ensure that a diagnostic workup is performed to detect any concurrent illness.

Obesity

Pathogenesis

Obesity is not uncommon in captive reptiles yet it may go undiagnosed by both veterinarians and owners. Sedentary captive reptiles are often fed high-fat diets and are fed too much and too often, resulting in energy intake significantly higher than energy expenditure (Figure 15.9). A thorough clinical examination of the patient and evaluation of

Figure 15.9 Obese captive frilled lizard (*Chlamydosaurus kingii*).

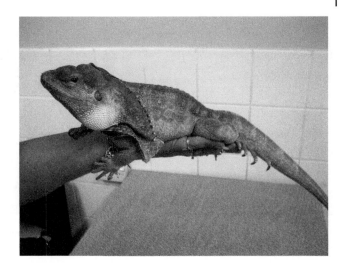

Figure 15.10 Large intracoelomic fat pads and hepatic lipidosis in obese central bearded dragon (*Pogona vitticeps*).

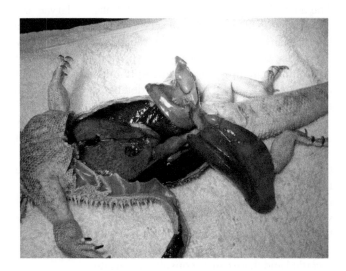

the captive diet and clinical history may indicate obvious signs of obesity. Excess intracoelomic fat will typically result in obvious coelomic distension (Figure 15.10). Some obese reptiles will have excessive fat stores in subcutaneous tissues or internal organs with resultant derangements, such as hepatic lipidosis. Clinical pathology may point towards organ dysfunction from fatty change and biopsy of affected organs. Other possible consequences of obesity include dystocia and decreased lifespan.

Treatment

Treatment of a reptile with obesity centres on ensuring that the animal is provided with adequate amounts and correct types of feed to enable safe weight loss. This is best undertaken slowly while monitoring the patient and evaluating clinical parameters. Specific treatment is required for any obesity related illnesses, such as hepatic lipidosis (see Chapter 19).

Prevention is aimed at educating clients regarding appropriate diets for captive animals and feeding frequency (Figure 15.11).

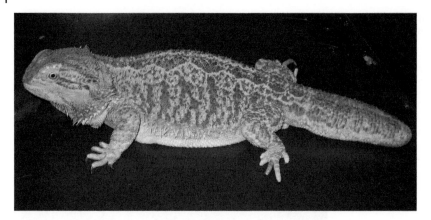

Figure 15.11 Treating an obese reptile is best undertaken by closely monitoring and a diet aimed at providing slow weight loss (courtesy of Brendan Carmel).

The nutritional requirements and metabolic rate of an individual reptile will vary, depending on many factors, such as sex, reproductive status, seasonal cycles and the vivarium environment (temperature gradient, humidity etc.; see Chapter 4 for further details of nutritional requirements). The effect of brumation, or lack thereof, on nutritional status of captive reptiles is unknown.

Although there is a lack of specific nutritional requirements for many captive reptiles, some general recommendations can be made to help to prevent obesity. Regular weighing of the reptile is a simple and effective method of monitoring condition. Some captive species have average body weights recorded and these can be consulted. Educate owners that captive reptiles lead predominantly a sedentary lifestyle, undergoing very little exercise, and are often fed food items high in fat. Owners should record the type and amount of food offered and its frequency and relate the diet fed to the natural diet of the species concerned. Overfeeding may be prevented in many cases by simply reducing the feeding frequency; for example, offering a thawed rat to an adult snake every two to three weeks rather than weekly. Carnivores should be fed lean prey, herbivores should be fed a diet high in fibre and insectivores should be offered food items low in fat. For example, mealworm (*Tenebrio molitor*)

larvae contain a much higher fat content than the adult mealworm beetle and would be best avoided or restricted as a food item for a bearded dragon.

It is not known whether increasing exercise will have a positive effect on an obese reptile or how practical this would be to initiate. Changing the habitat to encourage natural hunting, such as hiding food items and providing scent trails to follow, will help to encourage some reptiles to exercise.

Hypovitaminosis A

Pathogenesis

Hypovitaminosis A results from a diet lacking in vitamin A precursors/provitamins (carotenoids) and/or vitamin A (retinol, retinal and retinoic acid). It may take many months for a vitamin A deficiency to develop, as the liver can store vitamin A for long periods. Vitamin A is involved in many processes, including maintaining normal epithelial tissue. Hypovitaminosis A is most commonly seen in aquatic or semi-aquatic turtles; for example, the red-eared slider (*Trachemys scripta elegans*) and box turtles (*Terrapene* spp.), insectivorous reptiles (e.g. chameleons and geckos), young or reproductively active female lizards or turtles and crocodilians.

Herbivorous reptiles can endogenously synthesize vitamin A from dietary carotenoids. Vitamin A deficiency is uncommon to rare in these species, as many plants contain high amounts of carotenoids. Hypovitaminosis A would probably only occur if the animal were anorexic for several months. Vitamin A deficiency is also uncommon in carnivorous snakes fed whole prey items.

Clinical signs

Clinical signs can be non-specific but are typically related to the squamous metaplasia that occurs as a result of the deficiency, with the Harderian and lacrimal glands often affected. Classic signs in aquatic turtles and chameleons are swollen and closed eyelids. Other possible signs include blepharitis, blepharoedema, blepharitis, conjunctivitis, blindness from retinal damage, nasal discharge and respiratory disease. Nonspecific signs such as stomatitis, dysecdysis, stunted growth, anorexia and lethargy may also be present.

Diagnosis

Diagnosis is usually achieved by taking a good clinical history and conducting a thorough physical examination. Confirmation can be difficult, as vitamin A levels cannot be evaluated via blood sampling. Plasma retinol, one of the biologically active compounds of vitamin A, could be of use but interpretation can be challenging. Liver biopsy may be considered with hepatic vitamin A levels for carnivorous reptiles found to be greater than 1000 iu/g and are likely much less in herbivorous reptiles. Biopsy requires surgery, endoscopy or ultrasound-guided sampling and may not be practical in small reptiles. Response to therapy is often used to confirm the diagnosis. A full blood screen is advised to look for underlying issues.

Treatment

Treatment involves addressing any secondary issues, such as bacterial infections, and correcting the vitamin A deficiency, typically via supplementation for weeks to months. Any debris acclimated in the conjunctival sacs is removed and the eyes flushed with saline. Dose rates for vitamin A are mostly extrapolated from mammalian studies or from anecdotal reports. Oral supplementation is not necessarily safer as over-supplementation can occur regardless of the route of administration. Clinical improvements can take up to several weeks, depending on severity (see Hypervitaminosis A section for toxic effects of overdosing). Some reported dose rates for vitamin A in reptiles are given in Appendix 1 in this book.

Prevention

Prevention of hypovitaminosis A centres around providing an appropriate diet for the species. Feed carnivorous or omnivorous reptiles whole prey items such as rodents or whole fish. Commercial pellets are suitable for some species, such as aquatic turtle pellets. Invertebrates contain a low amount of vitamin A, so should be gut loaded and dusted with a supplement that contains vitamin A. Wild-caught invertebrates can be of excellent nutritional value, especially if part of the natural diet of the species. Herbivorous reptiles are unlikely to be vitamin A deficient if they are fed a broad-based diet of vegetables, as they are able to synthesize vitamin A from dietary carotenoids.

Hypervitaminosis A

Causes

Hypervitaminosis A is almost always caused by overzealous treatment with vitamin A, especially parenteral forms, but it can also occur if excessive amounts of raw liver are fed.

Clinical signs

Clinical signs are typically skin lesions, with characteristic flaking of skin, ulceration, blistering or sloughing seen. Secondary infections are common and depression, lethargy, anorexia and dehydration may also be seen.

Treatment

Treatment is based on supportive care, treating secondary infections if present, providing fluid therapy and assisted feeding where required, together with analgesia. Recovery may be prolonged.

Prevention

Prevent by avoiding vitamin A administration unless indicated (by evaluating the diet and patient). Do not give vitamin A at high doses or for prolonged periods. Note that herbivorous reptiles are extremely unlikely to develop hypovitaminosis A unless they are anorexic for long periods, so avoid administration of vitamin A to these species unless a vitamin A deficiency is confirmed.

Thiamine Deficiency

Thiamine, or vitamin B1, is a water-soluble vitamin part of the B complex required by all living organisms but only synthesized in bacteria, fungi and plants. All animals must therefore obtain thiamine from their diet.

Cause

Captive reptiles fed a large percentage of thawed fish are prone to thiamine deficiency. A slow thaw will result in a build-up of the thiaminase. The enzyme is not destroyed by the freezing process and depletes the thiamine present in the fish. Thiamine deficiency may also occur in herbivorous reptiles; for example, if the multivitamin supplement is lacking in thiamine, as thiamine is highly labile and may undergo rapid deterioration if the supplement is not used in a timely fashion or is stored incorrectly.

Clinical signs

Signs of thiamine deficiency relate to resultant nerve degeneration and neuropathy and typically include neurological signs such as tremors, incoordination, opisthotonus and torticollis. Diagnosis is typically based on the clinical history and clinical signs. Confirmation of the disease is via demonstrating the characteristic histopathological changes in the nervous system. Captive species of reptiles more likely to develop thiamine deficiency include semiaquatic turtles and crocodilians fed primarily a fish diet.

Treatment

Treatment is via administration of thiamine 50–100 mg/kg intramuscularly, subcutaneously or orally once daily or administering a vitamin B complex formulation which contains thiamine (Mans and Braun 2014). For crocodilians, thiamine can be administered in 30 g/kg of fish orally.

Postprandial Cardiac Hypertrophy in Pythons

Oxygen consumption by carnivorous reptiles increases enormously after they have eaten a large meal, to meet metabolic demands, and this places an extra load on the cardiovascular system. In the Burmese python (*Python molurus*) an extraordinarily rapid 40% increase in ventricular muscle mass occurs 48 hours after feeding, mainly due to increased gene expression of muscle-contractile proteins (Andersen 2005).

Hyperglycaemia in Bearded Dragons

Persistent hyperglycaemia associated with gastric neuroendocrine carcinoma in bearded dragons has been reported. Affected lizards may have a chronic history of anorexia, weight loss, depression and melaena. The neoplastic cells secrete somatostatin, inhibiting insulin release, which results in hyperglycaemia. Coelomic ultrasound may reveal the primary tumour in the stomach wall and metastases in the liver. The prognosis is poor and the diagnosis is often only confirmed at necropsy.

References

Hedley, J. (2012a) Metabolic bone disease in reptiles: part 1. *Companion Animal*, 17 (6), 52–54.

Mans, C. and Braun, J. (2014) Update on common nutritional disorders of captive reptiles. *Veterinary Clinics of North America Exotic Animals*, 17, 369–395.

Further Reading

Andersen, J.B., Rourke, B.C., Caiozzo, V.J. *et al.* (2005). Physiology: postprandial cardiac hypertrophy in pythons. *Nature*, 434 (7029), 37–38.

Carpenter, J.W. (2012) *Exotic Animal Formulary*, 4th ed. Elsevier Saunders, St Louis, MO.

Divers, S.J. and Cooper, J.E. (2000) Reptile hepatic lipidosis. *Seminars in Avian and Exotic Pet Medicine*, 9 (3), 153–164.

Frye, F.L. (1991) Common pathologic lesions and disease processes, in *Biomedical and Surgical Aspects of Captive Reptile Husbandry*, 2nd ed. Krieger, Malabar, FL, pp. 529–617.

Hedley, J. (2012b) Metabolic bone disease in reptiles: part 2. *Companion Animal*, 17 (7), 38–41.

Lyons, J.A., Newman, S.J., Greenacre, C.B. and Dunlap, J. (2010) A gastric neuroendocrine carcinoma expressing somatostatin in a bearded dragon (*Pogona vitticeps*). *Journal of Veterinary Diagnostic Investigation*, 22 (2), 316–320.

Mader, D.R. (2006) Metabolic bone diseases, in *Reptile Medicine and Surgery*, 2nd ed. (S.J. Divers and D.R. Mader, eds). Elsevier Saunders, St Louis, MO, pp. 841–851.

Ritter, J.M., Garner, M.M., Chilton, J.A. *et al.* (2009) Gastric neuroendocrine carcinomas in bearded dragons (*Pogona vitticeps*). *Veterinary Pathology Online, 2009* 46 (6), 1109–1116.

Simpson, M. (2006) Hepatic lipidosis in a black-headed python (*Aspidites melanocephalus*). *Veterinary Clinics of North America Exotic Animals*, 9, 589–598.

Wright, K.M. and Whitaker, B.R. (2001) Nutritional disorders, in *Amphibian Medicine and Captive Husbandry* (K.M. Wright and B.R. Whitaker, eds) Krieger, Malabar, FL. pp. 73–87.

16

Infectious Diseases and Immunology
Tim Hyndman and Rachel E. Marschang

Introduction

The collective knowledge of the infectious diseases of reptiles has been rapidly expanding in the last few years. Major breakthroughs have become commonplace. We now find ourselves in a golden age of new agent discovery and, as never before, we can detect a wide range of infectious agents with extraordinary sensitivity. Despite this, significant gaps still exist in our knowledge of infectious agents regarding routes of infection, pathogenicity, pathogenesis, treatment methods and prognoses. In spite of these limitations, however, several generalizations can still be made. It should be assumed that husbandry has played a part in all disease processes in reptiles. Inadequate husbandry will increase the susceptibility of reptiles to infection by viruses, bacteria, fungi and parasites. Mixed infections are commonplace in reptiles and the clinician should always be hesitant to conclude that a single aetiological agent is to blame for any disease process. The lack of detailed knowledge of the biology for many of these agents makes interpreting test results difficult. For example, a negative test result for an infectious agent should not be automatically interpreted to mean the animal is uninfected because it is often unknown how reliably that organism will be present in the part of the animal that was sampled. This overview is presented according to the anatomical location of the primary clinical complaint. Tables 16.1 and 16.2 provide summaries of the infectious diseases covered in this section and also serve to direct the reader to the relevant section of text.

Upper Respiratory Tract

Rhinitis and upper respiratory tract illness is most commonly seen in chelonians. In tortoises, mycoplasma, particularly *Mycoplasma agassizii*, is one of the most important causes of upper respiratory tract disease. Infected animals can develop palpebral oedema, conjunctivitis and rhinitis, although subclinical infections are also frequently reported. Infected animals remain persistently infected and may experience periods of recurring disease. These animals can shed mycoplasma, especially when they have nasal discharge (Figure 16.1). Mycoplasma have been repeatedly detected in aquatic turtles and sporadically reported in squamate reptiles, although their association with disease in those animals is not well understood. Testing for mycoplasma in chelonians is generally via polymerase chain reaction (PCR) using nasal lavages or oral swabs. In tortoises, detection of antibodies by enzyme-linked immunosorbent assay

Reptile Medicine and Surgery in Clinical Practice, First Edition. Edited by Bob Doneley, Deborah Monks, Robert Johnson and Brendan Carmel.
© 2018 John Wiley & Sons Ltd. Published 2018 by John Wiley & Sons Ltd.

Table 16.1 List of infectious agents mentioned in this chapter and clinically relevant information.[1]

Infectious agent	System most commonly affected[2]	Pathogenicity[3]	Infectivity[4]	Diagnostic test			Treatment		Other considerations
				Live animal	Serology[5]	Dead animal[6]	Environment[7]	Host	
Viruses:									
Adenovirus	Alimentary, liver > lower respiratory > neurological	0, +[1], ++	+, ++	PCR: cloacal swab	Virus neutralization	PCR: intestine, liver; Histology: liver, intestine	Difficult	None	–
Arenavirus/ inclusion body disease	Neurological, > lower respiratory, upper alimentary > skin, liver, blood	0, +[1], ++, +++	+	PCR: oesophageal swab, whole blood. Direct examination or IHC of whole blood/buffy coat smear	None	PCR: brain > liver, kidney; Histology: brain > liver, kidney	Routine	None	–
Bornavirus	Neurological, > upper alimentary	+, ++[1]	++	PCR: oral-cloacal swab	None	PCR: brain	Routine	None	–
Erythrocytic necrosis	Blood: > systemic	0, +, ++	0	Cytology: blood smear; PCR: blood	None	Histopathology, PCR: blood, liver	Routine	None (increase ambient temperature)	Probably transmitted by arthropods
Ferlavirus[8]	Lower respiratory > neurological	0, +, ++[1], +++	+++	PCR: lung wash, oral-cloacal swab	HI	PCR: lung > gut, liver, kidney, brain	Routine	None	–
Herpesvirus	Upper alimentary, upper respiratory > skin/shell, liver, neurological	0, +, ++, +++*	++	PCR: oral swab, lesions	Virus neutralization (some strains)	PCR: tongue, liver, brain, lesions	Routine	Aciclovir, ganciclovir, supportive therapy	Infectivity dependent on host species and virus strain; causes latent infections
Invertebrate iridoviruses	Skin	0*, +, ++	0, +	PCR: skin biopsy	None	PCR: skin, liver	Routine	None	–

Agent	Tissue distribution	Grade		Antemortem test	Serology	Postmortem test	Culture	Treatment	Comments
Nidovirus/coronavirus	Lower respiratory > upper alimentary	+, ++*, +++	++	PCR: lung wash, oral-cloacal swab	None	PCR: lung	Routine	None	–
Picornavirus[9]	Skin/shell, upper respiratory, kidney	0, +, ++*, +++	++	PCR and/or virus isolation: oral swab	Virus neutralization	PCR and/or virus isolation: tongue, oesophagus, intestine, trachea > other tissues	Difficult	None	–
Poxvirus	Skin	+*, ++*	+, ++	Cytology, PCR: skin	None	Histopathology, PCR: skin	Routine	None	–
Ranavirus	Upper respiratory, upper alimentary, liver, skin	0, +, ++*, +++	++, +++	PCR: oral swab, blood	None	PCR: liver, intestine, kidney, skin	Routine	None, increase ambient temperature	–
Reovirus	Lower respiratory > upper alimentary, alimentary, liver, neurological	0, +*, ++	?	PCR: oral-cloacal swab	Virus neutralization	PCR: lung, gut, kidney > brain	Difficult	None	–
Sunshinevirus	Neurological > lower respiratory, upper alimentary, skin, blood	0, +, ++*, +++	++	PCR: oral-cloacal swab	None	PCR: brain > kidney, lung	Routine	None	–
West Nile virus	Skin, blood	0*, +, ++, +++	+	PCR: Blood	ELISA	PCR: blood	Routine	None	Arbovirus, highly pathogenic in crocodilians, zoonotic
Bacteria:									
Chlamydia	Lower respiratory, liver > heart	+*, ++	?	PCR: tracheal wash, lesions	None	PCR: lesions, lung, liver	Routine	Systemic antibiotics	Some species are zoonotic

(Continued)

Table 16.1 (Continued)

Infectious agent	System most commonly affected[2]	Pathogenicity[3]	Infectivity[4]	Diagnostic test			Treatment		Other considerations
				Live animal	Serology[5]	Dead animal[6]	Environment[7]	Host	
Devriesea agamarum	Skin > systemic	0, +*, ++	+	Culture: skin scrapings, oral swabs	ELISA	Culture: skin	Routine	Ceftiofur 5 mg/kg IM for at least 12 days	–
Mycobacterium	Lower respiratory, liver > skin/shell, spleen, neurological > all other systems	0, +*, ++, +++	0, +	PCR, culture, cytology with acid-fast staining: lesions	None	PCR, culture, histopathology with acid-fast staining: lesions	Difficult	None	–
Mycoplasma	Upper respiratory > lower respiratory	0, +, ++*	+, ++*	PCR: nasal lavage > oral swab	ELISA	Nasal cavity	Routine	Systemic and local (nasal flush) antibiotics (especially fluoroquinolones (enrofloxacin), macrolides (clarithromycin) and tetracyclines); increased ambient temperature	Animals can remain persistently infected despite therapy
Fungi:									
Chamaeleomyces granulomatis	Liver, upper alimentary, skin, systemic	+, ++	+	Culture, cytology, PCR: oral-cloacal swabs, liver biopsy	None	Histology, culture, PCR: material from lesions	Routine	Nystatin, terbinafine	–

Nannizziopsis spp./ yellow fungus disease	Skin, liver	+, ++*, +++	++	Cytology, culture, PCR: skin scrapings, skin biopsy	None	Histopathology, culture, PCR: skin	Routine	Voriconazole	–
Ophidiomyces ophiodiicola	Skin	++, +++	++	Cytology, culture, PCR: skin scrapings, skin biopsy	None	Histopathology, culture, PCR: skin	Routine	Treatment as for *Nannizziopsis* spp. can be attempted	–
Yeasts (*Candida* spp.)	Alimentary	0, +, ++	0, +	Culture: cloacal swabs, faeces	None	Culture: intestine (interpretation with associated histology)	Routine	Nystatin, probiotics	Common in the environment and as commensals
Parasites:									
Acanthamoeba (protozoan)	Neurological, alimentary	0*, +++	+	Faecal exam: unstained, iodine stained	None	Histopathology: brain	Steam, heat	Treatment as for *Entamoeba invadens* can be attempted. No standard treatment reported	Intestinal forms non-pathogenic; neurological form only detectable post mortem
Choleoimeria spp. (protozoan)	Liver	+, ++*	++	Floatation: faeces	None	Histopathology: liver	Difficult	Some success reported with toltrazuril in combination with clindamycin over several days	–
Coccidia (e.g. *Isospora* spp.) (protozoan)	Alimentary	0, +*, ++	++	Microscopy, floatation: faeces	None	Microscopy, floatation: intestinal content	Difficult	Toltrazuril, hygiene	–

(Continued)

Table 16.1 (Continued)

Infectious agent	System most commonly affected[2]	Pathogenicity[3]	Infectivity[4]	Diagnostic test			Treatment		Other considerations
				Live animal	Serology[5]	Dead animal[6]	Environment[7]	Host	
Cryptosporidium spp. (protozoan)	Alimentary	++*, +++	++	PCR (and sequencing), microscopy, ELISA: faeces, gastric lavage (snakes), slime from surface of regurgitated food items (snakes)	None	Histopathology, PCR (and sequencing): stomach (snakes), intestine (lizards)	Difficult	Paromomycin, hygiene	Treatment does not eliminate the organism
Entamoeba invadens (protozoan)	Alimentary > liver, kidney	+, ++, +++*	++	Microscopy, iodine staining: faeces	None	Histopathology: intestine	Steam, heat	Metronidazole, paromomycin, increased ambient temperature, hygiene	–
Hexamita parva (protozoan)	Kidney < alimentary	0*, +, ++, +++	++	Microscopy: faeces, urine	None	Histopathology: kidney	Routine	Metronidazole	–
Intranuclear coccidiosis of tortoises (protozoan)	Alimentary, upper respiratory, liver, all other systems	+, ++*, +++	++	PCR: nasal lavage, oral-cloacal swab	None	PCR: Intestine, liver, kidney, pancreas > other tissues	Difficult	Toltrazuril, increased ambient temperature	–
Ophionyssus natricis (mite)	Skin	+, ++	+++	Visualization on skin	None	Visualization on skin	Difficult	Ivermectin, fipronil, pyrethroid	Environmental treatment is essential
Oxyurids (nematode)	Alimentary	0*, +, ++	++	Faecal examination, floatation	None	Microscopy: intestinal content	Difficult	Fenbendazole, hygiene	

Agent	System(s) affected[2]	Presentation[3]	Infectivity[4]	Antemortem diagnosis	Serology[5]	Post-mortem diagnosis[6]	Disinfection[7]	Treatment	Comments
Pentastomid (arthropod)	Lower respiratory > skin	0*, +, ++, +++	0	Endoscopy, radiography, faecal examination	None	Histopathology: lung, gut, skin nodules	Routine	Physical removal, macrocyclic lactone	Some species are zoonotic. Drug treatment can sometimes cause more harm than good due to the release of antigens from killed adult pentastomids
Strongylids, e.g. *Kalicephalus* spp. (nematode)	Alimentary	0, +*, ++	++	Faecal examination, floatation	None	Difficult	Difficult	Fenbendazole, hygiene	–
Spirometra (tapeworm)	Liver, skin, alimentary	0, +*	0	Faecal examination, floatation, skin swellings	None	Microscopy: intestinal content and skin swelling	Difficult	Praziquantel and surgical removal of skin nodules	–

[1] Controlled studies do not exist to support or refute much of this information. In these situations, the information provided has been based on anecdotal accounts or has been extrapolated from first principles knowledge of the biology of these infectious agents.

[2] System(s) most commonly affected; section of chapter to consult.

[3] Most common presentation: 0 subclinical, + mild, ++ moderate, +++ severe, * most common.

[4] Infectivity to conspecifics in captive environment: 0 non-infectious,? unknown, + low, ++ moderate, +++ high.

[5] Sample is always plasma or serum. Many of these serological tests are not widely available.

[6] Test for agent in dead animal; priority samples. A complete set of samples should be collected from all necropsies but extra attention should be paid to the organs listed.

[7] Routine treatment: household disinfectants; difficult: specialized disinfectants (Virkon, F10, bleach)

[8] Formerly ophidian paramyxovirus.

[9] 'Topivirus', virus 'x').

ELISA, enzyme-linked immunosorbent assay; HI, haemagglutination inhibition; IHC, immunohistochemistry; IM, intramuscularly.

Table 16.2 Agents most commonly implicated as primary disease of each system in chelonians, lizards and snakes.[1]

System affected	Chelonian	Lizard	Snake
Upper respiratory tract (rhinitis)	Mycoplasma, TINC, herpesvirus	–	Nidovirus
Lower respiratory tract (pneumonia)	–	–	Ferlavirus, nidovirus, arenavirus/IBD, pentastomids
Upper alimentary tract (glossitis and stomatitis)	Herpesvirus, ranavirus	*Chamaeleomyces*	Nidovirus, arenavirus/inclusion body disease
Alimentary tract (obstipation, diarrhoea, vomiting, regurgitation)	–	Adenovirus, coccidia, cryptosporidia	*Entamoeba invadens*, strongylids
Liver	Herpesvirus, ranavirus	Adenovirus, choleoeimeria	Arenavirus/IBD
Neurological system	Herpesvirus	Adenovirus	Arenavirus/IBD, bornavirus, Sunshinevirus, ferlavirus
Skin/shell	Herpesvirus, picornavirus	*Nannizziopsis* spp., *Devriesea agamarum*, mites	*Ophionyssus natricis*, *Ophidiomyces ophiodiicola*
Kidney/urinary tract	Picornavirus, *Hexamita parva*	–	–
Blood	–	–	Arenavirus/IBD

[1] Summaries of each agent are presented in Table 16.1. Secondary and tertiary causes of diseases, such as most bacterial and fungal infections, are not included in this table but will still often need to be treated.
IBD, inclusion body disease.

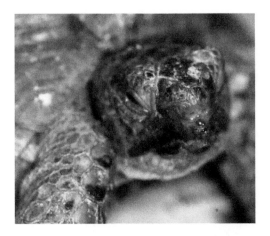

Figure 16.1 A spur-thighed tortoise (*Testudo graeca*) with nasal discharge indicative of rhinitis. This is often caused by infections with mycoplasma in tortoises but can also be associated with picornavirus or herpesvirus infections, as well as intranuclear coccidia.

(ELISA) can be helpful in detecting persistently infected animals (see Chapter 11). Ranaviruses have also been associated with rhinitis in tortoises but these viruses can also infect other reptiles, including aquatic turtles and various species of squamate reptiles. Ranavirus-infected animals may be anorectic and lethargic and may develop conjunctivitis, stomatitis, hepatitis, enteritis and pneumonia. Ranaviruses can be transmitted between reptile species and families, and even between reptiles, amphibians and fish. In live animals, ranavirus infections are generally diagnosed by testing oral swabs by PCR. In box turtles, blood can be used for virus detection. Picornaviruses have also been described as a possible cause of rhinitis in tortoises (see Skin/Shell Disease). Herpesviruses have been known to cause rhinitis in tortoises (see Upper Alimentary Tract Disease). Intranuclear coccidia have been described as a cause of rhinitis in various tortoise species (see Alimentary Tract Disease). A multitude of different bacteria can be involved in upper respiratory tract disease in reptiles. In general, these are involved in multifactorial disease processes.

Lower Respiratory Tract

The infectious causes of lower respiratory tract disease seen in reptile practice include viruses, bacteria, fungi and parasites. Disease of this system is common in all reptile species.

Ferlaviruses were previously reported in the literature as 'reptilian' or 'ophidian' paramyxoviruses. Ferlaviruses are seen far more commonly in snakes than lizards and chelonians. Clinically, infection can be characterized by dyspnoea, sometimes with open-mouth breathing, and oral secretions that are sometimes bloody (Figure 16.2). Nonrespiratory signs of disease, such as neurological signs, are also seen. It should be assumed that the virus can be transmitted from one snake to another through aerosols, so individual caging in the same room is not expected to form a barrier to infection. Current testing for this virus is through serology and PCR. Serological testing on a single blood sample can only inform on exposure to the virus. PCR testing on lung washes or combined oral–cloacal swabs is recommended. A positive result confirms the presence of infection and it should be assumed that clinically affected animals will not recover from infection and represent a source of infection for other animals.

Reoviruses have been detected in reptiles, mainly snakes and lizards, with respiratory disease but also in the presence of nonrespiratory clinical signs such as glossitis, papillomas, sudden death, enteropathy, hepatopathy and neurological disease. These viruses have also been detected in the absence of any clinical disease. Testing combined oral–cloacal swabs for these viruses by PCR is recommended.

In 2014, a novel nidovirus in the coronavirus family was detected. The virus was detected in the lungs of ball pythons (*Python regius*) with severe respiratory disease. Closely related viruses were subsequently detected in similarly affected snakes (many with stomatitis) in Europe and early indications suggest the virus is relatively common.

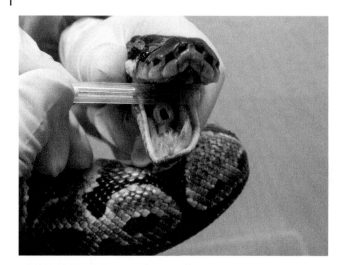

Figure 16.2 This ball python (*Python regius*) was infected with a ferlavirus and had small amounts of bloody mucous in the oral cavity as well as hyperaemia of the oral mucous membranes.

Transmission is expected to be through aerosols. PCR testing of pulmonary washes and oral swabs is recommended (Figure 16.3).

Inclusion body disease (IBD), which is probably caused by arenaviruses, has been associated with respiratory disease in snakes, as has sunshinevirus. These two viruses are covered in more detail in the section on neurological disease.

The vast majority of bacteria recovered from respiratory samples in animals with respiratory disease will either be commensals, playing no part in the disease process of that animal, or secondary pathogens. Two bacteria that can act as primary respiratory pathogens are worth mentioning, however. Chlamydia and mycobacteria have been associated with granulomatous disease in a number of tissues in a variety of reptile species. It is recommended that testing for these two agents is done using PCR and sequencing, especially considering that certain species are zoonotic.

Pentastomids are arthropods with worm-like or leech-like appearances. These parasites can create severe damage to the lungs and some species are zoonotic (Chapter 31).

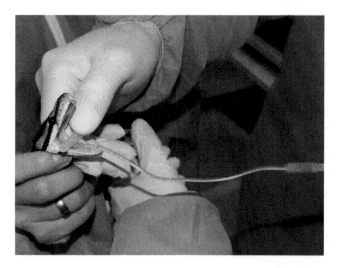

Figure 16.3 Tracheal washes can be used for the detection of many different pathogens of the lower respiratory tract. Tracheal wash fluid is often cloudy or flocculated in animals with lower respiratory tract infections. Fluid can be examined microscopically for cells, bacteria and fungi, can be used for isolation of bacteria and fungi and can be used for detection of various viruses, including ferlavirus and nidovirus.

Upper Alimentary Tract

Various severities of stomatitis are regularly observed in reptiles, especially tortoises, in association with various infectious diseases. Herpesvirus infections are frequently associated with severe, necrotizing stomatitis and glossitis, especially in tortoises (Figure 16.4). Affected tortoises are generally lethargic and anorectic. Chronically infected animals may also develop neurological signs and the upper and lower respiratory tracts, the alimentary tract and the liver may all be affected. The severity of disease, morbidity, and mortality depend on both the tortoise species and the virus strain. Diagnosis of acute infections should be by virus detection methods. PCR of oral swabs with material from the base of the tongue is recommended. Serological testing has also been described for some tortoise herpesviruses. Tortoise species that are resistant to disease, such as spur-thighed tortoises (*Testudo graeca*), are more likely to develop detectable antibody titres. Herpesviruses cause persistent latent infections and so any animal that survives infection or has antibodies against a herpesvirus must be considered a carrier. Herpesvirus infections with similar clinical signs have also been infrequently described in various lizard species. Reoviruses have also been described as a cause of stomatitis in tortoises and can also be diagnosed by virus detection (isolation in cell culture or PCR) from oral swabs. For more information, see the section on lower respiratory tract disease. Ranaviruses have been described in association with upper alimentary tract disease, mostly in turtles and tortoises but also in squamates. In animals with stomatitis, oral swabs can also be used for diagnosis. For more information, see the section on upper respiratory tract disease. In boas and pythons, IBD is frequently associated with a therapy resistant stomatitis, especially in boas. For more information on IBD and arenavirus infections, see the section on neurological disease. Nidoviruses have been described as a cause of pneumonia in pythons. A number of affected animals have also had stomatitis (see Lower Respiratory Tract section).

Multiple bacteria have been associated with upper digestive tract disease in various reptiles but most of these must be considered facultative pathogens that can belong to the normal flora of reptiles.

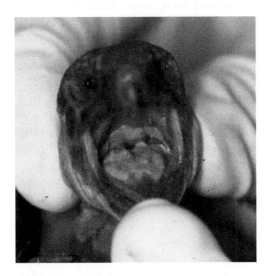

Figure 16.4 A Hermann's tortoise (*Testudo hermanni*) with sever diphtheroid-necrotizing glossitis as a result of a herpesvirus infection.

Lower Alimentary Tract

Multiple infectious agents have been associated with various signs of alimentary tract disease (obstipation, diarrhoea, vomiting and regurgitation). While various parasites are particularly important in diseases of this system, a number of viruses, fungi and bacteria have also been associated with disease.

Adenoviruses are most commonly found in lizards and snakes. Bearded dragons appear to be frequently infected. These viruses are mostly found in the liver and intestine of infected animals, where they can cause necrosis. Clinical signs associated with infection are variable and range from lethargy, anorexia, failure to thrive and wasting to neurological signs such as head tilt, opisthotonus and circling, as well as pneumonia, stomatitis and dermatitis. Chelonians have been increasingly reported with adenovirus infections. In this host, there appears to be a strong correlation between the genera of adenovirus and the clinical signs. Consequently, infected chelonians may be asymptomatic or they may be affected by severe disease with high rates of mortality. Testing cloacal swabs by PCR is the preferred method.

Bacterial and fungal infections of the alimentary tract can be very difficult to diagnose since the normal flora in reptiles can include multiple potential pathogens. Malnutrition, particularly a diet high in fruits, can result in dysbioses, such as yeast proliferations, that can lead to diarrhoea. This is most common in tortoises.

Multiple protozoal infections of the gastrointestinal tract have been described, some associated with severe clinical disease, while in other cases the infected animals may be clinically healthy. Many flagellates (e.g. trypanosomes, trichomonas, tritrichomonas and hexamita) are commonly detected in reptiles and are only associated with disease in the case of high parasite burdens or as secondary causes of disease.

Infections with the protozoan *Entamoeba invadens* have mostly been described in association with clinical disease in snakes and carnivorous lizards, while infections in herbivorous tortoises are often incidental. Mixing species in collections can lead to transmission and severe disease, and even death, in susceptible species. Clinical signs include anorexia, wasting, dysentery with mucus or blood in the faeces, vomiting and a firm swelling of the body from large intestine inflammation. *E. invadens* can also affect the liver and kidney. Affected animals often die relatively shortly after clinical signs are observed. Infection is via oral ingestion of cysts, which are resistant to inactivation or disinfection in the environment. Diagnosis is by direct examination of faeces and may be aided by iodine staining. Detection in necropsy tissues of affected animals is more reliable.

Coccidia (e.g. *Isospora* spp.) are often a problem in lizards in captivity. These have a direct lifecycle and can lead to high parasite burdens with corresponding clinical disease, particularly diarrhoea and anorexia. Diagnosis is by detection of oocytes in faecal material via floatation.

Intranuclear coccidia (tortoise intranuclear coccidiosis) is an important cause of disease in tortoises and box turtles and are associated with significant morbidity and mortality. Clinical signs associated with infection can include rhinitis, lethargy, wasting, dyspnoea and, in some cases, skin lesions. Tortoise intranuclear coccidiosis can be diagnosed by PCR and is most commonly found in the intestine, pancreas, liver and kidney. In live animals, it can be detected in cloacal swabs and nasal lavages.

Cryptosporidiosis, caused by *Cryptosporidium serpentis* and *C. saurophilum*, is an important cause of gastrointestinal disease in lizards and snakes. *C. saurophilum* causes an intestinal infection in lizards, leading to anorexia, wasting, lethargy, and death and has most often been described in leopard geckos. *C. serpentis* infection in snakes is associated with gastric dysplasia or hyperplasia with swelling of the stomach region of the body, regurgitation, and wasting. Diagnosis is by direct examination (with acid-fast staining), ELISA or PCR of faeces, mucous from regurgitated food items, gastric lavages or gastric biopsies. Since most methods can detect a range of cryptosporidia, including those of prey mammals, it is important to identify the cryptosporidium species, which is best done by sequencing PCR products.

There are many nematode parasites that can infect reptiles including strongylids, oxyurids and ascarids. Most will only cause disease of the alimentary tract when high numbers are present. Clinical disease generally includes anorexia and weight loss (see Chapter 31).

Liver Disease

Liver disease is relatively common in reptiles with many infectious agents, including viruses, bacteria, fungi and parasites capable of infecting the liver. Adenoviruses can cause liver damage and often also affect the alimentary tract. These are described in more detail in the section on the lower alimentary tract. Herpesviruses also commonly affect the liver, especially in aquatic turtles (see the section on the upper alimentary tract for details). The liver is one of the tissues most often infected by ranaviruses in many different reptile species. For more details see the section on the upper respiratory tract. In pythons, and especially boas, IBD is often associated with inclusions in hepatocytes, although these inclusions have not been associated with a specific pathology. IBD is discussed in more detail in the section on neurological disease.

Many bacteria have been detected in association with liver pathology. In general, these are facultative pathogens that can often belong to the normal bacterial flora of these animals and cause liver pathology following immune suppression or sepsis. Chlamydia (see Lower Respiratory Tract section) and various fungi have also been associated with granulomatous lesions in the liver, including members of the family Onygenaceae (e.g. *Nannizziopsis* spp., see section on skin and shell disease for more information). The fungus *Chamaeleomyces granulomatis* has been reported in association with liver lesions in chameleons in several cases and can be diagnosed in oral and cloacal swabs and liver biopsies by cultivation, PCR and cytology.

Multiple protozoan parasites can infect and damage the liver. The main text on these can be found in the section on the lower alimentary tract. In many cases, very high numbers of protozoa in the alimentary tract can lead to dissemination of these parasites into the liver. Entamoebae can also infect the liver, as can intranuclear coccidia in chelonians (see Chapter 19). *Choloeimeria* spp. are coccidian parasites with a direct lifecycle that can infect the bile ducts of lizards and snakes. Infection can lead to bile duct obstruction and hepatomegaly. Affected animals may be anorectic and lethargic and infection can lead to death of the animal. Diagnosis is via detection of sporulated oocysts in faeces (floatation). Helminths (e.g. the spargana of Spirometra tapeworms) and nematodes that wander through the body can also affect the liver and cause damage.

Neurological Disease

A number of infectious agents have been associated with neurological disease in reptiles, most of which are described in snakes. It must be stressed that for many of these neurological diseases, negative results of live-animal testing using minimally invasive samples, such as oral–cloacal swabs, can be misleading, as the agent will often be localized to the nervous system. This stresses the importance of collecting fresh samples from the nervous system during necropsy that are suitable for molecular testing, not just formalin-fixed tissues for histological examination.

IBD is an enigmatic disease that has been described in snakes and has neurological signs as its most common presentation. Traditionally, it has been diagnosed following the histological detection of numerous large intracytoplasmic eosinophilic inclusion bodies in a number of tissues (Figure 16.5). Following the groundbreaking work by Stenglein *et al.* (2012), it is now strongly suspected that arenaviruses cause this disease. However, it is still unknown what factors drive an arenaviral infection into a case of IBD, whether other agents can cause IBD and what factors are necessary for IBD to manifest itself into clinically detectable disease. IBD is found in pythons and boas and, anecdotally, pythons tend to develop clinical disease faster than boas. Testing oesophageal swabs and whole blood for arenavirus by PCR is probably the best test but cytological evaluation of blood or buffy coat smears is also valuable. Submitting oesophageal swabs for cytological examination and collecting liver biopsies for histological evaluation can also be considered. In live animals, the detection of arenavirus and inclusions is occurring more commonly in boas than pythons. It is recommended the clinician consults the most current literature on this disease, as new knowledge may suggest alternative testing recommendations.

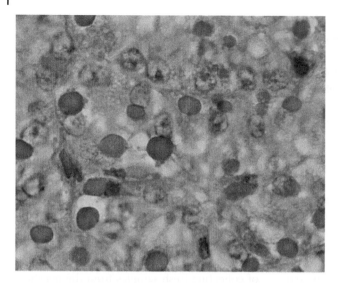

Figure 16.5 Multiple eosinophilic intracytoplasmic inclusion bodies in the pancreas of a boa constrictor with inclusion body disease (haematoxylin and eosin stain, 1000×; courtesy Kim Heckers, Laboklin).

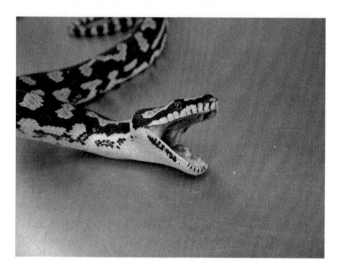

Figure 16.6 A jungle carpet python (*Morelia spilota cheynei*) with abnormal mouth gaping and incoordination, which could have been infected with a range of neurological infectious agents; for example, arenavirus/inclusion body disease, ferlavirus or, in this particular case, sunshinevirus (courtesy of Bob Doneley).

In 2012, a novel paramyxo-like virus was described in Australian pythons, which were primarily affected with neurological signs, but respiratory signs and non-specific signs of disease, such as lethargy and regurgitation, were also seen (Figure 16.6). The virus was named sunshinevirus after the geographical origin of the first isolate. It has been detected in a wide range of python species. Vertical transmission has been demonstrated and chronically infected animals have also been identified. Testing of combined oral–cloacal swabs by PCR is recommended.

The role of reptilian bornaviruses had been undefined for many years but, in Australia, a number of neurologically affected pythons have been found to be infected with highly divergent bornaviruses, many with neurohistopathology that is consistent with bornavirus infection in other species. Testing of combined oral–cloacal swabs by PCR is recommended. It is expected that this infection will become more significant as more information is obtained.

Ferlaviruses, adenoviruses and reoviruses have all been associated with neurological disease in reptiles, mostly snakes, and are described in more detail elsewhere in this chapter.

Bacterial infections of the neurological system are occasionally seen. Spinal osteopathies of bacterial origin (often secondary to skin trauma) can manifest as paresis and following sepsis, brain abscessation can occur. Also, multisystemic granulomatous disease (e.g. mycobacterium) can invade the central nervous system.

Parasitic causes of neurological disease include acanthamoebic meningoencephalitis and toxoplasmosis. It is suspected that acanthamoeba infections originate from water bowls and live animal testing for this parasite is very difficult, as infection is usually localized to the nervous system.

Skin and Shell Diseases

A number of related fungi have increasingly been shown to be important primary pathogens in squamate reptiles. First described as the *Chrysosporium* anamorph of *Nannizziopsis vriesii* in bearded dragons, similar pathogens have now been found in multiple species of lizards, including bearded dragons, iguanas, geckos and chameleons. Related fungi (*Ophidiomyces ophidiodiicola*) are considered an emerging pathogen in snakes causing severe disease and mortality in wild snakes in North America. Similar pathogens have also been described in crocodilians. Disease in bearded dragons has been called yellow fungus disease. Lesions consisting of yellow to brown crusts are often found on the head, but can also be found on other parts of the body, and infected animals can develop systemic disease. Diagnosis is by PCR or isolation of fungi using skin scrapings or biopsies as samples. Cytological or histological detection of fungi is also used diagnostically but this cannot identify the fungus to the level of species. Other fungi have also been described in association with skin lesions in reptiles, but are often secondary pathogens. Without cytological or histological evidence

of tissue invasion or active inflammatory responses to the fungi, the role of any detected fungi will remain speculative.

Picornaviruses have been associated with softening of the carapace in young tortoises, especially spur-thighed tortoises (*Testudo graeca*), probably as a result of kidney damage. Adult tortoises may be inapparent carriers or may develop various clinical signs, including rhinitis and ascites. Persistent carriers are common. Diagnosis is by virus isolation or PCR detection using oral swabs. Antibodies can be detected by virus neutralization tests.

Other viruses have also been associated with skin lesions in reptiles, including ranaviruses in lizards (Figure 16.7; see Upper Respiratory Tract section). Invertebrate iridoviruses, found commonly in insects sold as food items in the pet trade, have also been associated with skin lesions in insectivorous lizards in some cases. Papilloma-like lesions have been repeatedly described in various reptile species and have been associated with papilloma-like, reo-like and herpes-like viruses. Diagnosis is generally by skin biopsies and electron microscopic detection of virus. In sea turtles, herpesviruses have been associated with fibropapillomatosis and this is a cause of severe disease in several species throughout the world. Diagnosis in these cases is possible via PCR using tissue lesions. In crocodilians, poxviruses and herpesviruses have been associated with skin lesions in various species and can be diagnosed by histology or PCR using skin scrapings from lesions. West Nile virus has also been associated with skin lesions in infected alligators. This virus can also cause systemic disease and death in crocodilians and is zoonotic.

Many different bacteria have been associated with skin lesions in reptiles, mostly associated with poor hygiene and other husbandry issues. Examples include ulcerative shell disease of chelonians such as septicaemic cutaneous ulcerative disease in freshwater turtles. The bacteria that are involved are often secondary pathogens, and culture and sensitivity can help to guide treatment.

(a)

(b)

(c)

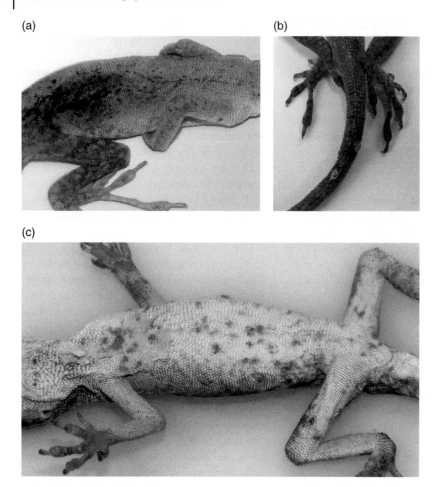

Figure 16.7 Skin alterations observed in ranavirus-infected green anoles (*Anolis carolinensis*; Stöhr et al. 2013).

The bacterium *Devriesea agamarum* has been shown to be a primary pathogen causing skin lesions (primarily around the mouth) and in some cases systemic disease and death in agamid lizards, particularly *Uromasytx* species. Other reptile species (e.g. bearded dragons) can carry the bacterium as part of their normal oral flora. Diagnosis is by isolation from skin swabs or scrapings and from oral swabs.

Numerous ectoparasites can affect reptiles and severe infestations can cause dermatitis. Haematophagous parasites can also weaken the animals, if they are present in large numbers. Mites are common in captive reptiles. The most common mite is the snake mite,

Ophionyssus natricis, which can infest lizards as well as snakes (see Chapter 31 for details).

Kidney and Urinary Tract Disease

Many infectious diseases of the kidney associated with bacterial infections have been described. These are generally secondary to other issues that either directly affect kidney function or the immune system of the affected animal. Picornaviruses in tortoises are believed to cause primary kidney disease, leading to various clinical signs including softening of the carapace in young animals (see Skin and Shell

Diseases). The flagellate *Hexamita parva* generally infects the gastrointestinal tract of chelonians without causing disease but, in young and immunocompromised animals, it can infect the kidney and cause nephritis and death. Detection of hexamites in faecal material is not necessarily indicative of kidney infection, and detection in urine, which can be slimy, should be attempted.

Blood Disease

Multiple infectious agents can cause inclusion body formation in blood cells and some can cause disease, including anaemia. Viruses known to cause inclusion bodies in erythrocytes include iridoviruses such as erythrocytic necrosis virus. These have most often been described in wild-caught reptiles in various parts of the world. Infections can cause anaemia and systemic disease in animals kept at suboptimal temperatures. Diagnosis is by visualization of inclusions in peripheral red blood cells followed by PCR to specifically identify the virus. IBD and sunshinevirus have also been shown to cause inclusions in erythrocytes and leucocytes of infected snakes, particularly boas (see Neurological Disease).

A number of endoparasites are capable of infecting erythrocytes, including trypanosomes and haemogregarines (e.g. *Hepatozoon* spp.).These generally require an invertebrate vector for transmission and are therefore found mostly in wild-caught reptiles. Diagnosis is by microscopic examination of stained blood smears.

Formulating a Plan

The biology of an infectious agent needs to be carefully considered once it has been definitively detected in a reptile. Several factors should be considered: pathogenicity, infectivity, host treatment, environmental treatment and other miscellaneous considerations.

Underlying the response to every diagnosis of an infectious agent should be a review of the husbandry of the animal(s) and, as mentioned earlier in this chapter, it should not be automatically assumed that the collection is affected by a single infectious agent as mixed infections are more common than single infections.

The pathogenicity of an organism is one of the most fundamental factors to consider. If an organism is not pathogenic or, even more pertinently, is actually beneficial to the health of the animal, any further management considerations, besides husbandry improvements, will often be unnecessary. There is evidence that pinworms play a supportive role in the digestive health of lizards. Conversely, ferlaviral outbreaks have been associated with mass mortalities and affected collections should be managed promptly and assertively. Euthanasia should be considered on welfare grounds for animals with highly pathogenic infectious disease that cannot be effectively managed.

Some infectious agents of reptiles are highly infectious, others are less infectious but, for most, the level of infectivity is unknown. Perhaps the best example of infectivity is provided by mites in snakes. Infestations in individual animals should be interpreted to mean that mites are widespread and therefore disinfection and treatment should be thorough. In contrast, the lifecycle of pentastomids means that single animals that were infected in the wild will not be infectious to their conspecifics in captivity.

Whether an animal is treated or not depends on a number of other factors: pathogenicity, infectivity, the value of the animal compared with the cost of treatment, owner consent, compliance concerns, drug toxicity and so on. For many agents, host treatments are not available. This is commonly the case for viral infections. For other infections, such as many intestinal nematodes, treatment of the infected animal will form the cornerstone of controlling the infectious disease.

The treatment of the environment also needs to be considered, requiring sound knowledge of the stability of the agent outside the host and how likely there will be significant loads of infectious agent present. For most instances, switching to nonparticulate substrates such as newspaper, changing the substrate often (sometimes daily) and using typical household disinfectants will be sufficient to address environmental contamination. For situations like mite infestations, more specific products, such as topical ivermectin, fipronil or pyrethroids, will be needed. Some infectious agents are remarkably resistant to disinfection. This includes nonenveloped viruses such as adenoviruses and reoviruses, cryptosporidium and bacterial spores. More specialized disinfectants such as biguanide–quaternary ammonium combinations (F10SC veterinary disinfectant) and peroxygen compound–surfactant–organic acid combinations (Virkon® S) should be used according to the label instructions that correspond to the most resistant agents. It is important to remember these substances may be highly toxic to reptiles, so thorough rinsing with clean water is necessary to avoid contact with animals. Replacement of porous (wooden) enclosures with non-porous (plastic) enclosures may need to be considered.

Following the definitive diagnosis of an infectious agent, there are a number of other considerations, such as whether there is a zoonotic potential for the agent (e.g. some mycobacteria, pentastomids) and whether the animal is a loved pet in a single-animal household or in a large breeding collection. These considerations influence the management decision making process.

For both large and small collections, closing the collection should be considered, so no animals are introduced or released from the collection for a time. Confidence to reopen a collection should come from multiple negative test results from surviving animals. Once the decision has been made to reopen a collection, strict biosecurity should be observed, including appropriate quarantining. There is growing evidence that some animals infected with certain infectious agents (e.g. sunshinevirus, tortoise picornaviruses) can remain asymptomatic for years. It cannot therefore be guaranteed that an asymptomatic animal that has been in quarantine for three months, six months, one year or even several years will be free of all pathogenic organisms. Because of this, it is strongly recommended that diagnostic testing should be performed during a quarantine period that is as long as is practically possible. The value of the individual animal in quarantine should be measured against the value to the collection when determining what testing will be performed on an animal while in quarantine. It is recommended that faecal samples are examined for parasites and PCR testing is performed on appropriate samples for the microbes of the most relevance to the local area. For agents known to cause persistent infections (herpesviruses, *Mycoplasma* and picornaviruses), serological testing should be considered as well. Testing should be repeated at least once.

Undiscovered Infectious Agents

This chapter has focuses on significant known infectious agents of reptiles. There is no question that there are many more to be discovered and that the overwhelming majority of these will be in animals that are first presented to private practitioners. The authors would like to embolden the readers to pursue interesting and atypical cases. It is recommended they make enquiries to find their nearest colleague that has the capacity (and motivation) to discover new agents and investigate the nature of these infections. Collaborations like these will always be worth more than any research grant.

Immunology

The immune system of reptiles is poorly understood. Nonspecific barriers such as skin form the first layer of defence from foreign materials. Nonspecific innate mechanisms such as the complement cascade serve as the second layer of defence and, finally, the adaptive immune system, made up of the components of humoral (antibody) immunity and cell-mediated immunity, provides antigen-specific responses. Although this system is said to be similar among all vertebrates, the components of the reptilian immune system have not been comprehensively defined in any species and it is likely that there are significant differences between taxa. In reptiles, the immune responses mounted against foreign antigens have not been fully mapped but it is suspected reptiles rely on nonspecific immunological defences more than mammals. However, virus neutralization assays for herpesviruses, ferlaviruses and adenoviruses prove that reptiles can produce humoral responses that can prevent in vitro infections. Information on the specific cell-mediated immune responses (e.g. cytotoxic cells) that reptiles produce is extremely sparse and incomplete. It is plausible that cell-mediated immune responses represent significant defensive mechanisms for reptiles and so results of humoral testing should be carefully interpreted. More specific information on the serological testing that is used in reptiles can be found in Chapter 11. It is broadly accepted that the innate and adaptive arms of the reptilian immune system function optimally at that animal's preferred optimal body temperature. Many reptiles are kept at suboptimal temperatures and so, often by simply warming them up, great improvements in their immunological defences can occur.

Reviews

For readers interested in more detailed overviews of the viral infections of reptiles, the reviews by Marschang (2011, 2014) are recommended. For an excellent review on the fungal infections of reptiles, the work by Paré (2014) should be read. For bacteriology and parasitology, the reviews by Paré at al. (2006) and Greiner and Mader (2006), respectively, are excellent. The most comprehensive review of all infectious diseases of reptiles was compiled by Jacobson (2007) and this text serves as an outstanding reference.

References

Greiner, E.C. and Mader, D.R. (2006) *Parasitology in Reptile Medicine and Surgery*, 2nd ed. Elsevier Saunders, St. Louis, MO, pp. 343–364.

Jacobson, E.R. (2007) *Infectious Diseases and Pathology of Reptiles*. CRC Press, Boca Raton, FL.

Marschang, R.E. (2011) Viruses infecting reptiles. *Viruses*, 3 (11), 2087–2126.

Marschang, R.E. (2014) Clinical virology, in *Current Therapy in Reptile Medicine and Surgery*, (D. Mader and S. Divers, eds). Elsevier Saunders, St. Louis, MO, pp. 32–52.

Paré, J.A. (2014) Update on fungal infections in reptiles, in *Current Therapy in Reptile Medicine and Surgery*, (D. Mader and S. Divers, eds). Elsevier Saunders, St. Louis, MO, pp. 53–56.

Paré, J.A. and Sigler, L., Rosenthal, K.L. and Mader, D.R. (2006) Microbiology: fungal and bacterial diseases of reptiles, in *Reptile Medicine and Surgery*, 2nd ed. (D.R. Mader, ed.). Elsevier Saunders, St. Louis, MO, pp. 217–238.

Stenglein, M.D., Sanders, C., Kistler, A.L. *et al.* (2012) Identification, characterization, and in vitro culture of highly divergent arenaviruses from boa constrictors and annulated tree boas: candidate etiological agents for snake inclusion body disease. *MBio*, 3 (4), e00180-12.

Further Reading

Hyndman, T.H., Shilton, C.M. and Marschang, R.E. (2013) Paramyxoviruses in reptiles: a review. *Veterinary Microbiology*, 165 (3), 200–213.

Jacobson, E.R., Brown, M.B., Wendland, L.D. *et al.* (2014) Mycoplasmosis and upper respiratory tract disease of tortoises: a review and update. *Veterinary Journal*, 201 (3), 257–264.

Miller, D.L., Pessier, A.P., Hick, P. and Whittington, R.J. (2015) Comparative pathology of ranaviruses and diagnostic techniques, in *Ranaviruses: Lethal Pathogens of Ectothermic Vertebrates* (M.J. Gray and V.G. Chinchar, eds). Springer, Vienna, pp. 171–208.

Stöhr, A.C, Blahak, S., Heckers, K.O. *et al.* (2013) Ranavirus infections associated with skin lesions in lizards. *Veterinary Research*, 44, 84.

17

Differential Diagnoses: A Problem-Based Approach

Helen McCracken, Brendan Carmel, John Chitty, Bob Doneley, Robert Johnson,
Angela M. Lennox, Deborah Monks and Annabelle Olsson

Introduction

The following lists provide a guide to the differential diagnoses of the most common presenting signs of disease in the four major reptile taxa: snakes, lizards, chelonians and crocodilians. Note that the lists include circumstances where the presenting sign represents a normal state for that group of reptiles. They also include the husbandry errors that will cause or predispose to these presenting signs. The lists are intended to give the clinician a starting point for the diagnostic process and should not be considered exhaustive.

Snakes

Anorexia

- Normal:
  - Before and during ecdysis.
  - Hatchling snakes.
  - Reproduction – gravid or brooding female, mating male.

- Decreased appetite associated with seasonal decreases in photoperiod and ambient temperatures.
  - 'Shy feeders' – these are snakes that prefer to feed while hidden and therefore refuse food offered in full view of the carer.
- Husbandry:
  - Suboptimal environmental temperature management, so cannot reach or maintain optimal body temperature for feeding.
  - Inappropriate photoperiod cycle, affecting stimulus to feed.
  - Maladaptation to new environment.
  - Environmental stress from enclosure mates.
  - Stress from increased frequency or duration of handling, including for management of a health:.
  - Disturbances in environment outside the enclosure.
  - Inadequate cage furniture to enable normal behaviour, such as basking, hiding, climbing, burrowing.
  - Inappropriate food item.

Reptile Medicine and Surgery in Clinical Practice, First Edition. Edited by Bob Doneley, Deborah Monks,
Robert Johnson and Brendan Carmel.

- Health:
  - Systemic infections including arenavirus (inclusion body disease) reported in pythons and boas, ferlavirus (ophidian paramyxovirus), reported in all snake families, predominantly in viperids and sunshinevirus, a paramyxovirus reported mainly in Australian pythons.
  - Antifungal drug toxicity (amphotericin B, griseofulvin, ketoconazole).
  - Toxicosis from ingestion of rodent killed by rodenticide.
  - Visual deficit, including due to cataracts.
  - Tongue or tongue sheath infection or trauma resulting in loss of olfactory function.
  - Occluded nares.
  - Pneumonia.
  - Stomatitis or oesophagitis or gastroenteritis.
  - Gastrointestinal tract parasites.
  - Gastrointestinal neoplasia.
  - Gastrointestinal obstruction (see 'Regurgitation').
  - Extra-intestinal inflammation or infection, neoplasia and other disease, including gout, hepatic lipidosis and other hepatopathies.
  - Dystocia.
  - Multiple rib fractures in constricting species (pythons and boas).
  - Pain.
- Weight loss
  - All causes of anorexia as above.
- Health:
  - Cardiac dysfunction.
  - Maldigestion or malabsorption (to date, no precise aetiologies are recognized for these:).
  - Nephropathy.

Distended Coelom

- Normal:
  - Gravid female.
- Husbandry:
  - Obesity due to overfeeding and inactivity; common in black-headed pythons (*Aspidites melanocephalus*) and royal or ball pythons (*Python regius*).
- Health:
  - Coelomitis.
  - Ascites.
  - Faecal impaction.
  - Dystocia.

Weakness, Decreased Muscle Tone, Lethargy, Reluctance to Move, Loose or Absent Coiling in Pythons

- Husbandry:
  - Inappropriately low or high environmental temperature.
- Health:
  - Non-specific sign seen with many disease processes, often coupled with anorexia.
  - Dehydration.
  - Systemic disease, including septicaemia, viral infection (ferlavirus, arenavirus, sunshinevirus).
  - Heavy external or internal parasite burden.
  - Neoplasia of any system.
  - Toxicoses, including organophosphate and carbamate insecticides, alcohol.
  - Visual deficits, including due to cataracts.
  - Head or spinal trauma.
  - Renal insufficiency.
  - Pain.
  - Early manifestation of all causes of neurological signs listed.
  - Haemorrhage.
  - Anaemia.
  - Visceral gout.

Increased Activity

- Normal:
  - Preparing for ecdysis.
  - Mate-seeking behaviour.
  - Gravid snake seeking nesting site.
- Husbandry:
  - Inappropriately high environmental temperature.
  - Inadequate or inappropriate retreat areas or cage furniture.
  - Environmental disturbance.

- Other:
  - Hunger or thirst.
  - Mite infestation.

Increased Time Spent Basking

- Normal:
  - Gravid female.
  - Behavioural thermoregulation to optimize postprandial digestion.
- Husbandry:
  - Decreased ambient temperature.
- Ill health.

Increased Time Spent Soaking In Water Bowl

- Normal:
  - Preparing for ecdysis.
- Husbandry:
  - Environment inappropriately dry or hot.
  - Mite infestation.

Dull, Dry, Pale or Discoloured Skin

- Normal:
  - Prior to ecdysis.
  - Stretched, pale skin over the mid-body bulge in a recently fed snake.
- Husbandry:
  - Inappropriately low environmental humidity.
- Health:
  - Fungal dermatitis (focal skin discolouration).
  - Scar at site of previous trauma or surgery (pale, smooth skin without scales).
  - Injection site of tissue irritant drug (e.g. enrofloxacin).

Dysecdysis (abnormal shedding): fully or partially retained slough

- Husbandry:
  - Inappropriately low environmental humidity
  - Failure to provide adequate water body for soaking (required by some species)
  - Inappropriately low environmental temperature
  - Lack of suitable cage furniture to initiate or assist shedding
- Health:
  - Malnutrition, dehydration, debilitation.
  - Concurrent illness.
  - Bacterial or fungal skin infection.
  - Mite or tick infestation.
  - Previous skin scarring from burn or trauma.

Dysecdysis: Increased Frequency of Sloughing

- Health:
  - Bacterial or fungal skin infection.
  - Mite or tick infestation.
  - Burns.
  - Hyperthyroidism.

Skin Hyperkeratosis, Granulomas, Proliferative Nodules, Papules, Pustules, Blisters, Ulceration

- Husbandry:
  - Inappropriately high environmental humidity, wet substrate, poor environmental hygiene (all predispose to bacterial or fungal dermatitis).
- Health:
  - 'Blister disease' caused by bacterial or fungal infection (fluid-filled skin vesicles most commonly involving the ventral scales).
  - Infection with *Chrysosporium* anamorph of *Nannizziopsis vriesii* (CANV) fungus.
  - Other bacterial or fungal dermatitis.
  - Sunshinevirus infection (blisters and dermatitis).
  - Nematodes, including Kalicephalus spp (blisters, pustules that rupture to form ulcers).
  - Thermal burns (blisters, crusting, ulcers, full thickness loss of epidermis).
  - Chemical burn from contact with concentrated disinfectants e.g. sodium hypochlorite.

Skin Abrasions, Thickening, Disruption

- Husbandry:
  - Mite or tick infestation.
- Trauma:
  - Stress-related rostral abrasion.
  - Traumatic wound (including bite from prey or enclosure mate).
  - Scar at site of previous trauma or surgery.

Cutaneous and Subcutaneous Swellings

- Iatrogenic:
  - Subcutaneous microchip (snakes are typically chipped caudolateral to the skull or craniolateral to the cloaca)
  - Injection site reaction.
- Health:
  - Subcutaneous abscess or granuloma (due to ectoparasite attachment, puncture wound, foreign body, injection site, poor environmental hygiene).
  - Soft tissue infection, abscess or granuloma as sequela of adjacent spinal osteomyelitis lesion.
  - Subcutaneous nematodes (visible under the skin).
  - Sparganosis (only in snakes that have consumed frogs or reptiles; lesions most commonly occur in the caudal half of the body).
  - Skin neoplasia.
  - Subcutaneous lipomas (most common in colubrids).
  - Bony swellings from focal vertebral osteomyelitis.
  - Rib fractures.

Eyes: Colour Change, Opaque or Dry Spectacle

- Normal:
  - Opaque spectacle associated with pre-ecdysis (normal).
- Husbandry:
  - Spectacle abrasion from constant face rubbing against solid objects due to peri-ocular mites, dysecdysis or dry skin caused by low humidity.
- Health:
  - Spectacle retention following ecdysis.
  - Indented spectacle due to previous case of retention.
  - Spectacle trauma or ulceration following incorrect treatment of retention.
  - Bacterial or fungal infection of eye or spectacle, including as extension from adjacent skin infection.
  - Subspectacular infection or abscess – most cases occur from ascending infection via the nasolacrimal duct secondary to stomatitis or respiratory tract infection.
  - Traumatic full or partial loss of spectacle.
  - Exposure keratitis following iatrogenic spectacle loss.
  - Cataract.

Eye or Spectacle Distension

- Spectacle:
  - Subspectacular infection or abscess (most cases occur from ascending infection via the nasolacrimal duct secondary to stomatitis or respiratory tract infection).
  - Subspectacular fluid accumulation due to blocked nasolacrimal duct ('pseudobuphthalmos').
- Globe:
  - Bacterial or fungal ocular infection (panophthalmitis) – most commonly from trauma.
  - Ocular neoplasia.
  - Traumatic eye injury.
  - Glaucoma (including secondary to cataract).

Periocular Swelling

- Health:
  - Periocular cellulitis or abscess.
  - Periocular mites or ticks.
  - Trauma.

Oral, Nasal and Choanal Discharge, Excessive Salivation, Mouth Gaping, Wheezing, Stridor, Dyspnoea

- Nares and nasal cavity:
  - Normal transient partial obstruction of nares during ecdysis, producing a wheezing sound.
  - Stomatitis (exudate or saliva may enter the choana, producing nasal discharge).
  - Complete or partial obstruction of nares by retained slough (mouth gaping, wheezing).
- Respiratory tract:
  - Obstruction of glottis by oral cavity foreign body or lesion, including abscess, neoplasia.
  - Rhinitis.
  - Pneumonia (may present with nasal discharge and/or exudate from glottis in oral cavity).
  - Aspiration pneumonia due to inexpert assist feeding or administration of oral medication.
  - Water aspiration (near-drowning), including in snakes unattended while soaking in buckets of water.
- Toxins:
  - Organophosphate, carbamate, pyrethrin and pyrethroid insecticide toxicosis (salivation, respiratory secretions, dyspnoea).
  - Toxicosis from ingestion of rodent killed by anticoagulant rodenticide (dyspnoea).
  - Inhaled irritants, including fumes of disinfectants and other chemicals.
- Systemic viral infections including ferlavirus (blood in oral cavity, stridor, dyspnoea), sunshinevirus and arenavirus (clear, viscous oral discharge, dyspnoea).

Gingival Inflammation, Ulceration, Petechiation, Exudation, Tooth Loss

- Health:
  - Hyperthermia.
  - Septicaemia (petechiation only).
  - Organophosphate toxicity.
  - Electrocution (petechiation only).
  - Stomatitis (bacterial or fungal).
  - Stress-related rostral abrasions – may extend deeply into oral tissues.

Tongue Lesions

- Health:
  - Bacterial or fungal infection of tongue or tongue sheath (erythema, ulceration, exudation).
  - Inability to protrude tongue due to adhesions within tongue sheath as sequela of trauma or infection.

Oral Mucous Membrane Colour

- White to very pale pink:
  - normal for most species.
- Pale green:
  - Hepatic disease.
  - Cholecystitis.
  - Bile duct obstruction.
  - Haemolysis.

Facial or Cephalic Swelling

- Infectious diseases:
  - Cephalic cellulitis as sequela of bacterial stomatitis.
  - 'Facial disfiguration syndrome' caused by *Ophidiomyces ophiodiicola* infection.
  - Venom gland abscess.
  - Abscess of other facial tissues, including due to puncture wound, ectoparasite attachment.
  - Osteomyelitis (bacterial, fungal).
- Trauma:
  - Fracture or soft tissue wound, including due to cage-mate trauma or bite from prey item.
- Bone or soft tissue neoplasia.
- Sialocoele.

Regurgitation, Vomiting

- Husbandry:
  - Suboptimal environmental temperature following feeding.

- Handling or other environmental stresses within 24–48 hours after feeding.
- Overfeeding.
- Inappropriate food item or inappropriate preparation of food item.
- Infection:
  - Systemic viral disease (arenavirus, sunshinevirus).
  - Bacterial or fungal gastroenteritis.
- Parasites:
  - *Cryptosporidium* spp. hypertrophic gastritis (most commonly seen in colubrids, elapids and viperids).
  - Other gastrointestinal parasites (notably cestodes, ascarids, *Entamoeba* spp.).
- Gastrointestinal obstruction:
  - Ingested foreign body (snakes will eat objects with the odour or remains of prey items on them (e.g. substrate material, mouse trap), neoplasia, granuloma, intussusception or faecal impaction.
  - Extraintestinal lesion.
- Hepatopathy.

Diarrhoea

- Normal:
  - Viperids produce semi-liquid faeces compared with other snake species.
- Husbandry:
  - Maldigestion and bacterial overgrowth due to suboptimal environmental temperature.
  - Overfeeding.
  - Recent diet change.
- Infection:
  - Ferlavirus (mucoid diarrhoea, malodorous stools).
  - Bacterial or fungal enteritis or colitis (including salmonellosis).
  - Protozoal enteritis or colitis (notably *Entamoeba* spp., flagellates).
  - Infestation with *Strongyloides* spp., hookworms or ascarids.
- Dysbiosis following antibiotic therapy or systemic illness.

Constipation, Reduced Faecal Output

- Husbandry:
  - Suboptimal environmental temperature.

- Dehydration due to low humidity environment or inappropriate delivery of drinking water.
- Insufficient exercise.
- Inappropriate food items (e.g. long-haired rodents).
- Incidental ingestion of enclosure substrate (pebbles, gravel, sand, bark).
- Health:
  - Gastrointestinal obstruction:
    - intraluminal (intussusception, neoplasia, foreign body).
    - Extraluminal (e.g. dystocia).

Mid-Body Swelling

- Normal:
  - Recently consumed food in stomach.
- Health:
  - *Cryptosporidium* spp. hypertrophic gastritis (most commonly seen in colubrids, elapids and viperids).
  - Gastric abscess or granuloma.
  - Gastric neoplasia.
  - Gastric foreign body.

Other Palpable or Visible Internal Swellings (Figure 17.1)

- Reproductive tract:
  - Folliculogenesis and atretic follicles.
  - Gravid female.
  - Oophoritis or salpingitis.
  - Dystocia.
  - Retained unfertilised eggs ('slugs').
- Cardiac:
  - Cardiomegaly (cardiomyopathy or pericardial effusion).
- Gastrointestinal tract:
  - Ingested foreign body.
  - Intestinal intussusception.
  - Faecal impaction.
  - Solid urate masses in colon.
- Generalized:
  - Abscess or granuloma of any internal organ or coelomic cavity, including *Mycobacteria* spp. infection.
  - Neoplasia or cyst of any internal organ or coelomic cavity.

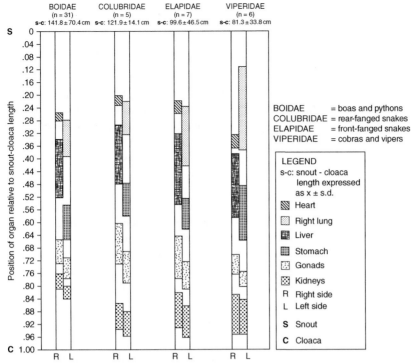

N.B.　Heart is located in the midline, not on the right-hand side as suggested in these graphs.

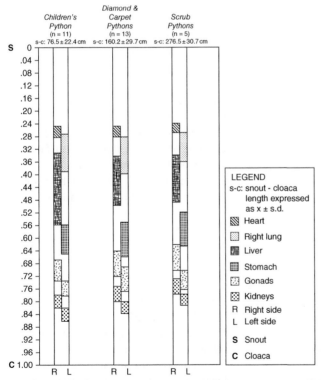

1. The sample size given (n) represents the total number of specimens examined for each species or family. The sample size for some mesurements is slightly less than this total because in a small number of specimens examined, some organs could not be measured due to pathological change.
2. The posterior pole of lung represented is the point of junction between alveolar lung and membranous air sac.

Figure 17.1 Identification of the location of internal organs in snakes by determining the distance from the snout, expressed as a percentage of snout–vent length (McCracken 1994).

- Inflammatory swelling of any internal organ.
- Steatitis.
- Gall bladder distension due to bile duct obstruction or bacterial or coccidial cholecystitis.
- Omphalitis (in hatchlings).

Diffuse Distension, Firmness or Puffiness in Caudal Half of Body Cavity

- Reproductive:
  - Folliculogenesis.
  - Gravid female.
  - Oophoritis or salpingitis.
  - Dystocia.
- Intestinal:
  - Ferlavirus (gaseous bowel distension).
  - Coelomitis (including yolk-related).
  - Steatitis.
  - Protozoal colitis (*Entamoeba* spp. or flagellates).
  - Intestinal or caecocolic neoplasia.
  - Faecal impaction.
  - Solid urate masses in colon or cloaca.

Swelling of the Cloaca or Hemipenal Region

- Health:
  - Protozoal colitis
  - Bacterial or protozoal cloacitis.
  - Hemipenal pocket infection.
  - Hemipenal trauma.
  - Mating trauma in female.
  - Oedema of cloacal mucosa secondary to tenesmus due to faecal impaction or dystocia.
  - Paracloacal gland infection.

Prolapse from cloaca

- Cloaca:
  - Generalized weakness (prolapsed cloaca, colon, bladder, oviduct or hemipenes).
  - Humid environment – predisposes to prolapse of cloacal tissue and terminal colon (most commonly in juvenile green pythons).

- Intestinal:
  - Gastrointestinal tract: parasitism, gastroenteritis, cloacitis or gut obstruction by faecal impaction, intussusception, neoplasia (prolapsed cloaca, colon).
  - Extraluminal gastrointestinal blockage, including neoplasia, abscesses (prolapsed cloaca, colon).
- Reproductive:
  - Dystocia (prolapsed cloaca, oviduct).
  - Prolapsed hemipenes, following probing for sex identification, traction during copulation, spinal injury, or contamination with substrate material or straining due to any of the causes listed.

Discoloured Urates

- Yellow:
  - normal variation of the usual white or cream urates
- Green (biliverdinuria):
  - Chronic anorexia or starvation.
  - Hepatic disease.
  - Cholecystitis.
  - Bile duct obstruction.
  - Haemolysis.
- Bloody:
  - Haemorrhage or inflammation of the kidneys, colon or cloaca.
  - Passage of abnormally hard faeces, causing blood streaking on surface of both faecal and urate masses.
  - Following manual palpation to resolve faecal impaction or egg retention.

Gravid Female not Commencing or Completing Parturition or Oviposition

- Normal:
  - Primigravid female.
- Husbandry and nutritional:
  - Environmental temperature or humidity not species appropriate.
  - Failure to provide suitable nest site.
  - Disturbance of parturition by cage mate or external stimulus.
  - Obesity due to overfeeding.
  - Malnutrition.

– Dehydration.
– Lack of fitness in chronically inactive snake.
● Health:
– Obstructive dystocia due to oversized or malformed egg or foetus, crushed egg, dead foetus, or pathology external to reproductive tract.

Salpingitis

● Health:
– Spinal disease.
– General debilitation due to other disease process.

Vertebral Swellings and Spondylosis

● Health:
– Vertebral osteomyelitis (generally focal).
– Bone neoplasia.
– Vertebral trauma.
– Proliferative spinal osteopathy (generally multifocal or diffuse, causing segmented fusion of adjacent affected vertebrae).
– Intervertebral articular gout.

Tail Necrosis, Missing Tail Tip

● Health:
– Trauma, or within two weeks of ventral caudal vein venepuncture (most likely due to iatrogenic vascular damage).
– Dysecdysis (tourniquet effect).
– Necrotising dermatitis.
– Spinal osteomyelitis.

Paralysis

● CNS lesions:
– Viral infections, including arenavirus, ferlavirus (flaccid paralysis).
– Other central nervous system infections, bacterial, fungal, viral or parasitic.
● Spinal lesions:
– Vertebral osteomyelitis.
– Bone neoplasia.
– Spinal trauma, including from handling, crushing by enclosure furniture.

– Pathological fracture (including as sequela of proliferative spinal osteopathy).
● Faecal impaction.
● Electrocution (flaccid paralysis).

Neurological Signs, Including Muscle Fasciculation, Incoordination, Ataxia, Writhing, Star-Gazing, Head Tilt, Opisthotonus, Convulsions

● Nutritional:
– Thiamine deficiency (notably in snakes fed frozen fish without vitamin B1 supplementation).
– Metabolic disease, including hypoglycaemia, hypocalcaemia.
● Toxicosis:
– Organophosphate, carbamate, pyrethrin and pyrethroid insecticide toxicity (ataxia, muscle fasciculation).
– Drug toxicity, including metronidazole, ivermectin and aminoglycoside antibiotics.
– Ingestion of disinfectants, including iodine.
– Ingestion of and exposure to fumes of household chemicals, including paint solvents, ethylene glycol.
– Plant toxicity, including cedar shavings.
● Central nervous system disease:
– Head or body trauma.
– Bacterial and mycotic encephalitis (including micro-abscesses secondary to septicaemia).
– Viral encephalitis including arenavirus, ferlavirus, sunshinevirus and bornavirus (reported mainly in pythons).
– Parasitic infections (including brain abscess due to *Entamoeba invadens*).
– Meningoencephalitis due to *Acanthamoeba* spp.
● Liver disease:
– Hepatic lipidosis.
– Hepatic encephalopathy.
● Renal failure and visceral gout.
● Disseminated infection or septicaemia.
● Electrocution (convulsions).
● Pain.

Loss of Righting Reflex, Abnormal Body Position and Movement, Inability to Strike at Prey

- Normal:
  - Gravid females frequently rest in dorsal recumbency.
  - Rolling and resting in dorsal recumbency may be normal behaviours for some individuals.
- Spinal disease:
  - Vertebral or spinal cord disease (infection, neoplasia, trauma).
  - Proliferative spinal osteopathy (may cause vertebral fusion and hence segmental rigidity, kinking or abnormal posture).
  - Congenital spinal deformities (lordosis, kyphosis, scoliosis).
- Thiamine deficiency (notably in snakes fed frozen fish without vitamin B1 supplementation).
- Organophosphate, carbamate, pyrethrin and pyrethroid insecticide.
- Systemic viral infections, including ferlavirus, arenavirus, sunshinevirus.
- Pneumonia (abnormal posture).
- Any cause of general debilitation.

Sudden Death

- Husbandry:
  - Hyperthermia from inappropriately high environmental temperature (e.g. thermostat failure or exposure to direct sunlight without opportunity to seek cooler area).
- Health:
  - Failure of carer to detect earlier signs of chronic illness.
  - Systemic infections including septicaemia and ferlavirus.
  - Leukaemia.
  - Organ failure (e.g. visceral gout).
  - Toxicities.
- Envenomation by cage mate.
- Toxicities including bufotoxin from ingestion of a cane toad.
- Trauma.
- Electrocution.
- Haemorrhage.
- Shock.

Lizards

Anorexia

- Normal:
  - Gravid female.
  - Males during breeding season.
  - Decreased appetite associated with seasonal decreases in photoperiod and ambient temperatures.
  - 'Shy feeders' – individuals that prefer to feed while hidden and therefore refuse food offered in full view of the carer.
- Husbandry:
  - Suboptimal environmental temperature management.
  - Lack of ultraviolet light or inappropriate photoperiod cycle, affecting stimulus to feed.
  - Maladaptation to new environment.
  - Stress from increased frequency or duration of handling, including for management of a health.
  - Disturbances in environment outside the enclosure.
  - Inadequate cage furniture to enable normal behaviour (e.g. basking, hiding, climbing).
  - Inappropriate food items (e.g. live insects are preferred over dead ones).
  - Environmental stress from enclosure mates.
- Health:
  - Metastatic soft tissue mineralisation due to excessive vitamin D supplementation.
  - Systemic infections including adenovirus (mainly in young bearded dragons).
  - Rodenticide toxicity, either primary from ingestion of bait pellets (herbivorous species) or secondary from ingestion of baited rodent (carnivorous species).
  - Sensual deprivation (e.g. loss of sight – cataracts, corneal lipidosis) or smell (severe upper respiratory tract infection).
  - Periodontal disease (agamids, chameleons).
  - Lesion of tongue sheath (monitors and chameleons) and tongue (all species) – affect food prehension.
  - Gastrointestinal tract infections, parasites, neoplasia or obstruction.

- Hepatopathy (including hepatic lipidosis).
- Nephropathy.
- Dystocia.
- Preovulatory follicular stasis.
- Pain.
- Visceral gout.

Weight Loss

- All causes of anorexia as above.
- Husbandry:
  - Dominance of food source or other resources by enclosure mate, together with the effects of hierarchical stress – may predispose to disease.
  - Malnutrition due to insufficient food quantity or inappropriate food items.
- Health:
  - Neoplasia of any system.
  - Coccidiosis due to *Isospora amphiboluri* (young bearded dragons, frequently as co-infection with adenovirus).
  - Cryptosporidial enteritis or gastritis.
  - Maldigestion or malabsorption – to date, no precise aetiologies are recognised for these problems.

Distended Coelom

- Reproductive:
  - Gravid female.
  - Preovulatory follicular stasis.
  - Post-ovulatory follicular stasis.
  - Dystocia.
- Other:
  - Obesity (common in blue-tongue lizards, bearded dragons and leopard geckos fat is stored in paired ovoid fat bodies in the caudal coelom).
  - Organomegaly (e.g. neoplasia, hepatic lipidosis).
  - Coelomitis (including yolk coelomitis, most common in bearded dragons and green iguanas).
  - Ascites (including from hypoproteinaemia due to anorexia, malnutrition, maldigestion, malabsorption, parasitism, hepatopathy, nephropathy).
  - Pneumocoelom due to ruptured lung(s).
  - Faecal impaction.

Lethargy, Weakness, Depression

- Normal:
  - Gravid female.
- Husbandry:
  - Inappropriately low or high environmental temperature.
  - Inappropriate light type or photoperiod cycle affecting activity levels.
  - Inadequate cage furniture to enable normal behaviour (e.g. basking, hiding, climbing).
  - Social stress from enclosure mates.
  - Hypocalcaemia due to chronic nutritional secondary hyperparathyroidism (NSHP) caused by dietary calcium or phosphorus imbalance and/or inadequate exposure to ultraviolet B light.
- Health:
  - Non-specific sign seen with many disease processes, often coupled with anorexia.
  - Hypocalcaemia due to renal secondary hyperparathyroidism (RSHP).
  - Dehydration.
  - Systemic infection including septicaemia and adenovirus (mainly in young bearded dragons).
  - Heavy external or internal parasite burden.
  - Neoplasia of any system.
  - Visual deficits, including due to cataracts, corneal lipidosis.
  - Renal failure (common in green iguanas).
  - Dystocia.
  - Preovulatory follicular stasis.
  - Vertebral and long-bone weakness and fractures as a result of NSHP or RSHP.
  - Pain.
  - Early manifestation of all causes of neurological signs listed.
  - Haemorrhage.
  - Anaemia.
  - Visceral gout.

Dull, Dry, Pale or Discoloured Skin

- Normal:
  - Prior to normal ecdysis (geckos only dull, pale skin).
  - During normal ecdysis (flaky, peeling skin as most lizards shed piecemeal).

- Behavioural or environmental skin colour change due to activation of chromatophores (normal in some species, including chameleons, anoles).
- Husbandry:
  - Stress-induced skin colour change (fine black dots over whole body) due to activation of chromatophores in some species, including chameleons, geckos, iguanas (common with handling).
  - Inappropriately low environmental humidity.
- Health:
  - Fungal dermatitis, notably with *Chrysosporium* anamorph of *Nannizziopsis vriesii* (CANV) (focal skin discolouration).
  - Scar at sites of previous trauma or surgery (pale, smooth skin without scales).
  - Site of injection of irritating substance, especially enrofloxacin.

Dysecdysis (Abnormal Shedding): Fully or Partially Retained Slough

- Husbandry:
  - Inappropriately low environmental humidity.
  - Failure to provide adequate water body for soaking (required by some species).
  - Inappropriately low environmental temperature.
  - Lack of suitable cage furniture to initiate or assist shedding.
- Health:
  - Malnutrition, dehydration or debilitation.
  - Hypovitaminosis A (chameleons).
  - Concurrent illness.
  - Bacterial or fungal skin infection.
  - Mite or tick infestation.
  - Previous skin scarring from burn or trauma.

Dysecdysis: Increased Frequency of Sloughing

- Health:
  - Bacterial or fungal skin infection.
  - Mite or tick infestation.
  - Burns.
  - Hyperthyroidism.

Skin Hyperkeratosis, Granulomas, Proliferative Nodules, Papules, Pustules, Blisters, Ulceration

- Husbandry:
  - Inappropriately high environmental humidity, wet substrate, poor environmental hygiene (all predispose to bacterial or fungal dermatitis).
  - Burns, including from contact with a heat lamp, wire mesh heated by an adjacent lamp or pieces of hot glass from a lamp shattered when spayed with water (blisters, crusting, ulcers, full thickness loss of epidermis).
  - Chemical burn from contact with concentrated disinfectants (e.g. sodium hypochlorite).
- Health:
  - 'Blister disease' (fluid-filled skin vesicles) caused by bacterial or fungal infection.
  - Infection with CANV ('yellow fungus disease' of bearded dragons causes coalescing necrotic hyperkeratotic epidermis on head, limbs, body).
  - Dermatophilosis (nodular hyperkeratosis).
  - Other bacterial or fungal dermatitis.

Skin Abrasions, Thickening, Disruption

- Mite or tick infestation.
- Scar at site of previous trauma or surgery.
- Stress-related rostral abrasion.
- Traumatic wound (including bite from enclosure mate).

Cutaneous and Subcutaneous Swellings

- Normal:
  - Subcutaneous microchip (lizards are typically chipped in the inguinal area, just cranial to the thigh).
  - Hemipenal bulge (normal, associated with onset of sexual maturity and breeding season).
  - Swollen hemipenal pockets due to seminal plugs.

- Health:
  - Hemipenal pockets distended with retained slough, generally due to low environmental humidity.
  - Subcutaneous abscess or granuloma (due to ectoparasite attachment, puncture wound, foreign body, injection site, poor environmental hygiene, dermatophilosis).
  - Soft tissue infection, abscess or granuloma as sequela of adjacent osteomyelitis lesion (most commonly of the digits of blue-tongue and shingleback lizards and mandible or maxilla of agamids and chameleons).
  - Cellulitis.
  - Subcutaneous nematodes and filaroid parasites.
  - Skin neoplasia.
  - Pseudoaneurysm or dissecting aneurysm in bearded dragons (fluctuant to firm subcutaneous swelling on the dorsolateral neck just caudal to the skull).
  - Impacted pores of secretory pre-femoral or perianal glands (generally due to suboptimal humidity).
  - Periarticular gout.
  - Injection site reaction.

Overgrown or Misshapen Nails

- Health:
  - Inadequate exercise and opportunity to wear nails, including climbing, digging, access to substrates of varying hardness or roughness.
  - Sequela to paronychia.
  - Chronic abnormal weight bearing due to injury, limb loss or degenerative joint disease.

Opaque or Dry Spectacle (in Geckos and other Lizard Species with Spectacles)

- Normal:
  - Opaque spectacle associated with pre-ecdysis.
- Husbandry:
  - Spectacle abrasion from constant face rubbing against solid objects due to

periocular mites, dysecdysis or dry skin caused by low humidity.
  - Spectacle retention following ecdysis (occurs less commonly than in snakes because geckos regularly lick their spectacles).
- Health:
  - Indented spectacle due to previous case of retention.
  - Spectacle trauma or ulceration following incorrect treatment of retention.
  - Traumatic full or partial loss of spectacle.

Eyes: Colour Change, Opacities

- Normal:
  - Arcus lipoides corneae (normal age-related change in monitors): partly or fully circumferential band of corneal opacity at limbus.
- Health:
  - Bacterial or fungal keratitis or corneal ulcer, including as extension from adjacent skin infection.
  - Keratitis or corneal ulcer due to trauma, foreign body or chemical exposure (e.g. hypochlorite bleach).
  - Exposure keratitis following iatrogenic spectacle loss (in species with spectacles).
  - Subspectacular infection or abscess (in species with spectacles).
  - Corneal lipidosis.
  - Cataract.

Eye or Spectacle Distension

- Health:
  - Bacterial or fungal ocular infection (panophthalmitis), most commonly from trauma.
  - Subspectacular infection or abscess (in species with spectacles most cases occur from ascending infection via the nasolacrimal duct secondary to stomatitis or respiratory tract infection, including with *Trichomonas* spp.).
  - Ocular neoplasia.
  - Traumatic eye injury.
  - Subspectacular fluid accumulation due to blocked nasolacrimal duct

(in species with spectacles; 'pseudobuphthalmos').
– Glaucoma (including secondary to cataract).

Blepharoedema, Blepharospasm, Ocular Discharge, Periocular Swelling

- Health:
  – Restraint behind the head may cause blepharoedema due to engorgement of periocular venous sinuses.
  – Hypovitaminosis A (chameleons, anoles).
  – Subcutaneous cellulitis or abscess – most commonly from trauma.
  – Bacterial or fungal conjunctivitis, including from ascending infection via the nasolacrimal duct secondary to stomatitis or respiratory tract infection.
  – Periorbital abscess, including as sequela of upper respiratory tract infection.
  – Periocular mites or ticks.
  – Periocular viral papillomas.
  – Ocular or periocular neoplasia, including squamous cell carcinoma in bearded dragons.
  – Ocular or periocular trauma.
  – Eyelid burns from heat lamp.
  – Conjunctival or subpalpebral foreign body, most commonly substrate material.
  – Cardiomegaly, pericardial effusion or mass in the pectoral region (causes bilateral periocular swelling likely due to partial occlusion of the venous return and lymph flow).

Ear Swelling

- Health:
  – Abscess (bacterial, fungal).
  – Ectoparasites – mites, ticks.
  – Neoplasia.

Nasal Discharge, Excessive Salivation, Open Mouth Breathing, Dyspnoea

- Normal:
  – Nasal salt gland secretions (clear liquid or dry white powder) in some species, including green iguana, shingleback lizard.
  – Inspiration or expiration in some species (including agamids) is exaggerated, may be mistaken for dyspnoea.
  – Transient partial obstruction of nares during ecdysis, producing wheezing sound (normal).

- Husbandry:
  – Open mouth 'panting' for thermoregulation (normal, but may indicate inappropriately high environmental temperature)

- Health:
  – Complete or partial obstruction of nares by retained slough.
  – Toxins:
    o organophosphate, carbamate, pyrethrin and pyrethroid insecticide toxicity (salivation, respiratory secretions, dyspnoea);
    o anticoagulant rodenticide toxicity, either primary from ingestion of bait pellets by herbivorous species or secondary from ingestion of baited rodent by carnivorous species (dyspnoea);
    o epistaxis due to haemorrhage from metastatic soft tissue mineralisation caused by excessive vitamin D supplementation;
    o inhaled irritants, including pollen and fumes of disinfectants and other chemicals.
  – Oral abnormalities
    o stomatitis (bacterial, fungal) – exudate or saliva may enter the choana, producing nasal discharge;
    o obstruction of glottis by oral cavity foreign body or lesion, including abscess, neoplasia.
  – Nasal:
    o infectious upper respiratory tract infection of unknown aetiology, including in juvenile blue-tongue lizards and 'bobtail flu' of shingleback lizards (nasal or oral discharge, epiphora, sneezing, dyspnoea);
    o rhinitis or sinusitis (bacterial, viral, fungal).

- Lower respiratory tract disease:
  ○ intracoelomic disease (including ascites, coelomitis, neoplasia, masses) may impede normal lung expansion, resulting in dyspnoea;
  ○ pneumonia (bacterial, fungal, viral, parasitic), including ferlavirus infection;
  ○ neoplasia, primary tumour or lung metastasis;
  ○ pulmonary oedema due to cardiac or hepatic disease;
  ○ aspiration pneumonia due to inexpert assist feeding or administration of oral medication;
  ○ water aspiration (near-drowning), including in lizards unattended while soaking in buckets of water.

Oral Discharge, Salivation, Gingival Inflammation, Recession, Ulceration, Hyperplasia or Exudation

- Health:
  - Stomatitis (bacterial, fungal, viral).
  - Chronic exposure gingivitis and ptyalism – due to traumatic lip defects or deformed mandibles or maxillae due to NSHP.
  - Periodontal disease in agamids, chameleons (includes gingival erythema, swelling, recession, ulceration, hyperplasia, exudation, mainly at the bone-gingiva junction).
  - Focal gingival infection following traumatic dental loss or fracture.
  - Oral neoplasia – may be ulcerated.
  - Stress-related rostral abrasion – may extend deeply into oral tissues.
  - Pneumonia (bacterial, fungal, parasitic) – may present with exudate from glottis in oral cavity.
  - Organophosphate, carbamate, pyrethrin and pyrethroid insecticide toxicity (salivation).

Dental Loss, Plaque or Calculus

- Normal:
  - Pleurodont species (skinks, geckos, iguanas, monitors): occasional missing

or shedding tooth – normal continuous tooth replacement that occurs throughout life in these species.
  - Acrodont species (agamids, chameleons): absence of teeth in all dental arcades – normal in aged individuals, as the teeth of these species progressively wear with age and are not replaced.
- Health:
  - Periodontal disease in agamids, chameleons (supragingival plaque and calculus, exposure of subgingival bone of mandibles or maxillae due to gingival recession, focal erosion and pitting of exposed subgingival bone).
  - Loose teeth in pleurodonts due to mandible or maxilla pathology caused by NSHP.
  - Trauma including from biting hard objects such as oral specula – transient tooth loss in pleurodonts, fractured teeth in acrodonts.

Tongue lesions

- Health:
  - Flaccid paralysis in chameleons (tongue droops from mouth, cannot be propelled for feeding) - common early sign of hypocalcaemia due to NSHP or RSHP.
  - Bacterial or fungal infection of tongue of all species and tongue sheath of monitors, chameleons (erythema, ulceration, exudation).
  - Inability to protrude tongue (monitors, chameleons) due to adhesions within tongue sheath as sequela of trauma or infection.

Oral Mucous Membrane Colour

- Normal:
  - White to pale pink: normal for most species.
  - Yellow-orange: normal for some bearded dragons and chameleons.
  - Dark purple to jet black: normal for some monitors, geckos and chameleons.
  - Dark pink: normal for some monitors.

- Health:
  - Erythema (generalised or focal): periodontal disease (agamids, chameleons); stomatitis.
  - Cyanosis: indicative of severe respiratory compromise.
  - Green (biliverdinaemia): pre-hepatic, hepatic or post-hepatic disease.

Facial or Jaw Swellings, Deformities

- Health:
  - Swollen or misshapen mandibles ('rubber jaw') due to fibrous osteodystrophy from NSHP.
  - Malocclusion, including overshot and undershot jaw, due to fibrous osteodystrophy from NSHP.
  - Subcutaneous abscess adjacent to osteomyelitis lesion of mandible or maxilla as a sequela of periodontal disease (agamids, chameleons).
  - Abscess of temporal gland of chameleons (positioned at the commissure of the mouth).
  - Abscess of other facial tissues, including due to puncture wound, ectoparasite attachment.
  - Cellulitis.
  - Fracture or soft tissue wound, including due to cage-mate trauma or bite from prey item.
  - Osteomyelitis (bacterial, fungal).
  - Bone or soft tissue neoplasia.
  - Gout.
  - Sialocoele.

Diarrhoea

- Husbandry:
  - Maldigestion and bacterial overgrowth due to suboptimal environmental temperature.
  - Sudden diet change (mostly affects herbivorous lizards).
  - Inappropriate diet for herbivorous lizards, including excessive fruit and insufficient fibre, fermented fruit or vegetables, selectivity for fruit.

- Inappropriate diet for carnivorous lizards, including dog food, meat parts and products instead of whole prey items.
  - Overfeeding.
- Health:
  - Bacterial or fungal enteritis or colitis (including salmonellosis).
  - Protozoal enteritis or colitis (including coccidia, *Cryptosporidium* spp., *Entamoeba* spp., flagellates).
  - Infestation with hookworms, ascarids, strongyles.
  - Dysbiosis following antibiotic therapy or systemic disease.
  - Polyuria, producing semi-liquid faeces due to mixing with urine.

Constipation, Reduced Faecal Output

- Husbandry:
  - Suboptimal environmental temperature, hence cannot reach or maintain optimal body temperature for normal gastrointestinal function.
  - Dehydration due to low humidity environment or inappropriate delivery of drinking water (e.g. some lizards will only drink from a spray bottle, or from droplets on leaves).
  - Insufficient exercise.
  - Insufficient fibre in diet of herbivores or omnivores.
  - Inappropriate food items (e.g. long-haired rodents, insects with heavy exoskeletons).
  - Overfeeding of beetle larvae ('mealworms') due to excess of indigestible chitin.
  - Ingestion of enclosure substrate (pebbles, gravel, sand, bark).
- Health:
  - Poor muscle tone and intestinal stasis due to hypocalcaemia from NSHP or RSHP.
  - Gut obstruction (e.g. intussusception, neoplasia).
  - Extraluminal gastrointestinal blockage (e.g. cystic calculi, dystocia).
  - Spinal neuropathy.

Palpable or Visible Internal Swellings

- Normal:
  - Gravid female; egg bulges may be visible through body wall.
- Health:
  - Abscess or granuloma of any internal organ or coelomic cavity, including *Mycobacteria* spp. infection.
  - Inflammatory swelling of any internal organ.
  - Neoplasia of any internal organ.
  - Ingested foreign body.
  - Faecal impaction.
  - Solid urate mass in colon.
  - Dystocia.

Swelling of the Cloaca or Hemipenal Region

- Health:
  - Increased production of hemipenal plugs due to hypovitaminosis A (chameleons).
  - Bacterial or protozoal cloacitis.
  - Hemipenal pocket infection.
- Trauma:
  - Hemipenal trauma.
  - Mating trauma in female.
  - Oedema of cloacal mucosa secondary to tenesmus due to faecal impaction or dystocia.

Prolapse from Cloaca

- General:
  - Poor muscle tone, intestinal stasis and bloating due to hypocalcaemia from NSHP or RSHP (prolapse of cloaca, colon).
  - Generalized weakness (prolapsed cloaca, colon, bladder, oviduct or hemipene).
  - Increased intracoelomic pressure due to coelomic distension (prolapsed cloaca, colon, bladder or oviduct).
- Gastrointestinal:
  - Tenesmus due to parasitism, gastroenteritis, cloacitis or gut obstruction by faecal impaction, intussusception, neoplasia (prolapsed cloaca, colon).
  - Straining due to extraluminal gastrointestinal blockage, including by tumour, abscess (prolapsed cloaca, colon).
- Urinary:
  - Straining due to bacterial cystitis, cystic calculi (prolapsed cloaca, bladder, colon).
- Reproductive:
  - Straining due to dystocia (prolapsed cloaca, oviduct).
  - Prolapsed hemipenes, due to traction during copulation, bite wounds from cage mates, spinal injury, contamination with substrate material, poor muscle tone from NSHP or straining due to any of the causes listed above.

Discoloured Urates

- Normal:
  - Yellow: normal variation of the usual white or cream urates.
- Health:
  - Green (biliverdinuria): chronic anorexia or starvation; hepatic disease; cholecystitis; bile duct obstruction; haemolysis.
  - Including frank blood: haemorrhage or inflammation of the kidneys, colon or cloaca; passage of abnormally hard faeces, causing blood streaking on surface of both faecal and urate masses; following manual palpation to resolve faecal impaction or egg retention.

Gravid Female not Commencing or Completing Parturition or Oviposition

- Husbandry:
  - Environmental temperature or humidity not species appropriate.
  - Failure to provide suitable nest site, including adequately deep substrate for burying of eggs.
  - Disturbance of parturition by cage mate or external stimulus.
  - Obesity due to overfeeding.
  - Malnutrition.
  - Exhaustion mid-lay due to poor fitness in chronically inactive lizard.

- Health:
  - Hypocalcaemia, including due to chronic NSHP or RSHP.
  - General debilitation due to other disease process, including systemic illness, dehydration, NSHP or RSHP.
  - Obstructive dystocia due to:
    ○ oversized or malformed egg or foetus, crushed egg, dead foetus;
    ○ pathology external to reproductive tract (e.g. cystic calculi, narrowed pelvic canal following fracture).
  - Salpingitis.
  - Preovulatory follicular stasis (these animals appear to be gravid).
  - Pelvic or spinal trauma.

Limb or Vertebral Swellings

- Health:
  - Bilaterally symmetrical swollen thighs due to fibrous osteodystrophy of the femoral diaphysis as a result of NSHP or RSHP.
  - Focal osteomyelitis of long-bone or vertebra due to trauma, spread from adjacent soft tissue infection or haematogenous spread.
  - Bone neoplasia.
  - Traumatic fractures, luxations and soft tissue injuries, including from handling and bites from cage mates.
  - Pathological long-bone or vertebral fractures due to NSHP or RSHP.
  - Septic arthritis.
  - Articular and periarticular gout (radiolucent uric acid deposits in and around joints).
  - Hypertrophic osteopathy (hypertrophic pulmonary osteoarthropathy).

Missing Digits or Tail Tip, Swellings, Constrictions

- Normal:
  - Partial tail loss and regrowth due to defensive autotomy (normal in many iguanas, skinks and geckos).
- Husbandry:
  - Slough retention on digits and tail tip due to low environmental humidity

resulting in tourniquet effect and avascular necrosis.

- Health:
  - Bacterial or fungal infection of digits due to poor environmental hygiene, overcrowding or trauma (digital swelling and loss due to osteolysis).
  - Cage-mate trauma.
  - Avascular necrosis of distal tail, digits due to crushing injury (caught in cage door, under rock).
  - Avascular necrosis of distal tail within two weeks of ventral caudal vein venepuncture (most likely due to iatrogenic vascular damage).

Lameness

- Health:
  - Osteomyelitis.
  - Septic arthritis.
  - Bone neoplasia.
  - Traumatic fractures, luxations and soft-tissue injuries, including from handling and bites from cage mates.
  - Pathological long-bone or vertebral fractures due to NSHP or RSHP.
  - Penetrating foreign body, plantar surface of foot.
  - Foot abrasion or ulceration due to contact with or pacing on rough substrate.
  - Degenerative joint disease.
  - Hypertrophic osteopathy.
  - Articular and periarticular gout.
  - Pseudogout (radiopaque calcium deposits in joints).

Gait and Posture Abnormalities

- Health:
  - Prone resting posture with ventrum not raised off substrate and limbs splayed from trunk, due to NSHP (agamids) (normal posture is with the limbs supporting the body, raising it at least partly off the substrate).
  - Ambulation with weight bearing on carpi and tarsi instead of on toes or feet, due to NSHP (iguanas).
  - Ossifying spondylosis, causing segmental fusion of adjacent vertebrae.

Paresis, Paralysis

- Neurological:
  - Adenovirus infections (mainly in juvenile bearded dragons).
  - Central nervous system infection, bacterial or fungal or viral or parasitic.
  - Electrocution (flaccid paralysis).
- Spinal:
  - Pathological vertebral fracture or collapse due to NSHP or RSHP.
  - Spinal trauma, including from handling, crushing by enclosure furniture, bites from cage mates.
  - Spinal osteomyelitis or abscess.
  - Bone neoplasia.
- Other:
  - Renomegaly.
  - Faecal impaction.
  - Dystocia.

Neurological Signs, Including Opisthotonus, Head Tilt, Circling, Ataxia, Muscle Fasciculation, Convulsions

- Nutritional:
  - Hypocalcaemia (causes muscle fasciculation and tetany mainly seen in conjunction with chronic NSHP).
  - Hypoglycaemia.
  - Thiamine deficiency (in lizards with a high proportion of un-supplemented frozen fish or vegetables in their diets).
  - Biotin deficiency (in lizards with a high proportion of unsupplemented raw eggs in their diets).
- Toxins:
  - Toxicoses from contact with insecticides (organophosphates, carbamates, pyrethrins and pyrethroids).
  - Toxicoses from ingesting *Photinus* fireflies (bearded dragons), snails killed by bait (blue-tongued lizards) or cane toads.
  - Drugs, including metronidazole, ivermectin, and aminoglycoside antibiotics.
  - Ingestion of marijuana.
  - Ingestion of nicotine in tobacco.
  - Ingestion of disinfectants including iodine.

- Ingestion of and exposure to fumes of household chemicals including paint solvents, ethylene glycol.
  - Ingestion of plant toxins including cedar shavings, lilies.
- Other:
  - Head or body trauma.
  - Bacterial and mycotic encephalitis (including micro-abscesses secondary to septicaemia).
  - Adenovirus (mainly in young bearded dragons).
  - Pain.
  - Electrocution (convulsions).
  - Visceral gout.

Sudden Death

- Husbandry:
  - Hyperthermia from inappropriately high environmental temperature (e.g. thermostat failure or exposure to direct sunlight without opportunity to seek a cooler area).
  - Failure of carer to detect earlier signs of chronic illness.
- Health:
  - Systemic infections including septicaemia and adenovirus (mainly in young bearded dragons); toxicoses from ingesting *Photinus* fireflies (bearded dragons), cane toads, nicotine or cyanogenic glycosides in seeds of apples, cherries, peaches and plums.
  - Aneurysm rupture (most commonly in bearded dragons).
  - Trauma.
  - Electrocution.
  - Haemorrhage.
  - Shock.
  - Organ failure (e.g. visceral gout).

Chelonians

Anorexia

- Normal:
  - Females during folliculogenesis, ovulation, oviposition.

- Males during breeding season.
- Decreased appetite associated with seasonal decreases in photoperiod and ambient temperatures.
- Husbandry:
  - Suboptimal environmental temperature management, so cannot reach or maintain optimal body temperature for feeding – this includes failure to insulate animals from overnight decreases in ambient temperature in colder seasons.
  - Inappropriate photoperiod cycle, affecting stimulus to feed.
  - Inappropriate humidity (too wet or too dry), affecting general health.
  - 'Post-hibernation anorexia' (land tortoises); multifactorial as sequela of incorrect hibernation management, including lengthy period of deprivation of heat, light, food and water.
  - Maladaptation to new environment.
  - Environmental stress from enclosure mates.
  - Stress from increased frequency or duration of handling, including for management of a health problem.
  - Disturbances in environment outside the enclosure.
  - Inadequate cage furniture to enable normal behaviour (e.g. basking, swimming, hiding).
  - Inappropriate food items (e.g. lettuce to a freshwater turtle; meat to a herbivorous land turtle).
- Health:
  - Hypovitaminosis A (mainly freshwater turtles).
  - Metabolic disease, including hypocalcaemia, dehydration.
  - Infection, neoplasia or organ failure of any system.
  - Sensory deprivation (e.g. loss of sight – cataracts, corneal lipidosis, frost injury) or smell (severe upper respiratory tract infection).
  - Gastrointestinal parasites, notably *Entamoeba* spp., *Hexamita* spp.
  - Gastrointestinal tract infections, neoplasia or obstruction.

- Dystocia.
- Follicular stasis.
- Pain.
- Visceral gout.

Weight Loss

- All causes of anorexia as above.
- Husbandry:
  - Suboptimal environmental temperature, so cannot reach or maintain optimal body temperature for digestion – note comment about overnight temperatures in Anorexia section.
  - Dominance of food source or other resources by tank or enclosure mate.
  - Malnutrition due to insufficient food quantity or inappropriate food items.
- Health:
  - Maldigestion or malabsorption – to date, no precise aetiologies are recognised for these: problems.
  - Endoparasites including amoeba, coccidia, *Cryptosporidium* spp., *Hexamita* spp., nematodes.
  - Foreign body ingestion, generally mistaken for food items, including plastic bags, fishing tackle, coins (mainly marine turtles).

Distended Coelom (Bulging Inguinal Fossae)

- Normal:
  - Gravid female.
- Husbandry:
  - Obesity due to inactivity and overfeeding (e.g. high-protein diet fed to omnivorous species; common in *Emydura* spp.).
  - Gastrointestinal bloating due to abnormal fermentation, including from suboptimal environmental temperature, inappropriate diet.
- Health:
  - Obesity due to hypothyroidism (anecdotal reports in giant tortoises due to low iodine or high goitrogen diets).
  - Ascites (see list of causes below).

- Coelomitis (including yolk coelomitis).
- Enlargement of any coelomic organ (e.g. neoplasia, granulomas, hepatic lipidosis).
- Cystic calculi (land tortoises).
- Dystocia.
- Follicular stasis.

Ascites, Subcutaneous Oedema

- Health:
  - Myxoedema due to hypothyroidism (anecdotal reports in giant tortoises due to low iodine or high goitrogen diets).
  - Renal failure due to hypovitaminosis A (axillary and inguinal oedema).
  - Systemic infection, including as a result of poor water hygiene.
  - Ranavirus infection (land tortoises and freshwater turtles) – severe subcutaneous cervical oedema.
  - Picornavirus infection (land tortoises) – ascites.
  - Herpesvirus infection (land tortoises) – cervical oedema.
  - Herpesvirus (freshwater turtles) – subcutaneous oedema, mainly of limbs.
  - Hypoproteinaemia due to anorexia, malnutrition, maldigestion, malabsorption, parasitism, hepatopathy, nephropathy.
  - Congestive heart failure or circulatory failure.
  - Excessive fluid therapy.

Lethargy, Weakness or Depression

- Normal:
  - Gravid female.
- Husbandry:
  - Inappropriately low environmental temperature, resulting in suboptimal activity.
  - Hypothermia due to lack of opportunity to thermoregulate to a higher body temperature (e.g. by basking) at times of sudden drop in environmental temperature.
  - Hyperthermia due to lack of opportunity to thermoregulate to a lower body

temperature (e.g. by soaking in water, entering shade) at times of high environmental temperature.
  - Inappropriate light type or photoperiod cycle, affecting activity levels.
- Health:
  - Hypocalcaemia due to chronic nutritional secondary hyperparathyroidism, NSHP, caused by dietary calcium or phosphorus imbalance and/or inadequate exposure to ultraviolet B light.
  - Hypocalcaemia due to renal secondary hyperparathyroidism (RSHP).
  - Hypovitaminosis A (mainly freshwater turtles).
  - Nonspecific sign seen with many disease processes, often coupled with anorexia.
  - Metabolic disease, including dehydration.
  - Systemic infection including septicaemia, viral disease.
  - Heavy parasite burden, notably *Entamoeba* spp., *Hexamita* spp.
  - Neoplasia of any system.
  - Toxicoses, including exposure to insecticides, inappropriate drugs or dosages.
  - Visual deficits, including due to cataracts, corneal lipidosis, frost injury.
  - Foreign body ingestion, generally mistaken for food items, including plastic bags, fishing tackle, coins, (mainly marine turtles).
  - Dystocia.
  - Follicular stasis.
  - Anaemia.

Inability to Submerge (Freshwater and Marine Turtles)

- Husbandry:
  - Inappropriately low environmental temperature, resulting in suboptimal activity and hence inability to dive normally.
- Health:
  - Weakness due to emaciation or any systemic illness, resulting in inability to dive normally.

- Pneumonia (bacterial or fungal).
- Lung, eye, trachea disease due to herpesvirus (green sea turtles) – bronchopneumonia.
- Pneumocoelom (air free in coelom), due to lung trauma.
- Gastrointestinal bloating due to abnormal fermentation, including from suboptimal environmental temperature, inappropriate diet.
- Bloat due to gas-producing gastrointestinal infection.
- Ileus due to intestinal impaction or obstruction (including ingested plastic bags in marine turtles), resulting in gas distension of bowel.
- Spinal trauma, resulting inability to dive normally.

Uneven Floating (Freshwater and Marine Turtles)

- Normal:
  - Gravidity (does not occur in all gravid chelonians).
- Health:
  - Any unilateral internal mass, including abscesses, granulomas, tumours, making one side of the body heavier than the other.
  - Pneumonia or lung abscess, or granuloma, making one lung less inflated then the other (may occur as sequela of lung injury and contamination associated with carapace fracture).
  - Asymmetric gas production (bloat), making one side of the body more buoyant than the other.
  - Dystocia.

Dry, Sloughing or Discoloured Skin

- Normal:
  - Ecdysis (flaky, peeling skin as chelonians shed piecemeal).
- Husbandry:
  - Abnormal shedding (increased or decreased), mainly in axillary and inguinal fossae, due to suboptimal environmental temperature or humidity.

- Dry skin due to inappropriately low environmental humidity or unsuitable water body (freshwater turtles).
- Health:
  - Hypovitaminosis A (mainly freshwater turtles) – hyperkeratosis.
  - Hypervitaminosis A (iatrogenic) – initially dry, flaky skin, then blisters, mainly on neck and limbs, progressing to necrotizing dermatitis and full thickness epidermal sloughing.
  - Deep bacterial or fungal infection – may cause full thickness epidermal sloughing.
  - Scar at sites of previous trauma or surgery (de-pigmented skin).
  - Burns (thermal, chemical) – may cause full thickness epidermal sloughing.

Skin Erythema or Petechiae

- Health:
  - Hypovitaminosis A (mainly freshwater turtles).
  - Septicaemia.
  - Burns.

Skin Abrasions or Ulcerations

- Health:
  - Septicaemic cutaneous ulcerative disease, caused by bacteria, including *Citrobacter freundii* and *Pseudomonas* spp. (freshwater turtles) – skin ulceration, sloughing, septicaemia, dehydration.
  - Other ulcerative bacterial or fungal dermatitis, including due to unsuitably high wetness or humidity (land tortoises), poor water hygiene or pool overcrowding (freshwater turtles).
  - Grey-patch disease due to herpesvirus infection (young green sea turtles) – epizootic of small circular papular lesions that coalesce into patches, then become ulcerated or necrotizing.
  - Trauma – bites on feet and neck from tank mates (freshwater turtles) and rats during hibernation (land tortoises).

- Abrasions, mainly on plantar surface of feet from contact with rough substrate (e.g. concrete pools, freshwater turtles).
- Burns (thermal, chemical).

Cutaneous and Subcutaneous Swellings

- Normal:
  - Subcutaneous microchip (chelonians are typically chipped in the inguinal fossa).
- Health:
  - Subcutaneous abscess or granuloma (due to ectoparasite attachment, puncture wound, foreign body, injection site, poor environmental hygiene) – notably on feet and neck in freshwater turtles due to bites from tank mates.
  - Soft-tissue infection or abscess, or granuloma, as sequela of adjacent osteomyelitis lesion.
  - Mycobacterial or fungal infection (nodular skin lesions).
  - Cellulitis.
  - Attached ectoparasites, including ticks, mites and leeches.
  - Myiasis due to botflies (mostly box turtles, mainly on neck, proximal limbs, axillary and inguinal fossae).
  - Fibropapillomas due to herpesvirus (common in green sea turtles also seen in other marine turtle species).
  - Other skin neoplasia, including epidermal papillomas.
  - Scar at sites of previous trauma or surgery (focal skin thickening).
  - Periarticular gout.
  - Injection site reaction.

Shell Fractures and Wounds

- Health:
  - Pathological fracture due to NSHP or RSHP.
  - Trauma, including motor vehicle, bite wounds from predators, garden tools, lawnmowers, falls (including being dropped), crush injury (including by enclosure rocks).

Soft Shell

- Normal:
  - Hatchlings and juveniles of many species (normally have soft shells).
  - Softshell turtles, pancake tortoises (normally have soft shells).
  - Box turtles (have hinged plastrons that may be mistaken as soft shells).
- Health:
  - NSHP (uniformly soft, 'bendy' shell).
  - Bacterial or fungal infections – focal areas of soft shell, hyperaemia, fibrinonecrotic debris ('shell rot').
  - Picornavirus (land tortoises) – softening of carapace in young animals.

Shell Deformity

- Health:
  - NSHP (distorted shell).
  - Trauma, including by heat, causing premature closure of shell growth plate(s).
  - Congenital deformity (mostly due to inappropriate incubation conditions).

Pyramidal Carapace

- Husbandry:
  - Possibly overly rapid growth in juveniles due to overfeeding or excess dietary protein.
- Health:
  - NSHP (due to fibrous osteodystrophy).

Shell Epidermis (Scute) Discolouration, Flaking, Thickening

- Normal:
  - Ecdysis (scutes are shed, one by one, from the carapace and plastron of some species).
  - Green algal growth on surface of scutes in freshwater turtles.
- Husbandry:
  - Dysecdysis (retained slough) due to suboptimal environment, including inadequate thermal management.

- Health:
  - Dysecdysis (increased frequency of sloughing) due to rapid growth, acute infections, hypo- or hypervitaminosis A.
  - Bacterial infection of dermal bone, causing fluid accumulation under scutes, creating pale foci.
  - Dermal bone (white) exposed by loss of overlying epidermal scute, including due to abrasions and other trauma.
  - Pitted or thickened scutes at sites of previous infection or trauma.
  - Scar at site of previous trauma or surgery (pale).

Shell Epidermis Erythema, Petechiae

- Health:
  - Bacterial or fungal lesions secondary to bite wounds, other trauma (including from abrasive substrates), inadequate environmental temperature management, poor water quality.
  - Septicaemia (diffuse erythema of scutes).

Shell Epidermis Ulceration, Abscessation

- Health:
  - Ulcerative shell disease of freshwater turtles, generally bacterial, may progress to septicaemia and death (septicaemic cutaneous ulcerative disease) – generally occurs as a result of suboptimal husbandry including inappropriately low water and/or basking site temperature, poor water hygiene, tank mate aggression and stress due to tank overcrowding.
  - Other bacterial or fungal infection, aka 'shell rot' (freshwater turtles, land tortoises).
  - Trauma, including bite wounds from other turtles, predators (such as domestic dog).
  - Burns.
  - Frost-induced necrosis.

Shell Epidermis Masses

- Health:
  - Fibropapillomas due to herpesvirus (common in green sea turtles also seen in other marine turtle species).

Overgrown or Misshapen Beak, Toenails

- Normal:
  - Long nails on hind limbs in females of some species for nest digging (normal).
  - Long nails on fore limbs in males of some species for mating (normal).
- Husbandry:
  - Overgrown toenails due to inadequate exercise and opportunity to wear nails, including digging, access to substrates of varying hardness or roughness.
  - Overgrown rhamphotheca (upper jaw) due to lack of exposure to hard or abrasive foodstuffs (land tortoises).
  - Possibly overly rapid growth in juveniles due to overfeeding or excess dietary protein.
- Health:
  - Overdevelopment of rhamphotheca due to NSHP (fibrous osteodystrophy).
  - Sequela of paronychia.
  - Chronic abnormal weight bearing due to injury or limb loss, or degenerative joint disease.

Eyes: Colour Changes, Opacities

- Normal:
  - Arcus lipoides corneae (normal age-related change) – partly or fully circumferential band of corneal opacity at limbus.
- Health:
  - Keratitis or corneal ulcer due to bacterial, fungal or viral infection.
  - Lung, eye, trachea disease due to herpesvirus (green sea turtles) – caseous keratitis, corneal ulceration.
  - Corneal fibropapillomas due to herpesvirus (common in green sea turtles also seen in other marine turtle species).

- Keratitis or corneal ulcer due to trauma, foreign body or chemical exposure (e.g. hypochlorite bleach).
- Lens opacity, hyphaema from frost damage due to hibernation outdoors in temperatures less than 0 degrees C (land tortoises).
- Corneal scarring post keratitis, frost damage.
- Corneal lipidosis.
- Cataract.

Exophthalmia

- Health:
  - Retrobulbar abscess or tumour.
  - Trauma.
  - Bilateral exophthalmia occurs with generalized oedema or vascular obstruction.

Blepharoedema, Blepharospasm, Conjunctivitis, Ocular Discharge

- Health:
  - Physical problems:
    - Restraint behind the head may cause blepharoedema due to engorgement of periocular venous sinuses.
    - Ocular or periocular trauma (eyelid trauma common in freshwater turtles from feeding frenzies).
    - Conjunctival or subpalpebral foreign body, including dust, sand, pollen.
  - Nutritional:
    - Hypovitaminosis A (mainly freshwater turtles) – palpebral oedema, caseous exudate underneath eyelids, blindness, nasal or ocular discharge.
    - Inflammatory.
    - Keratitis, corneal ulcer or panophthalmitis.
  - Infectious:
    - Bacterial or fungal conjunctivitis, including from ascending infection via the nasolacrimal duct secondary to stomatitis or upper respiratory tract infection.
    - *Mycoplasma* spp. upper respiratory tract infection – blepharoedema, conjunctivitis, ocular discharge.

  - Ranavirus infection (land tortoises, freshwater turtles) – conjunctivitis.
  - Picornavirus infection (land tortoises) – conjunctivitis.
  - Herpesvirus infection (land tortoises) – conjunctivitis.
  - Lung, eye, trachea disease due to herpesvirus (green sea turtles) – keratitis, conjunctivitis.
  - Tortoise poxvirus (land tortoises) – periocular papular skin lesions.
- Neoplasia:
  - Ocular or periocular neoplasia.
  - Periocular fibropapillomas due to herpesvirus (common in green sea turtles also seen in other MT species).

Loss of Vision

- Health:
  - Lens opacity, hyphaema, possible retinal injury from frost damage (due to hibernation outdoors in temperatures less than 0 degrees C (land tortoises).
  - Corneal opacity, including lipidosis.
  - Cataracts.
- Nutritional:
  - Hypovitaminosis A.
- Neoplasia:
  - Corneal or periocular fibropapillomas due to herpesvirus (common in green sea turtles but also seen in other marine turtle species).

Tympanic Membrane Bulge

- Health:
  - Middle ear infection or abscess (common in box turtles also seen in other freshwater turtle and land tortoise species).
  - Neoplasia.

Oral Inflammation, Ulceration, Abscessation

- Nutritional:
  - Hypovitaminosis A.
  - Hypovitaminosis C.

- Infectious:
  - Bacterial or fungal stomatitis.
  - Ranavirus infection (land tortoises, freshwater turtles) – stomatitis, tracheitis.
  - Picornavirus infection (land tortoises) – diphtheroid necrotising stomatitis
  - Herpesvirus infection (land tortoises) – diphtheroid necrotizing stomatitis, pharyngitis, glossitis, tracheitis (white plaque lesions).
  - lung, eye, trachea disease due to herpesvirus (green sea turtles) – diphtheroid necrotizing stomatitis (mainly periglottal), pharyngitis, tracheitis.
  - Loggerhead orocutaneous herpesvirus (loggerhead sea turtles) – ulcers, caseous plaques.
- Physical:
  - Chemical irritation, including from eating certain plants, household chemicals.
  - Penetration injuries or abrasions from food items (e.g. prickly branches).
  - Inflammation as sequela of food remnant putrefaction when chelonians are not fasted before winter hibernation.

Oral Mucous Membrane Colour

- Pallor
  - During hibernation (normal).
  - Inappropriately low environmental temperature.
  - Anaemia.
  - Cardiovascular disease.
- Erythema (generalized or focal):
  - Septicaemia.
  - Stomatitis.
- Cyanosis:
  - Severe respiratory compromise.
- Green (biliverdinaemia):
  - Pre-hepatic, hepatic or post hepatic disease.

Nasal or Oral Discharge, Nares Lesions

- Nutritional:
  - Hypovitaminosis A can predispose to secondary nasal sinus infections (mainly freshwater turtles).

- Infection:
  - Ranavirus infection (land tortoises, freshwater turtles).
  - Picornavirus infection (land tortoises).
  - Lung, eye, trachea disease due to herpesvirus (green sea turtles) – bronchopneumonia.
  - Herpesvirus infection (land tortoises) (mostly accompanied by whitish oral plaques) – rhinitis, pneumonia.
  - *Mycoplasma* spp. upper respiratory tract infection (land tortoises; not accompanied by oral lesions).
  - Other upper respiratory tract infections (viral, bacterial, fungal).
- Physical:
  - Excessive salivation, including due to stomatitis (saliva may enter the choana, producing nasal discharge).
  - Focal erosion or depigmentation of nares due to chronic upper respiratory tract disease.
  - Inhaled irritants, including pollen and fumes of disinfectants and other chemicals.
  - Foreign body, including grass seeds in upper respiratory tract or pharynx.

Tracheal Discharge

- Infection:
  - Pneumonia, bacterial, fungal, viral or protozoal, often secondary to chronically low environmental temperature.
  - Herpesvirus infection (land tortoises) – tracheitis.
  - Lung, eye, trachea disease due to herpesvirus (green sea turtles) – tracheitis.
  - Loggerhead genital–respiratory herpesvirus (loggerhead sea turtles) – tracheitis.

Dyspnoea, Abnormal Respiratory Sounds

- Nutritional:
  - Hypovitaminosis A.
- Infection:
  - Pneumonia, bacterial, fungal or parasitic, often secondary to chronically low environmental temperature.

- Upper respiratory tract infection due to Ranavirus (land tortoises, freshwater turtles), *Mycoplasma* spp. (land tortoises), other bacteria, viruses or fungi.
- Lung, eye, trachea disease due to herpesvirus (green sea turtles) – bronchopneumonia.
- Physical:
  - Neoplasia, primary tumour or lung metastasis.
  - Inhaled irritants, including pollen, chemicals.
  - Near drowning, including from head, limb or full body entrapment in fishing nets (marine turtles), pool furniture, uncovered drains or filters.
  - Aspirated foreign bodies, including grass seeds.
  - Aspiration pneumonia due to inexpert assist feeding or administration of oral medication.

Regurgitation or Vomiting

- Husbandry:
  - Suboptimal environmental temperature following feeding.
  - Excessive handling within 24–48 hours after feeding.
  - Overfeeding.
- Infection:
  - Septicaemia.
  - Bacterial or fungal gastroenteritis.
  - Gastrointestinal parasitism.
- Physical:
  - Gastrointestinal obstruction due to ingested foreign body, gastrointestinal neoplasia, granuloma, intussusception or faecal impaction.
  - Gastrointestinal obstruction due to extraintestinal lesion.

Diarrhoea

- Normal:
  - Semi-liquid faeces due to mixing with large volume of urine.

- Husbandry:
  - Maldigestion and bacterial overgrowth due to suboptimal environmental temperature.
  - Inappropriate diet, including fermented fruit or vegetables; selectivity for fruit.
  - Overfeeding.
- Infection:
  - Bacterial or fungal enteritis or colitis, including salmonellosis.
  - Parasitic enteritis or colitis, notably due to *Entamoeba* or *Hexamita* spp.
  - Dysbiosis following antibiotic therapy or systemic disease.

Constipation or Reduced Faecal Output

- Husbandry:
  - Suboptimal environmental temperature, so cannot reach or maintain optimal body temperature for normal gastrointestinal function.
  - Dehydration due to low humidity environment, inadequate pool or failure to provide water ad libitum.
  - Insufficient exercise.
  - Ingestion of enclosure substrate (pebbles, gravel, sand, bark).
  - Impaction with the chitinous and shell parts of prey (as sequela to ileus in wild marine turtles in rehabilitation care).
- Health:
  - Gastrointestinal obstruction (e.g. intussusception, neoplasia).
  - Extraluminal gastrointestinal blockage (e.g. cystic calculi, dystocia).
  - Spinal neuropathy.

Coelomic Masses Palpable or Visible at Inguinal Fossae

- Normal:
  - Folliculogenesis and atretic follicles.
  - Gravid female.
- Health:
  - Abscess or granuloma of internal organ or coelomic cavity, including *Mycobacteria* spp. infection.

- Neoplasia or cyst of internal organ or coelomic cavity.
- Inflammatory swelling of internal organ.
- Faecal impaction.
- Intussusception.
- Cystic calculi.
- Dystocia.
- Retained unfertilized eggs (slugs).

Cloacal Swelling

- Health:
  - Bacterial or protozoal cloacitis.
  - Myiasis, often as sequela of faecal soiling, diarrhoea (land tortoises).
  - Penile trauma.
  - Mating trauma in female.
  - Oedema of cloacal mucosa secondary to tenesmus due to faecal impaction or dystocia.

Bleeding From Cloaca

- Health:
  - Trauma, including phallus laceration, mating trauma in both males and females.
  - Haemorrhage from gastrointestinal tract, urogenital tract or cloaca due to infection, parasitism, neoplasia.
  - Cystic calculi (land tortoises).
  - Dystocia.

Intracloacal and Pericloacal Ulceration

- Health:
  - Loggerhead genital-respiratory herpesvirus (loggerhead sea turtles), including ulcers at base of phallus.

Phallic Prolapse (Large Pink, Purple, Tan or Black Mass with Spade-Shaped Tip)

- Normal:
  - Penile erection in male, retracts within several hours (normal).
- Health:
  - Inability to retract and retain phallus due to generalized weakness or poor muscle tone, including from systemic illness,

dehydration, hypokalaemia, hypocalcaemia from NSHP and RSHP.

- Coelomic distension, including due to obesity, causing prolapse by increased intracoelomic pressure.
- Tenesmus due to parasitism, gastroenteritis, cloacitis or gut obstruction by faecal impaction, intussusception, neoplasia.
- Straining due to extraluminal gastointestinal blockage, including by tumour, abscess, cystic calculi.
- Mating injuries, including forced separation during copulation
- Other trauma, including contamination of erect, protruded phallus with substrate material and bites from cage mates.
- Excessive libido (phallus becomes swollen and cannot retract).
- Spinal injury.

Prolapse of Other Organs from Cloaca (May be Urinary Bladder, Oviduct, Colon or Cloaca)

- Health:
  - Poor muscle tone due to hypocalcaemia from NSHP or RSHP.
  - Generalized weakness, including due to systemic illness, dehydration, hypokalaemia.
  - Coelomic distension, including due to obesity, causing prolapse by increased intracoelomic pressure.
  - Tenesmus due to parasitism, gastroenteritis, cloacitis or gut obstruction by faecal impaction, intussusception, neoplasia (prolapsed cloaca, colon).
  - Straining due to extraluminal gastrointestinal blockage, including by tumour, abscess.
  - Straining due to oviposition, dystocia, salpingitis.
  - Straining due to any other cause including dyspnoea, cystic calculi.

Gravid Female not Commencing or Completing Oviposition

- Husbandry:
  - Environmental temperature, humidity or lighting not species appropriate.

– Failure to provide suitable nest site, including adequately deep substrate for burying of eggs.
– Competition for nest sites by enclosure mates.
– Disturbance of parturition by cage-mate aggression or external stimulus.
● Health:
– Obesity, poor fitness.
– Hypocalcaemia, including due to chronic NSHP or RSHP.
– General debilitation due to other disease process, including systemic illness, dehydration, NSHP or RSHP.
– Obstructive dystocia due to oversized, malformed or crushed egg(s).
– Obstructive dystocia due to pathology external to reproductive tract (e.g. cystic calculi, narrowed pelvic canal following fracture).
– Ectopic egg(s), in coelom, urinary bladder, colon, pelvis.
– Reproductive tract infection.
– Pain or neurological deficits due to pelvic, spinal or shell trauma.

Swollen limbs

● Health:
– Fibrous osteodystrophy due to NSHP or RSHP, resulting in thickened bone shafts.
– Focal osteomyelitis due to trauma, spread from adjacent soft tissue infection or haematogenous spread.
– Bone neoplasia.
– Traumatic fractures.
– Pathological fractures due to NSHP or RSHP.
– Limb oedema or necrosis following entanglement (mainly marine turtles).
– Limb oedema or necrosis from frost damage due to hibernation outdoors in temperatures less than 0 degrees C (land tortoises).

Joint Swelling

● Health:
– Septic arthritis.
– Periarticular abscess.
– Osteomyelitis.

– Trauma, including fractures, luxations, cruciate ligament injury in land tortoises.
– Degenerative joint disease.
– Periarticular or articular gout.
– Pseudogout.

Missing Digits or Tail Tip

● Health:
– Avascular necrosis of digits as sequela of bacterial or fungal osteolysis due to poor environmental hygiene, overcrowding, trauma.
– Avascular necrosis of distal tail, digits following crushing injury (e.g. caught under rock), frost injury.
– Cage or tank-mate trauma.

Lameness, Gait Abnormalities

● Health:
– Osteomyelitis.
– Septic arthritis.
– Bone neoplasia.
– Traumatic fractures, luxations and soft tissue injuries, including from being dropped, crushed, bites from enclosure mates, bites from rats during hibernation.
– Pathological long-bone or vertebral fractures due to NSHP or RSHP (signs include inability to raise the body off the ground).
– Penetrating foreign body, plantar surface of foot.
– Foot abrasions or ulcerations due to contact with or pacing on rough substrate.
– Degenerative joint disease.
– Articular and periarticular gout.
– Cystic calculi.
– Dystocia.

Paresis or paralysis

● Normal:
– Gravidity or oviposition (may present with hind limb paresis).
● Health:
– Herpesvirus infection (land tortoises).
– Other systemic illness.

- Faecal impaction.
- Toxicosis from the products of ingesta putrefaction when chelonians are allowed to chill following feeding or are not fasted before hibernation.
- Renomegaly.
- Cystic calculi.
- Dystocia (egg retention).
- Follicular stasis.
- Spinal osteomyelitis or abscess.
- Bone neoplasia.
- Pathological vertebral fracture or collapse due to NSHP, RSHP.
- Spinal trauma, including from being dropped, crushed by enclosure furniture, carapace injury.
- Central nervous system infection, bacterial, fungal, viral or parasitic.
- Ivermectin toxicity (causes depression, paralysis, coma, death in chelonians).
- Visceral or intervertebral gout.
- Electrocution (flaccid paralysis).
- Iatrogenic spinal cord compression following injection of fluids or medication into dorsal tail vein (occurs occasionally).

Neurological Signs Including Ataxia, Hypermetric Gait, Circling, Convulsions

- Health:
  - Sequela of hibernation outdoors in temperatures less than 0 degrees C, hyperthermia or near drowning (possibly due to hypoxia-induced cerebral oedema or cerebellar injury).
  - Thiamine deficiency (in animals with a high proportion of unsupplemented frozen fish or vegetables in their diets).
  - Metabolic disease, including hypoglycaemia, hypocalcaemia.
  - Septicaemia.
  - Herpesvirus infection (land tortoises).
  - Toxicosis from contact with insecticides (organophosphates, carbamates, pyrethrins and pyrethroids).
  - Drug toxicity, including ivermectin, metronidazole and aminoglycoside antibiotics.

- Ingestion of toxic compounds, including pesticide residues on food, marijuana, nicotine in tobacco, disinfectants including iodine, snail or rodent bait.
- Ingestion of plant toxins including cedar shavings, lilies, oak leaves.
- Ingestion of and exposure to fumes of household chemicals including paint solvents, ethylene glycol.
- Otitis media or ear abscess.
- Joint luxation (ataxia, hypermetric gait).
- Bacterial and mycotic encephalitis (including micro-abscesses secondary to septicaemia).
- Central nervous system trauma or neoplasia.
- Hepatic encephalopathy.
- Pain.
- Electrocution.
- Visceral gout.

Sudden Death

- Husbandry:
  - Hyperthermia (from inappropriately high environmental temperature (e.g. thermostat failure or exposure to direct sunlight without opportunity to seek a cooler area).
  - Failure of carer to detect earlier signs of chronic illness.
- Health:
  - Systemic infections, including septicaemia.
  - Ingestion of toxic compounds, including nicotine, cyanogenic glycosides in seeds of apples, cherries, peaches and plums (land tortoises).
  - Ivermectin toxicity (this drug should not be used in chelonians).
  - Trauma.
  - Drowning, including from entrapment in fishing nets (marine turtles), pool furniture, uncovered drains or filters.
  - Electrocution.
  - Haemorrhage.
  - Shock.
  - Organ failure (e.g. visceral gout).

Crocodilians

Anorexia

- Husbandry:
  - Suboptimal environmental temperature management, so cannot reach optimal body temperature for feeding.
  - Inappropriate photoperiod cycle, affecting stimulus to feed.
  - Insufficient exposure to ultraviolet light.
  - Maladaptation to new environment.
  - Environmental stress from enclosure mates.
  - Stress from increased frequency or duration of handling, including for management of a health problem.
  - Disturbances in environment outside the enclosure.
  - Inadequate enclosure design to enable normal behaviour (e.g. basking, hiding).
- Health:
  - Systemic infections, including viral (herpes virus, adenovirus), bacterial (consider *Salmonella*, *Mycobacteria* and *Chlamydia* spp., as well as opportunists such as *Pseudomonas* and *Aeromonas* spp.), mycotic (particularly *Fusarium* spp.), parasitic (especially *Coccidia* spp. in hatchlings and yearlings).
  - Pneumonia.
  - Bacterial or fungal stomatitis, oesophagitis or gastroenteritis.
  - Gastrointestinal tract parasites.
  - Gastrointestinal neoplasia.
  - Gastrointestinal obstruction (see list of causes under Vomiting or Regurgitation).
  - Hepatopathy, including hepatic lipidosis.
  - Extraintestinal inflammation or infection, neoplasia and other disease, including gout.
  - Steatitis and fat necrosis due to vitamin E deficiency (in animals with a high proportion of frozen fish in their diet, as the vitamin E in fish is depleted during freezing, in its action as an antioxidant of polyunsaturated fatty acids).

Weight Loss, Suboptimal Growth Rate

- All causes of anorexia as above.
- Husbandry:
  - Suboptimal environmental temperature, so cannot reach or maintain optimal body temperature for digestion.
  - 'Runting' of some individuals housed in a group, likely due to competition for food, hierarchical stress – may predispose to disease.
  - Malnutrition due to insufficient food quantity or inappropriate food items.
- Health:
  - Neoplasia.
  - Cardiac dysfunction.
  - Mycobacterial infection (causes intestinal wall thickening, maldigestion, malabsorption).
  - Other causes of malabsorption and/or maldigestion.
  - Nephropathy.
  - Pain.

Distended coelom

- Normal:
  - Gravid female.
  - Recent large meal.
- Health:
  - Obesity due to inactivity and overfeeding, including dominant animal ingesting extra food.
  - Anasarca due to hypovitaminosis A (occurs when animals are not fed whole prey, without vitamin A supplementation).
  - Ascites.
  - Coelomitis.
  - Neoplasia of any coelomic organ, including lymphosarcoma.
  - Yolk sac retention in hatchlings, may include inspissation from secondary infection.

Changes in Behaviour

- Normal:
  - Posturing, vocalization, head and tail slapping (normal breeding ritual).

- Intraspecific aggression – breeding, territorial.
- Husbandry:
  - Intraspecific aggression due to over-crowding.
  - Stress associated with relocation.
  - Hypo- or hyperthermia.

Increased Time Spent Basking

- Normal:
  - Gravid female.
  - Behavioural thermoregulation to optimize postprandial digestion.
- Husbandry:
  - Decreased ambient temperature.
  - Decreased water temperature (cold shock).
  - Most causes of ill health.
- Health:
  - Pneumonia.

Increased Time Spent Submerged in Water

- Husbandry:
  - Environment inappropriately dry or hot.
  - Stress, lack of hides.
  - Dominant animal in enclosure occupying basking space.

Inability to Submerge, Floating Just Below Surface

- Normal:
  - Resting or observation position.
- Health:
  - Gas accumulation due to gut obstruction by ingested foreign body, enteric or colonic fibrosis or adhesions as sequel to infection, including with West Nile virus.
  - Gas accumulation associated with gastrointestinal infection or empty gastrointestinal tract.
  - Interdigital subcutaneous emphysema or oedema in hatchlings (bubble foot' – unknown aetiology).

Abnormal Swimming Motion, Posture

- Health:
  - Pneumonia (see list of causes under Mouth Gaping) – swimming in circles or tilted to one side.
  - Encephalitis (causes in Neurological Signs section) – head tilt, swimming in circles.

Skin Discolouration (Generalized or Focal)

- Normal:
  - White or patchy pigmentation (leucistic) – normal pigment variation due to recessive leucism gene.
  - Scar tissue from previous trauma, including propeller injuries, bites or rake marks from conspecifics.
- Health:
  - Septicaemia (pink or red discolouration especially seen on ventral scales).
  - *Dermatophilus* spp. infection (brown spot disease) – red or brown lesions, mostly between scales, mostly on the ventral skin.
  - *Chlamydia* spp. infection.
  - Lymphohistiocytic proliferative syndrome of alligators (PIX disease) – multifocal superficial dermal lesions (1–2 mm diameter), grey or red discolouration, mostly on the ventral mandibular, abdominal and tail scales (occurs in association with West Nile virus infection).
  - Sooty accumulations on skin, caused by unidentified *Trematode* sp.

Skin Hyperkeratosis, Granulomas, Proliferative Nodules, Papules, Pustules, Blisters, Ulceration

- Husbandry:
  - Poor environmental hygiene, including poor water quality management, predisposes to microbial dermatitis.
- Health:
  - *Dermatophilus* spp. infection – red or brown lesions, mostly between scales of the ventral skin, may include ulceration.

- *Erysipelothrix insidiosa* infection.
- Other bacterial dermatoses, mainly secondary to viral or fungal infections.
- Dermatomycoses, including *Chrysosporium, Paecilomyces,* and *Fusarium* spp. and *Candida albicans.*
- Interdigital subcutaneous emphysema or oedema (bubble foot – aetiology unknown) – *Trichophyton* or other fungi may be cultured from lesions.
- Herpesvirus infection (saltwater crocodiles) – crusty lesions on abdominal skin.
- Pox virus infection – white, grey, yellow or brown, circumscribed, raised, crusty foci of dermal necrosis (1–8 mm diameter) on head, jaws, eyelids, neck, limbs, trunk, which may coalesce and ulcerate (may occur as epizootic infection).
- Scars from healed pox virus dermal necrosis lesions – may cause skin contraction, deforming the head and mandible.
- Capillaria crocodilus skin lesions – zigzag shaped 'worm trail'.
- Pododermatitis, including due to *Trichophyton* spp. – hyperkeratosis, chronic proliferative lesions.

Skin Abrasions, Thickening, Disruption

- Husbandry:
  - Burns (including from contact with heat lamps or occasionally with electrostunning equipment).
  - Traumatic wounds, including bites from enclosure mates, fish hooks, entanglement injuries – may become secondarily infected, producing abscesses or draining sinuses.
  - Stress-related rostral abrasions.
  - Scar tissue from previous trauma, including propeller injuries, bites or rake marks from conspecifics.

Cutaneous and Subcutaneous Swellings

- Health:
  - Hypovitaminosis E – painful, swollen subcutaneous nodules due to steatitis, fat necrosis.
  - Excessive fibrocartilage deposition around long-bone or facial fractures

due to nutritional or renal secondary hyperparathyroidism (NSHP, RSHP).
  - Rib fractures.
  - Subcutaneous abscesses, including secondary to traumatic wounds.
  - Bony swellings due to focal osteomyelitis.
  - Soft tissue infection, abscess or granuloma as sequela of adjacent osteomyelitis lesion.
  - Omphalitis in hatchlings, including due to *Aeromonas* infection – swelling at site of yolk sac attachment on mid ventral body wall.
  - External yolk sac in hatchlings – due to premature hatching.

Eye Distension, Discharge, Conjunctival Swelling

- Health:
  - Eye trauma, including ocular rupture.
  - Blepharoconjunctivitis due to *Chlamydia* spp. infection – swollen eyelids, fibrinous discharge (typically seen as epizootics in young farmed crocodilians).
  - Opportunistic bacterial or fungal ocular infection.
  - Ophthalmia, including due to pox virus with secondary bacterial infection (*Streptococcus, Aeromonas* spp.) – periocular dermatitis, purulent or caseous ocular discharge, palpebral adhesions, hypopyon, uveitis.

Mouth Gaping

- Normal:
  - Basking position (aids in thermoregulation).
- Health:
  - Nasal disc and or or maxillary obstruction or injury.

Gingival or Oral Inflammation, Ulceration, Petechiation, Exudation

- Health:
  - Hyperthermia.
  - Hypovitaminosis A – nodular tongue lesions due to glandular squamous

metaplasia and hyperkeratosis (affected animals may also have similar pathology of the renal tubules).
– Trauma, including puncture wounds from conspecific bites, fish hooks.
– Electrocution (petechiation only).
– Septicaemia (petechiation only).
– Organophosphate toxicity.
– Bacterial stomatitis.
– Pharyngitis due to *Chlamydia* spp. infection – accumulation of fibrin in the oropharynx and on the gular valve, may obstruct airway (typically seen as epizootics in young farmed crocodilians.
– *Dermatophilus* spp. infection – focal, proliferative lesions.
– Fungal infections, including *Candida* spp.
– Pox virus infection – proliferative, crusty, white, grey, yellow or brown lesions on the tongue, palate, gingivae.
– Stomatitis, including due to *Aeromonas*, West Nile virus infection.

Tooth Loss or Damage

● Normal:
– Normal attrition (replaced regularly throughout life).
– Extreme age (absence of complete dentition).
● Health:
– Trauma (inconsequential).

Dyspnoea, Tachypnoea, Nasal Discharge

● Husbandry:
– Near drowning during capture, trapping or accidental net entanglement.
● Health:
– Aspiration pneumonia due to basihyoid valve malfunction, mostly in animals with generalized weakness from underlying illness.
– Rhinitis, pharyngitis, mainly bacterial, fungal.

– Pharyngitis due to *Chlamydia* spp. infection – accumulation of fibrin in the oropharynx and on the gular valve, may obstruct airway (typically seen as epizootics in young farmed crocodilians).
– Pneumonia due to *Mycoplasma* spp. – signs also include white ocular discharge, lethargy, weakness, paresis, oedema (facial, periocular, cervical, limbs).
– Pneumonia due to other bacteria, including *Staphylococcus aureus*, *Pasturella multocida*, *Pseudomonas*, *Aeromonas* spp.
– Fungal pneumonia, including due to *Paecilomyces*, *Fusarium*, *Aspergillus*, *Candida*, *Cephalosporium* spp.
– Parasitic lung lesions, including due to pentastomids.
– Granulomas and neoplasia of the upper and lower respiratory tracts.

Vomiting, Regurgitation (Uncommon)

● Health:
– Bacterial or fungal gastroenteritis, including due to *Candida* spp.
– Gastrointestinal obstruction due to ingested foreign bodies, including coins, polyvinylchloride pipe, components of the pool filtration or water treatment system.
– Gastrointestinal obstruction due to neoplasia, granuloma, intussusception, torsion or faecal impaction
– Gastrointestinal obstruction due to extraintestinal lesion.
– Hepatopathy.

Diarrhoea (Including Mucoid, Haemorrhagic)

● Health:
– Adenovirus enteritis, with secondary infections as detailed below.
– Bacterial enteritis in hatchlings, including due to *Salmonella*, *Aeromonas* spp., often as sequela of adenovirus infection.

– Coccidial enteritis due to *Eimeria*, *Isospora* spp. (often occurs together with *Aeromonas* infections as sequela of adenovirus infection.

Cloacal Swelling

- Health:
  – Bacterial or protozoal cloacitis.
  – Oedema of cloacal mucosa secondary to tenesmus due to faecal impaction or dystocia.
  – Phallic trauma.
  – Paracloacal gland infection.

Prolapse from Cloaca

- Health:
  – Cloacal mucosa, gut, phallus or oviduct due to generalized weakness, cloacitis, trauma.
  – Intestine due to parasitism or gut obstruction (faecal impaction, intussusception, neoplasia).
  – Oviduct, generally postpartum.
  – Phallus, generally post-mating or following trauma.

Gravid Female not Commencing or Completing Oviposition

- Normal:
  – Primigravid female.
- Husbandry:
  – Failure to provide appropriate environmental conditions, including suitable nest site.
  – Disturbance of parturition by enclosure mate or external stimulus.
  – Malnutrition.
  – Obesity.
- Health:
  – Exhaustion mid-lay due to poor fitness in chronically inactive crocodile.
  – General debilitation due to other disease process.
  – Dehydration.

– Obstructive dystocia due to oversized or malformed egg or pathology external to reproductive tract.
– Salpingitis.

Musculoskeletal Deformities, Swelling and Pain

- Normal:
  – Scute removal (routine marking method in farmed animals and in biological surveys of free-ranging animals).
- Health:
  – Congenital spinal deformities, including lordosis, kyphosis, scoliosis, due to egg incubation at inappropriately high temperatures.
  – Congenital deformities, including spina bifida, scoliosis, hydrocephalus, limb abnormalities, possibly due to maternal vitamin E deficiency.
  – Rubbery jaw, non-union long-bone fractures, skeletal demineralization, kyphoscoliosis, excessive fibrocartilage deposition, translucent teeth, due to RSHP or NSHP (from vitamin D, calcium and phosphorus imbalance, including inadequate exposure to ultraviolet B light).
  – Traumatic fractures, amputation (tail tip, limbs), luxations and soft tissue injuries, mainly from conspecific aggression.
  – Lactic acidosis or rhabdomyolysis associated with excessive exertion (fighting, mating, capture).
  – Polyarthritis due to *Mycoplasma* infection and secondary to systemic bacterial infection.
  – Polyarticular gout.

Necrosis or loss of tail, digits

- Health:
  – Avascular necrosis due to trauma.
  – Digital necrosis and sloughing due to pox virus.

– Necrotizing dermatitis.
– Spinal osteomyelitis.

Paralysis

• Health:
– Pathological fracture (including as sequela of NSHP, RSHP, proliferative spinal osteopathy).
– Electrocution or electrostunning (flaccid paralysis).
– Vertebral trauma.
– Vertebral osteomyelitis.

Neurological Signs Including Weakness, Lethargy, Muscle Tremors, Incoordination, Ataxia, Star-Gazing, Head Tilt, Opisthotonus, Convulsions

• Health:
– Thiamine deficiency (in animals fed frozen fish as a high proportion of their diet, without vitamin B1 supplementation, due to the action of thiaminases in the fish) - weakness, ataxia, muscle tremors, coma.
– Septicaemia.
– Hypoglycaemia, mostly as sequela of stress (notably from handling and restraint) or septicaemia (notably *Salmonella, Aeromonas* spp.) – muscle tremors, loss of righting reflex, mydriasis.
– Bacterial and mycotic encephalitis (including micro-abscesses secondary to septicaemia).
– West Nile virus infection – head tilt, swimming in circles, muscle tremors, opisthotonus, weakness, lethargy (mainly occurs as epizootic in juveniles).
– Chemical toxicity, including by iodine disinfectants and organophosphate or carbamate insecticides (predominantly in hatchlings).

– Heavy metal toxicity, including zinc, lead, mercury from ingestion of prey items killed with lead shot and metallic objects, including coins.
– Drug toxicity including metronidazole, ivermectin and streptomycin.
– Head or body trauma.
– Electrocution or electrostunning (convulsions).
– Hepatic encephalopathy, including due to hepatic lipidosis.
– Renal failure and gout.
– Pain.

Sudden Death

• Husbandry:
– Hyperthermia (from inappropriately high environmental temperature (e.g. thermostat failure or exposure to direct sunlight without opportunity to seek a cooler area).
– Cold shock (especially in hatchling farmed crocodiles).
– Stress response to handling (cause of death includes hypoglycaemia, see Health, but is not always understood).
– Failure of carer to detect earlier signs of illness.
• Health:
– Septicaemia.
– Hypoglycaemia, mostly as sequela of stress (notably from handling and restraint) or septicaemia (notably *Salmonella, Aeromonas* spp.).
– Trauma, including aggression from enclosure mates.
– Drowning during capture, trapping or entanglement in fishing nets, pool furniture.
– Electrocution.
– Haemorrhage.
– Shock.
– Organ failure (e.g. visceral gout).

Further Reading

DeVoe, R. (2015) Lacertilia (lizards, skinks, geckos) and amphisbaenids (worm lizards), in *Fowler's Zoo and Wild Animal Medicine* (M.E. Fowler and R.E. Miller, eds), Elsevier Saunders, St Louis, MO, Volume 8, pp. 52–60.

Flanagan, J. (2015) Chelonians (turtles, tortoises), in *Fowler's Zoo and Wild Animal Medicine* (M.E. Fowler and R.E. Miller, eds), Elsevier Saunders, St Louis, MO, Volume 8, pp. 27–38.

Fleming, G. and Fontenot, D. (2015) Crocodilia (crocodiles, alligators, caiman, gharial), in *Fowler's Zoo and Wild Animal Medicine* (M.E. Fowler and R.E. Miller, eds), Elsevier Saunders, St Louis, MO, Volume 8, pp. 38–49.

Funk, R., Barten, S., Boyer, T. and Nevarez, J. (2006) Differential diagnoses by symptoms, in *Reptile Medicine and Surgery*, 2nd ed., (D.R. Mader, ed.), Saunders Elsevier, St Louis, MO, pp. 675–714.

Lock, B. and Wellehan, J. (2015) Ophidia (snakes), in *Fowler's Zoo and Wild Animal Medicine* (M.E. Fowler and R.E. Miller, eds), Elsevier Saunders, St Louis, MO, Volume 8, pp. 60–74.

Marschang, R. (2014) Clinical virology, in *Current Therapy in Reptile Medicine and Surgery* (D.R. Mader and S.J. Divers, eds). Elsevier Saunders, St Louis, MO, pp. 32–52.

McArthur, S., Wilkinson, R. and Meyer, J., eds (2004) *Medicine and Surgery of Tortoises and Turtles*. Blackwell Publishing, Oxford.

McCracken, H. (1994) Husbandry and diseases of captive reptiles, in *Wildlife, Post Graduate Committee in Veterinary Science*, University of Sydney, Sydney, pp. 461–546.

Paré, J. (2014) Update on fungal infections in reptiles, in *Current Therapy in Reptile Medicine and Surgery* (D.R. Mader and S.J. Divers, eds), Elsevier Saunders, St Louis, MO, pp. 53–56.

Reavill, D. and Griffin, C. (2014) Common pathology and diseases seen in pet store reptiles, in *Current Therapy in Reptile Medicine and Surgery* (D.R. Mader and S.J. Divers, eds). Elsevier Saunders, St Louis, MO, pp. 13–19.

Wyneken, J., Mader, D., Weber, E. and Merigo, C. (2006) Medical care of sea turtles, in *Reptile Medicine and Surgery*, 2nd ed. (D.R. Mader, ed.). Saunders Elsevier, St Louis, MO, pp. 972–1007.

18

Disorders of the Integument

Linda Vogelnest

Anatomy and Physiology

See Chapter 2 for a review of anatomy and physiology of the integument.

Key Points

The skin is composed of two layers:
1) Epidermis.
   - Keratinizing continually renewing epithelial layer that is episodically shed throughout life (ecdysis).
   - Modified into scales in many body regions with the stratum corneum containing hard beta-keratins unique to birds and reptiles.
   - Scales vary in appearance (smooth, keeled), arrangement (tightly abutting, overlapping) and size (small, large sheets, called scutes) and are joined together by softer hinged regions, where the stratum corneum contains softer alpha-keratins, to enable flexibility.
2) Dermis.
   - Anchored firmly to the overlying epidermis; consists of connective tissue (collagen, elastin and ground substance), blood vessels, lymphatics, nerves and, in contrast to mammals, no hair follicles and very few glands.
   - Also contains some unique features, including chromatophore pigment cells (which, in addition to melanocytes in the epidermis, influence external colour and also impart ability to colour change), and osteoderms (bone deposits). Some osteoderms support overlying scales or scutes (chelonians, blue-tongued and bearded lizards) and others support body regions (ventral abdominal region of most lizards and crocodilians).
- It provides physical protection against dehydration, trauma, external pathogens, ultraviolet radiation.
- Skin also includes specialized display and defence structures in some species (e.g. spines, horns, keels and rattles).
- The appearance of the skin reflects general health status.
- The skin is frequently impacted by suboptimal environmental conditions and/or nutrition.
- Figure 18.1 shows examples of variation in reptilian epidermal colour and texture.

Reptile Medicine and Surgery in Clinical Practice, First Edition. Edited by Bob Doneley, Deborah Monks, Robert Johnson and Brendan Carmel.
© 2018 John Wiley & Sons Ltd. Published 2018 by John Wiley & Sons Ltd.

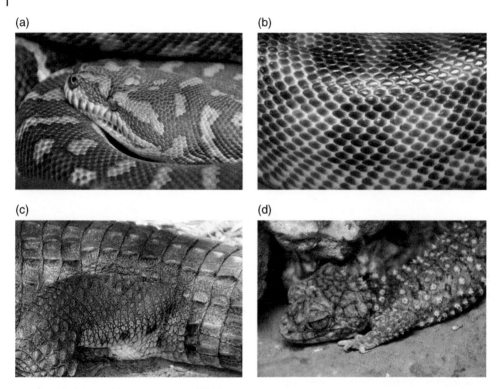

Figure 18.1 Examples of variation in reptilian epidermal colour and texture (courtesy of Larry Vogelnest, Taronga Zoo, Sydney Australia): (a) centralian carpet python; (b) scales on a black-headed python; (c) freshwater crocodile; (d) knob-tailed gecko.

Approach to Reptilian Skin Disease

Skin disease is one of the most common reasons that captive reptiles will be presented to veterinarians. Since a variety of different causal factors can produce similar clinical appearance, a sound approach to management is an invaluable clinical tool. As for dermatoses in any animal species, aiming to confirm a diagnosis or at least to narrow down to the most likely differentials will enable more successful treatment and management strategies for reptilian skin disease. A step-wise approach maximizes efficiency: gathering and collating clues from the history and clinical examination findings to formulate a preliminary prioritised differential diagnosis list and then choosing diagnostic tests and/or management plans accordingly.

Step 1: History Taking

Taking a history is the critical first step in a sound diagnostic approach to any dermatosis. As husbandry plays a central role in many reptilian dermatoses, collecting details on the cage or enclosure environment and current husbandry and feeding practices is vital (see Chapter 10 for more details). Metabolism, and thus development of disease, is notably slower than for mammals.

Step 2: Clinical Examination

Although many diseases with contrasting aetiology can produce similar clinical lesions, lesions can provide useful clues to suggest the more likely differentials, especially when considered together with history and test results. Primary lesions (e.g. vesicles, papules) are more useful clues and sampling sites

Figure 18.2 Adhesive tape impression with purple filamentous dermatophyte hyphae on pale blue keratinocytes (400× magnification; 40× lens).

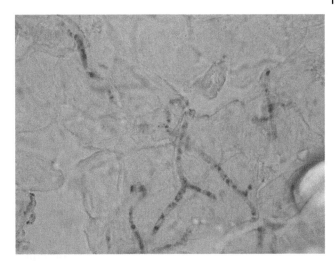

than secondary lesions (e.g. ulcers). It is important to examine all body systems, as systemic illness will commonly have cutaneous manifestation (see Chapter 10).

Step 3: Diagnostic Testing

Diagnostic testing is ideally guided by a list of the most likely differentials based on collation of history and clinical examination details. This enables the most appropriate tests to be initially chosen (see Chapters 11 12 for more detailed information). Common tests of value for reptilian dermatoses include:

- skin cytology
- skin scrapings
- skin biopsies
- microbial culture
- polymerase chain reaction testing.

Skin Cytology

Skin cytology is frequently indicated to evaluate for common bacterial and fungal infections, mites, and cell types (inflammatory, neoplastic):

- impression smears (moist lesions; Diff Quik® stain)
  Performed by pressing a glass slide firmly on to lesional skin.

- adhesive tape impressions (dry lesions; stained: no fixative)
  Performed by pressing an approximately 5 cm strip of 18 mm wide adhesive tape firmly on to lesional skin (Figure 18.2). Examine unstained for mites or stained for bacteria and fungi (e.g. Diff Quik or methylene blue placed on the glass slide under the tape and stain smeared out with a tissue wiped over the tape).

- fine-needle aspirates (nodules or swelling; Diff Quik stain)

  A 23–21 g needle and 5–10 ml syringe are used to collect a sample using negative pressure. The aspirated sample is forcefully sprayed on to a glass slide for staining as per impression smears.

Skin cytology:

- Bacteria:
  The presence of numerous bacteria on surface samples will mostly reflect surface overgrowth and not necessarily infection. Intracellular bacteria (within heterophils) are more consistent with infection, with bacilli more commonly opportunistic in reptiles.

- Fungi:
  Pathogenic fungi include environmental opportunists such as a range of moulds (e.g. *Penicillium, Aspergillus, Fusarium*),

Chrysosporium spp. (e.g. *Chrysosporium* anamorph of *Nannizziopsis vriesii*, CANV) or dermatophytes (e.g. *Trichophyton terrestre*). These moulds produce fungal hyphae within tissues: scattered surface spores can be normal surface contaminants, while the presence of fungal hyphae with tissue invasion and associated inflammation confirms infection.

- Mites:
Tape impressions are useful for evaluating for superficial mites; large body areas can be sampled simply. Tape samples can be stretched gently on to a glass slide and examined without staining.

Skin Scrapings

Skin scrapings can be useful for detecting mites but are often more difficult to perform on body regions with scales. All mites in reptiles are surface dwellers, so adhesive tape sampling that is readily performed on all skin regions including under lifted scales may be preferable.

Skin Biopsies

Skin biopsies can be collected under local anaesthesia using 2% xylocaine or lidocaine, with elliptical or excisional samples typically ideal. Punch biopsies can be collected from soft skin but not from areas with large scales. General anaesthesia is required for collection of shell biopsies from chelonians.

Microbial Culture

Microbial culture for bacteria or fungi should ideally be performed from fine-needle aspirates of mass lesions or from sterile tissue biopsies. For very superficial lesions, skin surface swabs can be collected after gentle surface cleaning with sterile saline but results may be difficult to interpret due to skin surface flora and contaminants.

Polymerase Chain Reaction

Polymerase chain reaction (PCR) testing is ideally performed from sterile tissue biopsy samples for most pathogens. Isolation from surface swabs does not confirm a role in disease for environmental organisms (e.g. many mycobacteria, *Flavobacterium* spp.).

Step 4: Collation of History, Clinical Examination and Diagnostic Test Results

Ensuring that the diagnostic test results make sense in light of the history and clinical findings is a vital last step in the diagnostic approach that is sometimes overlooked. If a diagnosis is not initially achieved, a review of all case details is important. Basic tests may need repeating if there are conflicting or unclear initial results, prior to consideration of additional testing.

Common Dermatoses

Diseases within this chapter are grouped based on the common clinical lesions they produce, with the important caveat that diseases will present with less characteristic lesions at times. Use this 'lesional clustering' of diseases as a guide only. Clinical lesions can provide helpful diagnostic clues but may also be misleading, so should not be considered in isolation from history and diagnostic test results.

Dermatoses Characterized by Abnormal Scaling or Colour Change

Abnormal or excessive scaling (sometimes called hyperkeratosis) and shedding abnormalities (dysecdysis) occur commonly and reflect changes to the outer epidermal layers with disruption of the normal keratinisation process. The major causes are suboptimal husbandry factors (environmental conditions and nutrition), often in combination with surface skin infections. Focal colour changes, including erythema, altered pigmentation and petechiae/ecchymoses, are often important hallmarks for developing systemic and/or cutaneous infections.

Dysecdysis

Dysecdysis refers to abnormal shedding of skin and is common in snakes and some lizards (e.g. bearded dragon). All healthy reptiles periodically shed their outer keratinized epidermal layers (ecdysis, see Chapter 2). Ecdysis takes approximately 14 days in lizards and snakes, during which time their appetite and behaviour may alter. Young growing snakes and lizards may shed every five to six weeks and adult snakes three or four times a year. Dysecdysis is usually associated with suboptimal environmental conditions and often one or more other contributing factors.

Aetiology

Low environmental humidity and low ambient temperature are considered the most important causal factors. Scars from previous wounds, a lack of appropriate substrates for rubbing and mite infections may also predispose. Systemic factors are important considerations, including any cause of dehydration, nutritional factors (e.g. hypovitaminosis A) and causes of immobility. Hyperthyroidism is reported to cause increased frequency of ecdysis (every 1–2 weeks) in older snakes.

Clinical signs

Retained sheets of shed skin are most common in snakes, either as localized (e.g. spectacles) or generalized forms, and some lizards (mostly localized; e.g. digits, spectacles, dorsal spine and tail). In lizards, normal fragmented sheets of shedding skin will be clear and flexible, while retained skin will be darker and dry (Figure 18.3). Chelonians are occasionally affected (typically localized to the digits). Circumferentially unshed portions of skin can form constricting rings around extremities (digits, tails), resulting in avascular necrosis. Unshed spectacles, producing a wrinkly or cloudy appearance to the eyes, can result in ocular disease.

Treatment

Affected individuals should be placed in a container of lukewarm water, where they can submerge but retain their head out of

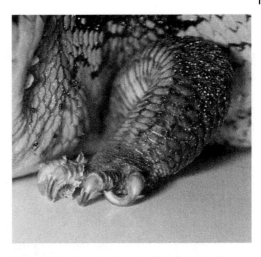

Figure 18.3 Dysecdysis and mite infestation in a blue-tongued lizard (courtesy of Larry Vogelnest, Taronga Zoo, Sydney, Australia).

water, for up to two hours daily for two to three days. Abrasive materials (e.g. wet towels) should be provided in the enclosure for rubbing against and also may be used with care to gently tease away persistent skin after soaking. Artificial tears applied several times daily can be useful to soften retained spectacles. A moist cotton bud can then facilitate gentle removal of the retained spectacle. It is important to address any other contributing factors or diseases (e.g. diet, mites). If necrosis of extremities has occurred, the affected areas should be amputated (Figure 18.4).

Prevention and Control

Optimizing environmental conditions is of major importance. Raising environmental humidity and/or temperature is often needed (e.g. for most snakes 50–60% humidity is ideal). Desert lizards (e.g. collared lizards, desert iguanas, horned lizards, thick tailed or leopard geckos) require low humidity and access to a moist area (e.g. plastic tub containing damp moss, cotton wool, or paper towels). Rocks and logs should be provided to rub against. See Chapter 5 for a more detailed discussion of vivarium requirements.

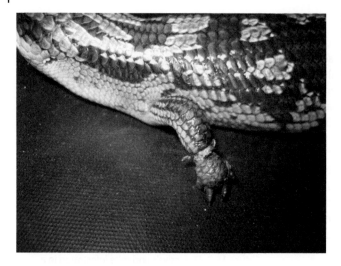

Figure 18.4 Dysecdysis and resultant avascular necrosis of the affected limb in a blue-tongued lizard (courtesy of Larry Vogelnest, Taronga Zoo, Sydney, Australia).

Key Points to Note about Dysecdysis

- Typically occurs due to low humidity and/ or ambient temperature, with or without complicating factors including previous scars, mites, and systemic illness.
- Treatment revolves around soaking and providing gently abrasive surfaces and addressing any other compounding factors.
- Prevention involves optimal enclosure environments.

Infections

Ectoparasites

Aetiology *Ophionyssus natricis* is a shiny black blood-sucking mite, with a two- to three-week lifecycle. It is the most important ectoparasite found on snakes and also occurs less frequently on a range of lizards, chelonians and crocodilians. Female mites live for up to 40 days, during which time they lay up to 80 eggs in dark, damp, warm niches within enclosures. A variety of other mites may also infect reptiles (see Chapter 31 for more details). Mites are contagious to other reptiles and occasionally people. Environmental parasites such as trombiculid mites (chiggers), ticks and leeches may also feed on reptiles.

Clinical Signs Irregular shedding cycles/ dysecdysis and pruritic behaviour are classical. Mites can be seen collecting in skin folds, including the gular fold (ventral neck) and legs, and inside the orbital rim (Figure 18.5). Anaemia may occur with severe infestations.

Diagnosis Diagnosis requires direct observation of mites (visible as minute moving dark spots) and microscopic identification from adhesive tape impressions.

Treatment Ivermectin and fipronil spray are commonly used. Thorough cleaning of the environment will help to hasten a response; eggs and mites may be found around water bowls. Pyrethrins and synthetic pyrethroids (e.g. permethrin) can be used in the environment and on snakes, and may be most suitable for large collections. See Appendix 1, Formulary, for more information.

Key Points for Mite Treatment

- All animals need treatment.
- Treat and disinfect the enclosure.
- Treat for adequate length of time: at least four to six weeks.

Figure 18.5 Mites visible inside the orbital rim (courtesy of Brendan Carmel).

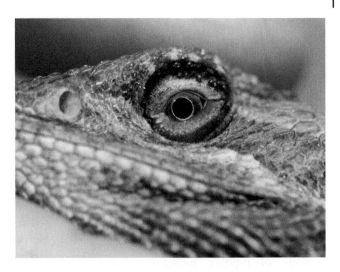

Fungal Infections

1) Yellow fungus disease

    Aetiology: CANV is now thought to be an obligate reptile pathogen. It is a keratophilic fungal species distinct from dermatophytes that may have previously been incorrectly labelled as a range of filamentous fungal infections, including *Trichophyton* spp. infections. An environmental source of this organism has not been determined, although infection has been linked to substandard husbandry and diet. Fresh food (e.g. crickets) or carrier animals may be sources of infection. Zoonosis has been reported, mostly in immunocompromised people, and contagion occurs to other reptiles. CANV has been isolated from captive reptiles in Asia, Australia, Europe and North America. The nomenclature and taxonomy of this fungus is currently under review.

    Clinical signs: bearded dragons and chameleons most commonly affected but also a variety of lizards, snakes and saltwater crocodiles. Typically, multifocal severe yellow scaling, progressing to regions of ulceration, necrosis, crusting and less commonly nodules. Necrotic black areas of skin with surrounding crusts are more typical in chameleons. Infections tend to expand from a central point, and may progress to systemic infection, which can be fatal.

    Diagnosis: histopathology, fungal culture and PCR testing are considered ideal for diagnosis, with PCR testing suggested as the most sensitive for detecting organisms; however, false positives may occur unless combined with histopathology showing fungal hyphae within in tissue. Fungal culture also confirms the presence of the organism but it can be difficult to culture (limited growth above 37 °C). Screening blood tests and evaluation for systemic disease are also indicated.

    Treatment: optimal antifungal therapies in reptiles have not been not determined and treatment has been ineffective in some cases. Combination topical and systemic antifungals are recommended. Ketoconazole has been used successfully (green iguanas) but it is no longer manufactured for humans. It has been superseded by safer efficacious alternatives (e.g. itraconazole, terbinafine, voriconazole; see Appendix 1 for dose rates, etc.). Raising the environmental temperature to between 37–39 °C may help during treatment if the affected reptile species can tolerate these temperatures.

2) Superficial fungal infections

    Dermatophyte infections, such as *Trichophyton terrestre*, occur in lizards (e.g. blue-tongued lizard) and can result in dysecdysis and resultant avascular necrosis and sloughing of digits or feet (Rose 2005). Surface infections with other environmental fungi may initially produce focal scaling regions or yellow, orange or brown lichenified skin in snakes and lizards. They will frequently progress to ulcers and necrosis or nodular granulomas if not diagnosed and treated early. See moist erythematous dermatoses, fungal infections for details. A variety of CANV-related *Chrysosporium* species has been reported as an emerging causes of ulcerative and nodular dermatoses in a range of reptiles, including iguanas, bearded dragons and rattlesnakes.

Bacterial Infections

1) Petechiae/ecchymoses
Discrete lesions of haemorrhage occur in chelonians and less commonly in other reptiles, associated with septicaemia. Affected reptiles are often weak, with poor body tone. Urgent aggressive antibiotic therapy, fluid-therapy, heating and support are required, but the prognosis is guarded.
2) Superficial bacterial infections
Aetiology: the Gram-positive rod-shaped coryneform bacterium *Devriesea agamarum* is an emerging cause of disease in captive desert lizards. It is part of the normal oral flora in some lizards (e.g. bearded dragons) and survives well in the environment in humid sand, water and shed crusts.
Clinical signs: severe scaling of the lip margins (e.g. cheilitis in spiny tailed lizards) or trunkal areas. Concurrent septicaemia is reported.
Treatment: third-generation cephalosporins (e.g. ceftiofur or ceftazidime), with or without topical chlorhexidine 0.1% baths, are reported as efficacious.

Viral Infections

Viral skin infections are rare in pet reptiles and occasional in wild reptiles, associated with reptile-specific and mammalian or avian-associated viruses. Both host and viral factors appear important in establishment of disease, and concurrent infections with multiple infectious agents, including multiple viruses, are recognized.

1) Poxvirus infections
Pox infections have been described in crocodilians (many species), lizards (tegu) and the Hermann tortoise. Multiple circular grey or white macules, papules or brownish wart-like lesions occur, more commonly on the face. Lesions tend to self-resolve in three to four months.
2) Herpesvirus infections
Herpesvirus is linked to small circular to coalescing papular grey lesions (grey patch disease) in young green sea turtles, with epizootic outbreaks in summer linked to high water temperatures, overcrowding and organic pollution. Electron microscopy has confirmed herpesvirus involvement. Herpesvirus has also been linked to more exudative cutaneous plaques in sea turtles and subcutaneous oedema in tortoises, both in association with signs of systemic illness.
3) Sunshinevirus infection
Sunshinevirus, a paramyxovirus seen in Australian pythons, has been associated with blisters on the skin of several pythons.

Hypovitaminosis A

Aetiology

Low levels of vitamin A in the diet, typically due to an all-meat diet, is a common cause of disease in chelonians (especially captive raised aquatic turtles), and also occurs in lizards.

Clinical Signs

Chemosis and blepharoedema of eyes is classical in chelonians. Dysecdysis, scaling or abscesses also occur in chelonians and lizards.

Diagnosis

Consistent clinical signs and history are usually diagnostic. Biopsy reveals hyperkeratosis and squamous metaplasia in the absence of infectious agents.

Treatment

Oral supplementation of Vitamin A is required; cautious incremental dosing is advised. Parental forms of Vitamin A should be used with caution as they can result in hypervitaminosis A (causing dry scaly skin progressing to widespread necrosis and sloughing of soft skin; see Appendix 1). Vitamin A levels must also be increased in the base diet.

Prevention and Control

Ensure that the animal has a supply of foods high in vitamin A, such as dark yellow vegetables (pumpkin/winter squash), and dark leafy green vegetables.

Beak and Claw Overgrowth

Beak and claw overgrowth occurs in chelonians, associated with a lack of sufficient abrasive substrates or foods, excessive dietary proteins or nutritional osteodystrophy in juveniles. Treatment involves trimming excessive growth (in stages when the overgrowth is severe), dietary changes and hard food items such as cuttlefish.

Moist Erythematous, Vesicular, Erosive/ Ulcerative and Necrotic Dermatoses

Suboptimal or inappropriate husbandry and diet is the most common underlying cause of moist erythematous, vesicular, erosive/ulcerative and necrotic dermatoses (see Chapters 4 and 5 for more information).

Environmental Factors

Traumatic Lesions

Skin abrasions occur in lizards, often on the rostral head but also on extremities, due to rubbing or repetitive pushing behaviour on abrasive surfaces. Wounds in snakes may occur from live prey. Cage-mate injuries are also common. General wound care principles apply. Bandaging can be helpful for large wounds.

Thermal or Chemical Burns

Thermal burns occur most frequently from direct contact with heat sources and mimic infectious causes of similar lesions. Careful placement, adjustment and protection from heat sources is the key. Heat sources are best located along the sides of tank rather than on the floor and should be screened to prevent direct contact. Chemical burns occur less frequently, associated with cleaning products used on enclosures. Treatment of both is similar, using the same principals as for mammals, including debridement of necrotic areas, wound care and dressings when the burns are severe. Silver sulfadiazine 1% cream can be helpful. Healing may lead to scarring, which may in turn interfere with normal ecdysis.

Infections

Bacterial Infections

1) Superficial bacterial infections
   Bacterial infections are very common causes and complications of reptile dermatoses, most typically causing erosive to ulcerative lesions. In snakes initial lesions with some infections are fluid-filled vesicles (blister disease).

   Aetiology: Most bacteria are Gram-negative environmental opportunists, invading when skin is damaged or weakened from other causes. In particular, they are associated with inadequate husbandry, especially high local humidity (particularly moist bedding or sub-floor heating), low environmental temperatures, poor cleaning of environment and poor water quality. Skin trauma and/or poor nutrition are often concurrent.
   - Lizards and snakes:
     – Aetiology: *Aeromonas, Pseudomonas, Citrobacter, Escherichia coli, Klebsiella, Proteus, Salmonella, Serratia,*

Flavobacterium, Morganella, Neisseria spp. all reported. Less frequently reported are Gram-positive bacteria, including *Staphylococcus, Streptococcus, Dermatophilus congolensis* or anaerobes including *Bacteroides, Fusobacterium, Clostridium* spp.

- Clinical signs: moist, exudative and erythematous lesions on the ventrum are most typical, with fluid-filled vesicles prominent in snakes, which may progress to crusts and ulceration.

• Chelonians:
- Aetiology: *Aeromonas, Citrobacter* and *Beneckia chitinovora* are most commonly implicated.
- Clinical signs include superficial shell erosions progressing to ulceration and are common in aquatic chelonians, often with a surrounding rim of hyperpigmentation. Deep abscesses may penetrate the full shell thickness. Ulcerative dermatitis of the feet, associated with *Pseudomonas* spp. has been reported in a captive breeding programme for western swamp tortoises.

Diagnosis: Consistent history, clinical signs and cytology (impression smears: heterophils, macrophages; intracellular bacteria: typically rods) supports involvement of bacteria. Bacterial culture can indicate causal species; pure growths are more supportive of a causal role.

Treatment: Correction of substandard husbandry is paramount; particularly providing dry bedding (e.g. newspaper) or improving water quality. Aquatic species may benefit from temporary restriction of water access to one hour twice daily. Surgical debridement is required to remove necrotic areas, repeated daily until resolving. For superficial lesions, twice daily soaks in chlorhexidine (2–3% solution for superficial lesions, avoiding contact with eyes and mucous membranes; 0.5% solution for deeper lesions) or povidone iodine 5–10% solution. Silver

sulfadiazine 1% cream or manuka honey can be helpful to limit infection and encourage healing. For deep lesions, systemic antibiotics are often required, ideally based on culture and sensitivity testing; enrofloxacin, cefotaxime or ceftazidime may be useful initial empirical choices while awaiting culture results. Treatment should continue for a minimum of three to four weeks, until one to two weeks beyond complete clinical resolution. In deep lesions in chelonians, radiographs can be helpful for initial assessment to determine the depth of involvement and to guide prognosis.

2) Systemic bacterial infections
Septicaemic cutaneous ulcerative disease (shell rot) occurs in aquatic chelonians, particularly soft-shelled turtles. Bacterial septicaemia in other reptilian species may also produce skin lesions.

Aetiology: *Citrobacter freundii, Beneckea chitinovora, Aeromonas hydrophilia* and *Serratia* spp. are most commonly implicated, although other Gram-negative bacteria can be involved. *Beneckea chitinovora* may be carried by crustaceans given as a food source.

Clinical signs: ulceration of the plastron, carapace and skin (irregular, caseated, crateriform ulcers), together with systemic signs (anorexia, lethargy). Petechiae and ecchymoses occur commonly in chelonians with bacterial septicaemia.

Diagnosis: Consistent history, clinical signs (cutaneous and systemic signs) and cytology (impression smears: heterophils, bacterial rods) is suggestive. Bacterial culture of commonly implicated bacteria helps to confirm a causal role; blood cultures are suggested as ideal when septicaemia suspected.

Treatment: The prognosis is guarded but can be successful with surgical debridement, antibiotics based on culture and sensitivity testing, supportive care and shell support with fibreglass and resin if the destruction is extensive.

Fungal Infections

Fungal infections are less frequent than bacterial infections and typically occur following injury and skin maceration. They may be more difficult to treat when established. Mixed bacterial and fungal infections are common. In aquatic chelonians, deep infections involving bone are reported. A range of opportunistic fungal may be involved.

Aetiology *Aspergillus, Basidiobolus, Beauveria, Geotrichium, Mucor, Saprolegnia, Candida, Fusarium, Trichosporon, Trichoderma, Penicillium, Paecilomyces* and *Oospora* spp. are reported. In aquatic and semi-aquatic turtles, the incidence of fungal infections may relate to water pH, as growth of most fungi is inhibited if the water pH is less than 6.5. CANV is responsible for yellow fungus disease, which is primarily seen in the bearded dragon (see Dermatoses Characterised by Abnormal Scaling or Colour Change section for details). Unlike other fungi, this appears to be a primary pathogen, and is contagious.

Clinical signs Scaly yellow, orange or brown lesions occur most typically on the lateral and ventral scales in snakes and lizards and may progress to ulcers, necrosis or nodules. In chelonians, exudative, erythematous ulcers and crusts are most common and fluffy or scaly white growths occasional.

Diagnosis Consistent history, clinical signs and cytology (impression smears: heterophils, macrophages, fungal elements) can be suggestive, with histopathology required for confirmation and fungal culture ideal to guide therapy. The major differentials are thermal or chemical burns, bacterial infections and dysecdysis. A Wood's lamp is generally not useful for reptilian fungal infections. It will fluoresce a subset of *Microsporum canis* dermatophytes only, which is a rare pathogen in reptiles. It will not detect other fungal species.

Treatment Topical antimicrobials (chlorhexidine, 2–3% solution or povidone iodine,

5–10% solution) or antifungals (miconazole, ketoconazole, nystatin) can be effective. Deep lesions require debridement and may require systemic antifungals. Oral itraconazole has been used in spiny lizards (23.5 mg/kg) and a corn snake (1.5 mg/kg every 36 hours).

Nutritional Factors

Hypovitaminosis E from high-fat diets is implicated in ulcerative, necrotic lesions related to underlying steatitis; reported more commonly in obese monitor lizards. Hypervitaminosis A occurs subsequent to subcutaneous administration of concentrated Vitamin A and causes focal to generalized necrosis and ulceration.

Papular and Swollen or Nodular Dermatoses

Infections

Bacterial Infections

1) Abscesses

   Abscesses may develop due to traumatic implantation or haematogenous spread of infectious agents and may be multifactorial in origin. They mostly occur because of trauma, bite wounds or at injection sites in chelonians. Wounds from live prey in snakes or following previous episodes of septicaemia also occur. Abscesses are common in lizards, typically associated with underlying husbandry issues.

   Aetiology:

   • Bacteria – common isolates include *Pseudomonas, Proteus, Aeromonas, Serratia, Providencia, Escherichia coli, Citrobacter, Salmonella, Serratia, Streptococcus* and *Neisseria* spp., and *Corynbeacterium pyogenes*; occasionally mycobacteria or anaerobes (e.g. *Bacteroides, Clostridium, Fusobacterium, Peptostreptococcus*).

   • Secondary nutritional hyperparathyroidism is multifactorial and can be attributed to a calcium/phosphorus dietary imbalance, lack of ultraviolet B exposure or vitamin D3, or poor husbandry. It more frequent in lizards and chelonians (see Chapter 15).

Clinical signs: localized soft to firm well-demarcated nodules, typically in subcutaneous location and more often on the head and extremities, containing thick caseous exudate (reptilian heterophils cannot form liquid purulent material). May ulcerate when very large and may involve deeper structures such as tendon sheaths, dental arcades, joints and bones.

Diagnosis is usually straightforward, based on typical lesions with caseous contents. Cytology of abscess contents can guide probable causal organisms, with bacterial culture (ideally of tissue; e.g. fibrous capsule) required for identification. Radiographs are important to screen for deeper invasion in larger lesions.

Treatment: full surgical excision is ideal. Wounds will often heal readily without suturing (Paré 2003) or may be sutured closed. Systemic antibiotics may be required for larger lesions not readily excisable, ideally based on culture and sensitivity testing. A third-generation cephalosporin (e.g. cefotaxime or ceftazidime), which has good efficacy against Gram-negative bacteria, may be a useful initial empirical choice.

2) Intermandibular cellulitis

A diffuse swelling of the lower jaw and throat occurs as a manifestation of acute severe sepsis in snakes, most typically associated with *Pseudomonas* or *Aeromonas* infection. Urgent aggressive antibiotic therapy, fluid therapy, heating and supportive care are required.

3) *Dermatophilus congolensis*

Aetiology: *Dermatophilus congolensis* is a facultatively anaerobic Gram-positive filamentous moisture-loving bacterium that survives for at least short periods of time in the environment, allowing it to readily transfer to other animals or humans. Lizards (bearded dragons, marbled lizards, green iguanas and chameleons), and crocodiles are most frequently infected following minor skin trauma (e.g. tick bites, skin abrasions) in association with moist conditions.

Clinical signs: initial scaling, erythema and necrosis may develop into subcutaneous nodules.

Diagnosis is usually straightforward based on clinical signs and cytology, with the characteristic appearance of filamentous zoospores lined up in double chains, with a 'railway track' appearance (Figure 18.6).

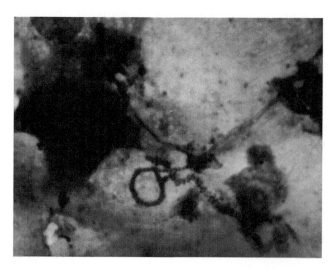

Figure 18.6 Adhesive tape impression with parallel rows of deep blue-staining *Dermatophilus* zoospores among nucleated and anucleate keratinocytes and scant degenerate neutrophils (upper right) (1000× magnification; oil immersion field).

Histopathology may be required to confirm some cases. Bacterial culture can be difficult and slow due to fastidious requirements.

Treatment: removal of crusted lesions, excision of abscesses, drying the environment and potentially systemic antibiotics (penicillin, amikacin) are effective. Topical povidone iodine (5–10%) or chlorhexidine (2–3%) can be helpful for surface regions.

Mycobacterial Infections

Subcutaneous nodules are reported rarely in chelonians and there is one report in a boa constrictor.

Fungal Infections

Fungal abscesses are less common than bacterial. They are typically associated with high humidity, low temperatures, poor nutrition, concurrent disease and opportunistic pathogens.

Aetiology *Aspergillus, Basidiobolus, Geotrichium, Mucor, Saprolegnia, Candida, Fusarium, Trichosporon, Trichoderma, Penicillium, Paecilomyces, Oospora, Trichophyton.*

Clinical signs Nodules with or without systemic signs.

Diagnosis Consistent history, clinical signs and cytology (impression smears; heterophils, macrophages and may see fungal hyphae) are suggestive. Fungal culture (tissue samples) and histopathology is confirmatory.

Treatment Complete surgical excision of abscesses can be curative. Ketoconazole 20–30 mg/kg once daily for two to four weeks has been effective in snakes but is no longer commercially available (see comments on treatment of scaling and moist fungal infections). Itraconazole has been used in lizards. Topical dilute povidone iodine (10%) has been used for superficial lesions.

Viral infections

Papillomas Squamous papillomas, attributed to papillomaviruses, have been reported in bearded dragons, green lizards and a number of chelonians, including Bolivian side-necked turtles. Lesions vary from small white to grey, raised, spherical papules to nodules that coalesce and may ulcerate. Papillomavirus has been detected by electron microscopy. Lesions have been reported to self-resolve.

Cutaneous fibropapillomatosis Papillomatous nodules are reported commonly in green turtles, other species of marine turtles and green lizards. Histologically, they are benign fibroepithelial tumours. Species-specific herpesviruses have been incriminated as the causative agent; they have been sequenced by PCR testing but virus particles have not been seen on electron microscopy studies and other viruses demonstrated in some cases may play a contributory role. Multiple verrucous epidermal proliferations occur on the neck, head and thighs; particularly in soft skin including flippers, neck, chin, inguinal and axillary regions and tail base. Fibromas can also develop in multiple internal organs including the lungs, kidneys, liver and intestines. Wide surgical excision is recommended.

Poxvirus Poxviruses have been detected in crocodiles, tortoises and other reptiles with skin lesions: in caimans (grey or white lesions), Nile crocodiles (brown macules to wart-like lesions), a Hermann's tortoise (papular periocular lesions) and a tegu lizard (brown papules).

Ranaviruses Most notably linked to outbreaks of morbidity and mortality in fish and amphibians, Ranavirus infections are also reported occasionally in chelonians, lizards and snakes. Lesions include ulcerated papules (1–4 mm diameter) with overlying yellow-grey crusting, severe subcutaneous oedema in association with oral erosions, ulceration and systemic illness and nodules. Transmission between several reptilian species can occur and the virus can survive long periods in water at low temperatures. Most viral lesions require electron microscopy studies for confirmation. PCR has been used for diagnosis of ranaviruses. Treatment by surgical excision (when possible) is often the treatment of choice, although some lesions may self-resolve.

Parasites

The larvae of *Dracunculus* spp. (free living in water) and *Filarioidea* (transmitted by arthropods) occasionally cause papular to nodular/draining lesions in wild-caught snakes and lizards, particularly chameleons and agamas.

Neoplasia

Nodular lesions, with or without overlying ulceration, may be neoplastic. Fibrosarcomas are reported as the most common neoplasm in snakes, developing in the intermandibular subcutaneous region most frequently, with potential metastasis to internal organs. Lipomas, liposarcomas, infiltrative lipomas, squamous cell carcinoma, melanomas, myxosarcoma, lymphoma and chromatophoroma are all reported in snakes, chelonians and lizards. A mast cell tumour requiring periodic acid–Schiff staining to detect granules and differentiate from fibrosarcomas is also reported. Squamous cell carcinoma, melanoma and liposarcomas are reported in lizards.

Miscellaneous Dermatoses

Nutritional Osteodystrophy

Inadequate diets with long-term deficiency of calcium or excess of phosphorus or lack of vitamin D3 and exposure to ultraviolet light can results in metabolic bone disease, characterized by either failure to mineralize a growing skeleton or demineralization of a mature skeleton (see Chapter 15).

Clinical Signs

Soft misshapen shells occur in chelonians, with upturned marginal scutes, irregular scutes, small shells or central sagging. Abnormal posture is characteristic in lizards, due to soft misshapen bones. Pathological fractures can occur.

Diagnosis

Visual inspection and palpation, together with radiographs, reveal reduced bone and shell density. Serum calcium and phosphorus levels are typically normal.

Treatment

The diet must be corrected, including a two to one ratio of calcium to phosphorus and ultraviolet light provided through exposure to sunlight or a broad spectrum artificial light within 60 cm of the reptile and without any filtration through glass or plastic. Severe deformities are not readily treated.

Appendix 18.1 Bacterial Species Involved in Reptilian Dermatoses

Presentation	Species	Clinical lesions	Common bacterial species	Major differentials	Treatment
Superficial	Chelonians (shell rot)	Shell (plastron) ulceration, loose scutes; hyperpigmented rim	Gram-negative opportunists: e.g. *Aeromonas, Citrobacter, Beneckia chitinovora*	Thermal or chemical burns, fungal infection	Reduce humidity, raise temperature, and improve cage sanitation, particularly bedding/water quality. Superficial: chlorhexidine soaks twice daily. Deep: systemic antibiotics (culture and sensitivity), 3–4 weeks minimum
	Snakes (bacterial dermatitis, blister disease)	Moist, exudative, erythema, oedema most commonly, or vesicles, crusts, ulcers (most commonly in snakes; frequently on ventrum)	Gram-negative opportunists: e.g. *Aeromonas, Citrobacter, Pseudomonas, Escherichia coli, Klebsiella, Proteus, Salmonella, Serratia, Flavobacterium, Morganella, Neisseria Aeromonas* or *Pseudomonas* spp. most commonly associated with vesicles		
	Lizards (bacterial dermatitis, blister disease)		*Actinobacillus, Arizona, Pseudomonas, Corynebacterium, Dermatophilus, Edwardsiella, Enterobacter, Flavobacterium, Flavomonas, Morganella, Salmonella, Serratia, Staphylococcus*		
	Desert dwelling lizards e.g. spiny tailed lizards	Cheilitis, trunkal scaling	*Devriesea agamarum*	Fungal infection	Above: ceftiofur 5 mg/kg once daily for 2–3 weeks (Hellebuyck *et al.* 2009)
	All, especially bearded dragons, turtles and shinglebacks	Exudative, non-healing bite wounds	Mixed	All of the above	Larger enclosures; reduce stocking density?
Deep	Chelonians (abscesses)	Localized soft to firm swellings, well-defined capsules, with thick caseous exudate	Gram-negative opportunists: *Pseudomonas, Proteus, Aeromonas, Serratia, Providencia, E. coli, Citrobacter, Salmonella, Corynebacteria* Gram-positives: *Streptococcus, Neisseria*	Neoplasia, fungal infection, hypovitaminosis A	Surgical excision of entire abscess if possible
	Aquatic turtles (SCUD)	Crateriform ulcers on shell and skin; systemic illness	*Citrobacter freundii* most commonly; other Gram-negative bacteria	Fungal infection	Surgical debridement, antibiotics (culture and sensitivity), supportive care, shell support

SCUD, septicaemic cutaneous ulcerative disease

Appendix 18.2 Common Dermatoses in Reptiles and Drug Contraindications

Reptile	Bacterial	Fungal	Parasitic	Nutritional/endocrine	Environmental/ Multifactorial	Neoplastic	Drugs
Chelonians	Superficial to deep ulcers/necrosis: shell rot, abscesses	Superficial scaling/ necrosis, abscesses	–	Hypovitaminosis A: scaly, lichenified skin; abscesses	Dysecdysis Thermal burns	Lipoma, SCC, melanoma	Ivermectin[1] Injectable Vitamin A[2]
Snakes	Superficial to deep: erythema, oedema, ulcers, necrosis: blister disease	Yellow-brown lichenified skin, scaling, necrosis, abscesses	Mites (*Ophionyssus natricis*, Trombiculids): pruritus, dysecdysis	Hyper- thyroidism: increased frequency of ecdysis	Dysecdysis	Fibrosarcoma	Systemic aminoglycosides:[2] neomycin, gentamicin, streptomycin, kanamycin Indigo snakes: ivermectin[1]
Lizards	Cheilitis in Agamids (e.g. spiny tailed lizard)	Yellow-brown, lichenified scaly skin, abscesses; yellow fungus disease (e.g. bearded dragon, chameleon); deep nodules, systemic illness	Mites (e.g. *Hirstiella* spp., *Ophinonyssus acertinus*): pruritus, dysecdysis	–	Dysecdysis (less common than in snakes)	SCC, melanoma, lipoma	Systemic aminoglycosides:[2] neomycin, gentamicin, streptomycin, kanamycin Skinks: ivermectin[1]

[1] Contraindicated.
[2] Use with care.

References

Hellebuyck, T., Pasmans. F, Haesebrouck F. and Martel, A. (2009) Designing a successful antimicrobial treatment against *Devriesea agamarum* infections in lizards. *Veterinary Microbiology*, 139, 189–192

Paré, J.A. (2003) Reptile dermatology, in Proceedings of the North American Veterinary Conference, Small Animal and Exotics, Orlando, Florida, USA, 18–22 January, 2003, pp. 1223–1224.

Rose, K. (2005) Reptiles, in *Common Diseases of Urban Wildlife (Australian Registry of Wildlife Health)*. Zoological Parks Board of New South Wales, http://arwh.org/common-diseases/reptiles (accessed 26 June 2017).

Further Reading

De Voe, R., Geissler, K., Elmore, S. *et al.* (2004). Ranavirus-associated morbidity and mortality in a group of captive eastern box turtles (*Terrapene Carolina Carolina*). *Journal of Zoo and Wildlife Medicine*, 35 (4), 534–543.

Goodman, G. (2007) Common dermatoses in reptiles. *In Practice*, 29, 288–293.

Harkewicz, K. (2002) Dermatologic problems of reptiles. *Seminars in Avian and Exotic Pet Medicine*, 11 (3), 151–161.

Hatt, J.M. (2010) Dermatologic problems in reptiles, in *Proceedings of the 35th Small Animal Veterinary Association Congress, Geneva, Switzerland, June 2–5 2010*, pp. 131–133, http://www.vin.com/apputil/content/defaultadv1.aspx?pId=11310&meta=Generic&id=4516323 (accessed 8 June 2017).

Hoppman, E. and Barron, H. (2007) Dermatology in reptiles. *Journal of Exotic Pet Medicine*, 16 (4), 210–224.

Johnson, R., Sangster, C.R., Sigler, L. *et al.* (2011) Deep fungal dermatitis caused by the *Chrysosporium* anamorph of *Nannizziopsis vriesii* in captive coastal bearded dragons (*Pogona barbata*). *Australian Veterinary Journal*, 89 (12), 515–519.

Latney, L. and Wellehan, J. (2013) Selected emerging infectious diseases of squamata. *Veterinary Clinics of North America Exotic Animal Practice*, 16, 319–338.

Literak, I. et al. (2010). Herpesvirus-associated papillomatosis in a green lizard. *Journal of Wildlife Diseases* 46 (1), 257–261.

Lukac, M., Robesova, B., Majlathova, V. *et al.* (2013) Findings of *Devriesea agamarum* associated infections in spiny-tailed lizards (*Uromastyx* sp.) in Croatia. *Journal of Zoo and Wildlife Medicine*, 44 (2), 430–434.

Maas, A. (2013) Vesicular, ulcerative, and necrotic dermatitis of reptiles. *Veterinary Clinics of North America Exotic Animal Practice*, 16, 737–755.

Marschang, R. (2011) Review: viruses infecting reptiles. *Viruses*, 3, 2087–2126.

Mitchell, M. and Walden, M. (2013) *Chrysosporium anamorph Nannizziopsis vriesii*. An emerging *fungal pathogen of captive and wild reptiles*. *Veterinary* Clinics of North America Exotic Animal Practice, 16, 659–668.

Nazir, J., Spengler, M. and Marschang, R.E. (2012) Environmental persistence of amphibian and reptilian ranaviruses. *Diseases of Aquatic Organisms*, 98, 177–184.

Palmeiro, B. and Roberts, H. (2013) Clinical approach to dermatologic disease in exotic animals. *Veterinary Clinics of North America Exotic Animal Practice*, 16, 523–577.

Reavill, D. and Schmidt, R. (2009) Review: pathology of the reptile integument. Proceedings of the Association of Reptilian and Amphibian Veterinarians. pp. 93–106.

White, S., Bourdeau, P., Bruet, V. *et al.* (2011) Reptiles with dermatological lesions: a retrospective study of 301 cases at two university veterinary teaching hospitals (1992–2008). *Veterinary Dermatology*, 22, 150–161.

Wyneken, J. and Mader, D. (2009) Review: reptilian dermatology. Proceedings of the Association of Reptilian and Amphibian Veterinarians. pp. 83-87.

19

Diseases of the Gastrointestinal System

Robert Johnson and Bob Doneley

Anatomy and Physiology

The reptilian gastrointestinal system is grossly similar to mammals, with significant physiological differences. See Chapter 2 for more information on the anatomy and physiology of the gastrointestinal tract.

Key Points

- Food intake and rate of digestion are determined by reptile size and metabolic rate.
- Snakes can swallow large prey items because of the unique anatomy of their jaws. The quadrate, maxillary and palatopterygoid arches are movable, while the rami of the lower jaw are connected at the symphysis by a very extensible elastic ligament.
- Acidic enzymatic stomach secretions help to prevent the putrefaction of large meals. The rate of gastric emptying is dependent on the

body temperature of the reptile and the meal size.
- Unlike mammals, the structure of the pancreas in the reptile is not always homogeneous. Variable secretions of pancreatic enzymes have been reported. In most snakes, the spleen and pancreas are closely joined to form the one organ mass, the splenopancreas.
- The gall bladder is located within the liver mass of Chelonia and lizards but is distinct from and caudal to the liver in snakes.
- Some species have specialized intestinal structures to aid digestion; for example, the green iguana (*Iguana iguana*) has a large sacculated colon to facilitate the fermentation of complex carbohydrates.
- The cloaca serves as a common exit chamber for the urinary, digestive and reproductive tracts. The slit-like exit is the vent.

Stomatitis and Dental Disease

Also known as mouth rot or canker, stomatitis is a necro-inflammatory condition of the mouth. The presence of purulent exudate on the glottis may lead to respiratory disease.

Aetiology

Predisposing factors for stomatitis include anatomy, diet and immunosuppression. Agamid lizards and Old World chameleons have acrodont teeth (attached to the alveolar ridge of the mandibular and maxillary bones with no sockets or roots) anchored in place

Reptile Medicine and Surgery in Clinical Practice, First Edition. Edited by Bob Doneley, Deborah Monks, Robert Johnson and Brendan Carmel.
© 2018 John Wiley & Sons Ltd. Published 2018 by John Wiley & Sons Ltd.

by a thin gum line along the lateral surface of the alveolar ridge. When this fragile gum tissue recedes or is damaged, the periosteum becomes desiccated and damaged, allowing bacteria to invade the underlying bone causing lysis and osteomyelitis. Inappropriate diet (e.g. feeding soft foods such as fruit and canned diets, lack of abrasive foods such as insect exoskeletons) can lead to the accumulation of plaque on the teeth, calculus, periodontal disease and gum recession. Tooth loss and osteomyelitis may result.

Immunosuppression is often associated with poor husbandry (e.g. suboptimal temperature and poor hygiene in the enclosure). This may change the bacterial population in the mouth from predominantly Gram-positive flora to Gram-negative populations (e.g. *Pseudomonas*, *Aeromonas*, *Citrobacter*, *Enterobacter*, *Eschericia coli* and *Salmonella*). These bacteria can become invasive following injury (e.g. striking at objects, bite wounds from live prey items) or primary viral infections (e.g. herpesvirus in tortoises).

Clinical Signs and Physical Examination Findings

Animals affected with stomatitis may be presented for inappetance (although often interested in feeding), halitosis (often severe), bleeding from the mouth and ptyalism. There may be discharge (purulent or mucoid) from the nares. Some animals will be presented for mouth breathing or respiratory noise; care must be taken to distinguish stomatitis from respiratory infections (remembering that they may be concurrent). In chronic cases that have progressed to osteomyelitis, there may be swelling of the bone and soft tissues of the jaw.

Careful examination of the mouth can be achieved by firstly reflecting the lips and then opening the mouth gently with a speculum. Care must be taken to avoid further trauma to an already painful mouth, and so metal specula are not recommended.

Diagnosis and Categorization

Diagnosis is usually made on clinical signs. Stomatitis may be graded as:

- Early – mild gingival swelling, pinpoint haemorrhages on the gums, and salivation (Figure 19.1).
- Moderate – swollen gums, calculus accumulation, mild gingival recession and occasional pockets or plaques of purulent material.
- Severe – abscessation and exposure of underlying bone. Occasionally there will be a generalized tissue infection and swelling of the whole head and neck (Figure 19.2).

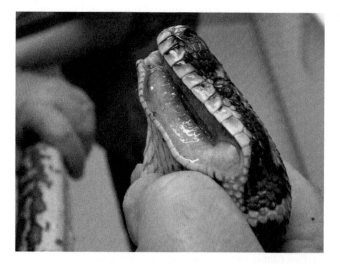

Figure 19.1 Early stomatitis in a carpet python.

Figure 19.2 Sublingual abscess in a carpet python.

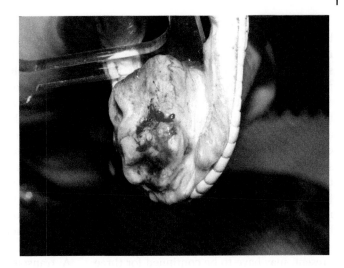

Culture and sensitivity can be used to identify the pathogenic organisms involved and to determine the most appropriate antimicrobial agent for treatment. Since mixed infections are common, both aerobic and anaerobic cultures should be taken. A sterile preparation should be performed over the site to be sampled and a sterile scalpel or needle should be used to collect a deep culture sample. Caution must be taken when interpreting the culture results, as it can be difficult to distinguish between pathogens and normal oral flora.

Biopsy of bone or associated soft tissue may be useful as a method for clarifying the disease process (e.g. distinguishing inflammation from neoplasia) or to identify pathogenic organisms not recoverable on culture.

Radiographic assessment of the mouth is usually unrewarding, owing to the superimposition of other skull bones, but it may detect osteomyelitis and determine its extent. With the advent of digital radiography and the availability of intraoral plates providing better resolution lytic lesions can be more clearly identified. Other modalities such as computed tomography and magnetic resonance imaging may be useful in detecting lesions not visible in radiographs (see Chapter 12).

Treatment

Treatment is often determined by the severity of the condition. Common to all treatments is attention to and improvement of husbandry. A small increase in the enclosure temperature above the reptile's preferred body temperature may facilitate an improved immune response. The enclosure substrate should be changed to newspaper or paper, and changed daily, and regular and effective disinfection carried out. Assisted feeding may be necessary in some cases, usually by stomach tube, as forced feeding of prey items may be painful. See Chapter 13 for more detailed information. Clean water bowls and fresh water daily are also recommended.

Early cases of stomatitis may respond to improvements in husbandry and the application of suitable topical nonsteroidal ophthalmic antibiotics or oral chlorhexidine-based gels. Mild cases may require injectable or oral antibiotics and, if present, gentle debridement of purulent material or periodontal pockets. Severe cases will require surgical debridement, fluid therapy and analgesia. Haematology and biochemical screening is recommended in these cases to determine the severity of the infection and to look for any underlying disease processes. Euthanasia may be necessary in severe cases.

Periodontal disease in agamids and chameleons will require dental scaling, debridement of necrotic gingiva and bone, and sometimes tooth removal. Many of these patients will require stabilization prior to aggressive dental therapy, including rehydration, assisted feeding and a broad-spectrum antibiotic regimen. Owing to the high incidence of mixed bacterial infections and the severity of osteomyelitis, a combination of two antimicrobials is recommended initially (e.g. enrofloxacin/amikacin and ceftazidime/metronidazole). This antibiotic regimen may be started while waiting for culture and sensitivity test results and, if osteomyelitis is present, may have to be continued for three to six months.

Mandibular and Maxillary Fractures

Mandibular and maxillary fractures are not uncommon in lizards and chelonians following trauma. They may also be secondary to osteomyelitis associated with stomatitis or osteopenia resulting from metabolic bone disease. Maxillary fractures may extend into the hard palate, warranting careful examination of this area.

As well as antibiotic and analgesic therapy, mandibular fractures in small to medium sized lizards can often be stabilized by moulding a suitable sized wire to the shape of the jaw and fixing it to the skin with a suitable cyanoacrylate adhesive. This external fixation can be replaced as required until the bone heals. If necessary, an oesophagostomy tube can be placed to facilitate feeding while the fracture heals. This is performed under general anaesthesia by choosing an exit site behind the head and infiltrating the area with local anaesthetic. After surgically preparing the site, a long curved haemostat is introduced through the mouth and the tip is pushed laterally against the exit site with enough pressure to displace any blood vessels. A small scalpel blade is used to cut down

on to the tip of the haemostats while they are forced through the oesophageal mucosa and overlying tissues. Once the haemostats are through the skin, the handle is opened just enough to grasp the oesophagostomy tube (usually a soft silicon or red rubber catheter) and the haemostat with tube attached is withdrawn through the mouth. The tube tip is then redirected back into the mouth and down the oesophagus to a premeasured length so that the tip is in the lumen of the reptile's stomach. A purse-string suture is placed around the incision and tube to seal off the incision, and a Chinese finger-trap suture is used to secure the tube to the skin. A transparent dressing is placed over the tube and around the neck to keeps the site clean. The oesophagostomy tube is capped and wrapped over the shell (chelonians, Figure 19.3) or body wall (lizards and snakes).

Oesophageal Foreign Bodies

Turtles, both marine and freshwater, not uncommonly swallow fishhooks and assorted marine debris. Diagnosis is made on clinical signs, diagnostic imaging and endoscopy. Surgical or endoscopic removal is usually required (Figure 19.4). Prognosis depends upon the chronicity of the problem, whether a viscus has been penetrated and the anatomical location of the obstruction. Complications include infection, gas build-up leading to floatation issues and gastrointestinal perforation.

Regurgitation

Regurgitation is often reported in captive pythons and less so in lizards and chelonians. This condition may be due to a variety of causes and poor husbandry is often involved. The swallowing and digestion of a food item is a complex physiological process that may take up to several weeks in some snakes.

Figure 19.3 Oesophagostomy feeding tube in a young turtle.

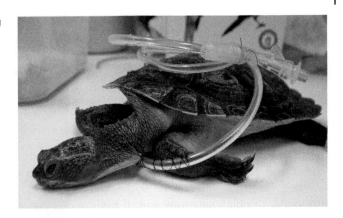

Figure 19.4 Endoscopic removal of an oesophageal foreign body in an eastern long-necked turtle (*Chelodini longicollis*).

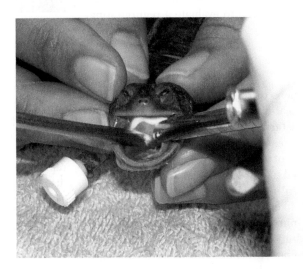

Aetiology

The causes of regurgitation can be grouped into husbandry issues, dietary issues, pathological processes and other causes. Husbandry issues include low environmental temperatures, excessive handling after eating and a lack of a hide for the reptile to lie quietly and undisturbed while it digests its meal. Excessively large (greater than 10–30% of the snake's body weight) or cold (thawed frozen rats and mice not warmed sufficiently) food items will frequently cause regurgitation. Pathological processes include gastrointestinal obstruction (intra- or extramural neoplasms or abscesses) and gastritis, such as viral infections (inclusion body disease in boids), *Cryptosporidia* and other protozoa or bacterial infections. Other causes include the administration of medications (e.g. parenteral enrofloxacin in tortoises), systemic disease, such as renal or hepatic disease, and toxins such as organophosphates and pyrethrins.

Clinical signs

The presenting complaint is usually finding fresh, digested or semi-digested food in the cage hours, days or weeks after food consumption. The reptile may or may not appear to be lethargic and depressed.

Diagnosis

Diagnosis of the cause of regurgitation starts with a thorough history, including a feeding history and enclosure conditions (size, temperature, handling, hides, hygiene, etc.). Careful palpation of the body may reveal swellings or discomfort. Haematology and biochemistry analysis is often useful to determine if systemic disease is present. Stomach washes and faecal analysis are useful for detecting parasitic infections. Radiology, ultrasound, flexible endoscopy and, if indicated, exploratory coeliotomy and biopsy of internal organs are other diagnostic tools that can be used to evaluate a regurgitating patient.

Treatment

Treatment of regurgitation begins with the identification and correction of husbandry and dietary issues. Warming the reptile's enclosure and reducing the size and frequency of the feedings may be all that is required to correct the problem, especially if acute in onset. More chronic problems are most likely associated with disease and the animal is often systemically unwell. Rehydration and patient warming are important supportive measures. Specific therapy can then be directed towards identified pathogens or disease processes.

Diarrhoea

The passage of loose, unformed faeces with increased water content is relatively common in reptiles. It should not be confused with polyuria. The clinician should be aware of species differences; for example, many colubrids have softer faeces than boids.

Aetiology

Diarrhoea can be due to infectious or non-infectious aetiologies. Non-infectious causes include change in diet, excessive feeding,

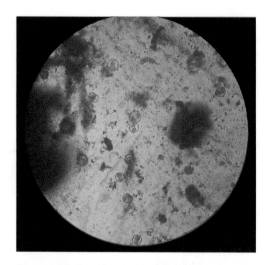

Figure 19.5 Coccidia oocysts in the faeces of a bearded dragon.

stress or foreign bodies. Infectious causes are more common and include bacterial, viral, fungal or parasitic infections (e.g. coccidiosis in bearded dragons; Figure 19.5). Although it is normal to see some flagellated protozoa in reptile faeces, overgrowth in a damaged or diseased gastrointestinal tract can perpetuate diarrhoea, even after the primary problem has been resolved. See Chapter 31 for more detailed information.

Clinical signs

Diarrhoea is a clinical sign, not a disease in its own right. It may be acute or chronic. Animals with acute diarrhoea may be minimally affected or may exhibit mild dehydration and lethargy. Chronic dehydration usually results on more obvious dehydration, weight loss and lethargy. As well as diarrhoea, there may be haematochezia and excessive mucus in the faeces.

Diagnosis

After thorough history and physical examination, faecal analysis – direct examination, flotation, cytology and culture – should be performed to help identify the aetiological agent involved. In some cases, polymerase chain reaction (PCR) may be needed to determine whether viral infections are present. If the animal is systemically affected, haematology and biochemistry profiles, as well as radiology and ultrasound, can be used to identify systemic disease or involvement.

Treatment

Supportive care (assisted feeding, fluids, and warmth) is beneficial for the patient, in addition to specific therapy directed towards the aetiological agent. Gastrointestinal motility modifying drugs such as metoclopramide or cisapride may also play a role in normalising intestinal function.

Intestinal Obstruction

Intestinal obstruction is often an acute and catastrophic event in reptiles.

Aetiology

Many reptiles are nonselective in their feeding habits and may ingest substrate or other items in their enclosure. Although the ingestion of foreign bodies (e.g. plastic items, sand, rocks) is the most common cause of intestinal obstruction, large masses of worms, neoplasia, abscesses, volvulus and intussusception can also be responsible for an intestinal obstruction.

Clinical signs

Animals with intestinal obstruction may present with an acute onset of lethargy, anorexia, vomiting or regurgitation, straining and occasionally diarrhoea. Melena and haematochezia may be present. With severe straining, cloacal prolapse may occur. Bloating of the coelom may also be seen. Partial or incomplete obstructions may be more insidious, with a chronic history of weight loss, reduced appetite and occasional vomiting/regurgitation.

Diagnosis

Careful palpation may detect a mass in the coelom, often tender when touched. In snakes, the organ involved can be determined by measuring its distance from the snout (see Chapter 10). Radiographs may demonstrate gas-filled loops of bowel proximal to the obstruction. Metallic foreign bodies; for example, fish hooks are readily detectable with survey radiographs but the detection of plastic and rubber foreign bodies may require contrast studies. Because of the slow gastrointestinal transit time in reptiles, contrast radiography may require hours, days or even weeks. Ultrasound can be an extremely useful diagnostic tool for imaging the intestinal tract and other coelomic organs.

Treatment

Intestinal obstruction is typically an emergency condition requiring surgery to confirm the diagnosis and relieve the obstruction. This may require an enterotomy or enterectomy.

Prognosis

The prognosis for an intestinal foreign body is always guarded, as ischaemic necrosis of the intestinal wall may be well advanced by the time that clinical signs are noted.

Colonic Impaction (Constipation)

Impaction of the colon, often accompanied by loss of appetite, is a common clinical problem of captive bearded dragons and occasionally other reptiles. The colon becomes impacted with indigestible material such as sand, rocks and chitin from insects.

Aetiology

There are many proposed causes of colonic impaction, including:

- pica associated with nutritional secondary hyperparathyroidism

- skeletal abnormalities preventing normal defecation (lizards with a history of metabolic bone disease appear to be more at risk of impaction, particularly if they have pelvic or spinal deformities)
- ingestion of loose substrate (e.g. sand or gravel)
- lack of dietary fibre (i.e. leafy greens)
- overfeeding insects
- low water intake
- stress (recent acquisition or recent changes in housing, over-handling, etc.)
- vitellogenesis
- extramural masses (abscesses, enlarged kidneys, neoplasia) obstructing the colon.

A variant of colonic impaction is the retrograde flushing of urates from the cloaca into the colon (urate impaction). This occurs most commonly in overweight, sedentary lizards that become subclinically dehydrated and are not defecating regularly due to variable food intake and suboptimal enclosure temperatures.

Clinical signs

Clinical signs may vary depending on the chronicity of the condition and include decreased or absent faecal output, inappetance, lethargy, straining, and occasionally cloacal prolapse. Severely affected animals may regurgitate food. There may be hind limb weakness. The coelom may become distended and, in chronic cases, there may be weight loss.

Diagnosis

Careful palpation of the coelom may reveal an enlarged and firm cylindrical structure consistent with an impacted colon. This must be distinguished from the coelomic fat pads, eggs or ovarian follicles. Radiology and ultrasound can help to make this distinction, as well as assessing other structures such as skeletal structure, reproductive activity and the presence of free fluid in the coelom. A warmed saline enema may assist in

diagnosing the aetiology of the impaction, as well as assisting in the treatment of the impaction.

A direct faecal examination is recommended to assess the parasite load, looking for flagellate protozoa, coccidia and nematode eggs. Examination of the cloaca using an otoscope or endoscope is useful in cases refractory to standard treatments.

Treatment

Many patients can be managed as outpatients. Daily soaking in warm water (35–40 °C) for 10–15 minutes daily will help with hydration and stimulate defecation. Daily spray misting to maintain a good state of hydration is recommended in susceptible animals. Any diagnosed underlying conditions should be treated, ensuring that adequate levels of supplemental calcium, heat and ultraviolet B lighting are provided. Increasing dietary fibre by assist feeding herbivore support diets (e.g. Critical Care®, Oxbow) is often effective and beneficial.

More severe cases will require hospitalization and parenteral fluids. If bathing does not stimulate the excretion, many will respond to cloacal stimulation using a well-lubricated cotton bud. In some cases an enema may be required, which is administered by inserting a lubricated catheter or crop needle into the cloaca, guiding it carefully into the proctodeum. Gently flush with 2–5 ml of a 50 : 50 mix of warm water (35–40 °C) and obstetrical lubricant. If the animal fails to respond to this treatment, an enterotomy to remove impacted foreign material or an exploratory coeliotomy or coelioscopy to assess an impinging coelomic mass may be necessary to resolve the impaction.

Cloacal Prolapse

Prolapse of the cloaca, bladder, lower colon or oviduct is a common problem in reptiles.

Aetiology

Causes of cloacal prolapse include:

- straining associated with intestinal disease such as colonic impaction (see above) or enteritis (intestinal obstruction, heavy parasitic burden or bacterial infections)
- dystocia
- urinary calculi or cystitis
- intestinal stasis secondary to hypocalcaemia and/or metabolic bone disease
- obesity and muscular weakness
- spinal trauma or deformity.

Diagnosis

Cloacal prolapses are readily identifiable (Figures 19.6 and 19.7). Close examination may help to evaluate which tissue has prolapsed since each has a unique appearance (although oedema and trauma may make identification difficult). Intestinal prolapses are usually identified by the smooth tubular appearance of the tissue. Sometimes faeces may be observed inside the prolapsed tissue.

Oviductal tissue appears similar to intestine, but has longitudinal striations and there are no faeces inside the prolapse. Bladder tissue is thin walled and often fluid filled.

Treatment

The prolapsed tissue should be gently cleaned with warmed saline or dilute chlorhexidine. Oedematous swelling can be reduced by the application of hypertonic saline or glucose and gentle massage. Once the swelling has resolved, the prolapsed tissue can be reduced with the use of a lubricated gloved finger or cotton-tipped swab. This may require sedation or general anaesthesia to prevent further straining while reducing the prolapse. The application of a local anaesthetic cream (e.g. EMLA® cream mixed with silver sulfadiazine cream at a ratio of one to nine) can also minimize this straining. Once the prolapse has been reduced, the tissue should be returned to its normal position by gentle probing. Transverse sutures are then placed through

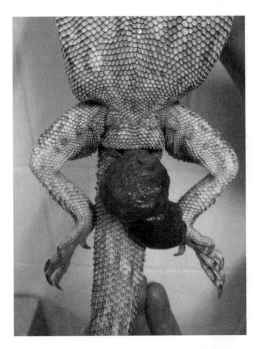

Figure 19.6 Cloacal prolapse in a bearded dragon.

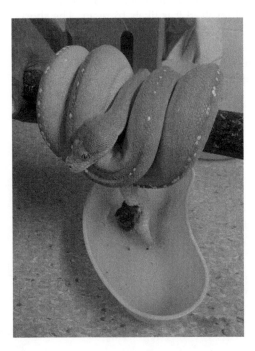

Figure 19.7 Cloacal prolapse in a green python (*Morelia viridis*).

the lateral margins of the vent to temporarily reduce the size of the vent. The centre of the vent should be wide enough for urine to pass while preventing recurrence of the prolapse. These sutures should be left in place for three to five days. In snakes, a percutaneous cloacopexy can be performed by passing a suture through the ventral skin into the cloaca (using a probe or small syringe case as a locater for the cloaca) and fixing the cloaca to the body wall. If this fails, a more aggressive approach (a coeliotomy and colopexy or cloacopexy) may be warranted.

Antibiotics and anti-inflammatories are often warranted. The application of EMLA cream mixed with silver sulfadiazine cream into the cloaca twice daily for several days can prevent further straining while the prolapsed tissues heal. The reptile should be kept well hydrated but not fed for several days to prevent defecation.

Prognosis

If the cause of the prolapse is not identified and resolved it is likely to recur. The short-term prognosis is determined by the underlying cause, the condition of the patient, the duration of the prolapse before treatment and the viability of the prolapsed tissue.

Cloacitis

Inflammation of the cloaca is occasionally seen in reptiles, especially snakes and lizards.

Aetiology

Cloacitis can be an extension of an enteritis (bacterial, fungal, viral or parasitic) or a secondary infection following urate impaction of the cloaca associated with dehydration or constipation. Inflammation may also occur after mating.

Clinical Signs

Early cases may present with a malodourous and/or bloody cloacal discharge (Figure 19.8), and oedema and ulceration of the vent lips. As the condition progresses, the cloaca and surrounding tissues become swollen (Figure 19.9). The cloacal wall is initially erythematous but may become swollen, haemorrhagic and covered with necrotic plaques. Inspissated purulent material and urates may be present in the cloaca (cloacoliths). Possible outcomes include an ascending infection of intestinal, urinary or reproductive tracts, leading to signs of systemic illness.

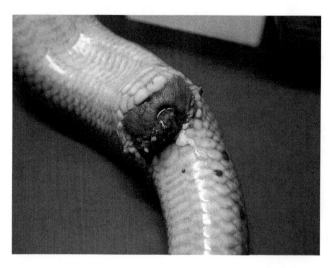

Figure 19.8 Cloacitis of unknown aetiology in a python.

Figure 19.9 A distended colon due to flagellate protozoal enteritis in a diamond python (*Morelia spilota spilota*).

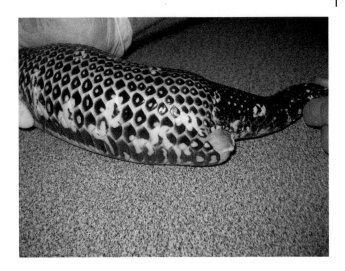

Diagnosis

A good history and physical examination will often reveal both the diagnosis and likely aetiology. Cloacoscopy using an endoscope or otoscope can demonstrate the extent of the lesions and allow biopsy for histopathology and culture and sensitivity.

Treatment

Treatment should include thorough but gentle cleansing with dilute chlorhexidine, topical application of an antibiotic cream and placing the animal on a nonadherent substrate such as newspaper or cotton towels. If the condition is severe, parenteral antibiotics and anti-inflammatory therapy are recommended.

Liver Disease

Liver disease is common in reptiles but often unrecognized until the disease is well-advanced.

Aetiology

Liver disease can be classified as acute or chronic, inflammatory (hepatitis) or degenerative (hepatosis). Table 19.1 shows the classification of liver disease. Hepatic lipidosis, the pathological increase in intrahepatic fat associated with overfeeding, obesity and lack of exercise, must be differentiated from physiologically normal hepatic fat associated with brumation or reproduction. Risk factors for hepatic lipidosis include age (it is uncommon in juveniles), lack of brumation opportunities and the lack of breeding opportunities for females. Large carnivorous reptiles (e.g. tegus, monitors and pythons) and bearded dragons appear to be most commonly affected.

Clinical signs

Most reptiles with liver disease show only subtle signs of disease:

- reduced appetite
- decreased activity
- weight gain (due to ascites) or gradual weight loss
- brumation problems, including post-brumation anorexia
- biliverdinuria
- diarrhoea
- polyuria.

These clinical signs may not be present all the time, only becoming apparent during episodes of increased physiologic demand (e.g., brumation, breeding or concurrent disease).

Table 19.1 Classification of liver disease.

Class	Inflammatory	Degenerative
Acute	Infectious: ● Bacterial (*Salmonella, Campylobacter, Chlamydia, Escherichia coli*) ● Viral (adenovirus in bearded dragons, ferlavirus and sunshinevirus in snakes) ● Fungal ● Parasitic (*Rhabdias* spp.) ● Coccidiosis (bearded dragons) Non-infectious: ● Leukaemia ● Trauma	Toxins: ● Ivermectin-induced hepatic lipidosis in chelonians ● Pyrethrin toxicity ● Organophosphate (pest strips)
Chronic	Chronic active hepatitis Cholecystitis Adenovirus in bearded dragons Herpesvirus (turtles) Mycobacteria *Nannizziopsis* spp. (CANV) Cryptosporidia *Caryospora* spp. (turtles) Parasitic (*Ophidascaris* spp.)	Metabolic: ● Hepatic lipidosis ● Gout ● Metabolic bone disease ● Renal metabolic bone disease Neoplastic: ● Primary neoplasia ● Metastatic disease, e.g. lymphoma

Diagnosis

Haematology and biochemistry analysis form the mainstay of the diagnosis of liver disease. It is important that blood samples are collected before fluid therapy and other supportive measures are initiated.

- Anaemia may be present in cases of chronic hepatopathy.
- Marked heterophilia and monocytosis suggest acute inflammation or necrosis of the liver.
- A normal white cell count does not rule out hepatitis, as chronic bacterial hepatitis and abscessation may not elevate the total white blood cell count.
- Liver enzymes such as aspartate aminotransferase, glutamate dehydrogenase and gamma glutamyl transferase must be interpreted carefully, as their significance in reptiles has not been fully evaluated. In reptiles, tissue distribution of many of these enzymes appears more widespread, making interpretation more difficult. In cases of chronic hepatopathy with little active damage, enzyme levels may remain normal.
- Bile acids have also not been fully evaluated but it appears likely that values above 60 μmol/l are indicative of hepatic dysfunction.

Radiology is of limited use in evaluating liver size but ultrasound is of much greater use, demonstrating liver size and echogenicity. Endoscopic or surgical liver biopsy can provide much needed information on the aetiology, extent and severity of suspected liver disease. Several samples should be collected for histopathology, culture and PCR.

Treatment

The objectives for the therapeutic management of liver disease are to support the patient while specific therapies aimed at treating the causative agent of the liver disease and repairing the damage done to the liver. This may take several weeks to many months.

Patient support includes correction of husbandry deficits (especially temperature), fluid therapy to correct dehydration and to improve perfusion of the liver and nutritional support (see Chapter 4). When providing nutritional support, it is important to consider:

- the patient's energy and nutritional requirements while recovering

- the patient's natural eating habits (herbivorous, omnivorous or carnivorous)
- the use of natural foods that may better meet the patient's nutritional requirements.

Specific therapy will be dictated by the results of the histopathology, culture and PCR testing. In many cases, an aetiological cause may not be determined; if this is the case, broad-spectrum antibiotic coverage is often indicated. Suggested hepatic supportive therapies include lactulose, carnitine methionine, ursodeoxycholic acid and silibinin.

Patients should be serially evaluated at three, six and nine months. Weight and food intake should be evaluated, as should liver enzymes and fasting bile acids. Ultrasound and endoscopic liver biopsies can be used to monitor response to therapy.

Further Reading

Divers, S.J. (2000) Reptilian liver and gastrointestinal testing, in *Laboratory Medicin: Avian and Exotic Pets* (A.M. Fudge, ed. WB Saunders, Philadelphia, PA, 205–209.

Divers, S.J. and Cooper, J,E. (2000) Reptile hepatic lipidosis. *Seminars in Avian and Exotic Pet Medicine*, 9 (3), 153–164.

McAllister, C.T., Upton, S.J., Jacobson, E.R. and Kopit, W. (1995) A Description of *Isospora amphiboluri* (Apicomplexa:Eimeriidae) from the inland bearded dragon, *Pogona vitticeps*

(Sauria: Agamidae). *Journal of Parasitology*, 81 (2), 281–284.

Mitchell, M.A. and Diaz-Figueroa, O. (2005) Clinical reptile gastroenterology. *Veterinary Clinics of North America Exotic Animal Practice*, 8 (2), 277–298.

Wright, K. (2008) Two common disorders of captive bearded dragons (*Pogona vitticeps*): Nutritional secondary hyperparathyroidism and constipation. *Journal of Exotic Pet Medicine*, 17 (4,) 267–272.

20

Diseases of the Cardiovascular System

Tegan Stephens and Alex Rosenwax

Anatomy and Physiology

Chapter 2 provides a more detailed review of anatomy and physiology of the cardiovascular system.

Key Points

- Crocodilian heart:
  A four-chambered heart with complete separation of the ventricles and atria. A small foramen (foramen of Panizza) persists in the interventricular septum and a left aortic arch allows for a right to left shunt during diving and prolonged submersion.
- Non-crocodilian heart (Figure 20.1a,b):
  Three-chambered heart including two atria, a single ventricle and a dorsal thin walled sinus venosus. The ventricle is functionally separated by a series of muscular ridges allowing separation of oxygenated and deoxygenated blood during contraction. The sinus venosus collects blood from the systemic circulation before entering the right atrium and acts as a cardiac pacemaker and blood pressure mediator.

- Renal portal system:
  Afferent renal portal veins are formed by the caudal vein from the tail and iliac veins from the hind limbs. The renal portal system perfuses the renal tubule cells and allows for continued blood supply to the tubules during periods of reduced glomerular filtration. Pelvic veins can allow blood to be redirected around the kidney via a valve. Postulated effects on drug distribution have been explored in a limited number of studies and shown variable results.
- Clinical implications:
  Pulmonary oedema generally develops before ascites during cardiovascular disease. Any reptile presenting with dyspnoea should be investigated for cardiac disease.
- Apnoea may be associated with vagal induced bradycardia, leading to anaesthetic complications and necessitating the use of intermittent positive pressure ventilation in all reptile anaesthesia.

Reptile Medicine and Surgery in Clinical Practice, First Edition. Edited by Bob Doneley, Deborah Monks, Robert Johnson and Brendan Carmel.
© 2018 John Wiley & Sons Ltd. Published 2018 by John Wiley & Sons Ltd.

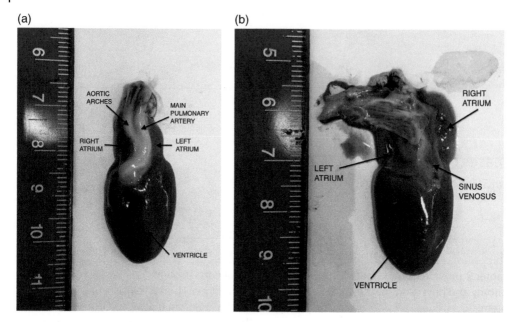

Figure 20.1 Python heart. (a) Ventral aspect. (b) Dorsal aspect.

The Cardiovascular Examination

History and Husbandry

An appreciation of husbandry is essential in all reptile disease investigations. Temperature, hydration, feeding history and access to ultraviolet light are all important factors in cardiovascular health in reptiles. Deficiencies in husbandry are a common initiating cause of disease.

It is useful to take baseline measurements of heart and respiratory rate at every routine annual health check. Values can vary greatly, even between individuals of the same species, and can vary with time of year, temperature, reproductive status and time of last feed. Where possible, cardiac examinations should be performed with the animal at its preferred optimal temperature zone. Take note of differences in activity levels between diurnal and nocturnal species. All measurement should be accompanied by notes regarding time of day, temperature, and pertinent husbandry points.

The most common reason for presentation of snakes with cardiac disease is a swelling in the cranial portion of the body. Other general causes of presentation are lethargy, inappetence or exercise intolerance. A history of open-mouth breathing may be noted.

Physical Examination

For further detailed information, refer to Chapter 10.

Mucous Membranes
Familiarity with normal mucous membrane colour is important when dealing with different species. Many reptiles have very pale or very dark normal oral mucosae. Cyanosis or ecchymosis can be seen with cardiovascular disease.

Heart Rate
Heart rate varies with body size, species, metabolic rate, season, time since last feed and respiratory rate. A predicted baseline heart rate for a reptile can be determined using allometric scaling (Sedgewick 1991):

$$= 33.4 \times (\text{weight in kg} - 0.25)$$

Reptiles with cardiac disease or those that have suffered blood loss may display tachycardia. Prolonged apnoea or pulmonary disease may be accompanied by bradycardia. The heart rate can often be determined by direct visualization of the heart movement under the ventral scales in snakes. Other species will require direct auscultation or Doppler examination to determine heart rate. A mark should be made over the heart with permanent marker if further monitoring or auscultation is required to allow it to be located quickly (e.g. during surgery or collapse).

It should be noted that the heart may beat in reptiles for minutes or hours following clinical death. This is an important point when considering monitoring procedures during anaesthesia and also when determining death following euthanasia.

Auscultation

Standard stethoscopes may not deliver adequate sound quality for assessment of reptile hearts due to friction on the scales and low amplitude heart sounds. Sound quality can be improved by placing a damp cloth between the scales and the bell of the stethoscope. More accurate auscultation may be achieved with a Doppler ultrasound probe.

Pulse

Peripheral pulse rates are difficult to determine in reptiles and no effective indirect blood pressure measurement method has been described. Surgically placed intra-arterial devices have been used to monitor pulse. In larger reptiles the intraoral vessels may be used to assess pulse quality but sedation of the animal is required.

Respiration

Measuring the respiratory rate, in conjunction with heart rate, is good practice. Respiratory rate will vary greatly with environmental changes and differences in activity levels.

General Signs

Swelling around the level of the heart, pleural or peripheral oedema, ascites, cyanosis and ecchymosis are all potential indicators of cardiac disease (Figure 20.2). Note that the size of a snake heart may enlarge up to 40% in the 48 hours following feeding. This is because of an increased gene expression of muscle contractile proteins. The heart returns to normal size once the meal is digested.

Laboratory Analysis

Fresh faecal and blood samples should be taken at the time of the consultation for examination and identification of haemoparasites,

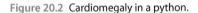

Figure 20.2 Cardiomegaly in a python.

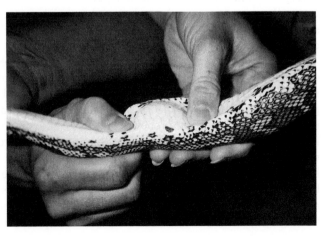

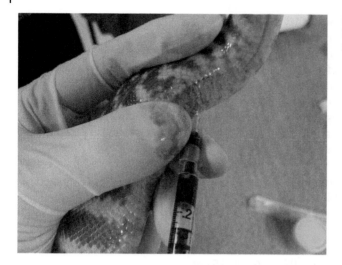

Figure 20.3 Cardiocentesis in a black-headed python (*Aspidites melanocephalus*).

endoparasites and haematological abnormalities. Blood samples may be obtained from the ventral tail vein in many species, from the jugular vein in many turtles or by jugular cutdown in snakes and lizards, and by cardiocentesis in snakes. Cardiocentesis should only be performed in animals larger than 300 g because of the risk of myocardial damage and haemorrhage in smaller animals. Using the ventrocaudal approach through the ventricular myocardium allows the needle to enter at a point where the wall is thicker and there is minimal twisting motion during contraction (Figure 20.3). Complications reported include atrophy, fibrosis and haemorrhage. See Chapter 13 for more detail on sample collection.

Very little information is available regarding cardiac enzymes in reptiles and no analysis has been done on their relationship to disease.

The use of pulse oximetry in reptiles is often not possible, owing to the heavily pigmented mucosa of many species and the presence of thick scales. In species with minimally pigmented mucosa, probes placed in the proximal oesophagus give the best results. The absorption wavelength of reptile haemoglobin and deoxyhaemoglobin have been shown to be roughly equivalent to mammalian levels. However, absolute value readings have not been validated in reptiles.

The oxygen carrying capacity of reptile erythrocytes varies greatly, most notably by being reduced during anaerobic glycolysis and the resulting acidosis experienced during periods of apnoea.

Doppler analysis gives a quantitative assessment of the intensity of the speed of blood traveling through the peripheral vessels. It is a sensitive way of monitoring changes in blood pressure quality during anaesthesia, despite not providing a quantitative reading. Doppler use in reptiles requires large amounts of coupling gel to remove the noise interference of air between the scales (Figure 20.4).

Imaging

We present the key points here. Refer to Chapter 12 for more detail.

Radiography

Radiography to assess the heart is generally not useful in reptile species, with the exception of snakes. There is significant overlap of the cardiac outline with the pectoral girdle in most lizards and the carapace and plastron in chelonian species. Cardiomegaly in snakes is determined by displacement of the trachea dorsally as well as distension of the body wall. Cardiac length may be easily compared to rib spaces. The best comparison of normal and

Figure 20.4 Doppler monitoring of a varanid to confirm death.

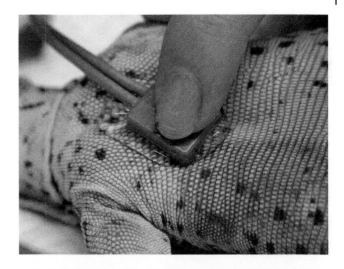

Figure 20.5 Ultrasound of a turtle heart.

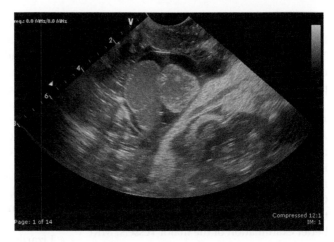

abnormal hearts can be made between animals of the same species and a similar size. While less useful for examining the heart itself, cranial coelomic radiographs can still be of benefit in assessing changes to the respiratory system.

Ultrasonography

Ultrasonography has many potential uses in investigating reptilian cardiac disease. Positioning is determined based on species and heart position.

- Snakes – directly through the midline acoustic window. Sedation and a water bath may facilitate imaging, otherwise copious amounts of coupling gel are required. Standard views include a sagittal plane with the heart in the long axis to identify chambers, major vessels ridges and valves and a 90-degree rotation to the short axis for a transverse view.
- Lizards such as agamids, with cranially positioned hearts at the level of the pectoral region and chelonians – images are obtained through the cervical window (Figure 20.5). In very small patients where the transducer cannot be placed directly on the acoustic window, a latex glove filled with water may be used as a standoff (Figure 20.6).
- Lizard species such as varanids, with hearts located caudally – the axillary window or a ventral approach.

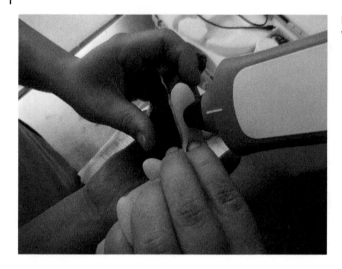

Figure 20.6 Ultrasound of small turtle with standoff.

Patient size limits usefulness, with better images obtained in patients over 1 kg weight. M-mode is generally not considered useful, owing to the spongy myocardium, which prevents accurate measurement.

Advanced Imaging

Advanced imaging, including computed tomography (CT) and magnetic resonance imagining (MRI), may have applications in investigation of cardiac disease in reptiles. CT provides much higher resolution imaging than standard radiography and may allow better examination of the major vessels. MRI provides very good contrast images of soft tissue and may be used to examine the heart itself and chambers, however the slow heart rhythm can disturb the image. These techniques are particularly valuable with chelonians, where the shell structure interferes with standard radiographic views. The disadvantages of CT and MRI include prolonged anaesthesia time in patients, which may already be poor anaesthetic candidates, cost and lack of availability.

Electrocardiography

Difficulties arise in reptiles due to small patient size, difficulty of conduction through thick scales, changes in depolarization with physiological state changes and the limited number of published normal values available. Reptiles lack the specialised Purkinje fibre-based conduction (pacemaker) system found in mammals. Contraction is initiated in the sinus venosus by the cardiac muscle fibres. Ventricular systole is long, and diastole is short. The best results may be achieved using metal crocodile clips with filed teeth in conjunction with coupling gel:

- Chelonians – cranial leads are placed on cervical or axillary skin folds and caudal leads on the skin folds caudal to the hind limb.
- Lizards – cranial leads are placed on the skin of the forelimbs, axilla or neck, caudal on the crural or popliteal fold.
- Snakes – a base-apex reading may be obtained with electrodes placed two heart lengths cranial and caudal to the heart on the lateral aspect.

Reptile electrocardiograms demonstrate a P wave, QRS complex and T wave pattern similar to mammals. An additional SV wave has been described representing the depolarisation of the sinus venosus. Normal findings include pleomorphism of the P wave, the QRS appearing as a single R wave and long repolarization phases (QT intervals). Abnormal findings include tachycardia, increased P or QRS amplitudes and heart blocks (Figure 20.7).

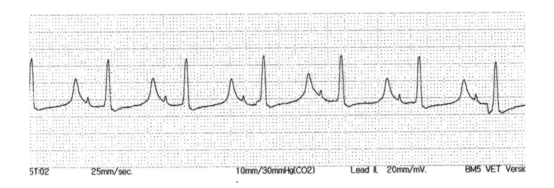

51:02   25mm/sec.   10mm/30mmHg(CO2)   Lead II. 20mm/mV.   BM5 VET Versio

Figure 20.7 Electrocardiogram trace of python under general anaesthesia.

Cardiovascular Disease

The clinical signs of cardiovascular disease in reptiles are generally nonspecific and rarely pathognomonic. These signs may include lethargy, inappetence, weakness, exercise intolerance, weight loss, swelling in the region of the heart, change in skin or mucous membrane colour and sudden death.

Congestive Heart Failure

While congestive heart failure is common in geriatric mammals; it is not commonly reported in reptiles. This may be because reptiles do not reach advanced ages in captivity owing to poor husbandry. Congestive heart failure has been described in a Burmese python (*Python bivittatus*; Jacobson *et al.* 1991), a mole kingsnake (*Lampropeltis calligaster rhombomaculata*; Barton 1980), a Deckert's rat snake (*Elaphe obsoleta 'deckerti'*; Jacobson 1979) and a carpet python (Rishniw and Carmel 1999). Despite advances in diagnostics available for reptiles, most cases are still identified post mortem. Changes may be seen in the cardiac muscle, valves, pericardium or major vessels.

Therapy for congestive heart failure in reptiles should follow similar protocols as for mammals, although the prognosis is considered poor, based on reports in the literature. There has been minimal evaluation of common drugs for congestive heart failure in reptilian species. While loop diuretics such as furosemide would seem to have little clinical application, owing to the absence of the loop of Henle in the reptilian nephron, numerous practitioners have anecdotally reported positive outcomes following their use. This may be due to a perceived action on the proximal tubules as noted in mammals. Cardiac glycosides, sympatholytics, vasodilators and diuretics may all be used with care. However, allometric scaling is recommended to determine optimal dose rates. Delivering medications, which are in most cases oral preparations, is also difficult in many reptile species and no information is available on oral bioavailability.

Congenital and Hereditary Disease

Congenital cardiac disease is uncommon in reptiles and generally reported on necropsy. Abnormalities may occur during embryo development and organ formation. Severe malformations generally will lead to death prior to hatching or birth, or soon after. Minor abnormalities may not be discovered for a significant time period (if ever) or may complete development postnatally, before signs are noticed.

Nutritional Disorders Affecting the Cardiovascular System

Hypocalcaemia affects all body muscle including cardiac muscle. Delayed cardiac depolarization can be seen on electrocardiogram (ECG) by increased ST and QT intervals. Secondary nutritional hyperparathyroidism is one of the more common causes of presentation of reptiles to veterinary clinics. Affected animals may display weakness, lethargy, depression, muscle tremors and seizures. While the changes to skeletal muscle are obvious, the affected cardiac muscle should not be forgotten and potential damage should be treated as an emergency. Nutritional hyperparathyroidism should be considered as a potential poor prognostic indicator when assessing anaesthetic risk. Diagnosis and treatment of nutritional hyperparathyroidism are discussed in Chapter 15.

Vitamin E deficiency may result in cardiac muscle abnormalities (white muscle disease) in reptiles as in mammals. More commonly affected species such as snakes, aquatic chelonians and crocodilians may have been fed a diet of excessively obese rodents or oily fish. Treatment with supplementary vitamin E (12.5 mg/kg) and selenium (0.05 mg/kg) is generally curative, except for severe cases.

Calcification of the tunica media of large vessels has been reported in reptiles. The aetiology is unknown. There have been some links made between this condition and both hypo and hypervitaminosis D.

Hypoalbuminaemia is a common finding in reptiles fed a suboptimal diet, with or without primary liver disease. Affected animals may present with oedema, ascites or anasarca as a result of fluid loss from the vascular space. These animals may present with tachycardia, compensating for fluid loss. Care must be taken with stress and handling until the hypoalbuminaemia and fluid deficits have been corrected.

Electrolyte imbalances are a potential cause of cardiac abnormalities. Hypokalaemia may occur in animals on suboptimal diets, where the potassium moves from the intracellular to extracellular space in order to preserve basic functions such as transmission of action potentials in nerve cells. Once glucose is provided, the potassium moves rapidly back into the intracellular space, which may result in the development of life-threatening arrhythmias. Primary hyperkalaemia is associated with renal disease and may cause arrhythmias. When arrhythmias are diagnosed, blood electrolyte levels should be measured. Calcium may be of benefit in conjunction with diuresis (hyperkalaemia) or supplementation of potassium to counter myocardial excitability.

Obesity is a contributing factor in some cases of cardiac disease in reptiles. Captive reptiles are more at risk of obesity than wild counterparts due to free access to prey and a predominance of high fat food items, together with a significantly decreased level of activity. A lack of hibernation has been postulated as a potential cause of obesity. As reptiles store excess fat in their coelomic cavity, this may lead to infiltration of the vital organs and subsequent health risks. Obesity should receive attention when assessing potential causes of cardiac issues in reptiles. Potential cardiovascular damage and increased cardiac workload should be considered when evaluating the obese patient.

Trauma

Animals that present following significant trauma or blood loss may display tachycardia. In cases of acute blood loss, fluid may shift from the intracellular to the extracellular space and so great care must be taken when selecting fluids to be used to expand the vascular space. A combination of lactated Ringer's solution or saline and dextrose allows for expansion of both the vascular space and intracellular spaces. Note that internal bleeding may be an insidious finding in cases of chelonian trauma due to falling from a height.

Neoplasia

Haematopoietic neoplasms are not generally detected until the later stages of disease. Diagnosis is based on leucocyte differential, bone marrow examination and cytochemical staining. Great variation exists in the reported incidence of these cancers; however, studies have shown the cardiovascular system to be the most commonly affected body system (Hernandez-Divers and Garner 2003).

Infectious Disorders

Bacterial Infections

Aetiology

Aerobic Gram-negative bacteria are the most common isolates to damage the cardiovascular system of reptiles. Bacteria found to have directly damaged the heart and vasculature include *Salmonella* spp., *Corynebacterium* spp., *Pseudomonas* and *Escherichia coli*. A chlamydial infection has been reported as the cause of myocarditis, pericarditis, pneumonia and hepatitis in puff adders (*Bitis arietans*; Jacobson *et al.* 1989). An outbreak of mycoplasmosis has also been reported in captive American alligators (*Alligator mississippiensis*), causing pneumonia, endocarditis and arthritis (Clippinger *et al.* 2000). Mycobacteria can cause granulomatous disease and potentially cause damage to the cardiovascular system.

Pathogenesis

Septic thromboemboli and secondary septic endocarditis are potential sequelae of systemic infection by the common Gram-negative aerobes. These commonly include *Aeromonas*, *Proteus*, *Pseudomonas*, *E. coli*, *Klebsiellla*, *Serratia*, *Enterobacter* and, while *Salmonella* is rarely associated with clinical disease in reptiles, it can develop into severe septicaemia with associated secondary complications. Reptiles debilitated from poor husbandry are more susceptible.

Clinical Signs

Similar to other causes of cardiovascular disease, the clinical signs of bacterial infections are generally non-specific. The reptile may present as lethargic, weak and/or anorectic or may suffer from apparent sudden death.

Diagnosis

Routine blood cultures and haematology should be performed on all cases of suspected sepsis. Imaging may indicate issues with the cardiovascular system; however, it is unlikely to determine the cause. Necropsy is the most common definitive diagnostic tool used in septic cardiac disease cases.

Treatment

Following a positive blood culture or suspicious haematology findings, appropriate antibiotic therapy may be initiated. Antibiotic choice should ideally be made following sensitivity testing. These cases are often systemically affected and other therapies may be indicated depending on clinical signs and other findings.

Prevention and Control

Most cases of septic cardiovascular disease are secondary to systemic disease; improper husbandry is a likely underlying cause in many cases. Where individual animals are likely to be suffering from immune suppression, the potential for transfer of infectious agents means appropriate quarantine procedures should be followed.

Parasitic Infections

Adult nematodes may live in the vascular system and release microfilaria into the circulation. While most infections are considered nonpathogenic, the adult worms may block major vessels and may lead to thrombosis, oedema and necrosis. Diagnosis is made by examining peripheral blood smears, where filarid worms are readily identified in heavily infected individuals. As these parasites require intermediate vectors, interrupting the life cycle is possible in captivity.

Treatment involves ivermectin at 0.2 mg/kg (not to be used in chelonians) or surgical removal of the adult worms.

Digenetic spirorchid flukes can be found in wild aquatic turtles or those housed outdoors. The adult flukes live in the heart and great vessels and, when eggs are released, terminal vessels may be occluded. Cardiovascular lesions may include endocarditis, arteritis and thrombosis. They are commonly associated with aneurysm formation. Enzyme-linked immunosorbent assay testing has been used effectively as a diagnostic tool in green turtles (*Chelonia mydas*). Praziquantel is recommended but its efficacy is unknown.

Haemoparasites are common in wild caught animals and, while most are nonpathogenic, malarial parasites (*Plasmodium* spp.) may produce haemolytic anaemia. Treatment involves use of chloroquine at 125 mg/kg orally every 48 hours for three treatments.

Viral Infections

McCracken *et al.* (1994) describe an erythrocytic virus causing anaemia in a diamond python (*Morelia spilota spilota*) and Jacobson *et al.* (2005) describes myocardial degeneration due to West Nile virus in American alligators. Viruses which can cause cardiovascular pathology in mammals (such as parvovirus) have been described in reptiles and may become a more recognized issue with further investigation.

References

Barton, S. (1980) Cardiomyopathy in a kingsnake (*Lampropeltis calligaster rhombomaculata*). *Veterinary Medicine Small Animal Clinics*, 75, 125–129.

Clippinger, T.L., Bennett, R.A., Johnson, C.M. *et al.* (2000) Morbidity and mortality associated with a new mycoplasma species from captive American alligators (*Alligator mississippiensis*). *Journal of Zoo and Wildlife Medicine*, 31, 303–314.

Hernandez-Divers, S.M. and Garner, M.M. (2003) Neoplasia of reptiles with an emphasis on lizards. *Veterinary Clinics of North America Exotic Animal Practice*, 6 (1), 251–273.

Jacobson, E.R., Gaskin, J.M. and Mansell, J. (1989) Chlamydial infection in puff adders (*Bitis arietans*). *Journal of Zoo and Wildlife Medicine*, 20, 364–369.

Jacobson, E.R., Ginn, P.E., Troutman, J.M. *et al.* (2005) West Nile virus infection in farmed American alligators (*Alligator mississippiensis*) in Florida. *Journal of Wildlife Diseases*, 41 (1), 96–106.

Jacobson, E.R., Homer, B. and Adams, E. (1991) Endocarditis and congestive heart failure in a Burmese python. *Journal of Zoo and Wildlife Medicine*, 22, 245–248.

Jacobson, E.R., Seely, J.C., Novilla, M.N. and Davidson, J.P. (1979) Heart failure associated with unusual hepatic inclusions in a Deckert's rat snake. *Journal of Wildlife Diseases*, 15, 75–81.

McCracken, H., Hyatt, A.D. and Slocombe, R.F. (1994) Two cases of anemia in reptiles treated with blood transfusions: (1) hemolytic anemia in a diamond python caused by an erythrocytic virus; (2) nutritional anemia in a bearded dragon, in 1994 Scientific Proceedings, Annual Conference of the American Association of Zoo Veterinarians 1994. American Association of Zoo Veterinarians, Pittsburgh, PA, (pp. 47–51).

Rishniw, M. and Carmel, B.P. (1999) Atrioventricular valvular insufficiency and congestive heart failure in a carpet python. *Australian Veterinary Journal*, 77 (9), 580–583.

Sedgewick, C.J. (1991) Allometrically scaling the data base for vital sign assessment used in general anaesthesia of zoological species. Proceedings of the American Association of Zoo Veterinarians 1991, pp. 360–369.

Further Reading

Gartner, G.E.A., Hicks, J.W., Manzani, P.R. *et al.* (2010) Phylogeny, ecology and heart position in snakes. *Physiological and Biochemical Zoology*, 83 (1), 43–54.

Holz, P., Barker, I.K., Burger, J.P. *et al.* (1997) The effect of the renal portal system on pharmacokinetic parameters in the red-eared slider (*Trachemys scripta elegans*). *Journal of Zoo and Wildlife Medicine*, 28 (4), 386–393.

Jensen, B., Abe, A.S., Andrade, D.V. *et al.* (2010) The heart of the South American rattlesnake, *Crotalus durissus*. *Journal of Morphology*, 271, 1066–1077.

Jensen, B., Nyengaard, J.R., Pedersen, M. and Wang, T. (2010) Anatomy of the python heart. *Anatomical Science International*, 85, 194–203.

Kik, M.J.L. and Mitchell, M.A. (2005) Reptile cardiology: a review of anatomy and physiology, diagnostic approaches, and clinical disease. *Seminars in Avian and Exotic Pet Medicine*, 14 (1), 52–60.

Latney, L.V. and Wellehan, J. (2013) Selected emerging infectious diseases of squamates. *Veterinary Clinics of North America Exotic Animal Practice*, 16, 319–228.

Mans, C. (2014) Update on common nutritional disorders of captive reptiles. *Veterinary Clinics of North America Exotic Animal Practice*, 17, 369–395.

Martinez-Jimenez, D. and Hernandez-Divers, S.J. (2007) Emergency care of reptiles. *Veterinary Clinics of North America Exotic Animal Practice*, 10, 557–585.

Mitchell, M.A. (2009) Reptile cardiology. *Veterinary Clinics of North America Exotic Animal Practice*, 12, 65–79.

Rush, E.M., Donnelly, T.M. and Walberg, J. (1999) Aortic aneurysm and subsequent cardiopulmonary arrest in a Burmese python (*Python molurus bivittatus*). Proceedings of the Association of American Zoo Veterinarians 1999, pp. 134–138.

Saggese, M. (2009) Clinical approach to the anaemic reptile. *Journal of Exotic Pet Medicine*, 18 (2), 98–111.

Schilliger, L., Chetboul, V. and Tessier, D. (2005) Standardizing two-dimensional examination in snakes. *Exotic DVM*, 7 (3), 63–74.

Schmidt, R. and Reavill, D. (2010) Cardiopulmonary disease in reptiles. 2010 Proceedings of the Association of Reptile and Amphibian Veterinarians, pp. 90–98.

Secor, S.M. and White, S.E. (2009) Prioritizing blood flow: cardiovascular performance in response to the competing demands of locomotion and digestion for the Burmese python, *Python molurus*. *Journal of Experimental Biology*, 213, 78–88.

Slay, C.E., Enok, S., Hicks, J.W. and Wang, T. (2014) Reduction of blood oxygen levels enhaces postprandial cardiac hypertrophy in Burmese python (*Python bivittatus*). *Journal of Experimental Biology*, 217, 1784–1789.

Taylor, E.W., Leite, C.A.C., Sartori, M.R. *et al.* (2014) The phylogeny and ontogeny of autonomic control of the heart and cardiorespiratory interactions in vertebrates. *Journal of Experimental Biology*, 217, 690–703.

Wyneken, J. (2009) Normal reptile heart morphology and function. *Veterinary Clinics of North America Exotic Animal Practice*, 12, 51–63.

21

Diseases of the Respiratory System

Melinda L. Cowan

Anatomy and Physiology

See Chapter 2 for more information on the anatomy and physiology of the respiratory system.

Key Points

- The glottis is located rostrally within the oral cavity in snakes and some carnivorous lizards. Chelonians and most lizards have a glottis positioned caudally in the oral cavity, at the base of a large tongue.
- The cartilaginous tracheal rings are complete in chelonians and incomplete in snakes and lizards.
- Lung anatomy varies and can be divided into single, transitional and multi-chambered. The lungs of most reptiles are sac-like and

paired, although in most snakes the left lung is vestigial or absent.

- The cranial lung in snakes participates in gas exchange and the caudal aspect of the lung forms a non-respiratory air sac. Some lizards have a similar lung structure.
- Gas exchange surfaces are ediculi and faveoli.
- Reptiles lack a diaphragm. Expiration and inspiration are therefore mostly active processes in most reptiles, although there are passive components to the respiratory cycle in snakes.
- Stimulus to breathe comes from low blood oxygen levels and increased oxygen demand is normally met with an increase in tidal volume, rather than respiratory rate.

Predisposing Factors to Respiratory Disease

The reptilian immune system shares many similarities with that of mammals and birds. Like other vertebrates, reptiles possess the innate and adaptive (cell-mediated and humoral) components and the efficacy of the overall immune response appears to decline with age. Compared with mammals, however, reptiles have a weaker and slower humoral response. The immune system in reptiles can also be directly influenced by other factors, such as the season, the animal's reproductive state and the environmental climate.

Being ectothermic, the most unique feature of the reptilian immune system is the response to variation in environmental temperature. In species that have been studied, peak immune performance occurs within a temperature range. When reptiles are exposed to environmental temperatures

Reptile Medicine and Surgery in Clinical Practice, First Edition. Edited by Bob Doneley, Deborah Monks, Robert Johnson and Brendan Carmel.
© 2018 John Wiley & Sons Ltd. Published 2018 by John Wiley & Sons Ltd.

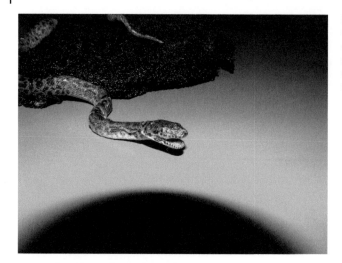

Figure 21.1 This spotted python (*Antaresia maculosa*) is exhibiting open-mouth breathing, which is likely secondary to dysecdysis and obstruction of the nasal passages (courtesy of Bob Doneley).

outside this range, impaired immune function is the consequence. While chronically low environmental temperatures are the most common scenario leading to disease, persistent overheating and acute, severe alterations in temperature can also impact the immune system in reptiles.

Reduced immune function secondary to the provision of inappropriate climatic conditions is the most common predisposing factor in the development of respiratory infections in reptiles. Other factors that can directly contribute to the development of respiratory disease include poor hygiene, irritating substrates (e.g. sawdust), substrates with high microbial concentrations (e.g. peat moss, mulch, potting soil) and transmission of disease through inadequate quarantine.

Aetiologies of Respiratory Disease

Respiratory disease in reptiles appears to be commonly caused by infectious organisms. Bacteria, fungi, viruses and parasites can all cause disease in susceptible animals. Other, non-infectious diseases of the respiratory tract have been reported in reptiles including trauma, foreign bodies, neoplasia and inhaled irritants (smoke, pesticides). Hypovitaminosis A is a well-recognized condition affecting

some reptile species. Clinical signs of respiratory disease can occur with occlusion of the nostrils from retention of skin after ecdysis (Figure 21.1).

Non-infectious Disease

Trauma

Captive reptiles can suffer from significant damage to the rostral maxillary region from repetitive collisions with enclosure walls. Lizards appear particularly prone to this type of trauma. Stress and small enclosure size are considered the main contributing factors. Although wild reptiles held in captivity are considered most at risk, this problem also occurs frequently in captive-bred lizards. It appears to be more common in anxious species, such as water dragons, Frill-neck lizards, monitors and some species of iguanas.

Wild reptiles frequently present to the veternarian with traumatic injuries caused by natural predators, domestic pets, vehicles and humans. Penetrating bite wounds can often involve respiratory tissue and can easily lead to both local infection and sepsis. Lawnmower blades are a common cause of severe lacerations in wild blue-tongued lizards in Australia. Often, these wounds are extensive and pulmonary tissue is exposed or exteriorized.

A common presentation in many captive reptile are wounds inflicted by other pets.

Cats and dogs can cause penetrating wounds to the thoracic region. The nasal cavity and nares are occasionally traumatized in lizards from fights between enclosure cohabitants. Snakes can suffer severe wounds when live rodent prey is offered.

Neoplasia

Various neoplasia affecting the respiratory tract have been reported in reptiles. These include cases of tracheal chondroma in ball pythons, a pulmonary melanophoroma in a Rio Fuerte beaded lizard (*Heloderma horridum exasperatum*), multicentric lymphoma, fibroma, fibroadenoma and adenocarcinoma. Metastases from a range of primary neoplasms have been documented. Retroviruses have been detected in neoplastic tissue and may be associated with the development of neoplasia in snakes. Clinical signs are dependent on the location of the disease within the respiratory tract.

Nutritional diseases

Hypovitaminosis A is well-recognized nutritional disease in chelonians, chameleons, bearded dragons and iguanas. Vague clinical signs include lethargy, anorexia and weight loss. Periorbital oedema, nasal discharge, ocular discharge, stomatitis and aural abscesses are reported clinical signs that appear to be due to squamous metaplasia of epithelium. Diagnosis can be difficult and is usually reliant on consistent clinical signs and response to treatment. Cytology and histology may demonstrate hyperkeratosis that support a diagnosis of hypovitaminosis A. Weekly treatment with parenteral vitamin A (see Appendix I) is recommended, although care must be taken to avoid iatrogenic hypervitaminosis A.

Infectious Diseases

Bacteria

Bacteria that have been isolated from the reptilian respiratory tract include *Pseudomonas*, *Klebsiella*, *Salmonella*, *Proteus*, *Aeromonas* species and *Morganella morganii*. The upper respiratory system and oral cavity in reptiles are normally colonized by some of these bacteria and others are also common environmental organisms. The presence of bacteria in the upper respiratory and digestive tracts is not necessarily indicative of infection, although isolation of them from the lower respiratory tract is more consistent with disease. Culture and sensitivities are recommended for diagnosis of bacterial infection and appropriate antibiotic therapy. Blood cultures and samples from bronchial lavage are warranted in cases of suspect pneumonia. Swabs and samples from nasal cavity flushing may be taken in cases of upper respiratory infection.

Mycoplasma

Respiratory disease in tortoises caused by *Mycoplasma agassizii* and *M. testudineum* can be particularly debilitating and potentially fatal. Wild and captive populations are affected and outbreaks are often reported. Environmental changes, especially those resulting in immunosuppression have been implicated in the development of infection and the conversion from subclinical to clinical disease. Rhinitis is the main feature of disease, although other manifestations, such as pneumonia, have been reported. Clinical signs include nasal and ocular discharge, lethargy, inappetance, periorbital oedema and conjunctivitis. Chronic cases can lead to erosion of the nasal cavity. Significant exudates can accumulate in the nasal and oral cavities, which may lead to dyspnoea and open-mouth breathing. Samples of this discharge can be used for culture of mycoplasma or polymerase chain reaction (PCR) testing. Material collected from swabs or flushing of the nasal cavity can also be used.

Mycoplasma has also been documented as a cause of respiratory disease in a variety of other reptile species, including crocodilians. Tracheitis and pneumonia have been associated with an undetermined species of mycoplasma in isolated cases in snakes. Mycoplasmas have also been reported in the green iguana, although their involvement in clinical disease is currently unknown.

Complete eradication of mycoplasma organisms is unlikely and infected animals often relapse after treatment. Antibiotics that have been used include fluoroquinolones, aminoglycosides, macrolides and tetracyclines.

Chlamydia

Chlamydiosis has been reported in captive and wild reptiles. *Chlamydia pneumoniae* appears to be the most widespread species and has been documented in snakes, crocodiles, chameleons and chelonians. Its detection is considered important since strains of *C. pneumoniae* are a common cause of respiratory and other chronic disease in humans. Unclassified organisms have also been detected. Infection results in granulomatous inflammation of the lungs, heart, liver and spleen, although asymptomatic carriers can occur. Treatment with doxycycline can be considered, although extensive granulomas will limit treatment efficacy.

Mycobacteria

A wide range of mycobacteria species have been associated with disease in reptiles, including *Mycobacterium chelonae*, *M. fortuitum*, *M. intracellulare*, *M. marinum*, *M. phlei*, *M. smegmatis*, *M. ulcerans*, *M. confluentis*, *M. haemophilum*, *M. hiberniae*, *M. neoaurum*, *M. nonchromogenicum*. *M. tuberculosis* complex has not been reported in a reptile. Owing to their ubiquitous presence in the environment, the development of infection often requires chronic immunosuppression of the host. Captive wild animals appear to be at greater risk, which may be associated with chronic stress. Lesions are typically granulomatous and because mycobacteria can colonize many tissues, clinical signs of disease are dependent on the system affected. Weight loss is a common nonspecific feature of disease. Reported clinical signs that reflect disease of the respiratory system include tachypnoea, increased respiratory effort and nasal discharge. Diagnosis of mycobacteria is based on detection of acid-fast organisms with Ziehl-Neelsen stain of affected tissues.

Broad range PCR followed by gene sequencing is important, as mycobacteria can have important zoonotic consequences. Euthanasia of affected animals remains the most appropriate course of action, although treatment protocols have been developed. Mycobacteria have also been detected in the faeces of asymptomatic pet reptiles, so strict hygiene is important when reptiles are kept in captivity.

Fungi

Mycotic infection of the respiratory tract was previously considered to be rare and required significant immunosuppression for disease to develop. While this is still considered true for saprophytic fungus, primary mycotic pathogens have more recently been identified as a major cause of disease in reptiles. It is possible that immunocompetent animals may develop infection if there is overwhelming exposure, particularly to an aggressive fungal species. This is more likely to occur in the confines of a captive environment, where predisposing factors include high humidity and poor hygiene. Both facultative and pathological species of fungi have also been shown to colonize normal reptilian skin. Mycotic disease appears to more commonly affect the skin than the respiratory tract, although there is considerable variation within reptilian species. Fungal lesions in the lungs have been reported in chelonians, snakes, crocodilians, chameleons. Mycotic respiratory infections in reptiles have included *Aspergillus* and *Fusarium* spp., *Cryptococcus neoformans*, *Trichophyton*, *Acremonium (Cephalosporium)*, *Beauveria*, *Chamaeleomyces* and *Chrysosporium* species. Fungal infection can be demonstrated by histopathology of lesions but species identification requires culture or PCR. Common antifungal agents include azoles (ketoconazole, itraconazole, clotrimazole, and miconazole) and polyene macrolides (amphotericin B, nystatin). Surgical debridement of granulomas is often required in addition to medical therapy.

Parasites

The types of parasites affecting reptiles are covered in Chapter 32. Those parasites that cause disease in the respiratory system include parasitic invertebrates (pentastomids), nematodes (lungworms, ascarids, oxyurids and filaroid nematodes), trematodes (spirorchids) and more rarely protozoan organisms (coccidia, flagellates).

Viruses

Ferlavirus, formerly known as ophidian paramyxovirus or OPMV, lies within the family Paramyxoviridae. Neurorespiratory disease is the main feature of ferlavirus infection in snakes. Nonspecific clinical signs include lethargy, food refusal, regurgitation and acute death. Respiratory lesions such as pneumonia are the primary pathology, with clinical signs including nasal discharge, increased oropharyngeal mucus, respiratory noise and open-mouth breathing (Figure 21.2). Neurological signs may include opisthotonos, loss of righting reflex, abnormal movements, tremors and flaccid paralysis. Asymptomatic infection and chronic, subtle infection can occur. Outbreaks of disease can occur, although these appear to be confined to captive populations with only sporadic reports of the presence of ferlavirus in wild snakes.

Sunshinevirus, also a paramyxovirus, has been identified in snakes from Australia. Similar clinical signs to ferlavirus have been reported in affected animals, although histopathological lesions are predominately found in the brain, rather than the respiratory tract. Dermatitis and stomatitis are other potential features of sunshinevirus infection. Chronic viral shedding has been documented in snakes with asymptomatic infection and vertical transmission has been documented. Diagnosis is based on PCR testing of blood and swabs of the oropharynx and cloaca.

Inclusion body disease has been associated with respiratory symptoms in snakes from the family Boidae. An arenavirus has been implicated in the disease and it appears likely that the immunosuppressive effects allow secondary infections, such as pneumonia, to occur. The disease appears to be progressive and chronic, characterized by weight loss, regurgitation and anorexia. Neurological symptoms include head tremors, incoordination, opisthotonos and loss of righting reflex.

Other important causes of respiratory disease in snakes include reovirus and a nidovirus, which appears to cause severe respiratory disease in captive ball pythons. The Iridoviridae family that includes the genera *Ranavirus*, has mainly been associated with disease in chelonians. Clinical signs

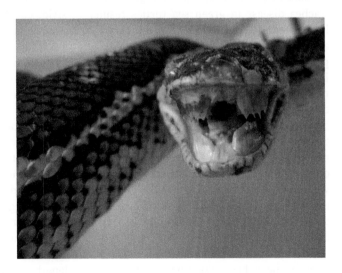

Figure 21.2 Typical open mouth posture of a dyspnoeic snake. This carpet python hybrid has evidence of stomatitis that is often a concurrent disease process (courtesy of Tegan Stephens).

that may be observed include nasal discharge, conjunctivitis and subcutaneous oedema of the neck. Pneumonia, stomatitis, hepatitis and enteritis have been reported with ranavirus infections. Ulceration of the nasal mucosa has been documented in green tree pythons, in addition to necrosis of the liver and pharyngeal region. Anorexia, lethargy, cloacal prolapse and sudden death have been reported in juvenile animals.

Herpesviruses have been documented in chelonians, snakes, lizards and crocodilians. Chelonians appear to be more commonly affected and the respiratory tract is frequently involved. Tortoises affected by testudinid herpesviruses can present with nasal and ocular discharge, caseous stomatitis, anorexia, lethargy and dyspnoea. Neurological signs, such as ataxia and paralysis, are occasionally observed. Diagnosis is based on PCR of swab or tissue samples. Acyclovir has been used with frequency in the treatment of these cases.

Painted turtles (*Chrysemys picta*), map turtles (*Graptemys* spp.) and Pacific pond turtles (*Clemmys marmorata*) have been documented with a herpesvirus that results in hepatic necrosis and pulmonary oedema. Lethargy, anorexia and subcutaneous oedema have been the observed clinical features. A variety of herpesviruses affect a number of sea turtle species. Lung, eye and trachea disease in green sea turtles results in caseous material in the eyes, oropharynx and trachea. Other clinical features include problems with buoyancy and dyspnoea. Loggerhead sea turtles have been documented with two herpesvirus-associated diseases known as loggerhead genital–respiratory herpesvirus (LGRV) and loggerhead orocutaneous herpesvirus (LOCV). Affected animals develop ulcers in the mucosal surfaces of the trachea and cloacal tissue in LGRV, while LOCV results in ulcers in the oral cavity and integument. Exudate adheres to the ulcers in LOCV and pneumonia has also been associated with infection.

Other viruses, such as flavivirus and adenovirus, have been documented to cause mild pneumonia, although infections result in more significant pathology in other organs.

Diagnosis of Respiratory Disease

Evaluating the respiratory system of the reptile can be challenging, primarily because of the thick, horny integument that limits auscultation and accurate localization of disease. Investigative methods include lung washes, multiple radiographical views, advanced imaging (computed tomography, magnetic resonance imaging), tracheoscopy and pulmonoscopy.

A thorough assessment of the respiratory system may include haematology, biochemistries and blood cultures. Exudates from the upper respiratory tract should be examined cytologically. Samples from the lower respiratory tract are best obtained with a tracheal or lung wash.

Sampling of the trachea or lung is best performed under sedation or anaesthesia, although it is possible to perform a cranial tracheal wash on a conscious animal. Care is taken to avoid touching the oral cavity mucosa as a sterile, flexible, plastic tube (such as a nasogastric feeding tube) is passed into the trachea (Figure 21.3). In small patients, an intravenous catheter without stylet can be used. The collecting tube can also be directed through a previously placed sterile endotracheal tube. The level of the tracheal bifurcation depends on the species. The catheter should be advanced to the level of the forelimbs in lizards and just caudal to the heart in snakes. Further advancement will facilitate sampling from the lung. A volume of sterile saline (5–10 ml/kg) is recommended for flushing. Cytology, microbial culture and PCR for viral aetiologies can be performed on samples.

The lung can also be accessed transcutaneously in snakes via the air sac portion of the lung (Figure 21.4). The entry point in the coelom is made 35–45% of the snout–vent length on the right side of the body; after

Figure 21.3 A sterile feeding tube has been passed into the glottis and trachea of this carpet python (*Morelia spilota*) for a tracheal wash (courtesy of Bob Doneley).

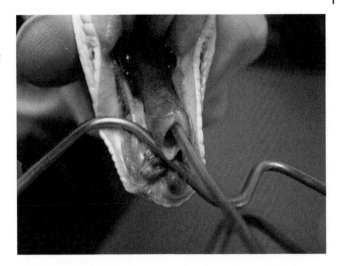

Figure 21.4 Endoscopic examination lower respiratory tract via the air sac in a spotted python (courtesy of Bob Doneley).

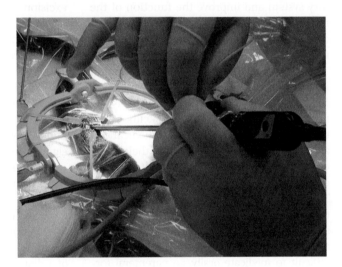

entering the coelom, the air sac of the right lung can be visualized and entered. Exudates, mucosal scrapings and biopsy samples can be taken. A coeliotomy can also be performed in snakes and lizards to access the lung. Access in chelonians is more difficult, with pulmonoscopy best performed via the pre-femoral region. It is critical to close the horizontal septum that is perforated when accessing the lung with this approach. A dorsal osteotomy over the affected area of lung can also be performed in chelonians for the collection of samples, but has limited value in terms of visualization of the architecture of the lung.

Principles of Treatment

Initial treatment and the requirement for hospitalization depends on the presenting clinical signs. A thermal gradient should be provided if a patient is hospitalized; supportive care may include fluid therapy and tube feeding. Although severe dyspnoea warrants oxygen therapy, it must be remembered that the stimulus for ventilation in reptiles is hypoxaemia. Chronic oxygen supplementation, especially at high levels, is therefore not recommended. Nebulization with saline can be employed to help reduce congestion in the upper respira-

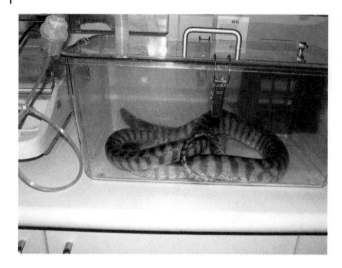

Figure 21.5 Nebulization of a black-headed python (*Aspidites melanocephalus*) in an oxygen chamber (courtesy of Bob Doneley).

tory system and improve the function of the respiratory mucosa. Nebulization can also deliver aerosolized antimicrobials to the lower respiratory tract (Figure 21.5).

Other methods of drug administration include parenteral, per os and topical routes. Medication supplied in drinking water is not recommended, owing to the likelihood of inconsistent intake. Injectable medications are preferred in snakes because of their infrequent feeding patterns and the potential for erratic absorption with oral administration. This should also be a consideration for all reptile species where digestion may be delayed or impaired, such as can occur with debility, brumation and hypothermia. Chelonians can be difficult to medicate orally, so parenteral formulations of medication are usually selected.

Granulomas and abscesses are common developments in reptile infections. Surgical excision of abscesses or debridement of caseous exudates is required to treat these infections effectively. While the upper respiratory tract is reasonably accessible, surgery of the lower respiratory tract is more difficult, especially in chelonians. Debridement of pulmonary lesions and biopsy of masses can also be performed with endoscopic guidance. Endoscopy is also useful in the removal of foreign bodies, pentastomids and other parasites.

The air sac component of the lung in many snakes and lizards can pose a significant challenge in treating respiratory infections. Exudates can accumulate in this portion of the lung and are unable to be cleared effectively. Clearance is impaired by the absence of a diaphragm and the subsequent inability to cough. It may be required in some cases to drain mucous or surgically remove caseous accumulations.

Further Reading

Jacobson, E.R. (2007) Parasites and parasitic diseases of reptiles, in *Infectious Diseases and Pathology of Reptiles* (E.R. Jacobson, ed.) CRC Press, Boca Raton, FL, pp. 571–666.

Mehler, S.J. and Bennett, R.A. (2006) Upper alimentary tract disease, in *Reptile Medicine and Surgery* (D.R. Mader, ed.) WB Saunders, Philadelphia, PA, pp. 299–322.

Lock, B.A. and Wellehan, J. (2015) Ophidia: snakes, in *Fowler's Zoo and Wild Animal Medicine* 8th ed. (R.E. Miller and M.E. Fowler, eds), Saunders, St Louis, MO, pp. 60–74.

Schumacher, J. (1997) Respiratory diseases of reptiles. *Seminars in Avian and Exotic Pet Medicine*, 6, 209–215.

Marschang, R.E. (2011) Viruses infecting reptiles. *Viruses*, 3, 2087–2126.

22

Disorders of the Reproductive System

Timothy J. Portas

Anatomy and Physiology

See Chapter 2 for a more detailed review of the anatomy and physiology of the reproductive system. See also Chapter 7 for general information about the management of normal reproduction.

Key Points

- Male chelonians and crocodilians have a single copulatory organ referred to as the penis, which is located on the cranioventral aspect of the cloaca.
- Male snakes and lizards have paired hemipenes located in the caudal cloaca and inverted into the ventral tail base.

- The copulatory organs do not contain a urethra.
- The paired testes are intracoelomic.
- Some female reptiles can retain viable sperm in their uterus for several years after copulation.
- All chelonians and crocodilians are oviparous.
- Some snakes and lizards are viviparous.
- All crocodilians and some chelonians, lizards and the tuatara (*Sphenodon punctatus*) exhibit temperature-dependent sex determination.

Dystocia/Post-Ovulatory Egg Stasis

Aetiology

Captive reptiles are commonly presented for veterinary evaluation and care as a result of dystocia. Dystocia occurs most frequently in oviparous reptiles but can also occur in viviparous reptile species.

Pathogenesis

Predisposing environmental and husbandry related factors include:

- inappropriate humidity, temperature and photoperiod
- absence of ultraviolet lighting
- inappropriate or insufficient nesting substrate
- lack of a nesting site in which the female feels sufficiently secure.

Host factors that can contribute to dystocia include:

- metabolic imbalances such as hypocalcaemia and hypovitaminosis A
- obesity and/or poor muscle tone
- nutritional imbalances
- salpingitis

Reptile Medicine and Surgery in Clinical Practice, First Edition. Edited by Bob Doneley, Deborah Monks, Robert Johnson and Brendan Carmel.
© 2018 John Wiley & Sons Ltd. Published 2018 by John Wiley & Sons Ltd.

- oviductal rupture
- coelomic cavity masses, including nephromegaly
- cystic and cloacal calculi
- gastrointestinal tract obstruction
- relative oversize or malformation of the egg(s)
- dehydration
- pelvic stenosis caused by nutritional secondary hyperparathyroidism or trauma
- concurrent disease.

Clinical Signs

The clinical signs of dystocia may vary from species to species and individual to individual. Clinical signs may be nonspecific or absent but may include reduced appetite or anorexia, dehydration, nesting behaviour, straining and cloacal or oviductal prolapse, weight loss, posterior paresis, coelomic cavity distension and lethargy. Coelomic cavity distension and partial or complete anorexia can occur normally during folliculogenesis and during advanced gravidity in some lizard species. The normal oviposition of a partial clutch with retention of one to two eggs can also occur and is most common in snakes.

Diagnosis

Dystocia can be challenging to diagnose in some cases. Some clinical signs exhibited during dystocia can be difficult to differentiate from those exhibited by gravid females progressing normally to oviposition or parturition, including coelomic cavity distension and anorexia. Additionally, chelonians can retain eggs for prolonged periods without apparent ill effect and snakes may retain eggs without systemic effects for variable periods of time. Multiple diagnostic techniques are often required to obtain a definitive diagnosis of dystocia and to develop an appropriate treatment plan. Eggs may be detected via palpation of the coelomic cavity. In chelonians, the shell limits coelomic cavity palpation but eggs may still be palpated or balloted via the inguinal fossa, although they must be differentiated from faecoliths and uroliths. Palpation of fetuses in viviparous species can be challenging and ultrasonography or radiography is indicated for definitive diagnosis of pregnancy.

Ultrasonography and radiography are an integral component of the diagnostic evaluation of the dystocic reptile. Both imaging modalities can be used to demonstrate the presence of eggs, although it should be noted that the presence of eggs alone does not indicate dystocia. Retained eggs in chelonians may develop abnormally thickened shells. In those species producing soft-shelled eggs (snakes and many lizard species), poor mineralization of the shell, particularly in the early post-ovulatory stage, results in a radiolucent shell which may be difficult to differentiate radiographically from preovulatory ova. Preovulatory ova are typically rounded in shape and tightly associated while post-ovulatory ova tend to be more oval and develop a linear association particularly as oviposition approaches. On ultrasound examination eggs have a hyperechoic perimeter equating to the mineralized shell and, in squamates, the albumin tends to be hypoechoic while the yolk is hyperechoic. The inguinal fossa of chelonians provides an appropriate acoustic window for ultrasonographic examination of the female reproductive tract.

Radiography is superior to ultrasonography in determining the size, shape, position and number of eggs present. Additionally, radiography can be used to evaluate the patient for the presence of underlying metabolic bone diseases, pelvic stenosis, cystic and cloacal uroliths, faecoliths and coelomic cavity masses. Radiography can also be used to detect the embryos of viviparous species in late stages of development.

Blood should be collected to assess underlying or concurrent disease. A complete blood count and full biochemical analysis (or at a minimum, serum calcium, phosphorous and uric acid values) should be determined as dehydration, hypocalcaemia, infection and renal insufficiency may all accompany dystocia in reptiles. Results should be interpreted in the light of other clinical findings, as elevations in serum calcium and phosphorous can occur during normal vitellogenesis in some lizard species as well as in dystocic patients.

Treatment

General Principles

Underlying physiological abnormalities must first be corrected and the patient stabilized before correction of the dystocia can take place. Dehydration is treated with intracoelomic, intravenous or intraosseous Ringer's solution for reptiles (one part lactated Ringer's solution, two parts 2.5% dextrose/0.45% saline solution) at 10–20 ml/kg every 24 hours. Hypocalcaemia is treated with oral calcium glubionate at 360 mg/kg every 6–24 hours. Parenteral calcium supplementation is generally avoided unless hypocalcaemic tetany is present, in which case parenteral calcium gluconate at 100 mg/kg may be administered until the patient is stabilized. A thermal gradient appropriate to the species in question should be supplied. Appropriate analgesia and antibiotic therapy, where indicated, should be provided. Empirical antibiotic therapy with ceftazidime at 20 mg/kg every 72 hours or piperacillin at 100 mg/kg every 48 hours may be used if the results of microbial culture and sensitivity are not available. The reader is referred to the relevant chapters within this text for managing underlying and concurrent disease processes.

In the early stages of non-obstructive dystocia, where the patient is otherwise clinically normal, correction of environmental and husbandry deficiencies may be sufficient. Providing an appropriate thermal gradient, correcting dehydration through warm water soaks or parenteral fluid administration and provision of a suitable nesting site may induce oviposition.

Medical management of non-obstructive dystocia may be attempted in reptiles without significant underlying or concurrent disease.

Following administration of oral calcium glubionate, intramuscular oxytocin (5–30 iu/kg) is administered. The dose may be repeated within 3–12 hours if there is no response to initial administration. Oxytocin is most effective in chelonians, less so in lizards, with snakes being the least responsive. Oxytocin therapy is most likely to be effective if administered within 48–72 hours of the onset of oviposition or parturition in squamates. The intravenous administration of oxytocin may result in more rapid induction and subsequent completion of oviposition than intramuscular administration. Oxytocin is contraindicated in cases of follicular stasis or obstructive dystocia. Arginine vasotocin is described in the literature as being potentially more effective than oxytocin it but is not available for routine clinical use. The use of prostaglandin F2 alpha has also been reported but with variable efficacy.

Cases of nonobstructive dystocia unresponsive to medical management and most cases of obstructive dystocia will require coeliotomy (or coelioscopic assisted surgery) and surgical correction. In viviparous species presenting with dystocia, a caesarean section is indicated (Figure 22.1). The reader is referred to Chapter 28 for a detailed account of surgical approaches to dystocia. Supportive care includes thermal support, fluid and nutritional support, antibiotic therapy and analgesia.

Management in Chelonians

In chelonians, eggs maybe retained for variable and prolonged periods without ill effect, so a decision to intervene must be based on the results of the physical examination and ancillary diagnostic tests (Innis 2002). Dystocia in chelonians is rarely a medical emergency, so correction of underlying environmental and husbandry related issues is a reasonable first step in otherwise clinically normal animals. Oxytocin can be administered every 3–12 hours, although treatment should cease if no eggs are produced in a 48-hour period. Oxytocin administration and supportive medical therapy

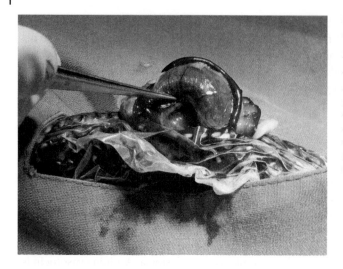

Figure 22.1 Caesarean section to correct dystocia in a broad-headed snake (*Hoplocephalus bungaroides*). The snake had given birth to two dead foetuses over the preceding 48 hours and was presented for evaluation for potential dystocia. Ultrasound examination revealed the presence of additional foetuses and a further three dead foetuses were removed by performing a coeliotomy and multiple salpingotomies.

may be continued over several days until all eggs have been deposited if there is no underlying pathology. Beta-adrenergic blockers such as propranolol and atenolol have been shown to potentiate the effects of oxytocin and their use prior to oxytocin administration has been advocated in chelonians (Chitty and Raftery 2013).

In cases of obstructive dystocia, per cloacal aspiration and collapse of eggs that have progressed to the junction of the oviduct and urodeum is possible, although cloacoscopy may be necessary to effectively and safely access the egg. If oversized eggs are not accessible per cloaca then surgical intervention is indicated.

Management in Lizards

In contrast to chelonians, dystocia in oviparous lizards often progresses rapidly and can be fatal without prompt and appropriate intervention. Cases of nonobstructive dystocia that are not responsive to medical therapy and most cases of obstructive dystocia will require surgery. Per cloacal aspiration of egg contents, followed by collapse and removal of the egg, is possible in lizards (Figure 22.2). Cloacoscopy and ovocentesis can be performed with readily available nonspecialized equipment, such as a standard domestic animal otoscope in many lizard species.

Percutaneous aspiration of egg contents for the correction of dystocia has also been described in lizards. Potential complications associated with per cutaneous aspiration of eggs include yolk coelomitis and penetration of viscera.

Management in Snakes

In the case of snakes with non-obstructive dystocia unresponsive to medical therapy, eggs may be gently manipulated, with the aid of adequate lubrication, towards the cloaca and removed under anaesthesia. Oversized eggs may require per cloacal or per cutaneous aspiration to collapse the egg shell and allow passage through the cloaca. Oviductal rupture and/or prolapse are potential sequelae to the physical manipulation of retained eggs and this approach should be used with caution (Stahl 2002).

Prevention and Control

Dystocia in captive reptiles is best prevented by ensuring appropriate environmental conditions and husbandry practices for the species in question, maintaining physically fit animals at appropriate body weights, careful breeding management and close behavioural monitoring and observation of breeding animals.

Figure 22.2 (a) Per cloacal aspiration of yolk and albumin from an oversized egg in a gila monster (*Heloderma suspectum*). (b) Following aspiration and lubrication of the cloaca, the collapsed egg is removed using alligator forceps.

(a)

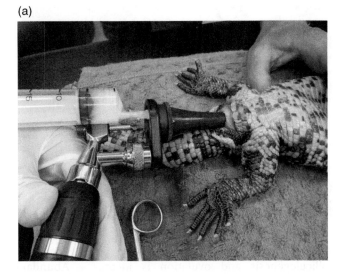

(b)

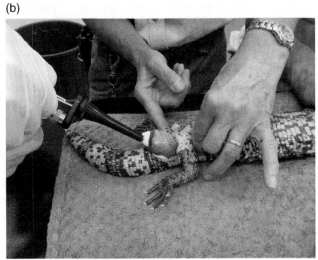

Preovulatory Follicular Stasis

Aetiology

Preovulatory follicular stasis occurs when a female undergoes vitellogenesis but then fails to ovulate or resorb the ova. The condition occurs most commonly in lizards, in particular iguanids, agamids, chameleons and varanids; it also occurs in chelonians but is uncommon in snakes.

Pathogenesis

The pathogenesis of preovulatory follicular stasis in captive reptiles in poorly understood. However, many of the same environmental and host factors that underlie the development of post-ovulatory egg stasis have been implicated in the development of preovulatory follicular stasis. Inappropriate environmental conditions (temperature, photoperiod) seem to be particularly important in some tortoise species held outside

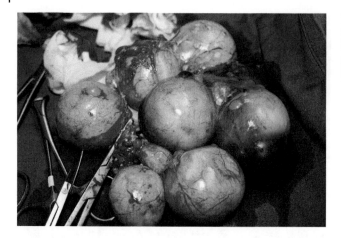

Figure 22.3 Inflamed, necrotic and ruptured follicles in an ovary removed from a female perentie (*Varanus giganteus*) with follicular stasis (reproduced with the permission of Timothy Portas and Reptile Publishers).

their natural range. The endocrinology of folliculogenesis and ovulation is incompletely understood in many reptile species and disruption of normal endocrine processes in captivity may underlie some cases of follicular stasis. The presence of a male has been shown to be necessary for follicular development and ovulation in some species (Sykes 2010). Static follicles may eventually become inspissated and necrotic or may rupture, liberating yolk material into the coelomic cavity (Figure 22.3).

Clinical signs

Clinical signs include coelomic cavity distension, reduced appetite or anorexia, dehydration and lethargy. In some cases, the reptile may be found dead without premonitory signs.

Diagnosis

While the clinical signs of coelomic cavity distension, anorexia, dehydration and lethargy are suggestive, follicular stasis must be differentiated from dystocia. Follicles can be detected via coelomic cavity palpation in some species, although care should be taken to avoid rupturing the thin-walled ovarian follicles. Follicles may be difficult to see radiographically and a contrast penumocoelogram can be performed using 10 ml of room air injected into the coelomic cavity to provide greater contrast (Funk 2002). Abundant vitellogenic follicles can also be readily detected via ultrasonography in most species, although follicles are of variable echogenicity depending upon the stage of development and species in question. Sequential ultrasound examinations can be used to track follicular development and demonstrate stasis (over a period of several weeks). With experience, developing and atretic follicles can be differentiated on the basis of echogenicity or ultrasonographic appearance (Figure 22.4). Coelioscopy under anaesthesia, while more invasive, provides for visualization of the ovaries and internal organs. Haematology and biochemistry may indicate systemic illness and further support the diagnosis. Potential abnormalities include heterophilia (with or without toxic changes), leucopenia, haemoconcentration, hypoproteinaemia, hyperalbuminaemia, hypercalcaemia, hyperphosphataemia and elevated alkaline phosphatase and creatine kinase (Sykes 2010, Chitty and Raftery 2013).

Treatment

While it is theoretically possible that female reptiles exhibiting follicular stasis may subsequently resorb these follicles, in the author's experience this is rarely, if ever, the case. Medical management of follicular stasis through attempted induction of ovulation are usually unsuccessful. Follicle-stimulating

Figure 22.4 Ultrasonographic appearance of a vitellogenic (a) and atretic (b) follicle in an Aldabran tortoise (*Aldabrachelys gigantea*).

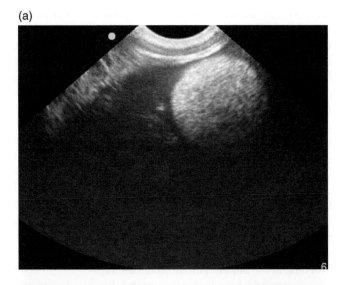

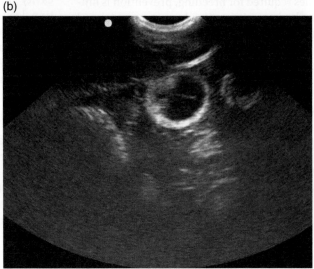

hormone, gonadotropin-releasing hormone II and progesterone followed by prostaglandin F2 alpha are ineffective in inducing ovulation in veiled chameleons (*Chamaeleo calyptratus*). Proligestone has variable efficacy in inducing follicular resorption in chelonians (Chitty and Raftery 2013). Treatment of follicular stasis is currently limited to coeliotomy (or a coelioscope-assisted approach in chelonians) for ovariectomy or ovariosalpingectomy. As with dystocia, the patient must first be stabilized and any underlying or concurrent disease processes managed prior to surgery. The reader is referred to Chapter 28 for a detailed account of surgical approaches to ovariectomy. Supportive care includes thermal support, fluid and nutritional support, antibiotic therapy and analgesia. Any concurrent disease, such as hepatic lipidosis, must also be managed.

Prevention and Control

Contraception of females, not required for breeding, either via surgical sterilization or the administration of exogenous hormones are currently the only preventative options. However, variable results have been observed with the administration of exogenous hormones for contraception. Administration of leuprolide acetate or medroxyprogesterone during the previtellogenic phase does not inhibit or delay follicular development in veiled chameleons. However implantation of the gonadotrophin-releasing hormone (GnRH) agonist deslorelin acetate appears to be effective in inhibiting the production of estrogen and progesterone and preventing follicular development in green iguanas (*Iguana iguana*). Further investigation into the application of deslorelin as a contraceptive implant for females not required for breeding is warranted. For those female reptiles required for breeding, prevention is limited to ensuring optimal environmental and husbandry conditions specific to the species and routine ultrasonography of follicular development during the breeding season.

Yolk-Associated Coelomitis

Aetiology

Yolk-associated coelomitis occurs as a sequel to follicular stasis or dystocia. It has been reported as a common problem in green iguanas, Fijian banded iguanas, various varanids, bearded dragons and various chelonian species (Jacobson 2003, Sykes 2010).

Pathogenesis

The physiology of vitellogenic follicle atresia and resorption in reptiles remains incompletely understood. However, it appears that spontaneous rupture of multiple large, atretic, vitellogenic follicles can overwhelm the coelomic resorptive capacity of yolk material, leading to coelomitis (Stacy *et al.* 2008). Liberation of yolk material into the coelomic cavity may also occur subsequent to trauma, overly rough palpation of follicles or per cutaneous aspiration of egg contents. The liberation of vitellin into the coelomic cavity incites a sterile inflammatory reaction leading to granulomatous coelomitis, serositis, extensive mesothelial proliferation of serosal surfaces and yolk embolism (Figure 22.5). Secondary bacterial infections are common.

Clinical Signs

As with dystocia and follicular stasis cases the clinical presentation can be variable, often nonspecific, and may include coelomic cavity distension, dehydration, inappetance, dark discolouration of the skin or death without premonitory signs (Figure 22.6).

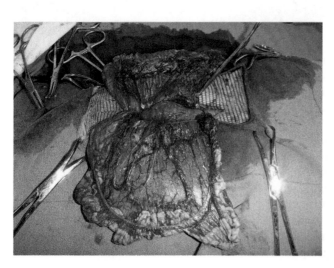

Figure 22.5 Intraoperative photograph of a female perentie (*Varanus giganteus*) with yolk coelomitis following ovariectomy and removal of yolk material from the coelomic cavity. The mesovarium and the serosal surfaces of oviducts and gastrointestinal tract are severely inflamed as a result of yolk material in the coelomic cavity.

Figure 22.6 Abundant yolk material removed from coelomic cavity of a female green iguana (*Iguana iguana*) that died of egg yolk coelomitis without exhibiting premonitory signs (courtesy of Claude Lacasse).

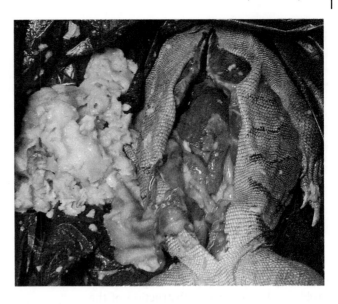

Diagnosis

Establishing a definitive diagnosis of yolk associated coelomitis can be challenging as the clinical signs are often nonspecific. Clinical pathological changes can be variable but may include hypercalcaemia, hyperphosphataemia, hyperuricaemia (and elevated blood urea nitrogen in terrestrial chelonians), heterophilia and elevated aspartate aminotransferase. Coelomic cavity ultrasonography can be used to demonstrate coelomic cavity fluid and guide coelomic cavity centesis for fluid analysis (Rivera 2008). Coelioscopy is a more invasive method but allows for direct visualization of the ovaries and coelomic cavity and definitive diagnosis.

Treatment

The prognosis is guarded as affected reptiles are typically profoundly unwell at the time of diagnosis and often have concurrent renal dysfunction. Patients must be stabilized before anaesthesia and surgical management. Treatment involves surgical management; ovariectomy or ovariosalpingectomy, removal of yolk material and copious coelomic cavity lavage. The reader is referred to Chapter 28 for a detailed account of surgical approaches to ovariectomy. Supportive care includes thermal support, fluid and nutritional support, appropriate antibiotic therapy and analgesia.

Prevention and Control

Prevention in breeding females involves ensuring optimal environmental and husbandry conditions specific to the species, close monitoring during the breeding season and routine clinical evaluation and ultrasonography of high risk patients. Females not required for breeding may be surgically sterilized or contracepted (see follicular stasis section).

Salpingitis

Aetiology

Salpingitis has been reported from various chelonian and squamate species but appears to be an uncommon finding.

Pathogenesis

Salpingitis may be the result of infection with a wide range of bacteria including *Pseudomonas* and *Salmonella* species. Infection may occur following oviposition or

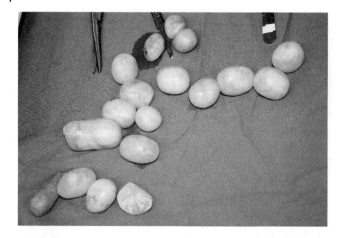

Figure 22.7 Eggs removed via salpingotomy to correct a dystocia in a female western brown snake (*Pseudonaja nuchalis*) with a *Pseudomonas aeruginosa* salpingitis. Note the thickened and deformed shells and the variable size of the eggs.

secondary to dystocia or other reproductive problems. In chelonians, obstruction of the pelvic canal by oversized or malformed eggs may result in the backflow of urine and faecal material into the oviducts resulting in salpingitis. Conversely, where salpingitis occurs as a primary disorder it may be a predisposing factor for dystocia.

Clinical Signs

The clinical signs of salpingitis may include infertility and dystocia. Affected reptiles may produce eggs with thickened, uneven shells, deformed eggs or eggs of variable size (Figure 22.7).

Diagnosis

Salpingitis may be diagnosed by demonstrating oviductal enlargement via ultrasonographic examination or coelioscopy. Haematology and biochemistry may provide further evidence of an infectious process.

Treatment

Therapy with appropriate antibiotics and anti-inflammatories may be effective in early cases but is unlikely to be successful in cases of advanced infection. Ovariosalpingectomy is indicated in advanced cases or those cases failing to respond to medical therapy.

Prevention and Control

As with other reproductive diseases for which the causes are incompletely understood, prevention is limited to ensuring appropriate species specific environmental conditions and husbandry practices.

Oviductal Prolapse

Aetiology

Oviductal prolapse is seen most commonly in snakes but can also occur in lizards and chelonians.

Pathogenesis

Oviductal prolapse occurs secondary to dystocia or other causes of straining such as constipation or cystic and cloacal calculi. Oviductal prolapse may also be iatrogenically induced following attempts to manipulate retained eggs in snakes.

Clinical Signs

The thin-walled oviduct, which may or may not contain eggs, is evident protruding from the cloaca (Figure 22.8). Depending upon the duration of the prolapse the oviduct may be oedematous, traumatized or necrotic.

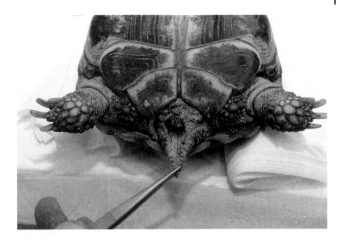

Figure 22.8 Prolapse of the oviduct in a Steppe tortoise (*Testudo horsfieldii*) subsequent to dystocia. Photo credit Zdenek Knotek.

Diagnosis

The prolapsed oviduct is generally self-evident but may need to be differentiated from prolapsed cloacal tissue, bladder or colon.

Treatment

Damage to the suspensory ligaments of the oviduct is highly likely following prolapse. Even with successful inversion and reduction of the prolapsed oviduct per cloaca, suspensory ligament damage will likely limit the ability of the oviduct to receive ovulated follicles in the future. Additionally, the prolapsed oviduct is frequently severely traumatized and compromised following prolapse. Surgical removal of the affected oviduct and its associated ovary is recommended. Retention of the contralateral ovary and oviduct preserves the breeding potential of the female if required. The underlying cause must also be addressed. Appropriate antibiotic therapy, analgesia and symptomatic support should be initiated in affected animals.

Prevention and Control

Ovariosalpingectomy via coeliotomy is recommended to prevent recurrence. Nonbreeding females may undergo elective ovariectomy or ovariosalpingectomy or contraception.

Phallus Prolapse

Aetiology

The term 'phallus' is used to encompass both the penis of crocodilians and chelonians and the hemipenis of squamate species in this section. Phallus prolapse occurs most commonly in chelonians; can also occur in snakes and lizards; but is uncommon in crocodilians.

Pathogenesis

Predisposing factors include:

- excessive breeding and breeding on particulate substrate
- inflammation and infection including from inappropriate probing techniques
- hemipenal abscessation
- nutritional causes such as hypovitaminosis A (lizards) and nutritional secondary hyperparathyroidism (young chelonians and lizards)
- straining secondary to endoparasitism, constipation or cystic and cloacal calculi
- trauma including autotomy close to the base of the tail in lizards
- neurological deficits of the retractor muscles
- gastrointestinal foreign bodies.

The prolapsed phallus is typically swollen, because of decreased venous and lymphatic drainage, and inflamed, preventing inversion or retraction into a normal anatomical position. It is likely to sustain physical trauma, including from conspecifics and become desiccated and necrotic with prolonged exposure.

Clinical Signs

The prolapsed phallus is evident protruding through the vent and may exhibit varying degrees of oedema, trauma and necrosis depending upon the cause and the duration of the prolapse (Figure 22.9).

Diagnosis

A prolapsed phallus is generally self-evident but may need to be differentiated from prolapsed cloacal tissue, bladder or colon.

Radiography may be useful to demonstrate spinal lesions such as scoliosis, kyphosis, fractures and other underlying causes which may be contributory.

Treatment

Under general anaesthesia, the prolapsed phallus is cleaned and debrided as required, lubricated and replaced into the normal anatomical position. If the prolapsed phallus has become extensively swollen, the application of hypertonic solutions, cold compresses and the use of topical and systemic anti-inflammatory drugs may be necessary to reduce swelling sufficiently to replace the prolapsed tissue. Care should be taken manipulating the phallus as the prolapsed tissue is frequently fragile and prone to further

(a)

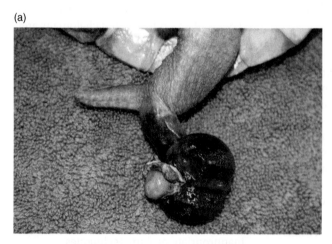

Figure 22.9 (a) Prolapse of the phallus in a Krefft's turtle (*Emydura macquarii krefftii*) following conspecific trauma during the breeding season. (b) Hemipenal prolapse in a Komodo dragon (*Varanus komodensis*) secondary to neurological deficits associated with a spinal lesion (reproduced with the permission of Timothy Portas and Reptile Publishers).

(b)

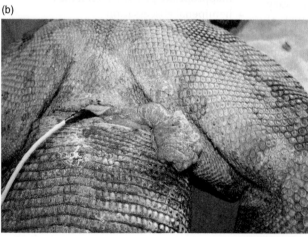

damage. Once returned to a normal anatomical position, the cloaca of chelonians may be sutured partially closed with a purse-string suture. In lizards and snakes, single interrupted sutures are more suited to the linear opening of the cloaca. Sutures can be left in place for up to two weeks. If the underlying cause of the prolapse is not identified and managed or resolved recurrent prolapse is a distinct possibility. Where there is extensive tissue necrosis or swelling, neurological deficit or where the phallus has repeatedly prolapsed surgical amputation may be performed as the phallus has no function in urination. The reader is referred to Chapter 28 for a detailed account of surgical approaches to phallus amputation. Amputation of a hemipenis in snakes and lizards does not preclude future reproduction. Systemic (and topical) antibiotic therapy and appropriate analgesia should be initiated.

Prevention and Control

The breeding activity of males should be limited to reduce the risk of trauma and prolapse associated with overuse of the phallus or hemipenes. Consideration should be given to appropriate substrates in breeding enclosures. Ensuring adequate nutrition, particularly for young growing chelonians and herbivorous or insectivorous lizards, is important to prevent nutritional secondary hyperparathyroidism and hypovitaminosis A, which may be contributory to the condition.

Hemipenal Plugs

Aetiology

Hemipenal plugs have a firm waxy consistency, are composed of seminal material, glandular material and sloughing epithelium and form within the lumen of the hemipenes in various lizard (iguanids, agamids and gekkonids) and snake species.

Pathogenesis

Hemipenal plug formation is a normal occurrence and plugs are typically shed when the hemipenes are everted during breeding. In some lizards, these plugs may fail to shed and become enlarged and impacted. Large plugs preclude the lizard from everting the hemipenes, inhibit defecation and may be associated with dysecdysis around the vent. Hemipenal abscessation and rupture can occur in severe cases. Potential causes include hypovitaminosis A associated squamous metaplasia, inappropriate humidity and reduced opportunities to breed.

Clinical Signs

Hemipenal plugs are evident as pale waxy material protruding from the inverted hemipenis into the caudal cloaca (Figure 22.10a,b). The cranial end of the plug may be covered in faecal material and/or urates. Large hemipenal plugs may cause pronounced hemipenal bulging and where abscessation has occurred there may be localised cellulitis.

Diagnosis

Hemipenal plugs are readily diagnosed on the basis of clinical examination.

Treatment

In mild cases, the plug may be removed from the conscious lizard using gentle traction and lubrication. For larger plugs or where there is significant impaction, general anaesthesia may be required to facilitate removal. Complete eversion of the hemipenis may be necessary to ensure that all of the plug material is removed.

Prevention and Control

Prevention is limited to ensuring appropriate species specific environmental conditions and nutrition. The caudal vent should be regularly inspected and hemipenal plugs removed before they become a problem.

Ectopic Eggs

Aetiology

Ectopic eggs are seen most frequently in chelonians but can also occur in squamates. Ectopic eggs may be located free in the coelomic cavity in all reptiles or in the urinary bladder of chelonians.

Pathogenesis

Ectopic eggs in the urinary bladder of chelonians can occur subsequent to oxytocin therapy; oxytocin administration is thought to result in the retrograde movement of cloacal eggs through the wide urethral opening into the bladder. Previous salpingotomy, without suturing of the thin-walled oviduct, may be a risk factor for ectopic eggs in subsequent breeding events. Nutritional secondary hyperparathyroidism and failure to provide appropriate nesting sites have also been postulated as potential causes in terrestrial chelonians.

Clinical Signs

The clinical signs associated with ectopic eggs are frequently nonspecific or absent all together.

Diagnosis

Differentiating ectopic eggs that are either free in the coelomic cavity or in the urinary bladder from those in the oviduct using radiography can be challenging. Eggs within the urinary bladder of chelonians may be identified by ultrasonography although if urine is not present in the bladder differentiation from the eggs in the oviduct is challenging.

(a)

(b)

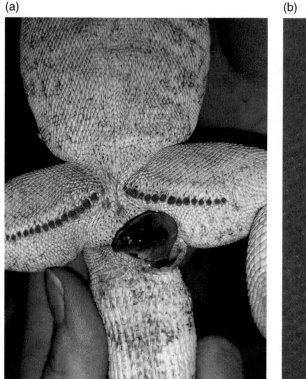 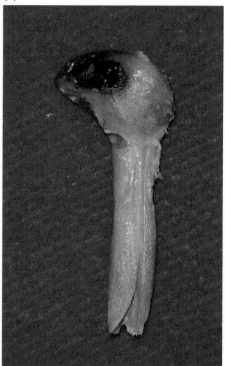

Figure 22.10 (a) Fijian crested iguana (*Brachylophus vitiensis*) with a hemipenal plug. (b) Hemipenal plug following removal.

Cystoscopy using saline infusion, for eggs located in the bladder, and coelioscopy, for eggs free in the coelomic cavity, can be used to obtain a definitive diagnosis.

Treatment

Coeliotomy is indicated for eggs free in the coelomic cavity. Ectopic eggs in the urinary bladder may be removed or cystotomy or via a cystoscopic approach in which the egg is snared or destroyed for removal (Di Girolamo and Selleri 2015). The reader is referred to chapter 28 for detailed accounts of these procedures.

Infertility

Potential causes of infertility in female reptiles include inappropriate environmental cues, malnutrition, underlying systemic disease and salpingitis. Options for evaluating infertile females include reviewing husbandry and nutrition, clinical examination to rule out underlying disease processes, ultrasonographic evaluation of the ovaries to confirm vitellogenesis, ultrasonographic evaluation of the oviduct for evidence of salpingitis, and endoscopic evaluation of the reproductive tract.

Potential causes of infertility in male reptiles include lack of interest in or inability to copulate and lack of spermatogenesis. Options for evaluating infertile males include analysis of serum testosterone or faecal testosterone metabolites, testicular biopsy via a coelioscopic approach and semen collection either postcopulation or via electroejaculation. However, normal values for testosterone concentration are unknown for many species and semen analysis has rarely been performed in reptiles, such that reference values for a given species are unlikely to be known.

References

Chitty, J. and Raftery, A. (2013) Essentials of Tortoise Medicine and Surgery. John Wiley and Sons Ltd, Oxford.

Di Girolamo, N. and Selleri, P. (2015). Clinical applications of cystoscopy in chelonians. *Veterinary Clinics of North America Exotic Animal Practice*, 18, 506–526.

Funk, R.S. (2002) Lizard reproductive medicine and surgery. *Veterinary Clinics of North America Exotic Animal Practice*, 5, 579–613.

Innis, C.J. and Boyer, T.H. (2002) Chelonian reproductive disorders. *Veterinary Clinics of North America Exotic Animal Practice*, 5, 555–578.

Jacobson, E.R. (2003) Biology, Husbandry and Medicine of the Green Iguana. Krieger Publishing, Malabar, FL.

Pimm, R.H. (2013) Characterization of Follicular Stasis in a Colony of Female Veiled Chameleons (*Chamaeleo calyptratus*). MSc Thesis, University of Guelph. https://atrium. lib.uoguelph.ca/xmlui/bitstream/ handle/10214/6678/Pimm_Robyn_201305_ Msc.pdf?sequence=1 (accessed 12 June 2017).

Rivera, S. (2008) Health assessment of the reptilian reproductive tract. *Journal of Exotic Pet Medicine*, 17, 259–266.

Stacy, B.A., Howard, L., Kinkaid, J. *et al.* (2008) Yolk coelomitis in Fiji Island banded iguanas. *Journal of Zoo and Wildlife Medicine*, 39, 161–169.

Stahl, S.J. (2002) Veterinary management of snake reproduction. *Veterinary Clinics of North America Exotic Animal Practice*, 5, 615–636.

Sykes, J.M. (2010) Updates and practical approaches to reproductive disorders in reptiles. *Veterinary Clinics of North America Exotic Animal Practice*, 13, 349–373.

23

Diseases of the Urinary Tract

Peter Holz

This chapter provides a practical approach to the diagnosis, treatment and prevention of urinary system disease in reptiles. It is not intended to be a comprehensive review of the reptilian urinary system, its disorders and treatments.

Anatomy and Physiology

Consult Chapter 2 for more detailed information on the anatomy and physiology of the urinary system, Chapter 11 for diagnostic testing and Chapter 13 for clinical techniques.

Key Points

- The fundamental structure and function of the reptilian urinary system is similar to mammals with several key variations:
- There is no loop of Henle. Reptiles cannot therefore produce hypertonic urine.
- Terrestrial reptiles excrete uric acid instead of urea.
- Reptiles have a renal portal system, which allows reptiles to shunt venous blood from the caudal part of the body through the kidneys during periods of water deprivation to prevent renal tubular ischaemia.
- A urinary bladder is present in chelonians, tuataras and some lizards (some skinks, geckos, iguanas and chameleons) but is lacking in snakes and crocodilians.
- Ureters connect directly with the cloaca, not the urinary bladder (where present).
- In most lizard species, the kidneys are located within the pelvis.
- Many of the standard blood and urine tests used to diagnose renal disease in mammals do not apply in reptiles.

Renal Disease

Diagnosis

Renal disease in reptiles is underdiagnosed, frequently presenting in conjunction with systemic illness. It can be difficult to recognize as signs are vague, nonspecific and many of the diagnostic tests used to detect renal disease in mammals do not apply.

As with all reptile disorders, it is important to obtain as thorough a history as possible. This should focus not just on the animal but also on the environment and husbandry. Has the patient been eating? What is its diet? Are protein type and levels appropriate for that species? Does it have access to fresh water in a form it will recognize? Chameleons, for example, only drink dripping water and will

Reptile Medicine and Surgery in Clinical Practice, First Edition. Edited by Bob Doneley, Deborah Monks, Robert Johnson and Brendan Carmel.
© 2018 John Wiley & Sons Ltd. Published 2018 by John Wiley & Sons Ltd.

dehydrate if water is put out in a dish. Is the humidity level appropriate for the species? Is the environment warm enough? Is there sufficient ultraviolet light and how often are the light globes replaced? Is there a history of exposure to poisonous plants or other possible toxins, including antibiotics? Obtaining a thorough background is vital to direct the clinician to a possibility of renal disease. For more information refer to Chapters 4, 5 and 6.

Often, particularly in acute renal disease, clinical signs are minimal. There may be non-specific signs such as anorexia, depression and weakness. If more chronic renal disease is present, signs may include chronic weight loss or emaciation, dehydration and general ill thrift. Polyuria and polydipsia are rare.

Published normal blood values for reptiles are often based on a small number of individuals and vary widely (Table 23.1). Consequently, it is best to establish normal values for the particular animal in question when it presents for its initial wellness examination. Blood should be drawn and, assuming that the animal is healthy at the time of examination, these results should be used as a comparison against future disease states. This will provide a more accurate representation of what is happening inside the patient than relying on published data collected on animals held in differing conditions. While diagnosis of renal disease via blood work is problematic, a few abnormalities may appear which can lead the clinician in that direction.

Early stages of renal disease may present with no haematological changes. The haematocrit may be increased because of dehydration. Nonregenerative anaemia has been reported, as have a mild leucocytosis with monocytosis or heterophilia.

Biochemistry is of limited use. Blood urea nitrogen and creatinine are poor indicators of renal function as terrestrial reptiles excrete uric acid, while sea turtles and crocodilians predominantly excrete ammonia. Only freshwater chelonians excrete significant amounts of urea and blood urea nitrogen may be of more use in these species. However, elevated levels usually indicate dehydration or increased protein catabolism rather than renal disease.

Uric acid is secreted by the renal tubules and is unaffected by glomerular filtration rate. Three times as much uric acid is excreted in a hydrated reptile compared with a dehydrated one. Once secreted into the tubule, uric acid complexes with protein and either sodium or potassium to form a suspension. A herbivorous diet leads to a greater amount of potassium complexing with urate, while a carnivorous diet favours sodium urate complexes.

Reptiles should be fasted prior to blood sampling as uric acid increases by 1.5–2 times the day after a meal, particularly in carnivores. Uric acid levels may be normal early in renal disease but increase with end stage renal disease. Hyperuricaemia or uraemia is generally a terminal event as it indicates that two-thirds or more of the functional renal mass has been lost. A single elevated value is not diagnostic but chronic elevations in herbivorous reptiles warrant further evaluation. Uric acid levels should be under 600 µmol/l for herbivorous reptiles. Hyperuricaemia greater than 900 µmol/l is usually associated with renal disease, with urate deposition occurring in tissues above 1500 µmol/l. More than twofold increases in uric acid generally signify renal disease or gout.

Total calcium levels may be low, normal or high. Phosphorus is frequently elevated, especially with advanced renal disease, and animals may have an inverted calcium to phosphorus ratio. The solubility index is calculated as the product of calcium (mmol/l) and phosphate (mmol/l) and is normally less than nine. If the solubility index rises above 12 then healthy tissue will start to mineralize, while if it is between 9 and 12, mineralization of diseased tissue (kidneys) occurs. Potassium may be elevated. Haemolysis will artificially increase both phosphorus and potassium. Aspartate aminotransferase is present in the proximal tubule cells and levels may be elevated if these are damaged. However, it is usually excreted into the urine rather than the blood. Total protein and albumin may be low.

Table 23.1 Blood parameters[a] in the red-eared slider (*Trachemys scripta elegans*), boa constrictor (*Boa constrictor constrictor*) and bearded dragon (*Pogona vitticeps*) used in the assessment of renal disease (Carpenter 2013).

Blood parameter	Diagnostic use
Total white blood cells	May be increased as a result of inflammation or infection
Heterophils	Usually increased with bacterial infection
Lymphocytes	May be increased with viral disease
Azurophils	Elevated during bacterial infections and necrosis
Monocytes	May be increased with chronic infections
Packed cell volume	May be increased with dehydration or decreased with anaemia
Red blood cells	Decreased with anaemia
Haemoglobin	Decreased with anaemia
Urea	Poor indicator of renal function; may be increased with dehydration and protein catabolism
Creatinine	Limited and variable production; not reliable
Uric acid	Raised during dehydration and with renal disease; affected by nutrition
Calcium	May be low, normal or high; affected by nutrition and albumin levels, decreased during chronic renal disease
Phosphorus	Increased during renal disease
Potassium	Often increased, especially in acute renal failure

[a] Please note that normal values vary with species, sex, nutrition, environment, season and reproductive status.

Unfortunately, urinalysis is not very helpful in diagnosing renal disease. Polyuria is rare and difficult to recognize, as the urine is often mixed with faeces. Urine specific gravity is of limited usefulness, as reptiles cannot produce a hypertonic urine as they lack loops of Henle. A low urine specific gravity reflects normal hydration. Herbivore urine should be alkaline, while carnivore and omnivore urine is acidic. Herbivorous tortoises will produce acidic urine during times of drought, at the end of hibernation, if they are anorexic or fed a high protein diet. After recovery the urine becomes alkaline again. Ureteral urine normally contains a large amount of protein. When it enters the urodeum the urine moves into the rectum by reverse peristalsis, where the protein is reabsorbed and recycled. Thus, voided urine should contain little to no protein. Glucose should also be absent. Bladder urine does not reflect renal function because water, sodium and bicarbonate are absorbed across the bladder wall while hydrogen is excreted. Unlike mammals, it is also nonsterile as it has passed through the urodeum. Urine should be clear or yellow. Green urine is indicative of starvation or hepatic disease because of the presence of biliverdin.

Radiography is an insensitive tool for the diagnosis of renal disease but may show soft tissue mineralization. Ultrasound can be used but it is difficult to visualize the kidneys, as they lie deep in the pelvis in turtles and most lizards, with the exception of monitors. Endoscopy is probably the most useful tool to diagnose renal disease, as it can be used to take a renal biopsy, which can be examined histologically and submitted for culture. However, if lesions are not uniformly distributed throughout the kidneys it is possible to miss them with a biopsy.

Aetiology

The causes of renal disease are many and varied. Some are specific to the urinary system while others cause a multisystem disease with renal manifestations.

Infection

As reptile kidneys have a relatively high blood flow and can receive additional blood from the caudal part of the body via the renal portal system, bacteria frequently localize to the kidneys and can often be cultured from the kidney. There are no specific bacterial

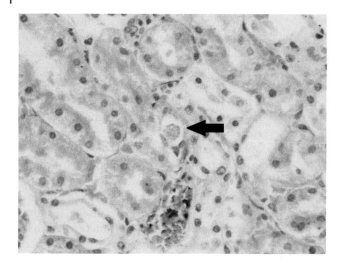

Figure 23.1 *Klossiella* sp. (arrow) in renal tubule; haematoxylin and eosin stain.

aetiologies of renal disease. Common Gram-negative bacteria that may be found in the kidneys as part of a systemic disease process include *Salmonella* and *Pseudomonas*. Similarly, systemic mycotic infections can produce renal granulomas. Evidence of viral infections, such as inclusion body disease, can be detected by the presence of inclusion bodies in the kidney.

Microsporidia were considered to be protozoa but have been reclassified as fungi. They have been found in snakes, turtles, and lizards, including bearded dragons where they can be associated with systemic disease. Signs include lethargy, anorexia and weight loss. Infections are probably opportunistic secondary to immunosuppression. No treatment has been described and diagnosis will likely be at post mortem.

Spironucleus (synonymous with *Hexamita*) appears similar to *Giardia*. Trophozoites are pyriform, with two anterior nuclei, four pairs of flagella and no adhesive disc. It is found in the urinary tract of chelonians and snakes and has a direct lifecycle. Signs include lethargy, anorexia and weight loss. Diagnosis is by finding the organism in fresh urine or faeces. Treatment is with 50 mg/kg metronidazole, repeated in two weeks. Prevention is via regular cleaning and disinfection of the environment to stop direct transmission. Cysts are destroyed by exposure to 70% ethanol or boiling water for one minute but are reasonably resistant to bleach, requiring contact for at least 24 hours before they are devitalized.

Klossiella is found in the kidney of boa constrictors. It has a direct life cycle. Infections are generally asymptomatic. Diagnosis is by histological demonstration of sporocysts in the kidney or in fresh urine/urates (Figure 23.1). Prevention is via cleaning and disinfection. Other protozoa such as *Entamoeba invadens* and *Eimeria* spp. can be found in the kidneys as part of a systemic disease.

Myxozoa have been found in the renal tubules of freshwater turtles, potentially associated with nephritis. Trematodes can occur in the renal tubules and ureters of snakes and crocodiles and the urinary bladder of sea turtles. Infections are generally asymptomatic. Diagnosis is by finding the characteristic yellow, 40 × 18 μm eggs in the urine or faeces. The lifecycle is unknown but probably involves an intermediate host. Infections in captivity should therefore be self-limiting.

Non-Infectious Aetiologies

As well as infectious causes of renal disease there are numerous non-infectious aetiologies. These include congenital or hereditary conditions, such as renal cysts and aplasia. Degenerative conditions, such as glomerulosclerosis, have been described in snakes and

Figure 23.2 Inland bearded dragon (*Pogona vitticeps*) with articular gout. Note swollen forelimb.

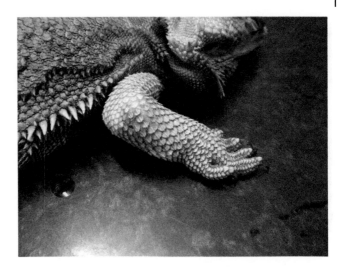

alligators. Glomerulosclerosis consists of fibrous tissue accumulations in the glomeruli. Amyloid-like material has been found in the glomeruli of a range of reptile species. While similar in appearance to amyloid microscopically the composition of this material has not be determined.

Various renal neoplasms have been described including adenocarcinomas in snakes, lizards and chelonians, myxofibromas in chelonians, renal adenomas in snakes and lizards and transitional cell carcinomas in snakes. Unfortunately, diagnoses are often made post mortem.

Inappropriate diet can result in renal disease. Hypervitaminosis D3 through over-supplementation or accidental ingestion of cholecalciferol rodenticides can cause nephrocalcinosis. Signs include depression, weakness and anorexia. Prognosis is poor. Treatment includes fluids and corticosteroids (prednisolone 5–10 mg/kg intramuscularly), which suppress bone resorption and intestinal calcium absorption and promote calciuresis.

One of the more common manifestations of renal disease is visceral gout, which occurs in uricotelic (fully terrestrial) reptiles only. It does not occur in aquatic or amphibious reptiles that excrete predominantly urea or ammonia. In terrestrial reptiles purine is metabolized to uric acid while, in aquatic reptiles, it is broken down to allantoin.

Predisposing factors for gout include low water intake, excessive dietary purine ingestion and nephrotoxic drugs. Renal disease, especially tubular disease (as uric acid is excreted by the tubules) can lead to decreased uric acid excretion and hyperuricaemia. High blood uric acid leads to precipitation in joints (articular gout; Figure 23.2), on serosal surfaces (e.g. pericardial sac) and in various tissues (visceral gout; Figure 23.3; see Case Report 1), particularly kidney, liver and lung. Urate crystals destroy kidney tubules (urate nephrosis) leading to renal failure (Figure 23.4). The characteristic lesions are white nodules called tophi, which consist of refractile, radiating, faintly basophilic urate crystals with fine spicules, in a tubule lumen, surrounded by heterophils and necrotic tubular epithelial cells during the acute phase, and by giant cells later. Urates dissolve during routine processing for histology but the tophi remain visible and are more obvious with silver stains.

Prognosis is guarded but hyperuricaemia can be treated with allopurinol, which decreases uric acid production by halting purine breakdown. 20–25 mg/kg/day or 50 mg/kg every three days has proven effective. Treatment is long term, over several months. Prevention focuses on not providing animal protein to herbivores, as it is high in purines. Minimize the feeding of peas,

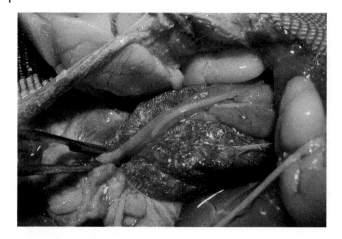

Figure 23.3 Visceral gout. Note pale streaks through kidneys, representing urates.

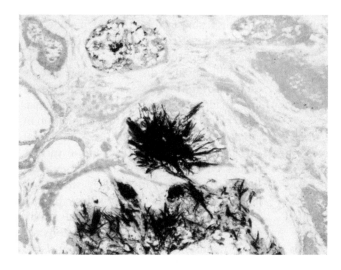

Figure 23.4 Urate tophi in renal tubules. Silver stain has stained urate crystals black.

spinach and cauliflower, as they are also high in purines.

Renal toxins include antibiotics and anti-fungals. High doses of aminoglycosides such as gentamicin and amikacin can cause renal tubule damage, particularly in dehydrated animals. Amphotericin B causes renal vaso-constriction, reduced glomerular filtration rate and renal tubule damage leading to acute tubular necrosis. Clinical signs are vague and include anorexia, lethargy and weight loss. Treatment involves discontinuation of the drug and fluid therapy.

Ingestion of oak leaves has been associated with renal tubular necrosis and death in tortoises. This is caused by tannic acid con-tained within the leaves.

Renal disease, once established, leads to a gradual deterioration of the patient that can result in hyperphosphataemia and renal sec-ondary hyperparathyroidism due to decreased phosphorus filtration. Increased phosphorus results in hypertrophy and hyperplasia of the parathyroid gland, which secretes parathyroid hormone to mobilize calcium from the osse-ous matrix, leading to an osteomalacia called renal osteodystrophy. The bones and shell become demineralized and soft with bones potentially increasing in girth due to the depo-sition of excessive fibrous tissue.

Prognosis and Treatment

Long-term prognosis for reptiles with renal disease is poor. As reptiles cannot produce a hypertonic urine, they conserve water by decreasing the number of filtering glomeruli, resulting in tubule collapse. However, uric acid continues to be secreted into the proximal tubules leading to tubule blockage. Restoring hydration is therefore vital to flush out the accumulated uric acid. Use an isotonic fluid, such as lactated Ringer's solution, delivered at 20–40 ml/kg/day intravenously or intraosseously. If this is not possible, administer a bolus of 5–10 ml/kg intravenously or intracoelomically twice a day.

Aluminium hydroxide given orally at 100 mg/kg once a day can be administered to treat hyperphosphataemia. B vitamins (10 mg/kg intramuscularly) and anabolic steroids (nandrolone 1 mg/kg intramuscularly), given every one to four weeks, may also be beneficial.

Aim to correct any husbandry issues. In cases of prolonged anorexia, lizards can be stomach tubed while chelonians will require oesophageal tube feeding.

Lower Urinary Tract Disease

Uroliths

Snakes and crocodilians lack urinary bladders. Chelonians, rhynchocephalians (tuataras) and some lizards (skinks, geckos, iguanas, and chameleons) have bladders. Uroliths have been found in lizards, turtles and snakes (in the distal ureter). Causes of urolithiasis include vitamin A or vitamin D deficiency, excess dietary protein or oxalates (e.g. spinach), bacterial infection, and dehydration. Animals are often asymptomatic but clinical signs can include straining, constipation, anorexia, paresis/paralysis and cloacal prolapse. If the animal is not experiencing signs then treatment may not be required but the urolith will probably continue to increase in size, potentially leading to haematuria, bladder wall irritation and thickening, and pressure necrosis.

Uroliths may be visible or palpable in the cloaca. They can also be diagnosed via radiography, ultrasonography or endoscopy. Urate stones are radiolucent but become radiodense when complexed with calcium or potassium. Blood uric acid levels are not elevated.

If the urolith is in the cloaca, it can usually be removed manually. The urolith will appear rough, white and crumbly. If a piece of it is placed on a slide with a drop of water, urate crystals should be visible. If the urolith is in the bladder, it may be possible to remove it endoscopically via the cloaca, otherwise a cystotomy will be required. Urolith prevention focuses on the provision of adequate hydration and excellent husbandry.

Case Report 1

A carpet python was referred with a history of inappetence. Clinical examination revealed an obviously swollen mouth. The gingiva appeared thickened, with petechial haemorrhages evident on the surface. A small amount of caseous material was present around some teeth. The referring veterinarian had diagnosed a case of necrotic stomatitis and treated the snake with high doses of gentamicin for two weeks.

The snake was extremely lethargic with poor muscle tone. It had not eaten for four months. A blood sample revealed extremely high uric acid levels. Given the history and blood result, renal disease was strongly suspected. The owner declined a renal biopsy and, given the snake's poor condition and prognosis, it was euthanized.

Necropsy revealed swollen and pale kidneys with white streaks, indicative of visceral gout. While gentamicin can be an excellent antibiotic for treating bacterial infections in reptiles, high and/or prolonged doses without the provision of fluid support, especially in an animal that is not eating, can frequently result in renal disease.

Case Report 2

A panther chameleon was presented with a one-week history of hind limb lameness. On examination, the chameleon could move both hind limbs but the movements were weak and poorly coordinated. There were no visible wounds or palpable fractures. Based on the clinical signs, a spinal lesion was suspected. Dorsoventral and lateral radiographs were taken. No spinal damage was visible but a large mass was apparent in the caudal abdomen. The chameleon was anaesthetized and a small incision was made in the paralumbar region, to allow endoscopic access. A large irregularly shaped mass was visible. Two biopsies of the mass were taken and submitted for histological evaluation. The diagnosis was renal adenocarcinoma, necessitating euthanasia of the lizard. This case highlights the fact that renal disease will not always present with symptoms relating to the urinary system.

Further Reading

Carpenter, J.W. (2013) *Exotic Animal Formulary*, 4th ed. Elsevier, St. Louis, MO.

Girling, S. and Raiti, P. (2004) *BSAVA Manual of Reptiles*, 2nd ed. British Small Animal Veterinary Association, Gloucester.

Mader, D.R. (2006) *Reptile Medicine and Surgery*, 2nd ed. Elsevier, Philadelphia, PA.

Mader, D.R. and Divers, S.J. (2014) *Current Therapy in Reptile Medicine and Surgery*. Elsevier, St. Louis, MO.

McCracken, H.E. (1994) Husbandry and diseases of captive reptiles. *Proceedings of the Post-Graduate Committee in Veterinary Science, University of Sydney*, 233, 461–545.

24

Diseases of the Nervous System
Hamish Baron and David N. Phalen

Anatomy and Physiology

See Chapter 2 for a review of the anatomy and physiology of the nervous system.

Key Points

- The reptilian nervous system is organised in a linear fashion. The central nervous system consists of the brain and the spinal cord, which extends virtually the entire length of the vertebral canal. The peripheral nervous system includes the cranial nerves and the spinal nerves.

- There are both subdural (beneath the dura mater) and epidural (above the dura mater) spaces within the brain case.
- There is no arachnoid mater or subarachnoid space in reptiles. There are two meninges which cover the brain and spinal cord; the outer dura mater is tough and largely avascular while the inner pia mater is more delicate and vascular and lies directly on the surface of the brain.
- Nerve function can be modified by temperature (heat and cold), medication, trauma, viral, bacterial, fungal, parasitic and metabolic disorders.

History and Husbandry

Malnutrition and improper management are leading causes of neurological disease. A detailed history of the feeding and care practices for the patient and collection will often reveal inadequacies. For more information on history and husbandry refer to Chapter 4. Infectious diseases are common causes of neurological signs and are more likely to occur in recently obtained animals or collections where animals have recently been introduced. A history of disease in other reptiles in the collection may also provide clues to the aetiology of the current reptile's condition.

The Neurological Examination

Distant Examination

The first step of the assessment of a reptile with neurological signs is the distant examination, observing natural and instinctive behaviours and movement. Snakes, lizards

Reptile Medicine and Surgery in Clinical Practice, First Edition. Edited by Bob Doneley, Deborah Monks, Robert Johnson and Brendan Carmel.
© 2018 John Wiley & Sons Ltd. Published 2018 by John Wiley & Sons Ltd.

and skinks should take an interest in their surroundings while turtles may be actively swimming or completely withdrawn into their shell. For additional information refer to Chapter 10.

Signs of central neurological disease in snakes include reduced frequency of tongue flicking, slow protrusion and withdrawal of the tongue and incomplete withdrawal of the tongue. Affected snakes often hold their head up at an angle with the mouth open. This behaviour can also occur in snakes having difficulty breathing. Abnormal movements or the absence of movement in any section of the snake is often the result of neurological disease. Generalized weakness, inability to support the weight of the body and muscle fasciculations are manifestations of neurological disease in lizards. Inability to use one or more legs may represent peripheral or spinal cord disease in lizards and turtles. Lizards and turtles with advanced neurological disease may present with severe weakness and may be obtunded. Secondary nutritional hyperparathyroidism can cause scoliosis and/or ventral or dorsal curvatures of the spine. Spinal fractures sometimes cause deviation of the vertebral column. Fractures across the midline of the carapace in a turtle, with the exception of its most caudal aspects, will generally result in hind limb paresis or paralysis.

Close Examination

The neurological examination is best done with the animal within its preferred optimum temperature zone. During the winter months, reptiles are likely to be cold on presentation. This can be assessed by touch or, more accurately, using a remote heat-sensing thermometer.

Cranial Nerves

The cranial nerve structure and function of reptiles is much the same as in small mammals, although it is more difficult to assess in reptiles. Table 24.1 outlines the cranial nerves that are able to be examined in reptile patients.

Assessment of Muscle Innervation

Snakes

Spinal reflexes are part of the reptilian nervous system control. Somatic spinal reflexes sense and control muscles, tendons and skin to maintain posture. Visceral spinal reflexes control cardiac muscle, smooth muscles of the digestive tract and blood vessels and glands. Generalized atrophy of the epaxial muscles suggests a disease of many months or more. A well-muscled snake is more likely to have an acute or subacute problem, although loss of condition may take many weeks. Segmental loss of epaxial muscles may also occur and may indicate a spinal cord lesion at the junction of the normal and abnormal musculature. Proliferative lesions of the vertebrae may compress spinal nerves, resulting in segmental muscle atrophy (Figure 24.1).

Healthy snakes are uniformly strong and responsive to handling or noxious stimuli. Weakness may be determined by holding the snake's tail off the table and observing how it uses the rest of the body. The righting reflex assesses both brain and spinal cord function. A normal snake will immediately right itself beginning head first if turned over (Figure 24.2). In snakes with spinal cord lesions, the portion of the body caudal to the lesion will be unable to right itself. Snakes with viral induced neurological dysfunction may be unable to right themselves or righting may be delayed (Figure 24.3).

Snakes have sensitive skin over the dorsum. The cutaneous nerves supply tissue caudal to their nerve root and so if the skin becomes nonresponsive to a pin prick, the spinal lesion is likely to be cranial to the point at which denervation is evident. Cloacal tone may be absent in some cases of spinal cord disease.

Lizards

Lizards normally have a strong withdrawal response and placing reflex. In some lizards, especially those with long legs, hopping reflexes and even the ability to wheelbarrow can be assessed. As with snakes, response to

Table 24.1 Nerves suitable for assessing cranial nerve function.

No.	Name	Innervation	Function	Assessment
I	Olfactory	Chemosensory	Olfaction	Place a cotton tip applicator soaked in alcohol beneath the nostrils; a healthy patient will show an aversive response.
II	Optic	Sensory	Vision	Reptiles with eyelids will display a menace response. Snakes and small lizards without eyelids can be placed in a novel environment and their ability to navigate can be assessed. Pupillary light response is not relevant in reptiles as iris diameter is voluntarily controlled by skeletal muscle.
V	Trigeminal	Sensory and motor	Motor function to the mandible; sensory around the eye	Reptiles with normal trigeminal nerve function will clamp their jaw tightly if an attempt to open their mouth is made. Stimulating the skin surrounding the eye using a blunted needle will cause animals with eyelids to close them and may cause other reptiles to exhibit an aversive behaviour.
VII	Facial	Motor	Motor function to structures of the face	In reptiles with eyelids, the facial nerve can be assessed using the palpebral reflex as with cranial nerve II. Otherwise, this nerve cannot be assessed.
VIII	Vestibulocochlear	Sensory	Audition	Most reptiles respond poorly to sound in the hearing range of humans and are more sensitive to low-frequency sound and vibrations. This makes assessment of the vestibulocochlear nerve very difficult. Diseases of the inner ear, however, can result in signs common in other animals such as head tilt and circling.
IX	Glossopharyngeal	Sensory and motor	Taste and motor function to the tongue, jaw and swallowing	The application of a bitter substance, such as lemon juice, to the tongue and the subsequent behavioural response indicates the ability of the reptile to taste. Observation of normal swallowing or eating indicates that cranial nerves IX, X and XI (the spinal accessory nerve) are intact.
X	Vagus	Motor	Parasympathetic innervation	Assessed as per glossopharyngeal nerve.
XII	Hypoglossal	Motor	Movement of the tongue, jaw and swallowing	The normal position of the tongue and the ability to withdraw the tongue into the mouth allows assessment of the hypoglossal nerve.

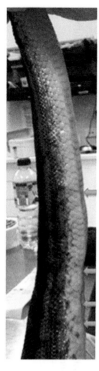

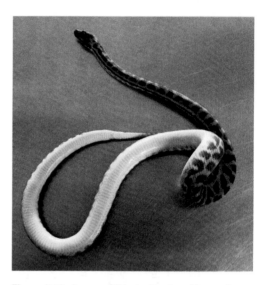

Figure 24.2 A normal Spotted python (*Antaresia maculosa*) performing righting reflex during a neurological examination. Note the normal head position, with the remainder of the body returning to ventral recumbency.

Figure 24.1 Segmental aplasia in a 14-year-old coastal carpet python (*Morelia spilota*) secondary to a proliferative spinal osteopathy. Note the muscle atrophy which is the result of nerve impingement and subsequent denervation (arrows).

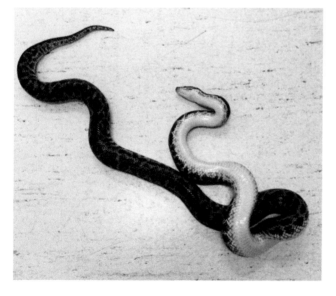

Figure 24.3 Spotted python (*Antaresia maculosa*) with central nervous system dysfunction. This snake was polymerase chain reaction-positive for sunshinevirus.

skin pricking can be assessed in those with loose skin (e.g. dragons) and in all lizards there should be cloacal tone. Lizards should rapidly right themselves if turned over. Denervation is one differential for localized muscle atrophy.

Chelonians

Healthy chelonians are strong and active or tightly withdrawn into their shell. The cloaca should have tone and will contract when pinched which may also cause the pelvic limbs to be brought together caudally. Chelonians placed on their back will right themselves using their head and neck. Stranded sea turtles with advanced disease exhibit nonspecific central nervous system depression. Localized brain disease may cause a head tilt, circling or infrequently nystagmus.

Crocodiles

While crocodiles are subject to a number of infectious diseases and disease syndromes that can involve the central nervous system, specific signs relating to central nervous system lesions are infrequently seen.

Diagnosis

The diagnostic work-up for neurological disease is much the same as for any unwell reptile (Table 24.2). Based on the history and clinical findings ancillary testing may be necessary to determine the location or locations of the neurological lesion and it(s) aetiology.

Congenital and Hereditary Disorders

Congenital abnormalities seen in other animal species may be encountered in reptiles, including polycephaly (having more than one head) in snakes and microphthalmia. The majority of congenital abnormalities are the result of poor maternal husbandry and improper incubation conditions. Many of these congenital conditions result in early embryonic or fetal death.

Non-Infectious Disorders

Nutritional Secondary Hyperparathyroidism

Aetiology and Pathogenesis

See Chapter 15 for the aetiology and pathogenesis of nutritional secondary hyperparathyroidism (NSHP).

Clinical Signs

Bone deformation and scoliosis (Figure 24.4) are common clinical presentations and are often presented concurrently with pathological fractures of long bones (Figure 24.5). NSHP occurs in lizards, especially bearded dragons and blue-tongued lizards. The lesions commonly involve the spine and may lead to cord compression and paresis or paralysis of the pelvic limbs. Cases may present with lameness of one or all limbs and may have an abnormal gait. When blood calcium levels cannot be maintained, animals will exhibit muscle fasciculation.

Diagnosis

Diagnosis is based on a thorough history, identifying incorrect husbandry and dietary practices, signs and radiographical and biochemical abnormalities.

Treatment

Initial therapy centres on stabilization of the patient, including correction of hypocalcaemia resulting in tetany and stabilization of pathological fractures. Parenteral administration of calcium is only indicated if presented with a reptile in acute hypocalcaemic crisis with muscle tremors and twitching. See Chapter 15 for further treatment options.

Prognosis

Once paralysis or paresis is present, the disease process is advanced and the prognosis for return to function is poor. The patient may

Table 24.2 Diagnostic work-up for neurological disease.

Diagnostic modality	Samples	Clinical application
Complete blood count	Blood heparin or fresh blood smear	Total white cell count and differential allows assessment of infectious or inflammatory changes in the white cell population. Refer to Chapter 11 for full haematological interpretation.
Plasma biochemistry (including electrolytes)	Blood in lithium heparin or serum clot tube (confirm with laboratory)	Assessment of organ systems and electrolyte imbalance. Refer to Chapter 11 for full biochemical interpretation.
Bacterial culture	Blood or CSF in EDTA	Organism isolation and identification as well as treatment susceptibility spectrum.
Fungal culture	Blood or CSF in EDTA	Organism isolation and identification as well as treatment susceptibility spectrum.
Viral PCR	Consult with laboratory regarding best samples for specific PCR	Sensitive and specific isolation of pathogen with the opportunity to sequence isolates.
CSF analysis	Direct smear CSF, centrifuged CSF and smear of sediment	CSF collection is challenging in reptiles. Reports exist of collection in a green iguana with osteomyelitis and American alligators (*Alligator mississippiensis*) but collection from Australian reptiles has not been reported.
Radiography	Full body radiographs	Allows visualization of the vertebral column, axial skeleton and spondylytic changes as well as fractures of the spinal column.
CT	Full body CT or skull CT	More useful at locating anatomical abnormalities, especially when assessing the skull.
Magnetic resonance imaging	Full body	Examination of microscopic structural changes associated with inflammation or vascular injury. Superior when imaging soft tissue such as the brain.
Ultrasonography	Coelomic cavity	Of limited use in determination of neurological disease in reptiles.
Diagnostic necropsy	Full body	Gross and histopathological examination of the brain, spinal cord. Facilitates tissue sampling for PCR, bacterial or fungal culture.

CSF, cerebrospinal fluid; CT, computed tomography; EDTA, ethylenediaminetetraacetic acid; PCR, polymerase chain reaction;

continue to live in a modified environment with a good quality of life. In cases where spinal fractures result in the inability to produce droppings, owners should be counselled regarding their pets quality of life and should consider euthanasia on humane grounds.

Prevention and Control

See Chapters 4 and 6 for detailed information on prevention and control.

Hypocalcaemia

Aetiology

Neurological signs due to low blood calcium are the result of an acute increased demand on calcium metabolism, such as during times of vitellogenesis or bone repair. In such cases, blood calcium levels become low prior to parathyroid hormone release and the subsequent mobilization of calcium from bone.

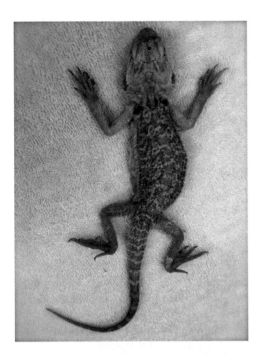

Figure 24.4 Bearded dragon (*Pogona barbata*) showing characteristic weakness, lethargy and scoliosis as a result of secondary nutritional hyperparathyroidism.

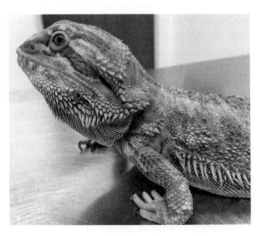

Figure 24.5 Bearded dragon (*Pogona barbata*) displaying clinical signs consistent with nutritional secondary hyperparathyroidism. Note the healed pathological fracture of the left forelimb and the undershot jaw.

Clinical Signs

Muscle tremors and fasciculation are the most common presenting complaint. The disease is progressive and, if left untreated, a single limb fasciculation may progress to become generalized tetanic spasms and result in the patient's death from heart failure.

Diagnosis

Diagnosis is based on history, examination, radiographs and biochemistry, which may show a mild hypocalcaemia or low normal calcium and an increased phosphorus level. See Chapter 15 for more detailed information.

Treatment

Treatment includes identifying and correcting the underlying cause and the administration of calcium intramuscularly or orally based on blood biochemical results. Administration of parenteral calcium without a biochemical panel may lead to hypercalcaemia.

Trauma

Carapace Fractures in Turtles

Trauma to the carapace may lead to spinal injury, as the spinal cord is contained within the carapace. The reptilian spinal cord contains locomotor control centres and the spinal cord has the capacity to regenerate to some degree. This gives reptiles with spinal cord or brain injuries a better prognosis than those same injuries in mammals. Fracture repair techniques for chelonians are discussed extensively in Chapter 29.

Spinal and Head Trauma

Head trauma may present as opisthotonus, seizures, paresis, profound depression or paralysis. Many blue-tongued lizards that present with head trauma will have their eyes closed and will be reluctant to open them. These animals will often have other signs of

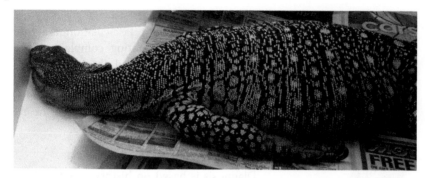

Figure 24.6 A lace monitor lizard (*Varanus varius*) mentally obtunded following a motor vehicle accident. With supportive care, this patient made progress but constantly circled to the left and was euthanized.

brain trauma, including lethargy and reduced response to stimuli (Figure 24.6). Although they appear to have a poor prognosis, with supportive care many will return to normal function.

Diagnosis and Treatment of Trauma-Induced Neuropathies

Diagnosis of neurological disease is based on history, signs and radiography. The treatment of these trauma-induced neuropathies involves stabilization of fractures, supportive care, analgesia, fluid therapy and antibiotics. Surgical intervention may be necessary for spinal cord injuries. Spinal fractures may be immobilised using external fixation such as casting.

Egg Binding

Egg binding may cause hind-limb paresis or paralysis in chelonians and in some lizard species. The hind-limb paresis is secondary to pressure from the internal organs or eggs engaged in the pelvic canal eliciting pressure on the sciatic nerves.

Neoplasia

In Australia, the majority of neoplastic diseases impacting the spinal cord are associated with the vertebral column of snakes. Both osteochondrosarcoma and osteosarcoma have been reported in snakes, often causing a flaccid paresis caudal to the lesion. There are few reports of primary central nervous system neoplasia in reptiles but these should be included as differentials in cases of neurological disease. Other reports of neoplasia causing neurological signs in reptiles are rare and there are very few cases of successful treatment of neurological neoplasia.

Toxicities

Drugs

The most common toxicities appear to be species specific such as ivermectin in chelonians, leading to general neuromuscular weakness, or metronidazole in various species of snake, resulting in vestibular disease with head tilt, circling and ataxia. Itraconazole, when used to treat fungal dermatitis in reptiles, is reported to cause hepatotoxicity, with neurological signs including lethargy and depression. Intoxication from a drug should be considered in any reptile exhibiting incoordination, circling, head tilt, opisthotonos or seizures.

Insecticides

Organophosphates are the most commonly reported toxicity in reptiles, although their use is declining. Overdose results in paresis, head tilt, circling, opisthotonos and convulsions. A history of treatment for mite infestation should cause the practitioner to consider insecticide toxicity as a differential. Treatment is aimed at removing the toxic substance and then providing supportive care, including fluid therapy and anticonvulsants if required.

Metal Toxicosis

Lead toxicity from ingestion of lead based paints is reported in chelonians. Animals exhibit ataxia, a head tilt and weakness. Treatment includes removing the lead from the gastrointestinal tract using gastric lavage and cathartics, alongside chelation therapy using calcium disodium edetate. Zinc toxicoses can result in weakness, anorexia and anaemia. Animals prone to ingesting foreign material while free ranging are susceptible.

Infectious Disorders

Bacterial Infections

Aetiology

Bacterial infection of the nervous system may be primary or secondary following septicaemia. Septicaemia may result in central nervous system infection or cause secondary skeletal abnormalities such as spinal osteopathy.

Pathogenesis

Commonly isolated organisms include *Salmonella*, *Staphylococcus*, *Mycoplasma* and *Mycobacterium*. Infection in the central nervous system is commonly the result of septicaemia following respiratory disease or other severe infection. Micro abscesses may form in the brain and the subsequent inflammatory response results in nonspecific clinical signs that vary in severity from altered mentation to terminal convulsions. Signs are dependent on the region of the brain where the bacteria localize.

Septicaemia, as well as penetrating wounds such as animal bites, may result in bacterial infection of the vertebrae and a subsequent osteomyelitis. The proliferative nature of the entheses or periosteal new bone results in compression of the spinal cord.

Localized bacterial infections in the ear of chelonians and lizards are relatively common.

Clinical Signs

Signs vary depending on the location of the underlying disease process. For example, an ear abscess results in head tilt, circling and swelling associated with the tympanic membrane, whereas spinal osteopathy secondary to bacteraemia causes damage to the spinal cord and leads to either acute onset or insidious and progressive flaccid paralysis, or paresis caudal to the lesion. Micro abscessation in the brain results in signs that are dependent on location of the lesion.

Fungal Infections

Fungal disease causing neurological clinical signs is uncommon in reptiles. Diagnosis of a fungal central nervous system infection would be challenging, possibly requiring cerebrospinal fluid analysis or advanced imaging. Treatment is likely to consist of systemic antifungals able to cross the blood–brain barrier and based on culture and sensitivity. Voriconazole appears safe and efficacious against a number of fungal infections.

Viral Diseases of Snakes

Sunshinevirus and two or more bornaviruses cause neurological disease in snakes in Australia. The ferlavirus and one or more arenaviruses can also cause neurological signs in snakes. Neurological signs caused by all of these virus infections are similar and reflect significant disease of the brain and, in many instances, spinal cord. They include a progressive paresis and paralysis that may be segmental or generalized, inability to right themselves, opisthotonos, head tremors and decreased or slow tongue flicking (Figure 24.7). Polymerase chain

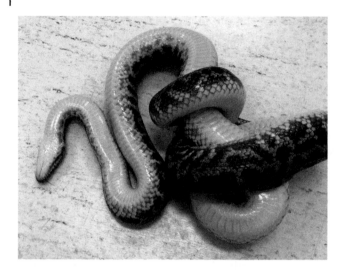

Figure 24.7 Spotted python (*Antaresia maculosa*) displaying classic signs associated with neurological viruses. Note the tight knots and inability to right itself.

reaction (PCR) diagnostics are available for all four of these viruses.

None of these viruses can be treated. Prevention and control is through prolonged quarantine of new snakes and the use of available testing. For more detail on infection control see Chapter 5 and Chapter 16 for information on reptile viruses and quarantine recommendations.

Arenavirus

Aetiology
Arenaviruses are enveloped RNA viruses with a segmented genome. They have been detected in snakes with neurological signs and inclusion body disease in the USA and the Netherlands.

Pathogenesis
Lesions in pythons are generally restricted to the brain and spinal cord. In other species of snakes, lesions can be more generalized and inclusions can be found in the oral mucosa, oral tonsils, pancreas and kidney. A correlation between arenavirus infection and cancer has been suggested, so testing tumours found on snakes for arenaviruses merits consideration.

Clinical Signs
Neurological signs occur mostly in pythons, where the disease has an acute onset and is rapidly progressive, resulting in death. In more chronic infections, animals may be lethargic, stop eating and lose condition.

Diagnosis
Arenavirus infection is a differential for any snake showing neurological signs. Definitive diagnosis is based on histopathological findings of eosinophilic intracytoplasmic inclusion bodies in the brain in pythons and liver, pancreas, kidney, oral epithelium or oral tonsils in other species. The PCR assay can be run on whole blood or serum.

Bornavirus

Aetiology
Bornaviruses are enveloped single stranded RNA viruses. Three genetically distinct bornaviruses have been identified in an African garter snake (*Elapsoidea loveridgei*) and pythons in Australia.

Pathogenesis
Bornavirus-positive Australian snakes that have been euthanized have had a nonsuppurative encephalitis.

Diagnosis
Diagnosis is made by finding the characteristic inclusion bodies in the brain and confirming infection by PCR of fresh brain tissue. Early results suggest that this virus will

not be consistently detected in oral and cloacal swabs, or in organs other than the brain.

Ferlavirus

Aetiology
Ferlavirus was previously known as ophidian paramyxovirus or OPMV.

Pathogenesis
Ferlavirus infection results in a nonsuppurative encephalitis and myelitis and a chronic active exudative pneumonia.

Diagnosis
Ferlavirus infection should be a differential in pythons that are unexpectedly found dead. Regurgitation is another nonspecific sign. Respiratory disease can be severe, so ferlavirus infection should be a differential for snakes that exhibit respiratory disease combined with neurological disease. Unlike in sunshinevirus, the material coming from the glottis is typically an exudate. A complete set of tissues from such snakes should be submitted to an experienced reptile pathologist, keeping back fresh frozen tissues for PCR diagnostics if necessary. Tissues most likely to be positive on PCR assay for ferlavirus are brain, kidney, lung and liver.

Sunshinevirus

Aetiology
Sunshinevirus (*Reptile sunshinevirus 1*) is a paramyxovirus.

Pathogenesis
Sunshinevirus causes neurorespiratory disease complex, resulting in spongiosis of the hind brain and, in some instances, an interstitial pneumonia. The virus has been isolated from oral and cloacal swabs and transmission is likely to occur via aerosol as well as cloacal secretions and faecal contamination. It has been isolated from blood. It is, therefore, possible that blood-sucking ectoparasites may act as a vector of transmission between snakes. Research is continuing into the possibility of vertical transmission after the virus was isolated from the allantois, amnion and embryonic tissues of a clutch laid by an infected dam.

Clinical Signs
Sunshinevirus infection should be suspected when neurological signs combine with respiratory signs including a clear discharge from the mouth and dyspnoea. Apparently healthy snakes have tested positive for sunshinevirus. The majority of these snakes have gone on to develop clinical signs over the ensuing years.

Diagnosis
Diagnosis of sunshinevirus is via PCR of swabs of the oral cavity and cloaca and by histological examination of intact brain for a sagittal section if the animal dies.

Adenovirus Infection in Bearded Dragons

Aetiology
Adenovirus infection is an Agamid atadenovirus, which spreads easily through direct contact and via contaminated hands and equipment.

Pathogenesis
Adenovirus is now considered to be endemic in Australia, Europe and the United States. Infected animals have extensive lesions in the liver and clinical signs may be the result of a hepatic encephalopathy.

Clinical Signs
Bearded dragons infected with adenovirus are characterized by poor growth rates, torticollis and opisthotonos (Figure 24.8). Affected animals range from 4 weeks up to 12 weeks of age and the onset of clinical signs is rapid.

Diagnosis
Diagnosis is via PCR from fresh liver or oral swabs and by characteristic histopathological findings that include intranuclear inclusion

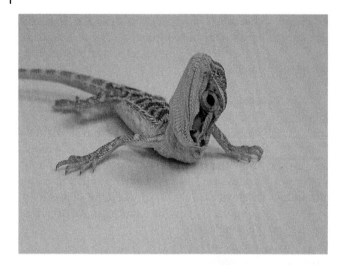

Figure 24.8 Bearded dragon (*Pogona vitticeps*) hatchling with adenovirus, showing classic torticollis and star gazing behaviour (courtesy of Bob Doneley).

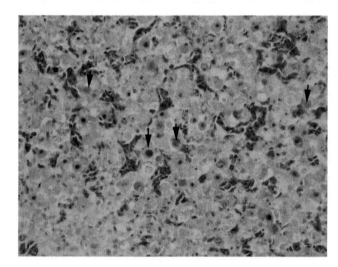

Figure 24.9 Bearded dragon (*Pogona vitticeps*) adenovirus inclusion bodies (40× haematoxylin and eosin staining. Arrows indicate adenovirus inclusion bodies.

bodies in the liver (Figure 24.9), oesophagus and gastric mucosa.

Treatment

There is no treatment available for adenovirus infections. Supportive care and nutritional support may help to prolong life.

Parasitic Infections

Systemic Coccidiosis in Green Turtles (*Chelonia mydas*)

Aetiology

Systemic coccidiosis is caused by a coccidian that morphologically resembles *Caryospora*

cheloniae. It has yet to be characterized genetically.

Pathogenesis

This parasite causes a mild to severe necrotizing enteritis and organisms can be found in other tissues including the brain and meninges. In the brain, it causes a lymphoplasmacytic and histiocytic encephalitis and meningitis with necrosis and malacia.

Clinical Signs

The majority of affected turtles are subadults. Outbreaks occur sporadically on the east coast of Australia. Outbreaks occur between September and February, with most turtles presenting in October, although outbreaks do not occur annually. Diseased animals are often found dead, dying or severely depressed. Some have a head tilt, swim in circles or, rarely, have nystagmus.

Diagnosis

Oocysts can be found in the faeces of live animals. Preliminary data suggest that some live animals may have schizonts in circulating blood cells. At necropsy, oocysts can be detected in scrapings of the diseased mucosa and diagnosis can be made by finding the characteristic microscopic lesions in haematoxylin and eosin stained tissues.

Treatment

Despite aggressive anticoccidial treatment and supportive care, most infected animals die or are euthanized.

Prevention

This appears to be an emerging infectious disease. Changing environmental conditions are postulated as being linked to outbreaks. At this time, there are no known preventative measures.

Spirorchid Flukes in Green Turtles

Aetiology

Multiple species of flukes in the Spirorchidae family can infect green turtles.

Pathogenesis

Adult flukes are found in the heart, large arteries and veins. Their eggs cause disease by lodging in capillaries and inducing microfocal granulomas. These parasites are also associated with formation of arterial thrombi. Septic aortic thrombosis may also occur with septicaemia. Lesions in the brain can be caused by egg emboli, the presence of trematodes in the meningeal vessels and bacterial meningitis secondary to septic aortic thrombosis.

Clinical Signs

Most infected animals do not exhibit clinical signs. Animals where disease is severe are generally found dead.

Diagnosis

Diagnosis is made at necropsy by finding the characteristic gross and microscopic lesions.

Treatment

Treatment in subclinically infected animals is not indicated.

Prevention and Control

No preventive or control measures are known.

Diseases of Unknown Aetiology

Systemic Lymphoid Proliferation and Non-Suppurative Encephalitis in Estuarine Crocodiles (*Crocodylus porosus*)

A disease syndrome, systemic lymphoid proliferation and non-suppurative encephalitis (SLPE), has been recognized in farmed estuarine crocodiles in the Northern Territory, Australia. Most animals are young growing animals. Disease occurs in outbreaks, with many animals in an enclosure affected. The only sign observed is a reduced growth rate. Microscopically, these animals have a lymphohistiocytic infiltration of multiple tissues. Gliosis and perivascular cuffing with lymphocytes and histiocytes is seen. The role of newly recognized herpesviruses of crocodiles in this syndrome is under investigation.

Bellinger River Turtle Mortality

In the autumn of 2015, large numbers of Bellinger river turtles (*Myuchelys georgesi*) were found dead or dying along a short section of the Bellinger River in northern New South Wales, on Australia's east coast, that comprised their entire range. The most prominent lesion was a severe conjunctivitis, keratitis and periocular cellulitis. Some animals also exhibited a posterior paresis. Microscopically, many animals were found to have severe necrotizing subacute encephalitis. Hydrocephalus was present in a small number of animals. This disease is suspected to have a viral aetiology.

Other Infections

Hypothermia resulting in central nervous system damage occurs commonly in chelonians following hibernation. It can result in blindness, circling or head tilt. It is thought that vasoconstriction leads to ischaemic brain injury and degenerative changes of the peripheral nerves. Hyperthermia may also result in neurological impairment as a result of a demyelinating peripheral neuropathy or central nervous system dysfunction, resulting in stupor, ataxia or coma. Treatment includes long-term supportive care, with initial slow correction of the patient's temperature and management of intracranial pressure. Antibiotics are indicated for secondary infections and tracheal intubation and ventilation as required.

Further Reading

Mans, C. and Braun, J. (2014) Update on common nutritional disorders of captive reptiles. *Veterinary Clinics of North America Exotic Animal Practice*, 17 (3), 369–395.

Wyneken, J. (2007) Reptilian neurology: anatomy and function. *Veterinary Clinics of North America Exotic Animal Practice*, 10 (3), 837–853.

Mariani, C.L. (2007) The neurologic examination and neurodiagnostic techniques for reptiles. *Veterinary Clinics of North America Exotic Animal Practice*, 10 (3), 855–891.

Hyndman, T.H. and Shilton, C. M. (2015) An update on Australian reptile viruses, in Unusual Pet and Avian Veterinarians Annual Conference 2015 (H.R. Baron, ed.) AAVAC, Sydney, Australia.

Hyndman, T. and Shilton, C.M. (2011) Molecular detection of two adenoviruses associated with disease in Australian lizards. *Australian Veterinary Journal*, 89, 232–235.

Hyndman, T.H., Shilton, C.M., Doneley, R.J.T. and Nicholls, P.K. (2012) Sunshine virus in Australian pythons. *Veterinary Microbiology*, 161, 77–87.

25

Disorders of the Musculoskeletal System

Adolf K. Maas

Anatomy And Physiology

Reptilian skeletal anatomy has many similarities to other clades, although there are key differences that are important for a clinician to understand. See Chapter 2 for a more detailed review of the anatomy and physiology of the musculoskeletal system.

Key Points

- The basic terraform tetrapod body plan is followed with key exceptions seen in snakes (loss of limbs) and turtles/tortoises (development of the shell).
- Uniquely, turtles and tortoises have their ribs external to their thoracic girdle, with most of them developing bone in the intercostal space to form the carapace and de

novo formation of bone in their ventral body wall to form the plastron.
- Snakes have lost their thoracic and pelvic girdles and limbs through evolution (except in rare species) and extended their thoracic vertebrae to make a long, fusiform body shape.
- Reptile bones do not have growth plates and although they will continually grow their entire lives, the growth occurs from endosteal ossification, whereby the bones progressively and gradually enlarge.
- Each clinician should undertake research appropriate to the species at hand so that they might be familiar with the unique variations of that reptile.

Congenital and Hereditary Disorders

Reptiles do not commonly have congenital disorders of the skeletal system, although there are a number of specific conditions reported. Axial deviation is likely the most commonly seen (scoliosis, kyphosis, lordosis) but has only rarely been reported. Skull deformities are not commonly identified but are well publicized and include bicephalism (Figure 25.1) and axial duplication, brachycephaly and cleft palate. The scientific literature has listed a number of axial skeletal conditions that are also seen in mammals, including hemivertebra, rib and vertebral duplication and intercalated half-vertebrae. Hind-limb paresis secondary to congenital spinal stenosis has been reported in a turtle.

Reptile Medicine and Surgery in Clinical Practice, First Edition. Edited by Bob Doneley, Deborah Monks, Robert Johnson and Brendan Carmel.

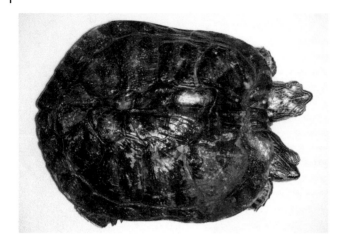

Figure 25.1 A two-headed red-eared slider turtle (*Trachemys scripta elegans*).

Variations in limb morphology are also reported including ectromelia and supernumerary limbs or digits.

The aetiology of these deformities has not been well assessed and they are assumed to originate similarly as in other clades. Genetic mutations, toxins and developmental infections all should be considered, but issues such as maternal health and nutrition (both deficiencies and excesses), incubation conditions and radiation exposure have been discussed as potential causes of congenital defects. As there can be significant connection to other disorders, genetic diseases should be considered as some of the most difficult to diagnose. Although seen primarily in young animals, they should still be considered a diagnosis of exclusion.

Non-Infectious Disorders

Metabolic and Nutritional Conditions

There are many causes of reptilian skeletal disorders that are neither primary congenital to the skeleton nor are infectious in aetiology. These primarily include nutritional, traumatic, degenerative and neoplastic disorders. Nutritional skeletal disorders among reptiles in captivity are well documented (Figures 25.2, 25.3 and 25.4). Maternal nutrition has been shown to be critical for fertility

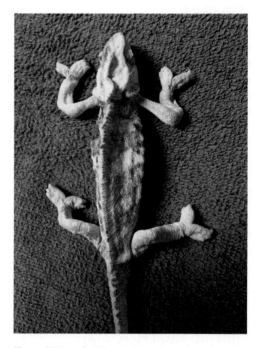

Figure 25.2 Veiled chameleon (*Chameleo calyptratus*) with advanced nutritional secondary hyperparathyroidism and multiple pathological fractures (courtesy of Todd Driggers DVM, Gilbert, AZ).

and very early development; it can be easily deduced to cause issues in neonate reptiles whose health depends on their maternally derived stores. Testing of the mother's general metabolic health and eggs for composition, as well as early testing of affected animals, may be necessary to diagnose these conditions.

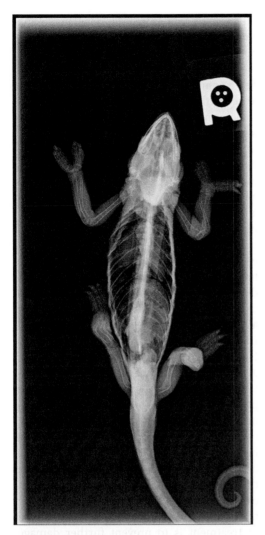

Figure 25.3 Radiograph of a veiled chameleon (*Chameleo calyptratus*) with nutritional secondary hyperparathyroidism and multiple pathological fractures (A.K. Maas).

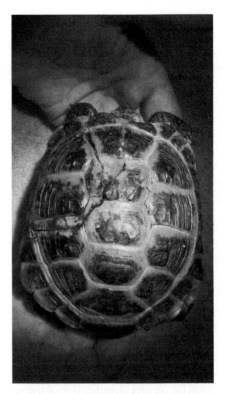

Figure 25.4 Russian tortoise (*Agrionemys horsfieldii*) with multiple trauma-induced shell fractures. This animal also was found to have moderately advanced nutritional secondary hyperparathyroidism, facilitating the fractures (A.K. Maas).

Once a reptile is no longer dependent upon its yolk supply, it becomes more susceptible to nutritional dyscrasias that cause skeletal disorders. Most commonly referenced are calcium deficiencies causing osteopenia, osteomalacia and hypomineralization. However, a singular calcium deficiency is not commonly responsible for many cases of nutritionally caused osteological disorders.

Metabolic bone disease is commonly named as an aetiology but, in all accuracy, this term is not a diagnosis. Rather, it is a collection of conditions that, although having a similar clinical presentation, have different causes, with often very different treatments and outcomes. A calcium deficiency is one form of metabolic bone disease but inappropriate levels of magnesium, phosphorus, vitamin D and vitamin A all fit under this umbrella description in reptiles. Renal disease, parathyroid disease and neoplasia, hypothermia and lack of appropriate ultraviolet B (UV-B) light all can produce conditions that can be categorized as metabolic bone disease.

Nutritional secondary hyperparathyroidism (NSHP) is one of the more common non-infectious skeletal conditions, often categorized as a metabolic bone disease. This is, again, a singular title for a condition with multiple aetiologies, including a low calcium and/or high phosphorus diet and/or hypovitaminosis D. Since many species of reptiles require UV-B exposure to convert 7-dehydrocholesterol to cholecalciferol, inappropriate (low) exposure levels of UV-B light can also be a cause. Additionally, as the isomerization of cholecholesterol to vitamin D3 requires heat, chronic hypothermia (inappropriate husbandry) will also cause hypovitaminosis.

Since kidney function is critical for the regulation of calcium (formation of calcitriol, retention of calcium, excretion of phosphorus), renal secondary hyperparathyroidism (RSHP) is also a common aetiology of reptile skeletal disease. Nephritis, nephosclerosis, hypovitaminosis A, toxins (including many commonly used medications) and chronic dehydration all need to be considered differentials for the aetiology of RSHP. Furthermore, NSHP and RSHP can occur concomitantly, exemplifying that plasma biochemistry analysis is critical for correct identification of these and similar conditions. It is easy to see that a diagnosis of any of these conditions without appropriate diagnostics is inappropriate and can easily lead to treatment failure (see Chapters 6 and 15 for further information).

Trauma

Traumatic skeletal disorders are commonly seen in practice. Fractures are seen in all reptile bones and can be both primary as well as secondary (pathological; Figures 25.3 and 25.4). As with any other patient, radiographs are essential to assess bone density and condition and, if an underlying infectious aetiology is suspected, aerobic and anaerobic culture should be performed with samples obtained by surgical biopsy or, if this is not feasible, a blood culture. Fractures secondary to osteopenia are exceptionally common in NSHP and related conditions due to low bone strength.

Luxations have been reported in multiple reptile cases but are not considered common. These injuries are believed to occur for the same reasons as in other quadrupeds and similar treatment options should be pursued.

To obtain an accurate diagnosis for a disorder, a complete review of the husbandry, followed with a further evaluation of the patient to determine whether additional or underlying conditions in other systems are contributing to the malaise of the patient. Standard diagnostic techniques should be employed, including plasma biochemistries, hormone and vitamin assays, radiographs, cytology and histopathology. Once aetiology is determined, treatment options are similar to in other quadrupeds. Dietary and husbandry issues must be corrected or successful resolution may not be possible. Bones of normal density can be reassembled and realigned using common surgical techniques or, if appropriate for the species, specific bone and fracture, external coaptation may be applied. It must be noted that reptilian healing occurs at slower rates than mammals and avian reptiles so treatment is likely to be much more protracted. As callus formation is not as pronounced, owing to endosteal regeneration, repeat radiographs should be taken to assess healing. In cases of pathological fracture, the underlying condition must be addressed at the same time or healing may be hampered or inhibited. Many defects (scoliosis, long bone valgus) will not be treatable, so the goal of treatment is to prevent further damage and improve the general health and welfare of the patient.

Neoplasia

Although once believed to relatively rare in reptiles, neoplasia occurs at similar frequencies to avian and mammal species. In general, bony tumours have been found to be non-metastatic in cases examined, while being locally invasive. In many cases, complete surgical excision is curative, although with the frequency that osteological neoplasias are found to be metastases from other primary tumours, appropriate diagnostic work-ups are warranted (Figure 25.5).

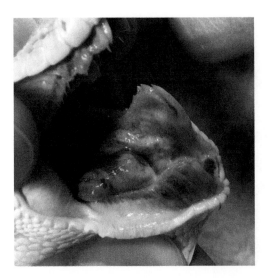

Figure 25.5 Oral mass in a green tree python (*Morelia viridis*) determined to be osteosarcoma (with permission from Bradley Waffa, DVM, Portsmouth, VA).

Infectious Disorders

Bacterial and Mycotic Infections

Infectious diseases, and particularly bacterial infections, are an exceptionally common cause of skeletal disorders in reptiles (Figure 25.6). The dissemination and localization of these infections into the bone is a frequent sequela and has been identified even in the fossil record. Based on clinical observations, osteomyelitis may occur at a much higher frequency than it does in higher vertebrate forms; this may be because preliminary studies have identified septicaemias in up to 5% of apparently healthy animals tested at random.

Osteomyelitis can result from any infection in the body, such as pneumonia, a bite wound, hepatitis, enteritis, bacterial translocation, nephritis and gingivitis. The infections themselves have been identified in long bones, joints, the spinal column and ribs. In most cases of both superficial and deep carapacial and plastronal disease of chelonians, the aetiology is infectious osteomyelitis. No single bacterial agent is responsible for a significant percentage of osteomyelitis cases.

Salmonella has been implicated to occur at greater frequency in *Crotalid* snakes and has been isolated in bony lesions in other species but by no means is it the only agent.

Mycotic osteomyelitis is reported in reptiles and pathogens include *Nannizziopsis*, *Aspergillus*, *Mucor* and other genera. The source of these bone infections is similar to that of bacterial infections – disseminated infections. These often originate as mycotic pneumonia but since fungal infections have been reported in all tissues, it can develop anywhere.

Both bacterial and fungal osteomyelitis are often insidious in nature. Clinical signs seen can range from none to swellings of the bone involved (most common on distal extremities and the maxilla and mandible) to the development of fractures, spinal deviations and even paralysis and death. Often, the first presentation involves a symptom unrelated to the bony lesions as anorexia may be present and the animal may be lethargic. Any symptom that may be associated with septicaemia should have osteomyelitis as a differential.

Diagnosing these conditions first requires a complete blood count and radiographs of suspected or affected areas. Radiographs can be variable in appearance but commonly have a mixed lytic/clastic appearance and often some degree of periosteal proliferation. A complete blood count may produce a granulocytosis and/or a monocytosis or a generalized leucocytosis. Alongside confirmation of disease, blood cultures (both aerobic and anaerobic) must be taken prior to initiating antimicrobial therapy, although a bone biopsy and culture and/or polymerase chain reaction (PCR) and/or histopathology may be necessary to identify mycotic and mycobacterial osteomyelitis. Collecting samples from the surface of chelonian shell lesions is a poor source, as it will always be contaminated with environmental agents while the primary pathogen may no longer be present. Repeat blood counts, radiographs and follow-up blood cultures are necessary to follow efficacy of treatment and the patient's immune system response.

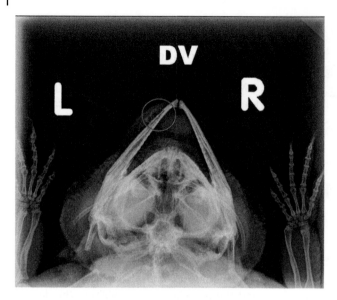

Figure 25.6 Bearded dragon (*Pogona vitticeps*) with a jaw mass and a radiographic lesions (circle). This was found to be a mycobacterial abscess (A.K. Maas).

Treatment should always be based on the results of diagnostic testing. In most cases, pure cultures from blood samples are a good indicator of the infectious agent, while multiple pathogens identified usually indicate a contaminated sample. Unfortunately, fungal, mycobacterial and some bacterial agents cannot be identified via blood cultures so, if the culture does not produce results, treatment should be based on the evidence produced by the blood count, radiographs and bone biopsy. Additional diagnostic tools such as enzyme-linked immunosorbent assay and PCR analysis of samples should be employed to obtain a diagnosis. Appropriate antimicrobial agents should be prescribed, depending on the type identified, response to therapy and the species of animal treated. Nonsteroidal anti-inflammatories are often indicated to improve general condition as most of these lesions are found to be painful in mammals and are likely so in reptiles.

Concurrent conditions can be diagnosed in the same animals. With weakened health from substandard husbandry, it is common to find secondary infections and there have been cases of animals that were diagnosed with both NSHP and osteomyelitis concurrently, causing severe skeletal deformities. Thus, despite common thinking to limit a condition to a single diagnosis, it is critical to collect and interpret all data sufficiently to allow for concurrent diagnoses.

As is the case in most reptile diseases, the best prevention is to provide the best possible husbandry, emulating the natural history conditions of the species in hand. In addition, since virtually any bacterial or fungal disease can develop into osteomyelitis, early identification, accurate and thorough diagnosis and aggressive, appropriate treatment of other infective processes will provide an excellent means of preventing infectious osteomyelitis in reptiles.

Parasites

Parasitic bone diseases are not as commonly seen as bacterial and fungal aetiologies but, as there are specific conditions seen, they should be considered in appropriate cases. Digenaean trematodes of the family Spirorchiidae inhabit the vascular system of many species of semi-aquatic and sea turtles, and release their ova within the vessels of the host. These ova can obstruct terminal arteries throughout the animal, with granulomas and abscesses developing in the carapace and plastron followed by the sloughing of superficial tissue. Oral infections of trichomonads are associated with abscess formation in the maxilla and mandible following deep gingivitis, both in extinct species as well as anecdotally in extant species of reptiles. Microsporidia is more commonly associated with myositis and disseminated infections in reptiles, but has been identified as the aetiology of skeletal defects in amphibians, so clinicians should consider it as a differential for skeletal pathologies in reptiles.

Diagnosing parasitic osteomyelitis and associated osteological disorders generally requires biopsies of affected bony tissues to obtain an accurate diagnosis. Trematode eggs can be identified on histopathology but diagnosis via blood samples or faecal analysis are generally unrewarding. Oral and faecal direct mount cytologies can be performed to identify Parabasalia-type protists but, again, these organisms only indicate association rather than infection, with the determination of infection based on other clinical information.

Effective treatment requires identification of the aetiological agent and administration of the appropriate anti-parasiticide. However, there are anecdotal reports of severe and extensive carapacial disease following treatment of pond turtles with praziquantel and fenbendazole. Extensive and acute die-off of embedded parasites can induce disseminated granuloma formation and tissue necrosis,

producing a serious health risk, for the patient. Concurrent with treatment appropriate sanitation must be administered to prevent both immediate and long-term reinfection, as there is likely little immunological protection developed.

Skeletal Disorders of Indeterminate or Mixed Origin

Spinal Osteopathy

The development of spontaneous spinal defects (spinal osteopathy) has been reported in all major orders of reptiles and has been anecdotally reported by reptile practitioners many times over (Figures 25.7 and 25.8). Despite this being not uncommonly seen in clinical practice, the specific aetiology of this condition has yet to be elucidated, with trauma, infectious agents, autoimmune conditions, toxins and degenerative metabolic conditions all believed to play a role. There are some distinctions within the classification of spinal osteopathy, such as osteitis deformans, and while each have histopathological differences they all have similar presentations in the patient. Morphologically, these lesions display irregular bone proliferation of the spine, often involving articular

Figure 25.7 Radiograph of a snake with osteitis deformans, showing irregular bone proliferation along the vertebral margins (with permission from Robert Schmidt DVM PhD DACVP).

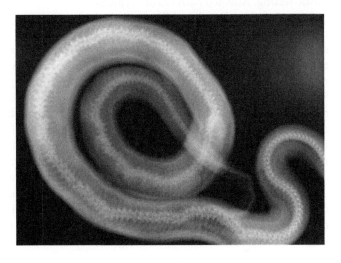

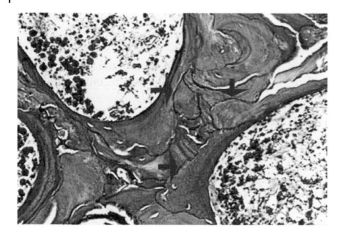

Figure 25.8 Generalized thickening of the bony trabeculae at the expense of the intertrabecular spaces and irregular patches of lamellar bone with a characteristic 'mosaic' pattern indicate osteitis deformans (courtesy of Robert Schmidt DVM PhD DACVP).

surfaces. There may or may not be active inflammatory processes and, if bacterial agents are present, they have been seen in all areas of affected tissue including joint spaces, superficial bone and new or established skeletal bone. A comparison to Paget's disease (osteitis deformans) has been made in published reports while, in other cases, the qualifications for this definition has not been met. Just as Paget's disease has been associated with a paramyxoviral infection in humans, there is some thought that there might be a viral induction of spinal osteopathy in reptiles. At this time, though, it is evident that more research is necessary to fully elucidate this condition.

Diagnosis of spinal osteopathy requires a combination of both clinical signs and diagnostic testing. Affected patients are typically presented with reduced mobility and flexibility of the vertebral column. On physical examination, portions of the spine are noted to be rigid and, in more advanced cases, regions of the spine will palpate as enlarged. Some cases will have paresis or paralysis caudal to the affected areas. Radiographs will confirm ankylosis of the hyperostotic regions intermixed with lengths of apparently normal spinal column. Fractures both adjacent and within area of spinal osteopathy are not uncommon. Bone biopsy, blood and biopsy cultures, haematological and plasma biochemical data, and serum vitamin D levels should be measured to confirm diagnosis

and identify additional correlating conditions. If it is available, nuclear bone scanning will provide information that correlates increased metabolic activity with sites of suspected spinal osteopathy.

At this time, there is no treatment modality that reverses the hyperostosis present at the time of diagnosis. This being said, the results of appropriate diagnostics can be applied to treat bacterial and fungal infections, nutritional deficiencies, husbandry issues and other pathological processes identified. As inflammation is often the limiting factor for quality of life in this condition, this should also be controlled; the author has had relative efficacy using long-term nonsteroidal anti-inflammatories, including meloxicam (refer to Appendix 1 for dosing recommendations).

Shell Deformities of Chelonia

Skeletal deformities are common in chelonians and are commonly categorized as distortions, pyramiding and 'flat' shell. Often referred to as a single condition, these disorders have been attributed to multiple aetiologies. NSHP and RSHP are known to cause abnormalities of bone formation, causing the carapace and plastron to form abnormally and of low density. These conditions often are associated with thickened bridges and peripheral shell margins. Low environmental humidity coupled with excessive protein or caloric intake has been postulated as a combinatorial aetiology, in that low humidity decreases the elasticity of the scutal keratin while diet increases the growth rate of the underlying carapacial bone. Increased nocturnal heat has been correlated with increased pyramid formation in leopard tortoises (*Stigmochelys pardalis*), providing strength to this argument. Fluoroquinolone administration in growing chelonians is also purported to cause shell deformities as a result of cartilage damage.

As these conditions are probably multifactorial, each case must be evaluated individually, including radiographs, plasma biochemistries, hormone and vitamin assays and, in some cases, shell biopsies may be necessary. Existing shell defects will not be able to be reversed, so the goal of diagnosis and treatment is to correct the metabolic abnormalities and husbandry shortcomings present in an effort to reduce (and possibly eliminate) the advancement of the condition as well as the development of secondary conditions.

Muscular and Soft Tissue Disorders

Congenital and Hereditary Disorders

There are few reports of congenital muscular disorders in reptiles. The few that are published appear to be associated with a litany of other defects, some with putative identification of a single-gene defect. It is likely that congenital connective tissue disorders could have the same aetiologies as seen in other terrestrial vertebrates.

Non-Infectious Disorders

As husbandry is the greatest underlying source of pathologies in captive reptiles, muscular abnormalities from nutrition aetiologies are the most common reported non-infectious disorders. Vitamin E deficiencies have been identified as an aetiology of steatitis in several species of reptiles of muscular degenerative disease in reptiles. Diets high in either polyunsaturated fatty acids and in vitamin A are known to increase vitamin E requirements, so reptiles fed large amounts of either component (fish oil, grain or seed-based diets, or rodents primarily fed grain or seed diets) should have higher supplementation of vitamin E.

Identification of these cases is often non-specific, with anorexia and lethargy being common identifying signs. In some cases, elevated aspartate transaminase (AST) was identified on plasma biochemistries. A diagnosis can be made with measurement of plasma alpha-tocopherol levels. Oral or parenteral vitamin E administration has been used for both suspected and confirmed deficiencies.

Tongue paralysis in old-world chameleons has been associated with vitamin A deficiencies, with recovery observed with parenteral administration of preformed vitamin A. No known clinical studies have been published, so it is not understood whether this is a musculoskeletal or neurological disorder caused by this deficiency.

Trauma

As soft tissue injuries occur in all species, they are also an issue in reptiles. Bites, wounds, burns and other muscular injuries all should be addressed and treated in any other terrestrial animals. With the unique issues encountered in skin anatomy and healing of reptiles, Chapter 18 should be reviewed for appropriate treatment.

Metabolic Disorders

Metabolic myopathies are specific enzymatic defects caused by hereditary muscle disorders (defective genes), such as glycogen or lipid metabolism disorders. No such myopathies have been reported in reptiles at this time.

Exertional or capture myopathy has been identified in reptiles and has been postulated in cases of routine handling. Also known as exertional rhabdomyolysis, this condition occurs in cases of exertion where there is additional fear or anxiety, excessive handling, shock, transport, extremes of age and other factors. In exertional rhabdomyolysis, the muscle tissue breaks down from depletion of ATP and increased production of lactic acid, leaking intracellular contents, eventually leading to cellular necrosis and death. Myoglobin is released into the circulation, causing renal necrosis and acute renal failure.

Identifying these cases is usually based on history with subsequent weakness and lethargy. Biochemistry profiles identify increased creatine kinase and AST, often with free myoglobinaemia and acidosis. Chelonians have displayed increased markers for exertional rhabdomyolysis in as little as 10–15 minutes of basic restraint for blood collection.

Treatment involves intravenous fluid administration and diuresis to increase vascular perfusion to affected tissues and prevent myoglobin accumulation in renal tissues. Nonsteroidal anti-inflammatories should be considered to reduce inflammation and discomfort but opiates, with both questionable efficacy in the various clades of reptiles and studies indicating opiate-induced exertional rhabdomyolysis in mammals, should be evaluated on a case-by-case basis.

Neoplasia

Few cases of myological neoplasias have been reported in reptiles. Rhabdomyosarcoma, has been reported in a captive Galapagos tortoise (*Geochelone nigra*) but the tumour was not further evaluated to assess possible aetiologies. A leiomyosarcoma has been reported in the coelomic cavity of a snake but it was not stated whether it was associated with the musculoskeletal system. Other cases of rhabdomyosarcoma, leiomyosarcoma and fibrosarcoma have been reported in reptile species.

Induction of a rhabdomyosarcoma by retroviral infection has been proposed in a corn snake (*Pantherophis guttatus*) and fibrosarcomas (and other neoplasias) are associated with retroviral infection in pythons.

Infectious Disorders

Although there are countless infectious agents identified in reptilian hosts, none is reported to be specific to the muscular system of reptiles.

Viral Infections

Retroviral infection has been associated with the formation of connective tissue neoplasia but no other specific muscular pathology has yet been identified with viral infections in reptiles. A complete blood count and plasma electrophoresis can be useful to help identify viral infections, but histopathology and electron microscopy of the tissue, with subsequent nucleotide sequencing for identification of the specific virus, is necessary to identify these infectious agents.

Bacterial and Fungal Infections

Any bacterial or fungal agent that can infect a reptile systemically has the potential to develop into a myositis. Inflammatory exudates in reptiles are typically solid, with granuloma formation expected as part of most inflammatory reactions. Localized inflammatory reactions are most common but diffuse inflammatory reactions are known to occur in *Mycoplasma* and *Helicobacter* infections. *Chrysosporium* anamorph of *Nannizziopsis vriesii*, although most commonly associated with dermatitis (see Chapter 18), has been identified in most tissues of affected animals and has been reported in cases of deep myositis.

Clinical signs depend on the dissemination of the disease. Systemic infections can present as acute or chronic decline, lethargy, anorexia, failure to thrive, erythema and vasculitis, diarrhoea, changes in behaviour or death. Localized infections may be seen as localized swellings, redness, changes in mobility, skin lesions or sloughing, bite or puncture wounds, with or without the generalized signs seen in disseminated infections. As in the case of any other bacterial or fungal disease, appropriate diagnostic tools are necessary to produce an accurate diagnosis (see Skeletal Disorders section).

Appropriate antimicrobial therapy should be started on the identification of disease, with modifications or changes pending blood and/or wound culture. Haematological analysis is recommended to assess involvement of other organ systems and to evaluate the immune system response to the infection. If abscesses are present, surgery is necessary for resolution since reptiles lack the enzymes necessary to liquefy purulent debris and the installation of drains typically results in additional tissue necrosis.

Parasitic Infections

Parasitic infections are common in reptiles, with a remarkable diversity of pathologies identified. Parasitic muscular disorders are less common but are well reported, involving a range of host species and both metazoan and protozoan parasites. Nematodiasis, common in the gastrointestinal tracts of reptiles, has also been identified in the skeletal muscles of tortoises. Filariasis, with subcutaneous and intramuscular migration and sparganosis, are commonly reported in wild caught reptiles.

Microsporidia, a class of parasitic intracellular fungus, is an emerging disease of concern that can involve the musculoskeletal system of reptiles. A bearded dragon (*Pogona vitticeps*) was identified as having a disseminated microsporidial infection involving the testes, trachea, right femur and associated musculature. *Heterosporis anguillarum*, a microsporidian species normally infecting eels, was associated with myositis having both extracellular and intracellular locations in a garter snake.

Identifying muscular parasitic infections can be challenging. The cases may present as primary problems, such as limb swelling or lameness, incidental such as focal masses unrelated to the presenting issue or as a conclusion to a work-up of non-specific signs. The clinician needs to maintain a perspective not to focus on a particular condition or symptom until a complete diagnosis is reached and to be complete in their use of diagnostic tools. In most cases, in addition to the collection of a minimum data base, radiographs, muscle biopsy and speciation of the parasite via PCR sequencing.

Caution must be used when treating disseminated metazoan infections. Muscular filariasis is often associated with coelomic migration as well as blood-borne microfilarial infections; thrombi formation and anaphylactic shock are associated with rapid die-off. Both these and other metazoan infections are best treated surgically to remove identified worms prior to systemic treatment, if systemic treatment is even indicated.

Microsporidial infections have yet to have a consistently effective treatment ascertained in reptile patients. Rabbits (infected with *Encephalitozoon cuniculi*) and fish infected with microsporidia have had good response to benzimidazole therapy, while most other agents (oxytetracycline/chloramphenicol, fluoroquinolones, monensin, metronidazole, toltrazuril, etc.) have produced equivocal or unconfirmed results in these and amphibian species. At this time, fenbendazole has been used by clinicians in the treatment of microsporidia in reptiles, with varying degrees of success, but a specific dose and treatment protocol have yet to be determined.

Further Reading

Bellairs, A.D.A. (1965) Cleft palate, microphthalmia and other malformations in embryos of lizards and snakes. *Proceedings of the Zoological Society of London*, 144 (2), 239–252.

Di Girolamo, N., Selleri, P., Nardini, G. *et al.* (2014) Computed tomography-guided bone biopsies for evaluation of proliferative vertebral lesions in two boa constrictors (*Boa constrictor imperator*). *Journal of Zoo and Wildlife Medicine*, 45 (4), 973–978.

Dierenfeld, E.S. (1989) Vitamin E deficiency in zoo reptiles, birds, and ungulates.

Journal of Zoo and Wildlife Medicine, 20 (1), 3–11.

Fransworth, R.J., Brannian, R.E., Fletcher, K.C. and Klassen, S. (1986) A vitamin E–selenium responsive condition in a green iguana. *Journal of Zoo Animal Medicine*, 17 (1), 42–43.

Frye, F.L. and Carney, J. (1974) Osteitis deformans (Paget's disease) in a boa constrictor. *Veterinary Medicine, Small Animal Clinician*, 69 (2), 186–188.

Girling, S.J. and Raiti, P. (2017) *BSAVA Manual of Reptiles*, 3rd ed. John Wiley & Sons, Ltd, Chichester.

Heinrich, M.L. and Heinrich, K.K. (2015) Effect of supplemental heat in captive African leopard tortoises (*Stigmochelys pardalis*) and spurred tortoises (*Geochelone sulcata*) on growth rate and carapacial scute pyramiding. *Journal of Exotic Pet Medicine*, 25 (1), 18–25.

Irizarry-Rovira, A.R., Wolf, A., Bolek, M. *et al.* (2002) Blood smear from a wild-caught panther chameleon (*Furcifer pardalis*). *Veterinary Clinical Pathology*, 31 (3), 129–132.

Isaza, R., Garner, M. and Jacobson, E. (2000) Proliferative osteoarthritis and osteoarthrosis in 15 snakes. *Journal of Zoo and Wildlife Medicine*, 31 (1), 20–27.

Jacobson, E., ed. (2007) *Infectious Diseases and Pathology of Reptiles: Color Atlas and Text*. CRC Press, Chichester.

Klaphake, E. (2010) A fresh look at metabolic bone diseases in reptiles and amphibians. *Veterinary Clinics of North America Exotic Animal Practice*, 13 (3), 375–392.

Raftery, A. (2011) Reptile orthopedic medicine and surgery. *Journal of Exotic Pet Medicine*, 20 (2), 107–116.

Richter, B., Csokai, J., Graner, I. *et al.* (2013) Encephalitozoonosis in two inland bearded dragons (*Pogona vitticeps*). *Journal of Comparative Pathology*, 148 (2), 278–282.

Rothschild, B.M., Schultze, H.P. and Pellegrini, R. (2012) Summary of osseous pathology in amphibians and reptiles, in *Herpetological Osteopathology: Annotated Bibliography of Amphibians and Reptiles*, Springer ,New York, NY, pp. 11–53.

Souza, S.O.D., Casagrande, R.A., Guerra, P.R. *et al.* (2014) Osteomyelitis caused by Salmonella enterica serovar derby in boa constrictor. *Journal of Zoo and Wildlife Medicine*, 45 (3), 642–644.

26

Diseases of the Organs of Special Senses
Alex Rosenwax and Tegan Stephens

Anatomy and Physiology

See Chapter 2 for further information on the anatomy and physiology of the organs of special senses.

Key Points

- The eyelids of all snakes and some geckos and lizards are fused and translucent, forming the spectacle. They are dermal in origin.

- Poor development of the rectus muscles means the movement of the eye in all reptiles, except chameleons, is limited.
- Chelonia do not have nasolacrimal ducts
- Reptiles are relatively resistant to the effects of mydriatics.
- Reptiles have an avascular retina.

The Eye

Physical Examination

There are many variations in the placement of reptilian eyes, making it difficult to determine whether the eye position is abnormal. The ophthalmic examination should begin with an assessment of the symmetry of the eyes to determine whether there is exophthalmos, enophthalmos or any swelling of either the eyes or the eyelids.

Ancillary Tests

The Schirmer tear test can be used to measure tear production in reptiles that do not have spectacles. Normal values are not known for many species. Samples may need to be taken from similar healthy species as an indication of normal tear production levels.

Fluorescein staining is useful for assessing corneal ulcers and nasolacrimal duct patency. In species with spectacles, the fluorescein must be injected through the spectacle, into the subspectacular space with a 27-gauge needle, while taking care to avoid damaging the cornea. In turtles, the absence of nasolacrimal duct leads to the fluorescein dye simply trickling down the side of the face.

Conventional mydriatics such as atropine and tropicamide are ineffective in reptiles, as the ciliary body muscles are mainly smooth muscle, preventing the parasympatholytic effect on pupillary dilation. Local anaesthetic drops can be used to assist in opening eyelids closed due to a response to pain.

Reptile Medicine and Surgery in Clinical Practice, First Edition. Edited by Bob Doneley, Deborah Monks, Robert Johnson and Brendan Carmel.
© 2018 John Wiley & Sons Ltd. Published 2018 by John Wiley & Sons Ltd.

Special Ophthalmic Instrument Examination

Many of the ophthalmic instruments used in mammals can be used in reptiles, with some modifications. A brief examination with a focal light source will establish if there is any cloudiness of the cornea or any adnexal problems. Pupillary light response is however not considered reliable, as the presence of striated muscle in the reptilian eye interferes with the autonomic control and can affect the pupillary light reflex. Reptiles also do not have consensual light reflex.

Magnification, and especially the use of a slit lamp (Figure 26.1), is essential to avoid missing subtle changes when examining the small reptilian eye. The slit lamp is also necessary to define subspectacular space, corneal depth and the anterior chamber. Magnification for fundoscopy is best performed in the nondilated eye with a panophthalmoscope or, if this is not available, with a 90-dioptre lens.

Tonometry can be performed on the eyes without anaesthesia. In animals without spectacles, both applanation and rebound tonometry have been used. Rebound tonometry is considered to be more precise in larger reptiles (Table 26.1) with neither method appearing to be precise in reptiles weighing less than 100 grams.

Table 26.1 Mean values for intraocular pressure in reptiles, using rebound tonometry.

Species	Pressure (mmHg)
Red-eared sliders (*Trachemys scripta elegans*)	6.1
Yellow-footed tortoise (*Chelonoidis denticulata*)	14.2
Bearded dragon (*Pogona vitticeps*)	6.16
Hermann's tortoises (*Testudo hermanni*)	15.74
Andros island iguana (*Cyclura cychlura cychlura*)	4.77–5.12

Ultrasound is used to determine the boundaries and constituents of periocular masses and to define fluid-filled areas in the subspectacular space.

Diseases of the Eye

Spectacle Disorders

The spectacle covers the eye and is formed from the fusion of transparent cells of the eyelids. Spectacles are found in all snakes, many geckos, *Pygopodidae* (legless lizards) and *Xantusiidae* (night lizard). Being of

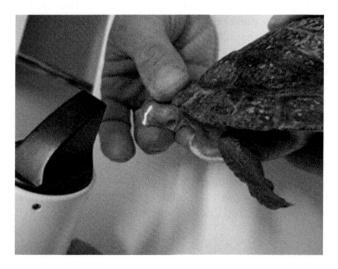

Figure 26.1 Murray river short-necked turtle (*Emydura macquarii macquarii*) eye examination with a slit lamp.

Figure 26.2 Python with retained spectacle.

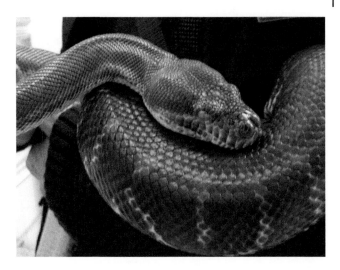

dermal origin, the spectacle is shed as part of the skin during ecdysis. It is not attached to the cornea and is separated from the cornea by the subspectacular space. Spectacles will usually become opaque prior to shedding; this is not a cause for concern and the spectacle will be shed with the skin. The spectacle may also appear slightly indented in snakes; this is normal and will generally resolve with the next shed.

Retained Spectacles

Retained spectacles are related to dysecdysis in snakes (see Chapter 18). The problem is most commonly related to dehydration, poor environmental conditions, poor nutrition and systemic disease. Scarring or trauma of the spectacle as well as any primary or secondary disease affecting the skin, such as mites, may lead to retained spectacles. Retained spectacles, especially in recurrent cases, may temporarily affect vision as the opaque skin debris builds up over the spectacle. This build-up of debris may also lead to secondary infection of the spectacle.

Diagnosis is relatively simple if examination of the snake's sloughed skin fails to find that the spectacle has been shed. It is not uncommon for clients to fail to realise there has been an incomplete shed and, as a consequence, they have not kept the sloughed skin for later examination. These snakes may present with a partial shed of the head, with the eyes appearing opaque. When multiple unshed layers are present, the opaque dried non-translucent spectacle is obvious (Figure 26.2). However, when only one extra layer of spectacle skin is present, after the rest of the cranial skin has sloughed, a slit lamp may be required to identify this thin extra layer.

To remove retained spectacles, soak the area with a moist cotton swab and then gently rub from the medial to lateral canthi with a moist cotton tip. If this fails to remove the retained tissue, add artificial tears five times daily to soften the spectacle and increase the enclosure's humidity before attempting removal of the retained spectacle with a cotton swab one to seven days later. Avoid using forceps to forcibly remove the retained spectacle as this can damage (Figure 26.3) or remove the healthy new underlying spectacle, leading to exposure keratitis.

Subspectacular Abscess

Infection may occur in the subspectacular space from penetrating spectacular wounds or bacteraemia, or via the nasolacrimal ducts. Subspectacular infections are usually bacterial

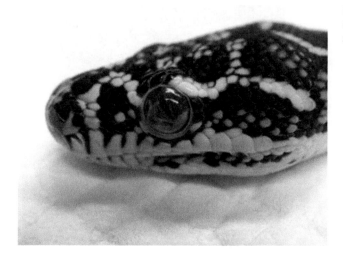

Figure 26.3 Indented spectacle, diamond python (*Morelia spilota spilota*).

or occasionally fungal in origin. Subspectacular nematodiasis has also been seen in ball pythons (*Python regius*).

Clinically, the spectacle will appear cloudy and discoloured, and may be distorted or distended and may appear similar to a blocked nasolacrimal duct. The two conditions can be differentiated by injecting fluorescein through the spectacle. The dye will drain into the choana and nares if the nasolacrimal duct is not blocked.

Treatment involves surgically removing a very small wedge section from the spectacle under general anaesthesia and flushing out the area with saline. Antibiotic eye drops (without corticosteroids) can then be applied into the eye via the resected wedge of the spectacle. A culture and sensitivity test can be used to determine appropriate antibiotics. Systemic antibiotics are often warranted unless unilateral localized trauma can be confirmed. Management as per traumatic spectacle loss is also necessary to avoid development of exposure keratitis.

Loss of Spectacle

The loss of a spectacle is most commonly related to iatrogenic trauma during attempts to remove retained spectacles. Infection, trauma, abrasion and bites by prey species (from the feeding of live rodents or cricket bites) can also cause spectacle trauma. The loss of a spectacle leads to the evaporation of the tear film and desiccation of the cornea. This may give the appearance of enophthalmos. Partial loss will lead to signs equivalent to epiphora, as the tears overflow through the traumatized area.

Treatment for complete spectacle loss includes topical antibiotics and commercial 'artificial tears' solutions applied regularly. Cut-down soft contact lenses, collagen grafts and oral mucosal flaps have been suggested as protective treatments for partial and total spectacle loss. As long-term resolution is difficult, enucleation may be necessary.

Eyelids

Tumours

Melanomas have been diagnosed on the eyelids of bearded dragons (*Pogona* spp.), related to artificial ultraviolet lights being in too close proximity (less than 30 cm) to the enclosure's basking area. These tumours may be amelanotic melanomas. Many other tumours have been seen on the eyelids of lizards and dragons, including squamous cell carcinomas and myxosarcomas. Viral fibropapillomatous tumours have also been reported in green sea turtles (*Chelonia mydas*).

Trauma

Eyelid trauma is often related to fighting in short neck turtles (*Emydura* spp.), red-eared sliders (*Trachemys scripta elegans*) and occasionally bearded dragons (*Pogona vitticeps*). Simple wounds will need cleaning with povidone-iodine. Only substantial wounds will require surgical intervention. Occasional more serious untreated cases will require systemic and/or topical ophthalmic antibiotics.

Swollen Eyelids and Associated Blepharospasm

Blepharoedema may be related to primary infectious agents, environmental irritants and Vitamin A deficiency. In reptiles with hypovitaminosis A, squamous metaplasia of the orbital glands and ducts develops, leading to xerophthalmia followed by a secondary blepharitis and conjunctivitis. Opportunistic bacteria can then invade. Diagnosis is made on clinical signs of swollen eyelids combined with dietary history of low vitamin A intake. Treatment for vitamin A deficiency may involve dietary or injectable supplementation, taking care to avoid iatrogenic hypervitaminosis A. Any primary or secondary infections will require systemic and topical antibiotics.

Periocular Area

Masses in the periocular region are usually found to be abscesses, although neoplastic lesions are also commonly encountered. Associated tissue swelling and exophthalmos

can easily be mistaken for periocular neoplasia. Melanomas, squamous cell carcinomas and adenocarcinomas have been seen in many reptile species, especially bearded dragons (*Pogona* spp.), often related to the basking area being too close (less than 30 cm) to the ultraviolet lights. A lacrimal cystadenoma in a Chinese box turtle (*Cuora flavomarginata*) and a myxosarcoma in a bearded dragon have also been reported to have caused periocular neoplasia and swelling.

Aspiration of the lesion for diagnosis may be unrewarding, as the caseous pus cannot easily be withdrawn through a needle. Ultrasound can be used to differentiate larger abscesses from neoplastic lesions. Surgery is then generally indicated to remove the caseous pus and determine whether neoplasia is involved. There are no bacterial infections specific to this area. Antibiotic coverage should be broad spectrum, including activity against anaerobes and *Pseudomonas* species until culture and sensitivity results are received.

Conjunctiva

Bacterial conjunctivitis is usually secondary to poor husbandry conditions. The eyelids are often semi-closed with dried caseous plaques (Figure 26.4) forming under or on the eyelids and within the conjunctival fornix. Infections may spread to cause

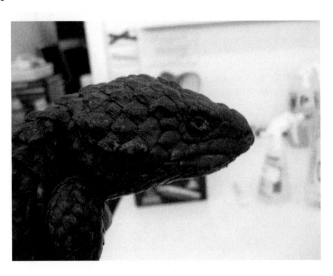

Figure 26.4 Shingleback lizard (*Tiliqua rugosa*) with conjunctivitis.

panophthalmitis and eventually septicaemia. Treatment involves removing plaques, flushing the eyes with sterile saline and the use of topical or systemic antibiotics against Gram-negative bacteria including *Pseudomonas* or *Aeromonas* species, as well as improving the predisposing husbandry issues.

Viral conjunctivitis (notably herpesvirus fibropapillomas in green sea turtles) has been recorded and is most likely to be diagnosed on biopsy samples. Parasites, including *Neophystoma* in a chelonian and *Chlamydia* in a case of conjunctivitis in a tortoise, have also been seen. In cases of unresolved conjunctivitis, a biopsy is required for diagnosis.

Foreign-body conjunctivitis may be related to the use of substrates such as corn husks, hay or sand. Treatment involves removal of the foreign body either under general anaesthesia or with the assistance of local anaesthetic ophthalmic drops. Antibiotics may be needed if secondary bacterial infection is present.

In all cases of conjunctivitis it is best to place non-aquatic species on plain sheets of paper or similar substrates to avoid foreign body conjunctivitis forming from small particles of the substrate adhering to the dried pus.

Nasolacrimal Duct

Nasolacrimal Duct Blockage

The nasolacrimal duct performs a similar function in reptiles as it does in all species, with the duct being absent in *Chelonia* species. In all reptiles without spectacles, blockage of or absence of the duct leads to epiphora. Nasolacrimal duct blockage is caused by ulcerative stomatitis, oral or nasal neoplasia, cranial granulomas, oral burns and scarring, cysts, as well as congenital blockage. The duct in any reptile may be closed by dacryocystitis. Abscessation and occlusion of the duct be may result from ascending oral bacteria or fungal infections, systemic infections as well as penetrating injuries to the spectacle in snakes. In reptiles without spectacles (most non-snakes), this will often be seen as a purulent discharge from the eyes.

Bullous Spectaculopathy (Pseudobuphthalmos)

In snakes with blocked nasolacrimal ducts, the spectacle does not allow excess tears to be shed externally. The excess clear fluid instead accumulates in the subspectacular space, resulting in a bulging of the spectacle (Figure 26.5). For diagnosis, a slit lamp can be

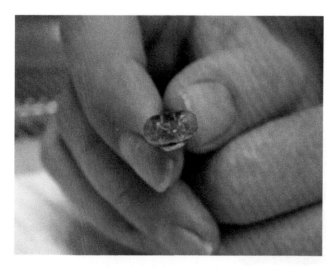

Figure 26.5 Nasolacrimal duct atresia in a juvenile eastern brown snake (*Pseudonaja textilis*).

used to demonstrate the increased distance between cornea and spectacle. Fluorescein staining can be used to investigate the lack of patency of the nasolacrimal duct. In snakes, this involves injecting fluorescein through the lateral canthus of the spectacle into the subspectacular space and observing whether the coloured dye drains out of the subspectacular space.

Temporary relief in chronic blockage cases can be achieved by cutting a small wedge section from the spectacle to allow drainage from the inferior quadrant of the eye. Another temporary treatment involves retrograde flushing of the duct with a 27-gauge cannula. However, blockage will often recur with these temporary methods. The continued blockage will lead to infection of the eye and pressure related pain. For a more permanent solution, surgical reconstruction of the duct has been advocated. However the long term prognosis post-surgery is unknown.

Cornea

Keratoconjunctivitis Sicca

Keratoconjunctivitis sicca has a similar presentation and aetiology as per all taxa and is related to poor tear production. Vitamin A deficiency may also be a predisposing cause. The dry eyes lead to metaplasia of the conjunctiva and corneal epithelium. Diagnosis is performed with a Schirmer tear test and treatment involves the regular and frequent use of 'artificial tears'. While taking care to avoid iatrogenic hypervitaminosis A, weekly vitamin A injections have also been advocated for four to six weeks.

Keratitis

White corneal masses from bacterial and fungal keratitis have been seen in tortoises and viral herpes papillomatous proliferative corneal lesions have been seen in green sea turtles. Fungal infections involving aspergillus have reported in tortoises. Bacterial infections are mostly caused by *Pseudomonas* and *Aeromonas* species. The raised corneal lesions should be removed under general anaesthesia, combined with concurrent use of local anaesthetic eye drops. Use a 25- or 27-gauge needle to elevate and pry the raised lesion off the cornea. Microscopic examination for fungi and bacteria should be performed immediately and the sample then sent for bacterial culture and sensitivity. Enrofloxacin eye drops can be used for Gram-negative bacterial infections and miconazole used topically for fungal infections prior to receiving the culture and sensitivity results.

Corneal Ulcers

Ulceration of the cornea is commonly caused by foreign body trauma, often related to the use of inappropriate substrate. It may also be related to intraspecies fighting or be secondary to keratoconjunctivitis sicca. Healed ulcers in reptiles may present with white scarring or slightly elevated areas of the cornea. In snakes, trauma to the spectacle should not be confused with corneal ulceration, as the spectacle is part of the dermis and is not part of the cornea. Diagnosis is made on positive fluorescein dye uptake. Full-thickness lacerations can be repaired with 8/0 or 10/0 sutures, preferably using an operating microscope. For minor ulcers, apply enrofloxacin eye drops. In addition, systemic antibiotics and nonsteroidal anti-inflammatory drugs should be prescribed for deep ulcers and lacerations. In cases of ulceration, remove any small particulate matter and, where possible, use plain paper or an equivalent non-irritant substrate until the lesion has healed.

Glaucoma

Glaucoma has rarely been reported in reptiles. Secondary glaucoma in reptiles has been seem with traumatic panophthalmitis (Figure 26.6). However, as normal intraocular pressure values for many species of reptiles are now becoming available, diagnosis of glaucoma is likely to become more common. When normal values are not available for a reptilian species, assess for glaucoma by measuring contralateral eye pressure or a similar species cage mates' intraocular pressure

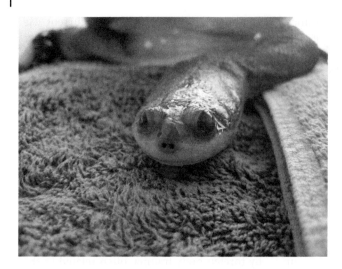

Figure 26.6 Eastern long-necked turtle (*Chelodina longicollis*) with unilateral panophthalmitis buphthalmos following trauma. The lens and anterior chamber are opaque.

values. The accuracy of intraocular pressure values in smaller reptiles have been affected by the inability to collect repeatable pressure results.

Lens

Cataract development is seen in aged reptiles and is assumed to have a similar aetiology to other taxa. Freezing during brumation has been associated with cataract formation in turtles and may be related to the softer fluid-like lenses of reptiles. Exposure to ultraviolet light has also been suggested to be a cause of cataracts. However, no direct links have yet been found between close proximity to ultraviolet lights and cataracts. The relatively soft lens has allowed successful treatment of cataracts in larger reptiles with phacoemulsification. In snakes, any cataract surgery also requires an incision through the spectacle.

Retina

When examining the reptilian retina, it is important to keep in mind that it is avascular. Blood supply is via the choriocapillaries. Reptiles are assumed to suffer similar retinal issues as per all veterinary patients, although these have rarely been reported in the literature.

Uvea

Uveitis in reptiles may be fungal, bacterial or viral. The infection can be local (often following trauma) or systemic in origin. When hypopyon is present, it is generally considered to be systemic in origin and a result of septicaemia. Freezing at brumation has also been associated with hyphaema and hypopyon in Chelonia. Blood tests for biochemistry, haematology and blood cultures should therefore be considered in cases of hypopyon. The treatment of uveitis requires the combined use of systemic nonsteroidal anti-inflammatories and antibiotics that cover for at minimum *Klebsiella* and *Pseudomonas* species.

Eye Shape and Position

Exophthalmos

Exophthalmos is caused by retrobulbar swellings or masses. The most common cause of exophthalmos is abscessation. Owing to the granulomatous nature of reptile abscesses, paracentesis may not always easily distinguish abscess from neoplasia. An aneurism in the retrobulbar vein following trauma has been reported as a cause of exophthalmos and a bearded dragon was reported to have exophthalmos and blepharoedema associated with congestive heart failure. Ultrasound can be used to determine the nature of the lesion but surgery is required for diagnosis and treatment. In snakes, exophthalmos needs to be distinguished from pseudobuphthalmos using either a slit lamp or ultrasound.

Enophthalmos

Enophthalmos is more commonly caused by emaciation and severe dehydration. Trauma may also give the appearance of enophthalmos and microphthalmia. Initial treatment involves an assessment for signs of dehydration and then, if necessary, rehydration of the reptile to see if the enophthalmos resolves.

Microphthalmia

Congenital microphthalmia has been reported in clutches of snakes. Suspected causes include genetics, incubation temperature and humidity with possible nutritional factors. It has been reported in red rattle snakes (*Crotalus ruber*) as well as Burmese (*Python bivittatus*) and ball pythons (*Python regius*). Presumptive anophthalmia has been used to determine whether a true anophthalmia is present or simply microphthalmia with scales covering the eye.

The Ear

Aural Abscesses

Aural abscesses are found in chelonians and occasionally lizards. Chelonians do not have an external ear. Instead, they have a superficial tympanic membrane and, medial to this, a relatively large tympanic cavity with a medial blind-ended sac. Abscesses in chelonians are generally formed from exogenous bacteria invading and colonizing the tympanic cavity of the middle ear. Abscesses are rare in snakes and lizards because, unlike turtles, they do not have a tympanic cavity.

The predisposition to aural infection appears to be related to poor husbandry and the subsequent invasion of opportunistic infections. The problem usually involves below preferred optimal temperature zone conditions for extended periods combined with poor nutrition and unsanitary conditions. When water is not changed regularly, there will be a build-up of faeces, with subsequent increased nitrates in the water, resulting in bacterial overgrowth in the pond or aquarium. This issue, combined with poor nutrition from inappropriate diets including poorly formulated commercial turtle dinner and pellets, will affect the immune system of the turtles. Dietary issues are especially common when commercial diets formulated for vegetarian turtles are fed to omnivorous turtles (such as Australian short-necked turtles, *Emydura* spp.) or carnivorous turtles (Australian long-necked turtles, *Chelodina longicollis*). Vitamin A deficiency has long been suspected of being the theoretical underlying cause of aural abscesses in vegetarian chelonians. Vitamin A deficiency will lead to squamous metaplasia within the middle ear and Eustachian tube. This results in swelling of cells in the tympanic cavity and the blockage of the cavity with dried exudate and exfoliated cells. The high bacterial load in water with high nitrate levels will overwhelm the already deficient immune system, allowing colonization of bacteria in the blind-ended tympanic cavity.

The poor blood supply to the centre of this lesion means antibiotics are unlikely to be effective. Bacterial infections in reptiles lead to a granulomatous reaction forming a semidried caseous pus that cannot easily drain out of the very short medial ear canal. This forms a hard dried often yellow-covered plug under the skin in the area of the ear and may have the initial appearance of a neoplastic lesion (Figure 26.7).

Diagnosis is made on the appearance and location of the lesion. Owing to the granulomatous nature of the lesions, paracentesis of the lesion is not likely to be rewarding and may simply lead to haemorrhage from the

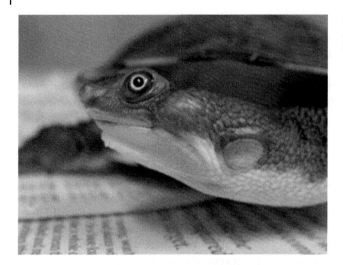

Figure 26.7 Swelling associated with an aural abscess in a turtle (courtesy of Bob Doneley).

needle insertion point. Water quality should be tested, using a sample collected from the turtle's normal enclosure, for pH, ammonia, nitrite and especially nitrate. A complete history of the diet, water changes, and water and air temperature should also be collected.

Treatment involves surgical incision. Before surgery, it is important to warm the patient to the correct optimal temperature and allow time for the antibiotic therapy to be effective. As it is assumed that aural abscesses are secondary to multiple husbandry issues, other organ or systems failure should be investigated before anaesthesia. Fluid therapy is also advised. Antibiotics, prior to culture and sensitivity of samples taken at surgery, should cover for both the water-borne bacteria *Aeromonas* spp. and for the anaerobes likely to be present within an abscess. Vitamin A injections may also be considered in susceptible species, while, taking care to avoid iatrogenic hypervitaminosis A.

Surgery involves the incision, shelling out and debridement of the lesion. Samples should be collected for culture and sensitivity. The area should be lavaged with dilute chlorhexidine and then packed with silver sulfadiazine, antibiotic-impregnated poloxamer-407 gel or at minimum with an steroid-free antibiotic ophthalmic ointment. Depending on the depth size and ability to effectively debride the wound, the area will need to be cleaned and repacked every one to three days. If it is possible to form an effective plug with poloxamer-407 gel, the area is more likely to require changing only every three days. Systemic antibiotics may not be effective in these localized lesions prior to surgery. However, once the wound has been debrided and inflamed, antibiotic therapy based on culture and sensitivity should be more effective.

The type of recovery enclosure will depend on the species. For turtle species that often spend long periods basking out of water, dry docking or dry docking with daily swims prior to wound cleaning are appropriate. For semi-aquatic or aquatic species dry docking for one to three hours once to twice daily may be more appropriate. Prevention includes regular water-quality testing and water changes, temperature regulation and dietary modification. Vitamin A injections may also be required until dietary changes are fully instituted. Initial success rate of treatment is high but abscess recurrence may also be seen.

Jacobson's Organ (Vomeronasal Organ)

The vomeronasal organ is an olfactory structure found on the roof of the mouth or choana of some reptiles. It detects pheromones and environmental cues. The organ is best developed in snakes and varanid lizards. In snakes and varanids, the flicking of the tongue brings air particles into direct contact with the organ. Any damage to the vomero-nasal system through trauma or oral infection may affect both mating behaviour and prey recognition, leading to possible anorexia. Studies on garter snakes with partial and full removal of the organ showed they could not follow prey trails and failed to display courtship behaviour.

Heat-Sensitive Receptors or Pit Organs

The heat pit sensors are found on some Boidae, Pythonidae (except womas and black-headed pythons, *Aspidites* spp.) and the *Crotalinae* (pit vipers). These heat sensors allow the snakes to make a visual picture using the infrared spectrum. This improves vision, as the snake can add infrared heat vision to their standard vision from their eyes. These 'infrared eyes' are termed 'pit organs' or simply 'pits' because they take the form of deep depressions in the skin of the head. The pit organs of Boidae (boas) and Pythonidae (pythons) are located in the rostral and labial scales. There may be 3–20 pits on each side, depending on the species. In some species of Boidae, the pits are not apparent but the sensors are still present. On clinical examination, the pits should be examined for mites, ticks, retained skin and fungus.

The ability to 'see' heat has been suggested as one of the causes of clients being bitten when feeding cold mice or rats to a snake, as the snake mistakes the client's heat for the prey.

Vestibular disease

The typical signs of vestibular disease in reptiles, including head tilt, rolling and twisting of the neck, may be caused by either central nervous system lesions or inner ear problems. Generalized systemic conditions often imitate the signs of vestibular disease (e.g. hypocalcaemia tetany and organophosphate toxicity). Viral infections affecting the nervous system (adenovirus in *Pogona* spp., inclusion body virus in pythons and paramyxovirus in snakes) as well as weakness from metabolic and musculoskeletal disease, will also mimic the signs of vestibular disease. If discrete cranial lesions are present, the head tilt or roll is usually to the side of the cranial lesion. Strabismus has been reported in reptiles with vestibular disease but nystagmus has rarely been seen.

If vestibular disease is suspected, it is best to initially rule out problems that may imitate vestibular disease. A detailed history is important including dietary calcium supplementation, enclosure temperature, appropriate exposure to ultraviolet light and any use of insecticides. If other generalized signs are present, including weight loss, anorexia and respiratory signs, it is also less likely to be a discrete cranial lesion. While flaccid paralysis or dyspnoea may suggest a generalized systemic condition rather than cranial vestibular disease. Samples should then be collected for PCR for viral infections, biochemistry for underlying systemic illness and bacterial blood cultures. Prognosis is more favourable in cases of nonviral systemic diseases that are imitating the signs of vestibular disease.

Further Reading

Brown, J.D., Richards, J.M., Robertson, J. *et al.* (2004). Pathology of aural abscesses in free-living eastern box turtles (*Terrapene carolina carolina*). *Journal of Wildlife Diseases*, 40 (4), 704–712.

Da Silva, M.A., Bertelsen, M.F., Wang, T. *et al.* (2015) Unilateral microphthalmia or anophthalmia in eight pythons (Pythonidae). *Veterinary Ophthalmology*, 18 (Suppl 1), 23–29.

Goris, R.C. (2011) Infrared organs of snakes: an integral part of vision. *Journal of Herpetology*, 45 (1), 2–14.

Hausmann, J.C., Hollingsworth, S.R., Hawkins, M.G. *et al.* (2013) Distribution and outcome of ocular lesions in snakes examined at a veterinary teaching hospital: 67 cases (1985–2010). *Journal of the American Veterinary Medical Association*, 243 (2), 252–260.

Labelle, A.L., Steele, K.A., Breaux, C.B. *et al.* (2012).Tonometry and corneal aesthesiometry in the red-eared slider turtle (*Trachemys scripta elegans*). *Journal of Herpetological Medicine and Surgery*, 22, 30–35.

Lawton, M. (2005) Reptilian ophthalmology, in *Reptile Medicine and Surgery* (S.J. Divers and D.R. Mader, eds). Elsevier Health Sciences, St Louis, MO, pp. 323–342.

Myers, G., Webb, T., Corbett, C.R. *et al.* (2011) Phacoemulsification for removal of bilateral cataracts in a black water monitor (*Varanus salvator macromaculatus*). *Journal of Herpetological Medicine and Surgery*, 21 (4), 96–100.

William, D.L. (2012) The reptilian eye, in *Ophthalmology of Exotic Pets* (David L. Williams, ed.). John Wiley & Sons, Ltd, Chichester, pp. 159–196.

27

Analgesia and Anaesthesia

Annabelle Olsson and Mark Simpson

Introduction

The general principles and analgesic and anaesthetic agents available to the general practitioner for more traditional patients are generally applicable to reptiles. Reptiles constitute an entire class of animals, for many of which there is scant quality evidence to guide analgesic or anaesthetic protocols. Practitioners should be aware of the significant differences in physiology and anatomy that may influence analgesia and anaesthesia in reptiles. Chief among these is ectothermy and its close relationship with metabolic rate. Reptiles should be maintained at the upper end of their preferred body temperature range throughout anaesthesia to properly metabolize anaesthetic agents.

Physiology

Various factors affect metabolic rate, the most influential being temperature. As temperature decreases, oxygen demand and metabolic requirements of tissues decrease, leading to increases in both the latency of onset and duration of effect of anaesthetic agent and time to recovery. Many reptiles can convert to anaerobic metabolism when placed in an oxygen deficient environment. This adaptive mechanism can make it impossible to induce anaesthesia with inhalation agents in some species, as they perceive the unfamiliar gaseous agent and become apnoeic, converting to anaerobic metabolism. Artificial ventilation, which mimics the frequency and depth of respiration in a conscious reptile, is essential to effectively manage an anaesthetized patient and help to combat hypoxia and hypercapnia.

The control of respiration in reptiles is more complex than in mammals. Both carbon dioxide and pH changes appear important for stimulating normal ventilation but there is evidence that, even under normoxic conditions, oxygen tension may play a role in normal ventilation. Generally, reptile respiration is an episodic pattern, with cycles of two or three rapid breaths followed by a longer pause. The respiration rate depends on the size of the animal, decreasing with increasing body mass. Ambient temperature has variable effects on the frequency, tidal volume and minute ventilation and due consideration should be given to maintaining the optimal temperature for a particular species.

The response of reptiles to inspired carbon dioxide is quite variable, as is the response to 100% oxygen. During anaesthesia, most reptiles are maintained with an inhalant anaesthetic delivered in 100% oxygen. High inspired oxygen may be responsible for some of the respiratory depression seen during gaseous anaesthesia. Reptiles appear to recover faster from isoflurane anaesthesia

Reptile Medicine and Surgery in Clinical Practice, First Edition. Edited by Bob Doneley, Deborah Monks, Robert Johnson and Brendan Carmel.
© 2018 John Wiley & Sons Ltd. Published 2018 by John Wiley & Sons Ltd.

if the animal is ventilated with room air rather than 100% oxygen.

While injectable anaesthetics generally have a long duration of action, with anaesthetic depth not changing rapidly or unexpectedly, depth and duration of gaseous anaesthesia are dependent on the rate of intermittent positive pressure ventilation (IPPV) and the concentration of gas delivered.

During anaesthesia, cardiac shunting can affect systemic arterial oxygen content and the uptake and elimination of inhaled anaesthetics. The size and direction of the shunts are ultimately controlled by pressure differences between the pulmonary and systemic circuits and washout of blood remaining in the vena cava. Changes in the level and direction of the shunts may account for the unexpected awakening seen in some reptiles anaesthetized with inhalant anaesthetics, emphasising the importance of careful monitoring of anaesthesia. Intracardiac shunts also have implications for patient monitoring, in particular airway gas monitoring and pulse oximetry. Post-anaesthetic monitoring is also critical in all reptiles since 'regression' apnoea can occur if animals are left unstimulated following administration of central nervous system depressants.

Although there is debate in the literature over the importance of the renal portal system on uptake, distribution and metabolism of drugs in reptiles, the system exists and it is therefore recommended that anaesthetic or sedative drugs be injected into the cranial half of the body.

As well as physiological features, there are anatomic idiosyncrasies among reptiles that especially influence the management of certain aspects of anaesthesia in those reptiles. Muscle relaxants, including most immobilization agents, interfere with the reflex closure of both the glottal and palatal valves in crocodilians. It is therefore important to be prepared to maintain the patency of the glottis by early placement of an endotracheal tube in crocodilians.

Intravenous Access

Intravenous administration of anaesthetic agents is the preferred choice. A sound knowledge of vascular anatomy is critical to effective venepuncture because it is frequently a blind technique (see Chapter 13). Added to this, many patients are very small and their veins can be extremely fragile and difficult to access. Aseptic preparation of the site is recommended to minimize the risk of infection or other complications.

Venepuncture in Snakes

Two commonly accessed sites in snakes are the ventral tail or coccygeal vein and the heart. The tail vein is accessed caudal to the cloaca, taking care to avoid hemipenal or hemiclitoral pockets. The needle is inserted 25–50% of the way down the tail on the midline. The needle is inserted between the scales, at an angle of 45–60%, and is advanced craniodorsally until it is inserted between the vertebrae.

Cardiac puncture requires excellent restraint, preferably with sedation or anaesthesia, to minimize the risk of significant cardiac trauma. The heart is located approximately 25–33% of the distance from snout to vent and is stabilized with one hand for ease of entry. The needle is introduced at 45% in a craniodorsal direction into the apex of the beating ventricle. Digital pressure for up to one minute following venepuncture is advised. It is reportedly safe for snakes from hatchlings to 150 kg and lymphatic contamination is less likely than with venepuncture.

Venepuncture in Lizards

The caudal tail vein is the venepuncture site of choice in most lizard species (Figure 27.1) and can be approached in a similar manner to snakes. An alternative approach is from the lateral aspect, inserting the needle at 45–90% in a craniomedial direction, just ventral to the coccygeal vertebrae. Lymphatic contamination is more likely with this approach. Other sites, such as the ventral abdominal,

Figure 27.1 The ventral coccygeal vein is an ideal route of administration for injectable induction agents for squamates such as this eastern blue-tongued lizard (*Tiliqua scincoides*).

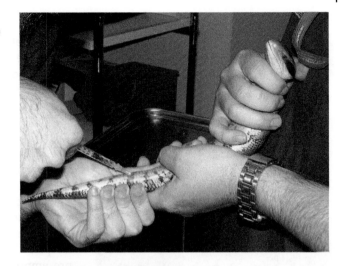

Figure 27.2 The jugular vein is reliably accessed immediately dorsal to the line of colour change on the neck in Australian long-necked turtles (*Chelodina* spp.).

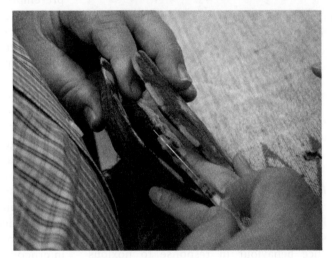

jugular vein and heart, are potentially useful but more difficult for the inexperienced clinician to access.

Venepuncture in Turtles

A variety of veins are accessible in most chelonian species. The most common site is the dorsal tail vein, accessed along the dorsal midline as cranially as possible. The technique is similar to that used in other reptiles. In long-necked turtle species, the jugular is accessible even in the conscious animal (Figure 27.2). The dorsal occipital sinus is relatively easily accessed in turtles but lymphoid contamination may occur.

In freshwater turtles, the sinus is accessed with the head flexed and the needle inserted just lateral to the dorsal midline. In marine turtles a more lateral approach is recommended.

Venepuncture in Crocodiles

In small crocodilians, the ventral and lateral tail veins can be accessed, as for lizards and chelonians. The dorsal occipital sinus is the venepuncture site of choice in larger crocodilians (Figure 27.3). While a midline approach is most commonly used, a paravertebral approach is also possible. Lymphatic contamination is possible at all sites.

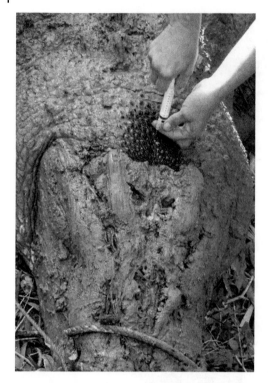

Figure 27.3 The dorsal occipital sinus is the venepuncture site of choice in larger crocodilians.

It is very important to note that an absence of clinical signs attributable to pain is not evidence of an absence of pain. Clinicians can reasonably assume that interventions likely to cause pain will do so in reptiles and can be treated accordingly.

Analgesia

Reptiles possess an endogenous opioid system. They are observed to display avoidance behaviour in response to noxious stimuli that is obtunded by administration of opioids. It is highly likely that pain perception in reptiles is analogous to that of mammals. There is, however, scant published evidence on pain and pain management in reptiles and many current practices may be altered as more evidence is established.

To manage pain effectively, it is first important to understand normal behaviour, to enable correct interpretation of changes associated with pain. Signs of pain can include resting in an abnormal or hunched position, restlessness, abnormal gait, increased respiratory rate and effort, aggression and anorexia.

The stress associated with pain responses can affect immune function, haematological and serum biochemical parameters and metabolic processes. Acute pain (surgery, trauma, acute infections) should be differentiated from chronic pain (arthritis, neoplasia). Acute pain is best managed pre-emptively, typically with potent analgesics such as mu-opioid agonists with demonstrated effect in the target species. There is currently very little evidence, from the few species studied so far, to support the use of the mixed agonist and antagonist opioids butorphanol or buprenorphine as analgesics in reptiles.

Most recent studies have indicated that much higher doses of mu-receptor opiate agonists are required to provide effective analgesia for acute pain (see Appendix 1). High doses can also lead to respiratory depression which can be critical in debilitated patients so caution should be exercised. Morphine is an effective analgesic in crocodilians, lizards and turtles, but in snakes the evidence is currently equivocal. Some initial research suggests fentanyl patches may be a useful analgesic modality in snakes. Methadone is metabolized to the same active opiate molecule as morphine, and anecdotal reports support extrapolation of its use for analgesia in lizards and turtles. Tramadol has recently been discussed as a suitable analgesic for reptiles. It is a weak mu-agonist with the advantage of minimal respiratory depression, at least in chelonians. There is some controversy about how effective tramadol is as an analgesic, and more study is required to confirm its role in analgesia for reptiles.

Any discussion of the use of opiates as analgesic agents in reptiles must conclude with the caveat that there is very little published evidence to guide our clinical decisions, and as that becomes available, some of the recommendations made herein may be reviewed.

Local anaesthesia is indicated for minor surgical procedures, such as skin laceration repair or abscess removal or as an adjunct to general anaesthesia for larger procedures. Lignocaine has a fast onset of action for topical or short-term analgesia, whereas bupivacaine has a longer duration of action for postoperative pain management.

Nonsteroidal Anti-Inflammatory Analgesia for Chronic Pain Management

There is limited information regarding the effectiveness of analgesia for chronic pain management in reptiles. Nonsteroidal anti-inflammatory drugs (NSAIDs) such as meloxicam appear to provide some degree of prolonged analgesia in all species of reptiles. Ketoprofen and carprofen (see Appendix 1) have also been used with some success. NSAIDs should be used with caution in animals suffering from dehydration, renal insufficiency or gastrointestinal disease.

Given the lack of published data for analgesic dose rates in reptiles, difficulty in assessing pain, and the likely high incidence of debilitation in painful patients, multimodal analgesia (where pain is treated with different modalities working at different levels of the sensory pathways) is likely to be the most successful strategy available to clinicians. Opioids given in conjunction with NSAIDs may be effective. Consideration should also be given to nonpharmacological interventions, such as splinting traumatized limbs or even the provision of suitable hides or refuges within enclosures to limit movement, which can considerably alter the development of pain.

Patient Assessment and Preparation for Anaesthesia

A detailed history, comprising medical aspects, as well as general husbandry and nutrition, is critical, since many health issues that impact on anaesthesia are the consequence of inappropriate husbandry or nutrition. A thorough physical examination, including a current body weight, is essential prior to anaesthesia. Physical examination should focus on the cardiopulmonary system (most effectively using a Doppler to record heart rate) and any signs of pathology. In particular, assessment of the rate and depth of ventilation can be crucial to anticipating and then identifying and correcting respiratory problems during anaesthesia. Pathological conditions such as a coelomic mass or ovarian follicular stasis can compromise ventilation and can therefore complicate anaesthesia. Since clinical signs of disease may not be readily apparent, a preanaesthesia complete blood count and plasma biochemistry profile is recommended. At a minimum, a blood sample should be collected to provide haematocrit, blood glucose and total protein. Assessment of hydration status and correction of any fluid imbalances is critical to management of a safe anaesthetic procedure.

Reptiles, as a rule, benefit from fasting before anaesthesia where possible. For most lizards and turtles, 24 hours is usually adequate. Snake anaesthesia should ideally be delayed for at least two to three days after the last meal, as the potential for regurgitation during or immediately after anaesthesia is high. Additionally, a large food mass in a tubular patient may interfere with normal cardiovascular or respiratory function.

Since they are ectotherms, it is essential that reptiles be maintained within their preferred body temperature range during anaesthesia where possible. This is important not only for proper immune and cardiovascular function but also provides a more predictable and repeatable response to anaesthetic agents. Monitoring of body temperature using an oesophageal or cloacal probe is strongly advised to prevent excessively high or low body temperatures.

Premedication

Premedication should serve the following purposes in an anaesthesia protocol:

- to render a candidate for anaesthesia more tractable for safer and easier handling
- to lower the anaesthetic induction and maintenance agent doses
- to provide additional or complementary analgesia.

Premedication protocol varies depending on the species and procedure being undertaken. Pre-anaesthesia analgesia is appropriate where painful or invasive procedures are planned. Opioids are the analgesics of choice (see previous section). These medications are often given in conjunction with a muscle relaxant, particularly in larger or more dangerous species. Extreme care must be taken when using local anaesthesia as part of the anaesthetic regimen, since overdosing can be fatal.

Hypothermia induces immobilization by lowering the metabolic rate. It does not provide muscle relaxation or analgesia and is not considered acceptable as a means of immobilization.

Benzodiazepines are useful premedicants for reptiles (see Appendix 1 for doses). Midazolam is advocated for all reptile species. It is useful in combination with dissociative and neuromuscular blocking agents. Antagonism of benzodiazepines with flumazenil is possible but usually unnecessary.

Neuromuscular blocking agents have historically been used for immobilization of large crocodilians, although they are inhumane when given alone and are largely outdated

now. They provide profound muscle relaxation but no analgesia or sensory deprivation. Their major advantage is the lack of sudden or unexpected recovery. Neuromuscular blocking agents can be antagonized with neostigmine methylsulfate.

Anticholinergics are not routinely used during reptile anaesthesia, except for procedures involving the oral or pharyngeal region where excessive salivation should be avoided.

Induction of Anaesthesia

The choice of an induction agent depends on the reptile species and the procedure being undertaken. Under hospital conditions, inhalational anaesthetics and advanced monitoring are usually available. Field immobilization requires a safe protocol using short-term or reversible, and usually injectable, immobilization agents. It is important to allometrically scale drug dosage rates for larger reptiles.

Commonly used medications and dose rates (listed in Appendix 1) vary, depending on the various species, and much of the information is anecdotal. Many agents result in prolonged recovery if used alone or at high doses. Barbiturates result in a long and unpredictable induction time and recovery period, and their use in reptiles is generally not recommended. Ketamine hydrochloride is a short-acting dissociative agent with analgesic properties used for immobilization in all reptilian orders. Ketamine given intramuscularly alone results in very effective chemical restraint, producing minimal respiratory depression and, except at high doses, minimal cardiac stimulation. However, it results in inadequate muscle relaxation characterized by the presence of uncoordinated voluntary muscle movement in response to external stimuli. This is not considered to be a surgical plane of anaesthesia. Bradycardia, respiratory arrest and even death have been reported at high doses. There is no antagonist agent and recovery can be very slow. It is common and highly preferable to use ketamine in combination with alpha-2 adrenergic agonists or benzodiazepines.

Zolazepam-tiletamine is a long acting benzodiazepine dissociative combined agent. Lower doses produce sedation without immobilization but higher doses (up to 100 mg/kg) provide prolonged surgical anaesthesia of up to 16 hours. Recovery from anaesthesia is up to 24 hours and deaths have been reported in a number of species.

Alpha-2 adrenergic agonists are sedatives and analgesics and have widespread effects on vertebrate physiology. The net clinical result of these effects varies with species, route of administration and time elapsed since administration. A major advantage of these agents is their ability to be antagonized. However, this also antagonizes their analgesic effects, so alternative analgesics may be required.

Medetomidine can be given intramuscularly in combination with local anaesthesia to perform minor surgery. It provides very effective sedation for mature reptiles, regardless of environmental temperature, and is readily antagonized by atipamezole. Dose rates vary depending on body size. Atipamezole is administered at an equal volume of medetomidine 1 mg/ml for reptiles less than 10–15 kg. For larger reptiles, the dose rate (5000 µg/m^2) is based on body surface area. Bradycardia and bradypnoea occurs following medetomidine administration but resolve within 15 minutes of administration of atipamezole. If not antagonized, immobilization is variable and can be prolonged. It is an extremely effective sedative for crocodilians.

Propofol is a commonly used induction agent in reptiles and can also be used as a continuous infusion for longer anaesthetic procedures (refer to Appendix 1). Its disadvantage is that it must be administered intravenously. Apnoea has been observed in some reptile species.

Alfaxalone is an injectable neuroactive steroid anaesthetic with a wide safety margin. It can be used intravenously, intramuscularly or intracoelomically. Its onset and duration of action are more variable by the intramuscular or intracoelomic route and higher dose rates are required. Alfaxalone is rapidly cleared and its metabolism is independent of organ function. Its safety and availability have led to frequent use among clinicians dealing with squamates and chelonians (refer to Appendix 1). It produces rapid induction but transient apnoea is common so prompt intubation is recommended. There may also be muscle fasciculations or tremors on induction but, generally, appropriate premedication controls these responses. Although it has reportedly produced surgical anaesthesia in crocodiles, severe muscle twitching and hyperexcitation experienced during recovery can be dangerous for inexperienced clinicians and staff.

Maintenance of Anaesthesia

Isoflurane is currently the inhalational anaesthetic of choice for reptiles. Inhalant anaesthetics undergo minimal metabolism before elimination by the lungs. Any underlying kidney or liver dysfunction therefore does not affect the clearance of inhalant anaesthetics. However, because of right-to-left cardiac shunting in reptiles, reduced lung perfusion can occur. Thus concentrations of inhalant anaesthetic gases in the lungs do not necessarily reflect concentrations in the blood and brain. Sudden changes in shunting direction of blood can lead to sudden changes in serum concentration of inhalant anaesthetic, which can prolong induction times, induce sudden changes in anaesthetic depth and increase or markedly decrease recovery times. Endotracheal intubation and assisted respiration are therefore recommended for inhalant anaesthesia in reptiles.

Most reptiles can sustain long periods of apnoea and are not suited to a mask induction. Anaesthesia is best induced using an injectable agent to allow for safe intubation, particularly in elapids (Figure 27.4). Once induced, the animal can be intubated (Figures 27.5a,b). In crocodilians, the top jaw is opened and a solid

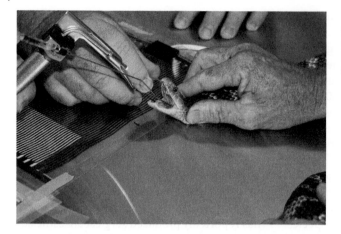

Figure 27.4 Use of a mouth gag facilitates visualization of the glottis in a tiger snake (*Notechis scutatus*). Elapids should be handled by experienced operators.

(a)

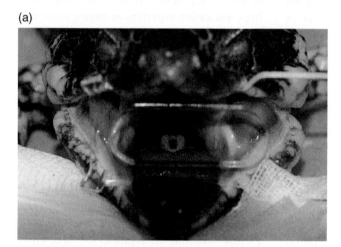

Figure 27.5 (a) The large, rostral glottis provides easy airways access in squamates such as this Shingleback lizard (*Tiliqua rugosa*). (b) Endotracheal tube in situ in an eastern water dragon (*Intellagama lesueurii*).

(b)

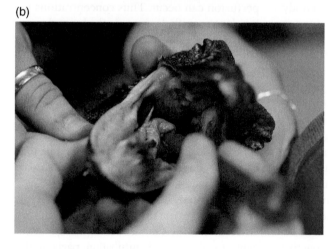

mouth gag is inserted between the jaws and taped in place. Before passing the tube, the palatal flap must be displaced rostroventrally to allow visualization of the glottis (Figure 27.6).

Unlike most reptiles, the trachea of crocodilians and chelonians is composed of complete cartilaginous rings, so intubation with an uncuffed tube is recommended.

Figure 27.6 The passive valve action of the palatal and, visible here, glottal folds means early airway access and control is important in crocodilians.

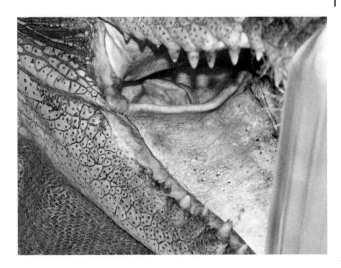

Inhalational anaesthesia is maintained using positive pressure ventilation. A non-rebreathing system is indicated for animals under 5 kg and a circle system for animals over 5 kg. Since oxygen consumption in reptiles is less than that of mammals an oxygen flow of 1–2 litres/minute for larger animals is usually adequate.

Anaesthetic Support

Mechanical/Assisted Ventilation

Reptiles, which lack a diaphragm, are dependent on skeletal muscle activity for ventilation to permit adequate gas exchange and oxygenation. Recumbency may cause viscera to place pressure on the simple lungs. As a consequence, reptiles are best artificially ventilated in all but the shortest of anaesthetic procedures. IPPV must be performed very gently owing to the fragile nature of the pulmonary tissue. Careful observation of the extent of ventilatory excursions of the thoracic wall in the conscious reptile before induction is valuable in indicating the amount of pressure required during IPPV. IPPV can be performed manually at 4–12 breaths/minute to effect induction and then most reptiles can be maintained at 2–6 breaths/minute. IPPV is generally reduced to once a minute during recovery until spontaneous ventilation resumes. Room air is preferably used during recovery. A number of mechanical ventilators suitable for reptile anaesthesia, such as the Vetronics Small Animal Ventilator VT-9093 (BASi Vetronics) are available. These are typically set with pressures of 6–10 cm of water, adjusted to cause identical chest excursions to those noted in the conscious patient. Monitoring of reptiles being maintained under anaesthesia by IPPV is critical as an overdose of anaesthetic is possible due to the forced delivery of gas to the patient.

Thermal Support

Appropriate thermal support is important for reptile patients undergoing anaesthesia to maintain body temperature within the preferred optimal temperature zone. Hypothermia significantly affects some drug performances. Body temperature is measured with a cloacal thermometer or thermistor (Figure 27.7). Ensuring that the reptile patient is at the preferred optimal temperature before induction makes it much easier to maintain the body temperature rather than trying to raise it once the animal is hypothermic. Electrical heating mats and hot water bottles or 'wheat bags' have largely given way to forced-air warming devices, conductive fabric (resistive polymer), electric warming (HotDogR Patient Warming SystemR) and radiant heat lamps as safer and more effective

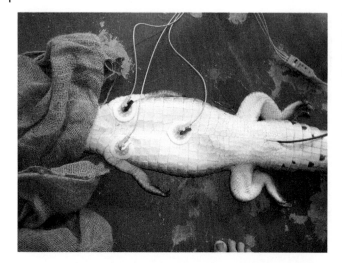

Figure 27.7 A small estuarine crocodile (*Crocodylus porosus*) with electrocardiogram leads attached to the thorax and thermal probe inserted cloacally.

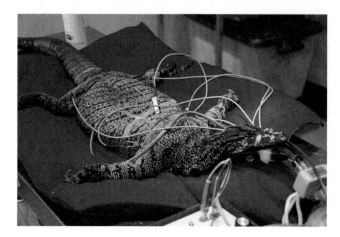

Figure 27.8 An anaesthetized lace monitor (*Varanus varius*) being monitored by electrocardiogram, oesophageal thermal probe, pulse oximetry and capnography, and being thermally supported by a forced air warmer as well as being mechanically ventilated.

methods of protecting anaesthetized patients from hypothermia (Figure 27.5).

Fluid Support

Hydration status is difficult to assess in most reptile patients. Where indicated by history or clinical presentation, appropriate fluid therapy with normal saline or Ringer's solution should be administered by the subcutaneous, intracoelomic, intravenous or intraosseous route, depending on the size and species of the reptile patient and the ease of venous access. In most cases, fluids are administered subcutaneously or intracoelomically. Intravenous or intraosseous fluids are usually given at a rate of 2 ml/kg/hour.

Monitoring of Anaesthesia

Monitoring Parameters

Physiological monitoring equipment includes stethoscope (may be of limited value), pulse oximeter, Doppler blood flow transducer, electrocardiography, ultrasound and blood gas analysis (Figure 27.8). It is of the utmost importance to develop good observational skills for assessing depth of immobilization and to correctly interpret changes in physiological parameters. A monitoring protocol should be developed for each species commonly encountered and should be sufficiently flexible depending on the individual situation (Figure 27.9).

Figure 27.9 A wooden tongue depressor can be used to stabilize endotracheal tubes and Doppler ultrasound probe against the patient during anaesthesia, as in this eastern bearded dragon (*Pogona barbata*).

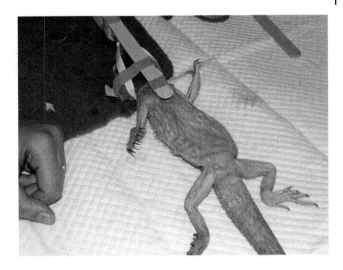

Anaesthetic depth is evaluated using signs including the limb withdrawal reflex, cardiac rate, righting response and bite and corneal reflexes. Other useful signs include tail 'flick' or withdrawal reflex, respiratory rate and depth and palpebral reflex. Mucous membrane colour is not particularly helpful but a degree of cyanosis is frequently observed due to changes in peripheral blood flow. Intermittent positive pressure ventilation is advised to reduce shunting mechanisms from being triggered and to maintain aerobic respiration.

Blood Gases

Blood gas measurements in reptiles are difficult to interpret because variables such as temperature, feeding and sample site (arterial, venous or a combination of both) influence the results. Blood gas measurements in reptiles are difficult to interpret because variables such as temperature, feeding and sample site (arterial, venous or a combination of both) influence the results.

Capnography

Capnography is the measurement of end-tidal carbon dioxide in expired air and provides useful information on quality of ventilation and pulmonary perfusion. While it has not

been validated for reptiles, and there are concerns about how the intracardiac shunting (especially of aquatic reptiles) will affect capnography, there is a growing bank of data to suggest that it will indeed become a useful additional monitoring modality for anaesthetized reptiles.

Pulse Oximetry

There is conflicting information as to the usefulness of pulse oximetry as a monitoring technique in reptiles. Reptile haemoglobin differs from mammalian haemoglobin. Pulse oximeters are calibrated to measure relative arterial saturation in humans so absolute values will not relate to the values in the reptile. However, pulse oximetry can be used on a comparative basis. In most reptiles, an oesophageal probe level with the carotid artery or a rectal probe can be used, although probes may not be validated for reptiles and for these locations.

Doppler

Doppler blood flow detection is a very reliable method of obtaining heart rate and rhythm. The probe is placed over the heart or a large blood vessel, such as the ventral coccygeal, brachial or femoral artery. Blood flow in the optic arteries may be detected by placing the probe against the globe with the eyelid or third eyelid closed. Alternatively, a dorsally directed probe placed in the cloaca may detect arterial blood flow.

Electrocardiogram

The electrocardiogram (ECG) and reference values have been described for the American alligator (*Alligator mississippiensis*). The three ECG leads are attached by 2.5-cm needles passed through the skin, alligator clamps or adhesive ECG pads on the skin of the ventral body (Figures 27.7 and 27.8). Depressed reptilian heart rates under anaesthesia may trigger bradycardia alarms in machines manufactured for use in mammals.

Recovery and Post-Operative Management

Any animal which has been anesthetized requires monitoring during recovery. It is imperative that regular voluntary respiration, in conjunction with movement of the limbs, is established since re-sedation may occur if the animal is not continually stimulated and apnoea can occur. Apnoea increases intrapulmonary pressure, diverting oxygenated blood away from the brain and heart, and reduces metabolic rate. Intermittent ventilation with room air simulates voluntary respiration and allows oxygenated blood to be directed to the brain and heart, increasing metabolic rate and assisting in recovery. The gular fold relaxes in crocodilians under immobilization. Post-anaesthetic monitoring of crocodilians is required until normal gular fold function occurs. Temperatures outside preferred optimal temperatures will potentially affect the rate of clearance of any drugs from the system. Under field conditions, it is extremely important to know how an adverse environmental temperature will impact on the anaesthesia and recovery. Semi-aquatic and aquatic reptiles which have undergone immobilization should be denied access to water until they can protect their airway, surface to breathe and protect themselves from danger.

Further Reading

Bradley, T. (2001) Pain management considerations and pain-associated behaviors in reptiles and amphibians, in Proceedings of the Association of Reptilian and Amphibian Veterinarians and American Association of Zoo Veterinarians, Orlando, FL. pp. 45–49.

Carpenter, J.W., Klaphake, E. and Gibbons, P.M. (2014) Appendix 3: Reptile formulary and laboratory normal, in *Current Therapy in Reptile Medicine and Surgery* (D.R. Mader and S.J. Divers, eds). Elsevier Saunders, St Louis, MO, pp. 382–410.

Heard, D.J. (2007) Monitoring, in *Zoo Animal and Wildlife Immobilization and Anesthesia* (G. West, D. Heard and N. Caulkett, eds). Blackwell Publishing, Ames, IA, pp. 83–91.

Hernandez-Divers, S.M., Schumacher, J., Stahl, S. *et al.* (2004) Reptile clinical anesthesia: advances in research. *Exotic DVM*, 6, 64–69.

Mosley, C.A. (2005) Anesthesia and analgesia in reptiles. *Seminars in Avian and Exotic Pet Medicine*, 14, 243–262.

Olsson, A.R. and Phalen, D.N. (2012) Preliminary studies of chemical immobilization of captive juvenile estuarine (*Crocodylus porosus*) and Australian freshwater (*C. johnstoni*) crocodiles with medetomidine and reversal with atipamezole. *Veterinary Anaesthesia and Analgesia*, 39, 345–356.

Ramsey, I. (2008) *Small Animal Formulary,* BSAVA Press, Gloucester.

Schumacher, J. and Yelen, T. (2006) Anesthesia and Analgesia, in *Reptile Medicine and Surgery* (D.R. Mader, ed.). Elsevier, St Louis, MO, pp. 442–452.

Sladky, K.K. (2014) Analgesia, in *Current Therapy in Reptile Medicine and Surgery* (D.R. Mader and S.J. Divers, eds). Elsevier, St Louis, MO, pp. 217–228.

Sladky, K.K. and Mans, C. (2012) Clinical anesthesia in reptiles. *Journal of Exotic Pet Medicine,* 21, 17–31.

28

Surgery

Zdeněk Knotek and Stacey Leonatti Wilkinson

Introduction

In reptiles, standard surgical methods apply, although the unique anatomy of reptiles and the huge variety in patient size are important factors to consider.

Patient Assessment and Preparation for Surgery

Preoperative physical examination is vital. Pre-anaesthesia blood work, such as a complete blood count and chemistry panel, are ideal. Diagnostic radiography, ultrasound, computed tomography (CT) and magnetic resonance imaging (MRI) are useful in both presurgical patient assessment and surgical planning. Reptile patients generally do not require fasting for surgery, as they are not prone to regurgitation under anaesthesia, nonetheless, fasting (lizards 1–2 days, snakes 2–3 days, tortoises 3–5 days) is recommended for elective surgery on the gastrointestinal tract.

Pre- and Perioperative Care

Many surgical procedures are not true emergencies and the patient may need to be hospitalized for supportive care measures prior to surgery. Thermal support is provided to the reptile patient before, during and after surgery. Before surgery, the patient is given analgesia (e.g. a combination of opioids and nonsteroidal anti-inflammatory drugs, NSAIDs) and fluids (see Chapter 27 and Appendix 1). After 30–45 minutes, anaesthetic drugs are given and the patient is prepared for intubation. After successful intubation, the patient is placed under inhalation anaesthesia using isoflurane or sevoflurane and oxygen.

Positioning

Most lizards and crocodilians are positioned similarly to mammals (e.g. ventral, lateral or dorsal recumbency). Chameleons are best positioned in lateral recumbency. For surgery involving the coelomic cavity, snakes are best positioned in right lateral recumbency (left lateral approach) to avoid the incision of the right air sac. Turtles and tortoises, when placed in dorsal recumbency, can be placed in the middle of a towel rolled into a ring.

Patient Preparation

Plastic adhesive drapes are recommended to aid visibility of the surgical field. Alternatively, spray adhesives may be used on standard

Reptile Medicine and Surgery in Clinical Practice, First Edition. Edited by Bob Doneley, Deborah Monks, Robert Johnson and Brendan Carmel.
© 2018 John Wiley & Sons Ltd. Published 2018 by John Wiley & Sons Ltd.

drapes. Standard patient surgical preparation is undertaken. When shell repair is necessary for chelonian patients, the surface of the shell must be prepared by cleansing and degreasing the surface, to enable restorative material to adhere to the shell.

Instruments

Small reptile patients necessitate the use of fine ophthalmological surgical instruments (e.g. micro haemostats, iris scissors), while large chelonians or crocodilians may require special equipment; for example for orthopaedic surgery. Haemostatic clips are useful where application of ligatures is difficult. Absorbable gelatin sponges should be used for controlling haemorrhage in reptiles (Figure 28.1). Eyelid retractors work well as wound retractors. Lone Star Veterinary Retractor Rings (type 4407G or 4405G, with retractor hooks, Cooper Surgical) are ideal for middle-sized and large reptile patients.

Sutures, Radiosurgery and Surgical Laser

Most reptiles do not traumatize surgical incisions. This makes closure with a continuous pattern safe and efficient (Mader *et al.* 2006). In the reptile, synthetic absorbable suture materials are absorbed very slowly. Recommended suture materials for the reptile patient are monofilament thread (e.g. Caprolon®, a copolymer of lactic acid and caprolactone), nylon or polypropylene (Mader *et al.* 2006). Wound healing is slow in reptiles and suture removal is generally scheduled four to six weeks after surgery. Skin closure is best accomplished with an everting suture pattern such as horizontal or vertical mattress. Radiosurgery is useful in reptile patients for skin incision, body wall incision, organ biopsies and a variety of other procedures. Bipolar forceps allow fine coagulation of vessels. Surgical lasers are used for precise cutting through reptile skin to minimize blood loss (Hodshon *et al.* 2013).

Soft-Tissue Surgery

Skin Wounds and Burns

Many wounds will heal by second intention with appropriate topical wound care and antibiotic use. However, some are large enough that repair is needed. Large wounds will eventually granulate and heal but may take months of care for full healing. Wounds on the chelonian shell can take up to one year or more to fully heal (Mader *et al.* 2006, Alworth *et al.* 2011).

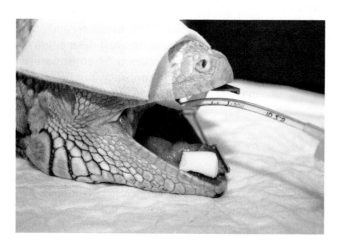

Figure 28.1 Absorbable gelatin sponges are useful for controlling haemorrhage in reptiles.

Subcutaneous Abscess Removal

There are different options for surgical management of abscesses in reptiles (Figure 28.2). One option is to lance the abscess, remove the caseous material inside and leave the wound open to heal by second intention (Mader *et al.* 2006, Alworth *et al.* 2011, Huchzermeyer and Cooper 2000). The cavity is then flushed daily with dilute chlorhexidine or povidone iodine and antibacterial creams or ointments are used to pack the capsule. Poloxamer gel infused with antibiotics may also be used. Another option is to remove both the inner caseous material and the entire fibrous capsule as well (Mader *et al.* 2006, Alworth *et al.* 2011). The resulting wound can be left open (to heal by second intention and should be cleaned daily and topical antibacterial creams applied if needed) or sutured closed.

Aural Abscesses

Aural abscesses are common in chelonians, specifically aquatic turtles and box turtles. The swelling over the ear is lanced and the caseous material removed. The skin over the ventral half of the ear is removed to keep the cavity open and allow it to heal (Murray 2006). The cavity is flushed with saline, appropriate antibiotic therapy is prescribed and any husbandry deficiencies corrected.

Subspectacular Abscess

Subspectacular abscess typically develops from bacteria that ascend the nasolacrimal duct from the mouth and colonize the subspectacular space but it can also arise from a penetrating wound to the eye or haematogenous spread (Alworth *et al.* 2011). An incision is made in the ventral half of the spectacle and a 30–90-degree wedge of the spectacle is removed (Alworth *et al.* 2011, Lawton 2006). A sterile swab in inserted to remove material for cytology and culture, then a small catheter (such as an intravenous catheter) is inserted and the area flushed with saline. Antibiotics can be flushed inside the spectacle and systemic antibiotics are often indicated, ideally chosen based on culture and sensitivity results (Lawton 2006). Within 24 hours, a hyaline proteinaceous plug and inflammatory debris fills the defect, sealing the subspectacular space and providing a barrier while healing progresses. This plug may need to be gently disrupted daily to apply topical antibiotics to the subspectacular space. By 21 days, healing has typically progressed such that the snake will have a multilayered regenerating spectacle and will have re-established subspectacular space. By three months, the spectacle is usually fully healed.

Figure 28.2 Surgical curettage of a mandibular abscess in a green iguana (*Iguana iguana*).

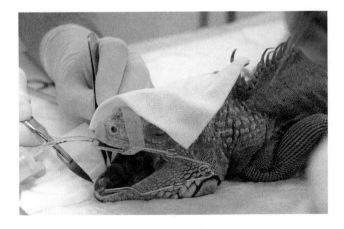

Nasolacrimal Duct Obstruction and Pseudobuphthalmos

Blockage of the nasolacrimal duct is most commonly encountered in snakes and geckoes (Alworth *et al.* 2011, Lawton 2006). As with an abscess, a wedge in the ventral aspect of the spectacle can be removed to allow the fluid to drain. Fluid should be collected from the subspectacular space and cytology performed to rule out other causes of fluid accumulation, as flagellates have been reported (Lawton 2006). If the problem recurs, a conjunctivoralostomy can be performed by inserting an 18-guage needle at the medial aspect of the inferior fornix of the subspectacular space and emerging on the roof of the mouth between the palatine and maxillary teeth. A fine silicon tube is threaded through the needle, the needle removed and the tube sutured in place on the periorbital scales and left in place for at least six weeks (Alworth *et al.* 2011, Lawton 2006, Millichamp *et al.* 1986).

Enucleation

In species with eyelids, the globe and all ocular tissue are removed and the eyelid margins are removed and sutured together (Alworth *et al.* 2011). In snakes or lizards with a spectacle, a circular incision is made around the entire circumference of the spectacle and all ocular tissue is removed. Vessels can be ligated with small suture, vascular clips or radiosurgery, or a gelatin sponge or direct pressure can be applied for haemostasis. The wound is left open to heal by second intention (Alworth *et al.* 2011, Lawton 2006).

Eyelid Surgery

There are many species in which one eyelid is more moveable than the others (the lower lid in lizards and chelonians and the upper lid in crocodilians). This needs to be accounted for when performing surgery and considering the function of the eyelids postoperatively (Lawton 2006). Snakes do not have eyelids.

Tracheal Resection and Anastomosis

Chondromas arising from the tracheal cartilage have been reported in snakes and can grow large enough to obstruct the airway and cause significant dyspnoea. Resection and anastomosis of the trachea is the treatment of choice. The anaesthetized patient is intubated with a long polypropylene or rubber catheter to the level of the mass. Stay sutures using a fine monofilament suture are placed and the affected area of the trachea removed. The catheter is advanced into the distal part of the trachea, both to help to realign the trachea for closure and to maintain anaesthesia. The absorbable sutures should encompass at least one or two tracheal rings on each side of the incision. All sutures are preplaced and then tightened. Care should be taken not to damage the dorsal tracheal membrane during the procedure. The trachea is tested for leaks by dribbling saline on the incision and watching for bubbles (Mader *et al.* 2006).

Surgery of the Tongue

In chameleons, small wounds of the tongue can be managed by putting the tongue back in its sheath and suturing. Serious or prolonged tongue injuries may involve complete or partial amputation of the tongue. The veins and tongue are carefully ligated rostrally, just before the attachment to hyoid apparatus, and the damaged part is snipped off. The cartilaginous apex of the hyoid bone should be adequately shortened to reduce the risk of perforation of the tongue stump. The patient may require hand feeding long term, although snakes have managed to eat normally after tongue amputation (Brendan Carmel, personal communication).

Oesophagostomy Tube Placement

Placement of an oesophagostomy tube is most commonly indicated in chelonians and can be placed in a similar manner in lizards. A tube should be premeasured and marked so that it can be inserted the distance from the cranial rim of the plastron to the junction of the pectoral and abdominal scutes. A curved pair of hemostats is inserted into the oral cavity. The hemostats are pushed laterally in order to 'tent' the skin on either side of the neck and allow the vessels on the neck to 'roll' out of the way so as not to be damaged. An incision is made on the lateral aspect of the neck where it meets the shoulder, just large enough to pass the tips of the hemostats out of the incision. The distal end of the feeding tube is grasped and pulled through the incision and back out of the mouth; it is then redirected and passed down the oesophagus into the distal oesophagus or proximal stomach. The tube is secured in place at the skin with a purse-string suture and, ideally, a Chinese finger-trap suture is placed around the tube with nonabsorbable material. Finally, the tube is taped or sutured in place along the animal's dorsum. Radiographs or endoscopy can be used to confirm proper placement. When removal is necessary, the sutures and tube can be removed and the surgical site left to heal by second intention (Alworth *et al.* 2011).

Coeliotomy

Coeliotomy has a wide range of applications (Mader *et al.* 2006, Alworth *et al.* 2011; Figure 28.3). Indications include reproductive disorders, gastrointestinal disease, urinary system dysfunction and exploration for obtaining organ biopsies. In all species, a nonabsorbable suture material is used for closing the skin in a continuous everting pattern. Sealing the incision site with tissue glue may help prevent postoperative infection. Plastron or carapace fixation should remain for approximately six months before removal. For at least 10–14 days postoperatively, the patient should remain in a warm and dry environment. Antibiotics and fluid therapy may be required. If the patient is anorectic, forced feeding may be required.

Coeliotomy in Lizards

Most lizards are positioned in dorsal recumbency, except chameleons, which are placed in the lateral recumbency, with the head and hind legs fixed to the drape. The skin is incised along the curvature of the ribs (chameleons) or in paramedial line of the abdominal wall (other lizards). Lone Star Veterinary

Figure 28.3 Coeliotomy in a green iguana (*Iguana iguana*).

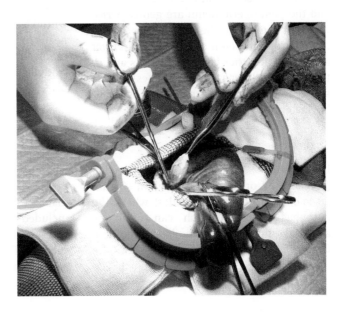

Retractor System may be used for improved access to the surgical field and better visibility of organs. The skin is separated from the muscle layer. The muscle layer and pleuroperitoneum are incised along the curvature of the ribs (in chameleons) or in the paramedial line (other lizards). In chameleons, the surgeon must be careful not to damage small veins located around the ribs. In chameleons, pause IPPV before entering the body cavity; if this is not done, air sacs may sharply protrude into the surgical incision. In other lizards, entering the body cavity is much easier. Take care to avoid the ventral abdominal vein by performing a paramedial incision or by starting caudally and incising the skin cranially on the midline. The muscle layer and pleuroperitoneum are closed (together in small patients and as two separate layers in large lizards) with 3-0 4-0 guage absorbable sutures in a simple interrupted pattern. Thereafter, 3-0 or 4-0 absorbable material or 3-0 non-absorbable material is used for closing the skin, as previously described.

Coeliotomy in Snakes

The snake is positioned in right lateral recumbency and fixed to a sterile drape. The incision is made between the first and second row of lateral skin scales. The muscle layer and the pleuroperitoneum are gently perforated. At the end of the surgical procedure, the pleuroperitoneum and the muscle layer are closed (together in small patients and as two separate layers in large snakes) with a single simple continuous pattern of absorbable material.

Coeliotomy in Chelonians

In chelonians, a plastronotomy is needed to reach the organs in the coelom (Figure 28.4a,b,c), except in sea turtles, where the oesophagus and stomach can often be accessed through an axillary incision. Oscillating saws or small circular saws are ideally suited for cutting through shell. The blades must not be overused, as a dull blade does not cut well and prevents proper healing. With careful handling, the same blade can be used for two to three patients before requiring disposal.

Ovariectomy

Ovariectomy is a common surgical procedure in lizards and chelonians. Once the coelom is entered, the fat body and the ipsilateral ovarium with follicles are exteriorized. In chelonians, this can be done through a pre-femoral incision or plastronotomy. An avascular area of ovarian interfollicular connective tissue is selected for placement of finger or grasping forceps, taking care to avoid rupture of ovarian follicles. Gentle traction is applied and the ovary is cautiously retracted toward the coelom incision. The ovarian vasculature is ligated with suture or haemostatic clips and the mesovarium is transected. Care must be taken not to accidentally remove the adrenal gland. The ligation sites are examined to verify haemostasis and to confirm complete excision of all ovarian tissue. The second ovary is exteriorized and resected in the same way as the first. The surgeon should ensure that all follicles are removed. If very small follicles (smaller than a pinhead) are overlooked, they can dramatically enlarge within few weeks or months and the surgery needs to be repeated. If the ovaries are being removed for prophylactic reasons and the oviducts are healthy, the latter can be left in place.

Salpingectomy

Salpingectomy is usually indicated in cases of postovulatory egg stasis in lizards and chelonians, removing the entire oviduct, eggs included. The distal part of the oviduct and veins in the mesosalpinx are ligated with sutures (Figure 28.5) or haemostatic clips and the mesosalpinx is transected close to the cloaca and removed.

Figure 28.4 (a) Tortoise positioned in dorsal recumbency for plastronotomy. (b) A square segment of plastron is gently elevated to provide excellent exposure for a cystotomy. (c) A sound seal over the surgical wound is essential for good healing after a plastronotomy.

(a)
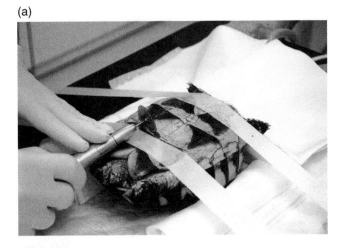

(b)
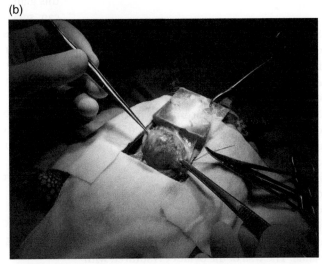

(c)
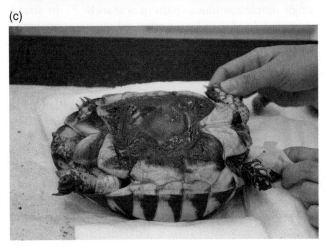

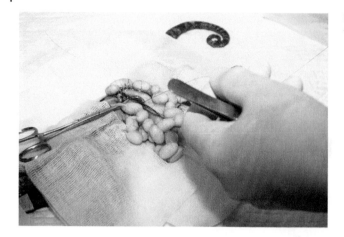

Figure 28.5 Ligation of the ovarian vasculature in a chameleon.

Salpingotomy

Salpingotomy is the same regardless of species. Surgical intervention is usually required for causes of dystocia in snakes (Alworth *et al*. 2011). The oviduct is gently elevated out of the coelom and assessed. Two absorbable fixation sutures are made in the wall of the oviduct and the central part of the oviduct wall is incised. An incision is made over the eggs. To decrease the distance between the eggs, they are gently massaged closer to the incision from the proximal and distal parts of the oviduct. Eggs are gently withdrawn from the lumen of the oviduct and the mucosa washed with warm sterile saline. The wall of the oviduct is sutured with a single simple continuous pattern of absorbable material and the pleuroperitoneal cavity is then evaluated and examined for any local complications (Mader *et al*. 2006, Alworth *et al*. 2011).

Orchidectomy in Lizards

The surgical technique is similar to that described for ovariectomy. The gonads are tightly adhered to adjacent structures, so excellent exposure is vital for successful removal. The right testicle is attached to the vena cava by very short vessels while the left adrenal gland sits between the testicle and its blood supply. Avoid removing or damaging this gland during surgery, although a patient can survive if it is inadvertently removed. The testes are gently elevated to expose the vasculature; a fine suture can be placed in the capsule to aid this if needed. The vessels ligated with haemostatic clips and the testicle removed. It is vital that all areas are ligated properly before cutting, as marked haemorrhage can occur. It is also important to ensure all testicular tissue is removed, as it can regrow if cells are left behind (Mader *et al*. 2006, Alworth *et al*. 2011).

Gastrotomy and Gastrectomy

In lizards and chelonians, the stomach is anchored tightly, making it difficult to fully exteriorize; however, it is much more mobile in snakes. In chelonians, a plastronotomy is needed to reach the stomach, except in sea turtles, where the oesophagus and stomach can often be accessed through an axillary incision. The stomach is isolated on saline-soaked laparotomy pads. Stay sutures are placed and an incision made in an avascular area. In the case of a mass removal or gastrectomy, the affected part of the stomach wall is removed. Closure is routine with a double layer inverting pattern (Mader *et al*. 2006, Alworth *et al*. 2011). Removal of foreign bodies from the stomach is also possible using endoscopy.

Enterotomy

Once the coelom is entered, the intestine is exteriorized. The colon (which is black in some lizards) can be used as a guide for recognizing the organs of the body cavity. The affected part of intestine is gently elevated and placed on saline soaked laparotomy pads to assess the extent of any pathological changes. Two absorbable fixation sutures are placed (Figure 28.6a) and the central part of the intestine wall is incised. Foreign body and faeces are gently withdrawn (Figure 28.6b) from the lumen and the mucosa is flushed with warm sterile saline. The wall of the intestine is closed with absorbable suture material in two layers. The first layer is a simple interrupted pattern and the second a continuous inverting pattern. The coelomic cavity is then carefully examined for any abnormalities. The coelom is then cleaned by repetitive irrigations with sterile saline solution and antibiotics.

Surgery of any of intestinal segment in larger lizards and snakes is usually uncomplicated; however, in chelonians it can be difficult. Complications arise particularly in the transverse colon and the functionality of the intestine after enterotomy cannot be always ensured. Enterotomy and colostomy (especially in the transverse colon) through the pre-femoral fossa is rather difficult, although in some aquatic chelonians it may be more accessible.

Figure 28.6 (a) Stay sutures placed in the intestine to assist surgical access. (b) Faeces are gently massaged out of the intestine through an enterotomy wound.

(a)

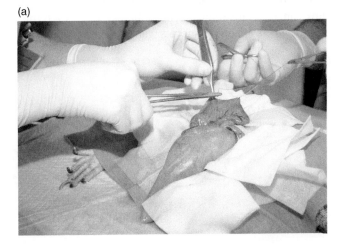

(b)

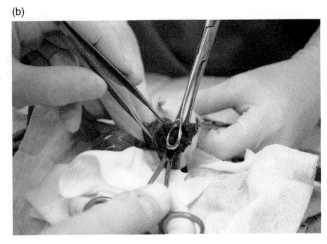

Complete or Partial Liver Lobectomy, Liver Biopsy

In snakes, the affected part of the liver is gently elevated out of the coelom cavity to assess any pathological changes. Temporary vascular clamps are placed cranially and caudally to the affected part of the organ. Ligatures are then placed allowing complete excision of the affected part of liver. Finally, the vascular clamps are released and occlusive ligatures tightened and examined. The cut surfaces of the remaining parts of the liver are rinsed with a sterile 0.9% sodium chloride solution to locate any bleeding.

In lizards and chelonians, an entire lobe can be removed if needed; the lobe is isolated and the blood vessels and bile duct double ligated and removed. The use of haemostatic clips can facilitate removal. Liver biopsy is performed as in other species via surgery (laparoscopy), minimal invasive surgery (endoscopy) or under ultrasound guidance.

Cystotomy

In most lizards, the bladder is readily elevated out of the coelom (Figure 28.7a,b,c). In chelonians, it can be accessed via a plastronotomy or though the pre-femoral fossa. The bladder wall is usually thickened if cystitis present. For small stone removal, retrieve with a lens loop or small forceps. Larger stones can be grasped and broken in situ if needed and the pieces removed. After the stone has been removed, the exteriorized bladder should be copiously flushed with sterile saline. A standard two-layer closure is generally recommended, then the coelom cavity irrigated with warm, sterile saline.

(a)

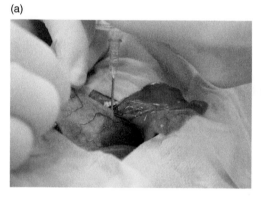

(b)

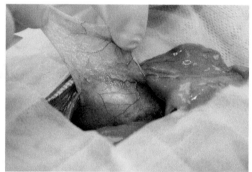

(c)

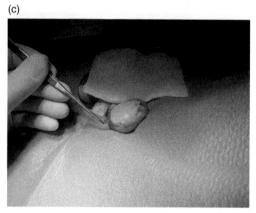

Figure 28.7 (a) Prior to cystotomy, urine is aspirated from the bladder. (b) The urolith is visible through the bladder wall. (c) Urolith surgically removed from the bladder of a tortoise.

Nephrectomy and Renal Biopsy

Nephrectomy is mostly straightforward in snakes and is usually indicated in cases of neoplasia. The kidney or mass is bluntly dissected out and the vessels supplying it and the ureter ligated and the kidney removed. In males, the seminiferous tubule may need to be bluntly dissected off and preserved (Vasaruchapong and Chanhome 2012). In lizards, the kidney is located within the pelvis, so complete nephrectomy is extremely difficult without transection of the pelvis and is not commonly performed. Endoscopy is the preferred method for obtaining biopsies but can also be obtained with a Tru-Cut device through a coeliotomy or an incision between the tail base and the rear leg in lizards.

Prolapsed Hemipene or Phallus

A prolapsed hemipene or phallus should be attended to as soon as possible, keeping the tissue moist, otherwise necrosis will occur. The prolapsed organ should be cleaned and any lacerations repaired. Tissue swelling can be reduced using sugar or other hypertonic solutions. The organ is then replaced and a horizontal mattress suture placed on either side of the cloaca. It is important to make the suture tight enough to prevent further prolapse but still allow the passage of faeces and urates. This suture can be removed after seven days. The underlying cause must be addressed and systemic antibiotics are indicated if infection is present. If necrosis is present or the hemipene or phallus has re-prolapsed multiple times, amputation may be necessary (Mader *et al.* 2006). For snakes and lizards with hemipenes, as long as one hemipene remains, the animal is still able to breed. To perform amputation, one or two transfixing sutures are placed at the base of the organ for haemostasis, the tissue transected and removed. The stump can be oversewn with a simple continuous suture if necessary. The tissue stump will usually retract easily into the cloaca. Postoperative antibiotics are recommended if there is evidence of infection.

Orthopaedic Surgery

Principles of Fracture Repair and Bone Healing

External coaptation, internal fixation and external fixation methods have all been used in reptiles. The method of repair is chosen based on the location of the fracture, the size of the patient, the ease of application and tolerance by the patient, the owner's ability to manage the patient postoperatively, financial concerns and the surgeon's comfort level. Complete healing from a traumatic fracture can take 6–18 months (although fixation is usually only needed for 6–12 weeks), although fractures due to nutritional secondary hyperparathyroidism (NSHP) seem to heal much faster, as long as the underlying problem is corrected. If significant damage to the soft tissues and vascular supply has occurred, amputation may be necessary.

External Coaptation

External coaptation involves the use of splints, slings or bandages to immobilize a fracture. Fractures with minimal displacement that are not compound tend to heal well with this technique. For patients with NSHP, this is the treatment of choice, as the bones are not strong enough to support additional hardware. The limb should be splinted in a normal walking position so that the patient can still ambulate and to avoid the potential for disuse atrophy or decreased range of motion in the joints after the bandage is removed. In lizards, a modified spica splint crossing over the pelvic or pectoral girdle to the limb on the opposite side can be used, particularly for fractures of the humerus and femur. This method keeps the limb in a normal position.

Alternatively, the pectoral limb can be pulled caudally and taped to the body or the pelvic limb taped to the tail. The disadvantage to this method is that the limb being held in extension but the results are usually acceptable. In small chelonians with a humeral or femoral fracture, the limb can be flexed up inside the shell and taped in place.

External and Internal Fixation

Intramedullary pins and cerclage wire are commonly used for internal fixation in smaller reptiles. Pins can also be tied in to an external skeletal fixator to provide additional stability. For external fixation, common injection needles or K-wires can be used, which are threaded transversely through the affected bone under and above the fracture and fixated from outside on both sides by an infusion tube filled with quick-setting cement or a light-weight casting material (Figure 28.8). In large chelonians, bone plates can be used to stabilize fractures of the long bones (Mitchell 2002). The same principles apply when using these techniques in reptiles as in other animals. Complications can occur such as premature pin loosening, infection, damage to joints, and so on. In the case of non-union fractures, bone grafts can be harvested and placed at the fracture site to stimulate healing.

Grafts can be collected from the humerus, femur, a rib or the wing of the ilium.

Amputation

Tail

Tail necrosis is common in lizards and partial amputation of the tail is often required. A ring block with lidocaine or bupivacaine is performed or the procedure performed under sedation or general anaesthesia. The tail is cut straight through with a scalpel blade. Pressure is applied for haemostasis and the end of the tail is left open to granulate in, so that the tail can regenerate; the skin can be closed in patients without natural tail autonomy (for instance chameleons, bearded dragons, green iguanas). The end of the tail should be kept clean and dry and the patient kept on nonparticulate substrate until the wound heals. When the diameter of the tail is large, primary closure should be used.

Limb or Digit

Determining when to amputate a limb or digit is based on how the species will use the limb postoperatively; sometimes leaving a stump for ambulation is preferable.

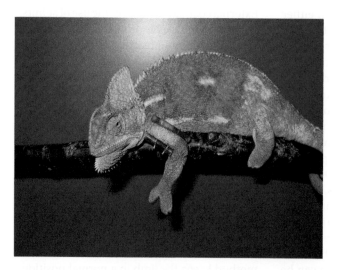

Figure 28.8 Repair of a forelimb fracture in a chameleon using segments of infusion tube filled with quick-setting cement and fine pins.

Regardless of the site, enough soft tissue should be left to pad the end of the bone. A skin flap should be created ventrally so that, when the incision is closed, it will lie on the dorsal aspect of the limb and not on the walking surface; healing is not delayed and the possibility of contamination of the incision is greatly reduced (Mader *et al.* 2006, Alworth *et al.* 2011). In chelonians, the prosthesis can be placed on the ventral aspect of the plastron postoperatively so that the patient does not fall to one side when walking. It usually needs to be replaced over time. The amputation of digits can be performed at an interphalangeal joint leaving healthy tissue and the skin closed routinely.

Skull and Facial Bone Fractures

Common principles of fracture repair are used for fractures of the maxilla or mandible in reptiles (Mader *et al.* 2006, Alworth *et al.* 2011, Tuxbury *et al.* 2010). If enough normal bone structure remains, hypodermic needles can be used to drill holes. Cerclage wire is passed through the needle, the needle is removed and the wire tightened to stabilize the fracture (Figure 28.9a,b,c). The use of external fixators has also been described. A 'bridge' over a fracture site should be created using a fibreglass and epoxy patch as one would use to repair shell fractures.

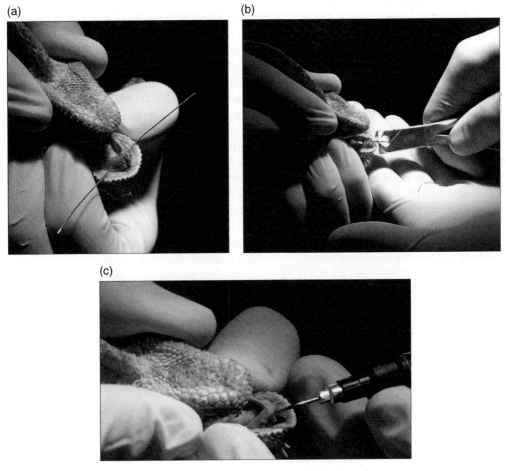

Figure 28.9 (a) Wiring of a mandibular symphysis fracture in a chameleon. (b) Gentle tension band wiring incorporating the transverse fixator. (c) Resin is applied to the sharp ends of the wires.

Venomoid Surgery

Owners of venomous species may request this surgery to make their venomous reptile less dangerous, but this reason must be actively discouraged. To provide such surgery is against the law, against the principles of animal welfare and unethical. Venomoid animals must still be treated as venomous for the safety of all involved and, in many Australian states these animals are legally still considered venomous (Johnson 2011). There may be limited situations where venomoid surgery is deemed appropriate. Once the snake is fully anaesthetized, the snake is placed in dorsal recumbency and the jaws are opened wide. An incision is made in the oral mucosa between the teeth and lip margin and the gland and duct are dissected out and carefully discarded. Sterile silicone prosthesis is placed in the surgical site and the mucosa closed with absorbable suture (Mader *et al.* 2006). After surgery, the snake is fasted for several weeks and must only be fed dead prey.

References

Alworth, L.C., Hernandez, S.M. and Divers, S.J. (2011) Laboratory reptile surgery: principles and techniques. *Journal of the American Association of Laboratory Animal Sciences*, 50, 11–26.

Hodshon, R.T., Sura, P.A. and Schumacher, J.P. et al. (2013) Comparison of first-intention healing of carbon dioxide laser, 4.0-MHz radiosurgery, and scalpel incisions in ball pythons (Python regius). *American Journal of Veterinary Research*, 74, 499–508.

Huchzermeyer, F.W. and Cooper, J.E. (2000) Fibriccess, not abscess, resulting from a localised inflammatory response to infection in reptiles and birds. *Veterinary Record*, 147, 515–517.

Johnson, R. (2011) Clinical technique: handling and treating venomous snakes. *Journal of Exotic Pet Medicine*, 20, 124–130.

Lawton, M.P.C. (2006) Reptilian ophthalmology, in *Reptile Medicine and Surgery*, 2nd ed. (D.R. Mader, ed.). Elsevier, St. Louis, MO, pp. 323–342.

Mader, D.R., Bennett, R.A., Funk, R.S. et al. (2006) Surgery, in *Reptile Medicine and Surgery* (D.R. Mader ed.). Saunders, St. Louis, MO, pp. 581–630.

Millichamp, N.J., Jacobson, E.R. and Dziezyc, J. (1986) Conjunctivoralostomy for treatment of an occluded lacrimal duct in a blood python. *Journal of the American Veterinary Medicine Association*, 11, 1136–1138.

Mitchell, M.A. (2002) Diagnosis and management of reptile orthopedic injuries. *Veterinary Clinics of North America Exotic Animal Practice*, 5, 97–114.

Murray, M.J. (2006) Aural abscesses, in *Reptile Medicine and Surgery*, 2nd ed. (D.R. Mader, ed.). Elsevier, St. Louis, MO, pp. 742–746.

Tuxbury, K.A., Clayton, L.A., Snakard, E.P. and Fishman, E.K. (2010) Multiple skull fractures in a captive Fly river turtle (*Carretochelys insculpta*): diagnosis, surgical repair, and medical management. *Journal of Herpetological Medicine and Surgery*, 20, 11–19.

Vasaruchapong, T. and Chanhome, L. (2012) Surgical treatment of renal gout in monocellate cobra, *Naja kaouthia*. *Thai Journal of Veterinary Medicine*, 42, 383–386.

29

Turtle Shell Repair

Jane Roffey and Sasha Miles

Introduction

There are approximately 250 species of turtles and tortoises in the world (Boyer and Boyer 2006). Shell injuries are common in wild chelonians but are also seen in captive animals. Causes of shell trauma include road trauma, predator attacks, falling, being trodden on, lawn mower injuries, boat propeller strikes and hailstone strikes (Figure 29.1). Shells may also require repair due to disease such as infection and abscess. Management of shell repair may be a prolonged process.

Anatomy

The turtle shell consists of two main sections: the dorsal carapace and ventral plastron, connected laterally by the bridges. The shell consists of about 60 dermal bone plates and these are covered externally by keratinized scales called scutes (Horowitz *et al.* 2015, O'Malley 2005). The scutes form from the epidermis and are the equivalent to scales in other reptiles. The position of the scutes does not correspond to the underlying bone plates of the shell, which acts to strengthen the shell (Barten 2006). Both the dermal bone plates and scutes are innervated and vascular (O'Malley 2005).

As well as the shell, the bone plates also form the modified pectoral and pelvic limb girdles, trunk vertebrae, sacrum and ribs (Horowitz *et al.* 2015). The trunk vertebrae and sacrum form part of the shell structure, as they are attached to the ribs, which in turn are fused to the dermal bone plates. The pectoral and pelvic girdles are situated internal to the ribs which mean they act to give additional strength to the shell in a vertical plane. Both these girdles attach to the plastron and carapace by pectoral and pelvic musculature (O'Malley 2005). Because of this structure, limb movement can be affected by some shell fractures and contraction of these muscles can sometimes cause movement of fractured shell segments (Vella 2009a).

Triage

Turtles presenting with shell damage should be triaged promptly. Evaluation of the patient's condition over the first few hours will determine which individuals should receive treatment and which require euthanasia. Wild turtles that will not be able to be returned to the wild in a fully functional state will need to be euthanized immediately. The time and resources required for rehabilitation are important factors to consider, particularly for wild turtles. Some turtles may require many months of treatment.

If a transverse fracture of the carapace is present then further work-up is required to assess for damage to the spine; for example, radiographs and/or computed tomography

Reptile Medicine and Surgery in Clinical Practice, First Edition. Edited by Bob Doneley, Deborah Monks, Robert Johnson and Brendan Carmel.
© 2018 John Wiley & Sons Ltd. Published 2018 by John Wiley & Sons Ltd.

(Abou-Madi *et al.* 2004, Fleming 2014). Further work-up is also required if turtles demonstrate neurological disorders. An initial assessment of all patients should include a neurological examination including assessment of gait, proprioception, sensation, withdrawal reflexes, deep pain, bladder and rectal function (Innis 2008). Evaluation of sensation and deep pain may assist in determining the extent of the injury (Fleming 2008). Five prognostic categories have been developed to assess shell injuries and these are detailed in Table 29.1 (Fleming 2008, 2014).

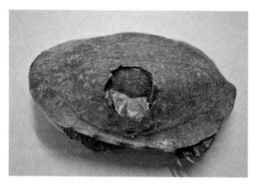

Figure 29.1 Multiple, depressed fractures of the carapace caused by hailstone trauma.

Supportive Care and Stabilization

Turtles with treatable shell injuries will require stabilization and supportive care as soon as the triage has been performed. The following steps should be taken:

- provide analgesia
- control haemorrhage

Table 29.1 A guide to the five prognostic categories for turtles with shell injuries.

Prognostic category	Characteristics	Expectations of treatment
Excellent	• Single fracture • Hairline fracture • Fracture that does not involve the spine • Minor road rash	• Supportive care • Often do not require surgical stabilization • Short term hospitalization (may only be a few days)
Good	• Multiple fractures • Unstable fractures • Open fractures (i.e. coelom visible) ± minor pieces of shell missing • Shell punctures (e.g. dog bite)	• Supportive care • Surgical stabilization of the fractures • Several months of treatment
Fair	• Multiple fractures involving pectoral and/or pelvic areas (can lead to ambulation difficulties) • Coelomic penetration • Fractures involving the bridge/s • Open fractures with large pieces of shell missing	• Supportive care • Surgical stabilization of the fractures • At least several months of treatment
Guarded	• Open fractures with damage to viscera • Gross contamination of the coelom	• Further diagnostics warranted (e.g. computed tomography and endoscopy) • Difficult to treat successfully
Grave	• Multiple comminuted fractures • Unable to stabilize shell • Internal injuries • Head injuries (including eye and jaw injuries) • Fractured spine • Paralysed limbs	Euthanasia advised

- provide warmth
- give antibiotics and fluid therapy
- stabilize fractures and protect wounds
- radiography and computed tomography (CT).

Analgesia

The turtle should be weighed and appropriate analgesia provided, depending on the severity of the injuries. Local anaesthetic splash blocks or infiltration can be administered. Opioid analgesia should also be administered in all but the mildest of cases. Butorphanol has been shown to be ineffective in one species of chelonian, whereas methadone, morphine and tramadol have shown more promising study results in terms of efficacy in reptiles including chelonians (Baker *et al.* 2011, Sladky *et al.* 2007). Morphine has been associated with significant respiratory depression so should be used with caution (Sladky *et al.* 2007). Nonsteroidal anti-inflammatory drugs can also be used in hydrated patients who are not experiencing shock. Meloxicam is widely used in reptiles based on anecdotal evidence (Fleming 2014). Refer to Chapter 27 for further information on analgesia.

Control Haemorrhage

If active bleeding is occurring from fracture sites, haemostasis can be achieved with a variety of methods including digital pressure, a pressure bandage, vessel ligation, absorbable gelatin sponges (e.g. Gelfoam®, Pfizer) and electrocautery.

Warmth

Turtles should be provided with an appropriate temperature gradient by maintaining them at 24–26 °C on a moist towel. This should be continued for the time that they are unable to be immersed in water. Fluid therapy and support feeding may be required during this time as many turtles will not eat while dry docked. The time the turtle will need to be kept out of the water will depend on the severity and location of the shell wounds and whether or not the coelom is penetrated.

Antibiotics

Almost all turtles with shell lesions will require antibiotics. Initially, an antibiotic with a broad Gram-negative spectrum is preferred, as most infectious bacteria in reptiles are gram negative (Fleming 2008). The third-generation cephalosporin, ceftazidime, is commonly used and it is given at 20 mg/kg intramuscularly every three days (Raftery 2011). It has a wide spectrum of activity against Gram-negative bacteria, including *Pseudomonas aeruginosa* (Gregory 2008). Alternatively, fluoroquinolones have a wide activity against both Gram-positive and -negative bacteria but limited spectrum against anaerobes (Gregory 2008). Enrofloxacin can be given at 10 mg/kg intramuscularly or orally every second day. This medication is associated with pain and tissue necrosis at the injection site and should be diluted with sterile water to reduce this effect (Fleming 2008). The choice of antibiotic for long-term use, with chronic wounds or abscesses, should be guided by culture and sensitivity (Fleming 2014).

Fluid Therapy

Turtles with shell injuries have often lost fluids and are not maintaining normal fluid uptake so can be considered mildly (less than 5%) to moderately (7%) dehydrated in most cases (Chitty *et al.* 2013, Fleming 2014). Dehydration can be indicated by sunken eyes, skin tenting, a dry mouth, thick oral mucus, a slow or faint heartbeat, minimal or no urination, a poor demeanour and increasing serial packed cell volume and total protein measurements (Norton 2005). Fluids should be warmed and can be given intravenously, intraosseously, subcutaneously, epicoelomically or intracoelomically in the initial phase, depending on the patient's requirements (Vella 2009a). Fluid maintenance rates are 15–25 ml/kg/day in most species (Norton

2005). Fluid therapy should be calculated based on this and the estimated deficit. After three or four days of parenteral fluids, most patients can often be switched to oral fluid therapy (Fleming 2008).

Initial Fracture Stabilization and Wound Protection

Displaced fractures may be temporarily stabilized to prevent further contamination and to assist with analgesia. An adhesive dressing tape can be used for this purpose, until the animal is stabilized and can be anaesthetized for repair (Figure 29.2). Any coelomic penetration or other wounds should also be bandaged to prevent any further contamination, until cleaning and irrigation can occur.

Radiographs

All turtles should be radiographed within the first 24 hours for a detailed assessment of injuries and to determine whether the turtle is gravid. The limbs, spine, pectoral and pelvic girdles should be assessed for damage. Occasionally, fractures to the bone plates of the carapace or plastron are not apparent as the overlying scutes are still intact (Fleming 2014). Three radiographic projections are required: dorsoventral, lateral and craniocaudal (Figure 29.3). Bridge fractures can be superimposed on dorsoventral views (Fleming 2008).

Computed Tomography

Some fractures may not be apparent on plain radiographs and computed tomography has been used as a more sensitive diagnostic tool (Abou-Madi *et al.* 2004). It may also be useful for assessing internal injuries.

Wound Care

Wound care should commence within a few hours of presentation and may need to be continued in the long term. Flushing of shell lesions should be performed with a 2% solution of chlorhexidine initially, and then followed by copious volumes of warm, sterile saline. Ensure the foreign material is flushed out, instead of into the wound, by holding the wounds ventrally. Depending on the severity of contamination, flushing may have to be repeated daily for the first few days and then reduced to every other day or weekly if required (Fleming 2008, Mitchell and Diaz-Figueroa 2004, Vella 2009b). If there is coelomic penetration, saline should be used for wound flushing, not chlorhexidine. Depending on the degree of coelomic penetration, endoscopy or a coeliotomy may be

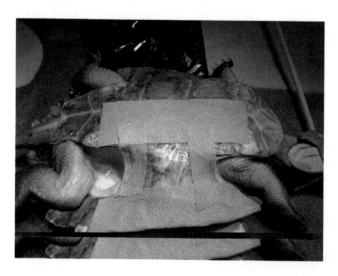

Figure 29.2 A clear adhesive dressing adhered to the shell with adhesive tape.

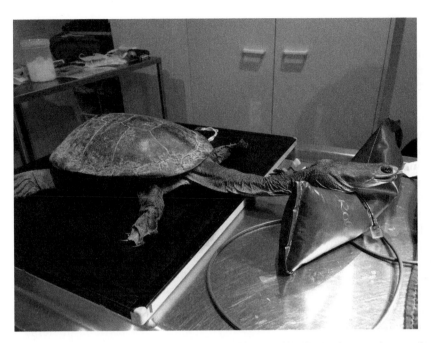

Figure 29.3 Performing a dorsoventral radiograph on an anaesthetised eastern long-necked turtle (*Chelodina expansa*).

Figure 29.4 Severe, multiple bridge and carapace fractures with shell deficits. The wound is grossly contaminated and has necrotic tissue present.

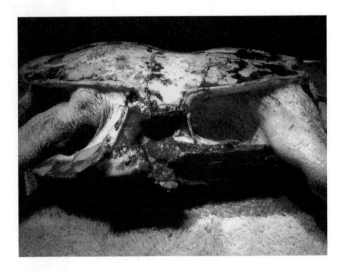

required to assess for potential internal bleeding and organ trauma. Coelomic lavage may be required if there is contamination; however, gross contamination of the coelom is associated with a poor prognosis. Fractured shell sites may need to be cleaned with brushes, cloths or sponges. Topical anaesthesia can be provided during this time with splash blocks of lignocaine and/or bupivacaine.

Some cases will require debridement and excision of necrotic tissue (Figure 29.4). Depending on the severity, this can be performed under local or general anaesthesia. If required, various tools can be used to debride the shell and these include needles, scalpels, rongeurs and electric high-speed burrs. The shell should be debrided until light bleeding occurs (Vella 2009b).

Wet-to-dry bandages are commonly placed after irrigation to facilitate the removal of debris and prevent further contamination (Mitchell and Diaz-Figueroa 2004). These bandages can be attached to the shell with an adhesive tape. Wet-to-dry bandages usually are used until wound exudate is controlled and from there non-adhesive dressings can be used. In cases of severe infection, silver-impregnated dressings can be used as the primary layer (Fleming 2014, Norton 2005). Closed fractures can be treated with bandaging alone to prevent contamination and encourage granulation tissue formation (Fleming 2014). For shell fractures that require surgical fixation, bandages are applied until the turtle is stabilized and the wound is clean enough to undergo surgery (Chitty and Raftery 2013).

In the case of shell deficits, which cannot be closed surgically, bandaging will need to be continued for many months. Generally two weeks of wet-to-dry bandaging is performed and then nonadherent bandages are used until a thick granulation tissue bed is present. This process takes at least six to eight weeks. Once a thick granulation tissue bed has formed, the area can be left unbandaged but monitored closely and kept clean (Fleming 2014).

Vacuum-Assisted Wound Closure

An alternative to wet-to-dry bandaging, vacuum-assisted wound closure or negative pressure wound therapy, is becoming increasingly common in human and veterinary medicine (Atay *et al.* 2013; Howe 2015). It has been shown to promote and expedite wound healing by increasing blood flow to the wound bed, increasing the rate of granulation tissue formation, reducing bacterial tissue counts and by removing exudates and reducing oedema (Marin *et al.* 2014, Morykwas *et al.* 1997). Contraindications for negative pressure wound therapy include the presence of local malignancy, undebrided osteomyelitis, active bleeding, concurrent anticoagulant therapy and the use over exposed vessels, nerves, tendons, ligaments or unprotected organs (Howe 2015).

Fracture Fixation

Fractures can be permanently fixated once the turtle has been stabilized and wounds have been treated appropriately. All repairs are performed under sedation or general anaesthesia (Figure 29.5). See Chapter 27 for further information on analgesia, sedation and general anaesthesia. There are currently many different techniques and materials used in the repair of shell fractures. Methods of repair discussed are sometimes used in conjunction with each other.

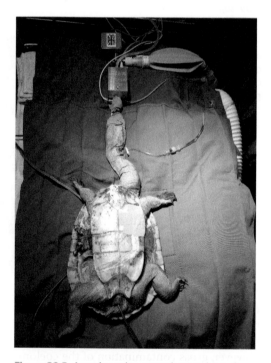

Figure 29.5 A turtle under general anaesthesia for shell repair. Note the placement of an intravenous catheter delivering intravenous fluids, an endotracheal tube (which is attached to a ventilator) and a rectal temperature probe.

Adhesives

The use of epoxies and fibreglass to completely cover shell fractures has fallen out of favour for the repair of traumatic and infected wounds, because of the risk of sealing in infection and the inability to manage wounds once this has been placed. This method of repair may also interfere with wound healing and growth (Bogard and Innis 2008, Fleming 2008, 2014, Vella 2009b). Epoxy products can generate a high degree of heat during placement and can damage soft tissue and live bone (Mitchell 2002); however, epoxy and other adhesives, such as resins, glues, cements and acrylics can still

be used as suitable materials for repairing nondisplaced fractures and for elective plastronotomy closure (Figure 29.6). When no longer required, these materials should be removed from young chelonians to prevent growth impediment and deformity (Fleming 2014). Adhesives can also be used to secure devices to the shell, as discussed in the section on bridging methods.

Glass ionomers have been used to seal fissures in the shell, cover small open wounds and seal areas that have not been completely closed by orthopaedic fixation (Figure 29.7). This material is used in human dentistry for permanent tooth fillings. The silicate cement

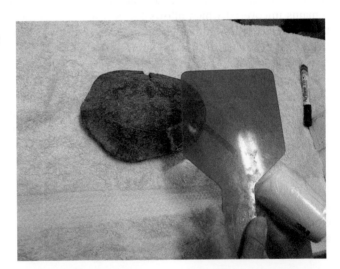

Figure 29.6 Ultraviolet light curing of a methyl-methacrylate repair (courtesy of Robert Johnson).

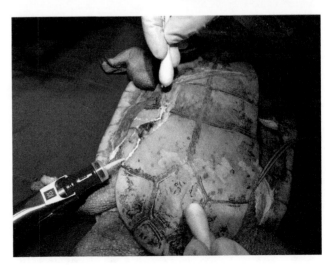

Figure 29.7 Filling small fissures in the shell with a dental acrylic.

in the product releases fluorine which provides a local antibacterial effect and increases precipitation of calcium in the surrounding tissue (Fowler and Magelakis 2004). This material should only be used at sterile or sterilized wound sites. Glass ionomers are usually shed with the scutes (Wilson and Burns 2000).

Bridging Methods

A bridging method involves securing various devices to the shell, on either side of the fracture to achieve compression and apposition of the fracture segments. A major advantage of this method is that the fracture site itself remains uncovered which allows for access to the wound and monitoring of the healing process. This method is also cost effective, minimally invasive and easy to perform. Disadvantages of this method include the possibility of the device detaching from the shell due to poor placement and that it generally does not provide the same degree of stabilisation as orthopaedic repair (Fleming 2014).

Many fixation devices can be purchased from hardware and haberdashery shops, including saddle clamps, wall hanging hooks, clothing hooks (Figure 29.8), curtain hooks and cable ties (Chitty and Raftery 2013, Divers 2011, Fleming 2014, Forrester and Satta 2005, Lloyd 2007, Vella 2009b). These devices may be placed once or many times along the fracture line, depending on the length of the fracture. Hook-like devices will need to be linked and tightened to reduced and stabilize the fracture. Suitable materials for this purpose include stainless steel wire and suture material (Bogard and Innis 2008, Fleming 2014, Vella 2009b). Saddle clamps are U-shaped clamps used to attach pipes to flat surfaces. These can be bent and cut to the contour of the shell and then attached with an adhesive (Vella 2009b). When using cable ties, a cable tie mount is adhered to the shell on either side of the fracture. A cable tie is then placed through both mounts and secured in place at one end with another cable tie. Once adequate tension is achieved, the ends are trimmed short (Divers 2001, Forrester and Satta 2005). A method using a human device designed for stretching skin called the TopClosure® Tension Relief System has also been described (Horowitz *et al.* 2015).

Metal plates have also been used to bridge fracture sites. Orthopaedic bone plates or metal plates from hardware shops can be used. These are particularly useful for plastron fractures as their low profile can allow for ambulation (Fleming 2014, Richards 2001). The plate should be cut and moulded

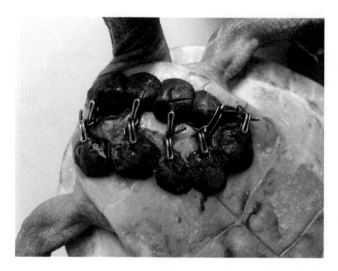

Figure 29.8 A bridging method of plastron fracture repair using clothing hooks and Knead-IT® (Selleys Australia & New Zealand).

to the shaped of the shell and if possible, a central arch will allow for increased wound management and visualization (Chitty and Raftery 2013).

Suitable adhesives for attaching these fixation devices to the shell include epoxies, polymethyl methacrylates, including dental acrylics and strong glues or adhesives including cyanoacrylates from hardware shops (Bogard and Innis 2008, Chitty and Raftery 2013, Horowitz *et al.* 2015, Vella 2009b). The keratin at the site of attachment can be roughened with a high speed burr or hand tool to improve adhesion (Bogard and Innis 2008, Horowitz *et al.* 2015). If wiring or suturing is required to attach the devices, then in most cases it is best to allow the adhesive to set for 12 hours prior to tightening. During this time, the fracture can be temporarily stabilized with adhesive tape (Bogard and Innis 2008). Care should be taken that adhesives do not come into contact with soft tissue or live bone during placement (Fleming 2014).

Once the fracture has healed, the devices can generally be removed with gentle rotational force applied by a grasping tool or by using a periosteal elevator or chisel to pry them from the shell (Divers 2011, Bogard and Innis 2008). There is generally little trauma to the underlying scutes using this method (Bogard and Innis 2008).

Orthopaedic Fixation

All orthopaedic repairs are performed under general anaesthesia using strict aseptic techniques (Mitchell 2002, Vella 2009b). The shell and surrounding soft tissue is aseptically prepared prior to fixation (Fleming 2014). Implants must be constructed from stainless steel as galvanized metals can release zinc systemically. Stainless steel screws can be purchased in a variety of sizes from hardware shops and then sterilized (Fleming 2014). Orthopaedic repairs may be used in combination with bridging and adhesive methods.

Advantages associated with this repair method include the ability to reduce complex fracture and increased fracture stability, particularly in larger chelonians. Disadvantages include increased costs, potential introduction of infection, requirement for general anaesthesia and the potential for implant failure (Vella 2009b).

One of the simplest methods of orthopaedic fixation involves drilling a hole on either side of the fracture and tightening Kirschner wires or cerclage wires through the holes (Figure 29.9). This method is repeated along the length of the fracture (Heatley 2011, Mitchell 2002, Barten 2006). Holes can be drilled using a Kirschner wire, power tool or electric drill. Care should be taken as damage

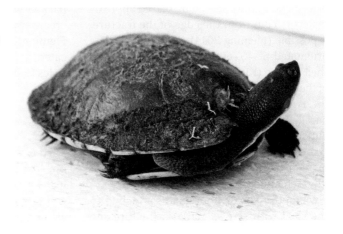

Figure 29.9 Peripheral carapace fractures have been repaired here using metal sutures (courtesy of Robert Johnson).

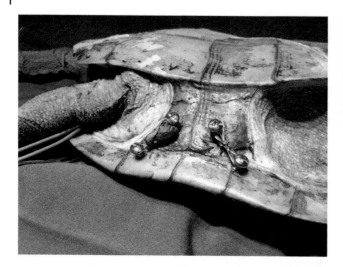

Figure 29.10 Stainless steel screws have been placed in the shell and orthopaedic wire has been applied in a figure of eight pattern to stabilize this bridge fracture. Note that the wire on the left side of the photo has been covered in an adhesive to protect soft tissue from trauma during ambulation.

to the internal organs and surrounding soft tissue can occur during drilling, wire placement and tightening. Depending on the location, placement of wires can be difficult. Wires should be covered to prevent tracking of infection into the bone and/or coelom (Heatley 2011, Kishimori *et al.* 2001).

A variation of this method involves placing orthopaedic or stainless steel screws on either side of the fracture line and connecting them with orthopaedic wire in a figure of eight pattern (Figure 29.10). This is repeated along the fracture line as required. The wire will need to be tightened to provide close apposition of the fracture segments (Chitty and Raftery 2013, Kishimori *et al.* 2001). Pilot holes are made with a drill bit slightly smaller than the size of the screw, prior to screw placement. Screws should be placed approximately 0.5 cm from the edge of the fracture, if possible (Fleming 2014). Screws should be orientated at 45–60 degrees to the healthy shell surface (Kishimori *et al.* 2001). The knot of the cerclage wire should be located between the two screw heads and this can be bent parallel with the shell or covered with epoxy putty or bandaging material (Fleming 2014). Damage to the internal organs and surrounding soft tissue is also a risk associated with this technique (Heatley 2011).

Metal bridges or bone plates attached to the shell with screws across a fracture site can also be used as a repair method (Chitty and Raftery 2013). This method is helpful for plastron fractures as it can allow for normal ambulation. Care should be taken as a large portion of the fracture site is likely to be covered by the plate which means wound monitoring and care is inhibited (Fleming 2014).

To remove any external fixation, the shell should again be aseptically prepared. This can generally be performed under sedation but in some cases general anaesthesia may be required. Screws are removed using an appropriate screw driver (Fleming 2014). The remaining holes will need to be kept clean and protected until they heal. Healing can take from four to eight weeks (Chitty and Raftery 2013). The holes can be bandaged, filled with a water proofing ointment or packed with a silver sulfadiazine-containing cream twice a week (Chitty and Raftery 2013, Fleming 2014). A course of antibiotics is indicated if there are a large number of screw holes (Fleming 2014).

Post-Surgical Care

Turtles should be kept warm and dry docked on moist towels after surgery. As turtles usually require immersion in water to eat and drink, dry docking is only continued for as long as it is necessary. It will need to be continued until there is sufficient epithelialization of the fracture and any wounds that may also be present. This time period can vary between two weeks for simple fractures and one to two years for a severe fracture with shell deficits (Fleming 2008, Vella 2009a). In some cases the fracture site may be able to be covered with a waterproof dressing to allow a 30–60-minute swim each day (Figure 29.3). This will assist in maintaining hydration and allow for food intake, urination and defecation. Turtles without plastron damage can be placed into a container of shallow water to allow water absorption though the cloaca. If a turtle is unable to be placed into water for many weeks or months, then nutritional support will be required. Tube feeding with an orogastric tube or placement of an oesophagostomy tube are possible options. Fluid therapy is also likely to be required for these turtles.

All fixation devices should be checked regularly to ensure that they remain intact and stable. Healing generally occurs between 4–8 weeks but in some cases can be up to 30 months (Fleming 2014, Mitchell 2002). Staged removal of the fixation devices is recommended for complex fractures. Callus formation is not often visible on radiographs so palpation for stability is often the best guide in assessing fracture healing (Fleming 2014).

References

Abou-Madi, N., Scrivani, P. V., Kollias, G. V. and Hernandez-Divers, S. M. (2004) Diagnosis of skeletal injuries in Chelonians using computed tomography. *Journal of Zoo and Wildlife Medicine*, 35 (2), 226–231.

Atay, T., Burc, H., Baykal, Y.B. and Kirdemir, V. (2013) Results of vacuum assisted wound closure application. *Indian Journal of Surgery*, 75 (4), 302–305.

Baker, B., Sladky, K. and Johnston, S. (2011) Evaluations of the analgesic effects of oral and subcutaneous tramadol administration in red-eared slider turtles. *Journal of the American Veterinary Medical Association*, 238, 220–227.

Barten, S. (2006) Shell damage, in *Reptile Medicine and Surgery*, 2nd ed. (D.R. Mader, ed.), Elsevier Saunders, St Louis, MO, pp. 893–899.

Bogard, C. and Innis, C. (2008) A simple and inexpensive method of shell repair in Chelonia. *Journal of Herpetological Medicine and Surgery*, 18 (1), 12–13.

Boyer, T. and Boyer, D. (2006) Turtles, tortoises, and terrapins, in *Reptile Medicine and Surgery*, 2nd ed. (D. Mader, ed.). Elsevier Saunders, St Louis, MO, pp. 696–704.

Chitty, J. and Raftery, A. Fractures of the shell, in *Essentials of Tortoise Medicine and Surgery*. John Wiley & Sons, Ltd, Chichester, pp. 216–221.

Divers, S. (2011) Zip-tie closure for turtle shell fractures: quick, simple and cheap! in NAVC Conference Proceedings, Orlando, FL.

Fleming, G.J. (2008) Clinical technique: Chelonian shell repair. *Journal of Exotic Pet Medicine*, 17 (4), 246–258.

Fleming, G.J. (2014) New techniques in Chelonian shell repair, in *Current Therapy in Reptile Medicine and Surgery* (D. Mader and S. Divers, eds). Elsevier Saunders, St Louis, MO, pp. 205–212.

Forrester, H. and Satta, J. (2005) Easy shell repair. *Exotic DVM*, 6 (6), 13.

Fowler, A. and Magelakis, N. (2004) Shell fracture repair using glass ionomer cement in the long neck turtle, in Proceedings of the Australian Veterinary Association Conference, Canberra, pp. 137–139.

Gregory, J. (2008) Clinical technique: chelonian shell repair. *Journal of Exotic Pet Medicine*, 17, 246–258.

Heatley, J. (2011) Chelonian shell repair, in American Board of Veterinary Practitioners Conference Proceedings, St Louis, MO.

Horowitz, I.H., Yanco, E. and Topaz, M. (2015) TopClosure System adapted to Chelonian shell repair. *Journal of Exotic Pet Medicine*, 24 (1), 65–70.

Howe, L. (2015) Current concepts in negative pressure wound therapy. *Veterinary Clinics of North America Small Animal Practice*, 45 (3), 565–584.

Innes, C. (2008) Restraint and physical examination of chelonians, in NAVC Conference, pp. 1780–1782.

Kishimori, J., Lewbart, G., Marcellin-Little, D. *et al.* (2001) Chelonian shell fracture repair techniques. *Exotic DVM*, 3, 35–41.

Lloyd, C. (2007) Alternative method for cable tie shell repair in chelonian. *Exotic DVM*, 9, 9–10.

Marin, M.L., Norton, T.M. and Mettee, N.S. (2014) Vacuum-assisted wound closure in chelonians, in *Current Therapy in Reptile Medicine and Surgery* (D.R. Mader and S.J. Divers, eds). Elsevier Saunders, St Louis, MO, pp. 197–204.

Mitchell, M.A. (2002) Diagnosis and management of reptile orthopedic injuries. *Veterinary Clinics of North America Exotic Animal Practice*, 5 (1), 97–114.

Mitchell, M.A. and Diaz-Figueroa, O. (2004) Wound management in reptiles. *Veterinary Clinics of North America Exotic Animal Practice*, 7, 123–140.

Morykwas, M.J., Argenta, L.C., Shelton-Brown, E.I. and McGuirt, W. (1997)

Vacuum-assisted closure: a new method for wound control and treatment: animal studies and basic foundation. *Annals of Plastic Surgery*, 38 (6), 553–562.

Norton, T.M. (2005) Chelonian emergency and critical care. *Seminars in Avian and Exotic Pet Medicine*, 14 (2), 106–130.

O'Malley, B. (2005) Tortoises and turtles, in *Clinical Anatomy and Physiology of Exotic Species*. Elsevier Saunders, St Louis, MO, pp. 41–56.

Raftery, A. (2011) Reptile orthopaedic medicine and surgery. *Journal of Exotic Pet Medicine*, 20, 107–116.

Richards, J. (2001) Metal bridges: a new technique of turtle shell repair. *Journal of Herpetological Medicine and Surgery*, 11 (4), 31–34.

Sladky, K., Miletic, V., Paul-Murphy, J. *et al.* (2007) Analgesic efficacy and respiratory effects of butorphanol and morphine in turtles. *Journal of the American Veterinary Medical Association*, 230, 1356–1362.

Vella, D. (2009a) Management of aquatic turtle shell fractures. *Lab Animal (NY)*, 38 (2), 52–53.

Vella, D. (2009b) Management of freshwater turtle shell injuries. *Lab Animal (NY)*, 38 (1), 13–14.

Wilson, G. and Burns, P. (2000) The use of a low exothermic-curing dental acrylic to repair turtle shell injuries. *Australian Veterinary Practitioner*, 30, 63–66.

Further Reading

KCI Animal Health (2012) *V.A.C. Therapy for Veterinary Use User Manual*. San Antonio, TX, KCI Licensing.

Kirchgessner, M. and Mitchell, M., (2009) Chelonians, in *Manual of Exotic Pet Practice*

(M.A. Mitchell and T.N. Tully, eds). Saunders Elsevier, St Louis, MO, pp. 207–249.

30

Necropsy
Catherine M. Shilton

Introduction

A diagnostic necropsy is the dissection of an animal after death to inform the cause of morbidity or mortality. The two main components are detailed systematic gross examination of organs to look for clues and sampling for further ancillary testing. A necropsy offers the opportunity for the clinician to compare necropsy results to clinical data and to add to the expanding field of reptile medicine and disease diagnosis.

Preliminary Considerations

Maximize Carcase Quality

Poor carcase quality will decrease the amount of information that can be gained from both gross examination and histopathology, and may limit interpretation of other tests (Table 30.1). Many reptiles are kept in proximity to a heat source, which hastens decomposition, resulting in significant degradation of carcase quality within a few hours of death. Decomposition can be minimized by refrigeration of the carcase for up to four days, after which it should be frozen. In an outbreak of disease in a reptile collection, carcasses for necropsy should be of the best quality, representative of the disease or syndrome of interest and performed on multiple affected individuals, so that a consistent pattern in necropsy findings can be discerned.

Necropsy Safety

Although there is a long list of theoretically possible reptilian zoonoses, with the exceptions of *Salmonella* species and pentastomes, actual transmission under natural circumstances is either rare or has never been documented (Johnson-Delaney 2006). However, opening the carcase of a diseased reptile may increase risk of human exposure to a variety of opportunistic or pathogenic organisms. This risk can be mitigated by use of disposable gloves and antiseptic hand wash for personal protection and hospital-grade disinfectant for equipment clean-up. Any wounds incurred by the dissector during necropsy should be immediately disinfected and bandaged. After necropsy, freezing the carcase in a designated carcase freezer is a good interim measure prior to disposal by deep burial or incineration, depending on disposal services available. When dissecting a venomous snake, the head should never be handled directly with fingers but always with instruments. The head should be removed as the first step of the necropsy and placed in formalin for complete fixation prior to detailed examination or brain removal.

Reptile Medicine and Surgery in Clinical Practice, First Edition. Edited by Bob Doneley, Deborah Monks, Robert Johnson and Brendan Carmel.
© 2018 John Wiley & Sons Ltd. Published 2018 by John Wiley & Sons Ltd.

Table 30.1 Post-mortem factors that may impact necropsy findings.

Change	Definition	Necropsy consequences
Hypostatic congestion	Fluid accumulation in tissues due to gravity	Artefactual appearance of congestion and oedema of tissues on side of carcase that was lowest at death.
Suffusion of pigment	Passage of pigment to surrounding tissues	Reddening of tissues near blood vessels or highly perfused organs by haemoglobin pigment may mimic haemorrhage (Figure 30.2d). Green tinge to tissues surrounding gall bladder due to bile pigment. Indicative of at least moderate decomposition.
Autolysis	Degradation of tissues by autogenous enzymes	Red-tinged watery fluid accumulation in body cavities and leakage from orifices. Loss of fine cellular detail (renders cytology nondiagnostic and reduces accuracy of histological interpretation of subtle lesions).
Putrefaction	Bacterial degradation of tissues, primarily due to anaerobes from the gastrointestinal tract	Colour change of tissues, generally towards pallor and/or green/grey tinge. Eventually results in gas production (artefactual emphysema) in organs. Progressive loss of histological detail. May confound meaningful bacterial and fungal culture and/or interpretation of results. May inhibit virus isolation and/or molecular testing.
Freeze-thaw cycle	Freezing and subsequent thawing of carcase	Generalized reddening of tissues due to suffusion of haemoglobin pigment from lysed red cells. Accumulation of red-tinged fluid in body cavities at thawing. Proliferation of putrefactive bacteria during thawing (minimize by thawing under refrigeration). Histological interpretation is severely confounded. Advantage is decomposition is greatly slowed so carcase is relatively well preserved for some ancillary tests (culture and molecular testing).
Euthanasia solution artefact	Due to caustic effect on tissues of concentrated pentobarbital	Discoloration, necrosis and mineralization of tissue perfused with pentobarbital. Histologically, tissues exhibit artefactual coagulation necrosis and loss of cellular detail. Minimize by using appropriate dose of pentobarbital, preferably injected intravenously rather than intracoelomically.

Necropsy Equipment

Being well equipped and having tools and sampling materials easily accessible during the necropsy will greatly facilitate dissection, thorough examination and optimal sampling (Figures 30.1a,b).

Necropsy Procedure

A list of differential diagnoses should be formed before the necropsy, based on the history and clinical record. The necropsy should involve a thorough examination of all body systems, plus detailed targeted examination and/or sampling of other components as required based on the list of differential diagnoses. Grossly appreciable abnormalities relate to organ size, shape, colour, texture and presence of exudates. For most organs, there is a wide range of 'normal' in reptiles, depending on the species, its age and metabolic status, which precludes the use of dogmatic descriptions for normal reptilian organ appearance. Images have been provided to exemplify the types of changes to look for

(a)

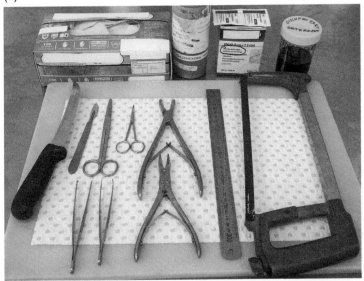

(b)

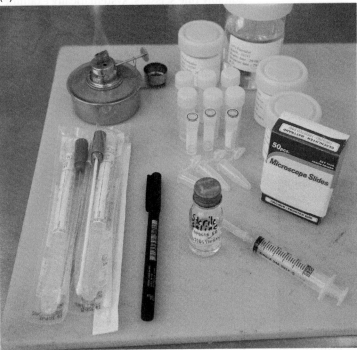

Figure 30.1 Necropsy equipment. (a) Sharp knife, scalpel, scissors and rongeurs (various sizes), forceps, hacksaw and ruler displayed on a disposable waterproof mat and underlying plastic cutting board. Disposable gloves, antiseptic hand wash, bandages, antiseptic and hospital-grade disinfectant displayed along the top. (b) Sampling supplies, clockwise from upper left: flame for sterilizing instruments before samples are taken, jars of 10% buffered formalin of various sizes for histology samples, sterile jars and vials of various sizes for individual fresh samples, glass slides for cytology impressions, syringe and needle for injecting formalin into tissues (unopened intestine, eyes) for histology, normal saline to moisten plain swabs or small fresh tissue samples, permanent marker for labelling, plain swab and swabs with bacterial transport media.

and the wide variation possible in reptiles, but each dissector will need to gain familiarity with the normal appearance of organs in the species they most commonly necropsy. If in doubt about the gross appearance of an organ, record it and sample the organ for histology.

External Examination of the Carcase

Record size (e.g. snout–vent or carapace length), weight and body condition (poor, fair, good, obese). Examine the skin, eyes, ears, oral cavity, take note of any oral, nasal or cloacal discharges and any asymmetries of body parts (abnormal size/shape of joints/bones, abnormal bulges in skin or body cavity) (Figures 30.2a–d).

Opening the Carcase

For snakes, lizards and crocodilians, a ventral midline incision is made from the jaw to immediately cranial to the cloaca (Figure 30.3a). Increased exposure of the organs in the body cavity can be obtained by reflecting back or removing the ventral skin and body wall (Figure 30.3b) using scissors or rongeurs to cut through the ribs and pectoral girdle. In chelonians, the plastron is removed (Figures 30.3c–e). It is at this stage, with the organs in the body cavity freshly exposed, that fresh samples should be taken aseptically for possible bacterial culture.

Examination of the Major Organ Systems

Organs are initially examined in situ but may then be removed to facilitate a more thorough examination, either by removing individual organs or, in small or medium-sized reptiles, the entire visceral mass in one piece (Figure 30.3b).

Cardiovascular System

Take note of any oedema, ascites, petechial or ecchymotic haemorrhages that could suggest heart failure, increased vascular permeability or vasculitis. Examine the pericardium for haemorrhages (Figure 30.4a) and incise the pericardium. There may normally be a small amount of clear, colourless to slightly yellow pericardial fluid. Reptiles with septicaemia may develop cloudy pericardial exudate, which is an excellent sample for bacterial culture (Figure 30.4b). In visceral gout, urates may accumulate in the pericardial sac. Examine the surface of the epicardium for haemorrhages (Figure 30.4c), pale streaking (which could be fibrosis or mineralization) or other abnormalities. Remove the heart, including the first few millimetres of the large vessels at the base of the heart. Using suitably fine scissors, systematically examine the inside of the heart, including the endocardial surface, heart valves and intimal surface of the large arteries, for abnormalities. Any blood clots in the heart that formed post mortem will be easily removable with forceps and not tightly adherent to the endocardium or valves, which suggests an organized (ante mortem) thrombus (Figure 30.4d). For histology, in small reptiles, the entire heart can be submitted in formalin; otherwise, sample a 1-cm transverse section across the ventricles, plus any lesions.

Respiratory System

Incise the lung(s) along their length and inspect the lumen and mucosal surface. Normal reptile lungs at necropsy are pink to pale red (depending on how congested with blood they are) and spongy with a central lumen free of any exudate. In reptiles that have been euthanized with pentobarbitone, died an agonal death, are septicaemic or have heart failure, the lungs may be dark red (markedly congested) and contain watery to foamy, possibly blood-tinged fluid (oedematous).

Figure 30.2 External examination of the carcase. (a) Patchy reddening of the skin in a snake with bacterial septicaemia. Note also caseous oral exudate. (b) Superficially intact plastron in which a layer of keratin overlies severe caseous necrosis (inset). Note also patchy reddening of the skin suggesting concurrent bacterial septicaemia. (c) Flaky, brown keratin in a snake with superficial fungal skin infection. (d) Unilateral submandibular swelling in a lizard. Dissection reveals a large, aged, chronic, inflammatory focus of caseous exudate with typical laminated appearance (inset). Note also the generalized reddening of other tissues of the neck due to suffusion of haemoglobin pigment in this moderately autolysed carcase.

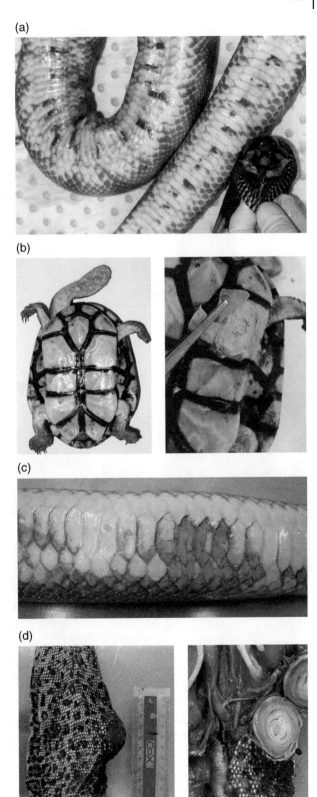

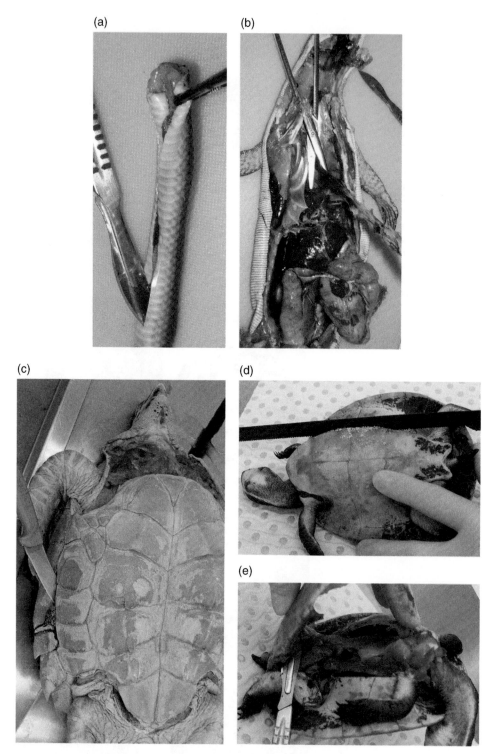

Figure 30.3 Opening the carcase. (a) Venomous or unidentified species of snakes should have the head removed as the initial step of the necropsy. The scalpel is turned upward during ventral midline incision to minimize the chance of inadvertently cutting into underlying organs. (b) Lizard opened ventrally with body wall removed. The internal viscera are being removed in one piece by placing traction on the dissected neck structures and using scissors to cut through dorsal connective tissue attachments. (c) Plastron removal from a large sea turtle by cutting the skin at the junction with the plastron and using knife to sever connective tissue attachments of the lateral plastron to the carapace. (d) Sawing through bony lateral plastron attachment of a freshwater turtle. (e) Once the skin and lateral connective tissue or bone attachments of the plastron are severed, the underlying tissue attachments are cut close to the plastron as it is elevated.

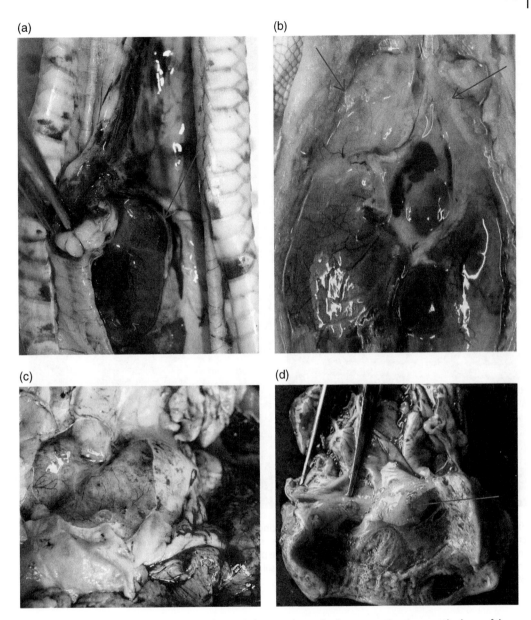

Figure 30.4 Cardiovascular system. (a) Ecchymotic haemorrhages in the connective tissue at the base of the heart (arrow) in a snake with acute Gram-negative septicaemia. (b) Fibrinopurulent pericardial exudate in a crocodile with subacute Gram-negative septicaemia. The pleura (arrows) and hepatic serosa are moist, cloudy and thickened. (c) Cloudy, moist epicardium with petechial haemorrhages in a sea turtle with Gram-negative septicaemia. (d) Multiple irregular, fibrinous nodules adherent to the atrioventricular valves (arrows) in a sea turtle with bacterial septicaemia.

If exudate or nodules are noted on initial incision of the lung (Figures 30.5a–c), a swab or tissue for bacterial and/or fungal culture should be taken aseptically from an unopened portion of lung. Incise the air sacs (if present) and inspect for thickenings or exudate. Palpation of the lungs is a good method to detect inconspicuous nodules or fibrous scarring (Figure 30.5c). Use fine scissors to cut along the length of the trachea to the

(a)

(b)

(c)

(d)

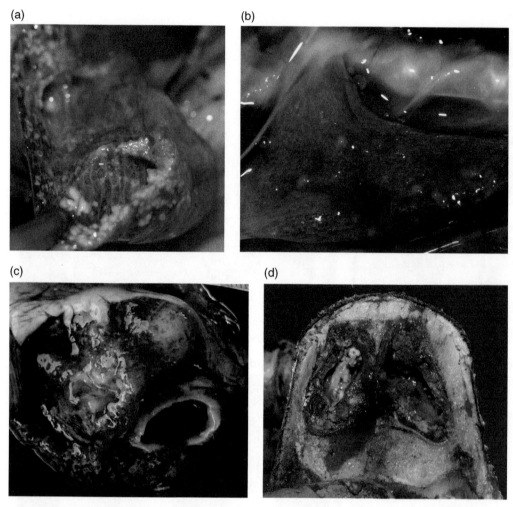

Figure 30.5 Respiratory system. (a) Multifocal to coalescing caseous foci in pulmonary infundibulae in a crocodile with fungal pneumonia. (b) Scattered, discrete, small granulomas in a crocodile with pulmonary mycobacteriosis. (c) Two large, irregular foci of firm white pulmonary fibrosis in a sea turtle with chronic mycobacterial infection. (d) Transverse section of the nasal cavity revealing copious yellow exudate in left side of nasal cavity in a sea turtle with fungal rhinitis.

glottis, looking for haemorrhage, exudate or obstructions. If there is a suspicion of abnormalities of the nasal sinuses, these can be exposed using rongeurs or a hacksaw and sampled for culture or molecular testing using a swab (Figure 30.5d). An intact section of the sinuses (large reptile) or the entire head (small reptile) should be included for histological evaluation.

Liver and Biliary System

The normal colour of the liver can vary considerably depending on the metabolic status of the reptile, the degree of hepatic congestion and the state of decomposition (Figures 30.6a,b). Thin reptiles will often have a relatively dark red-brown liver, owing to hepatocellular atrophy and absence of

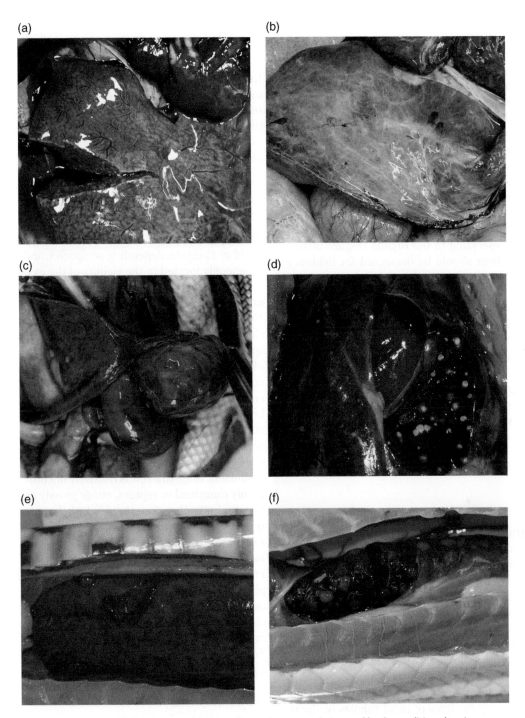

Figure 30.6 Liver and biliary system. (a) Liver of a captive sea turtle in good body condition showing reticulated pattern due to combined effect of diffuse moderate lipidosis (pale pink colour) and mid-zonal congestion (darker pink colour). (b) Dark green, atrophic liver of a thin, chronically injured free-ranging sea turtle. (c) Markedly enlarged gall bladder and adjacent bile duct due to cholelithiasis in an aged lizard. Histologically, the adjacent liver exhibited lipidosis and mild fibrosis but appears grossly dark owing to moderate numbers of parenchymal melanomacrophage clusters. (d) Multiple, small, caseous hepatic foci in a crocodile with embolic fungal infection. (e) Pale, indistinctly mottled, friable, fibrinonecrotic liver of a snake with overwhelming acute Gram-negative septicaemia. (f) Numerous discrete, raised, pale hepatic nodules in snake with hepatic neoplasia.

glycogen and lipid. A mild to moderate degree of hepatocellular lipid is usually considered within physiological normal in reptiles and imparts a light brown or pink colour to the organ, sometimes with a zonal pattern (Figure 30.6a). Congested liver appears redder than it would otherwise. With decomposition, the liver may take on a pale greyish-brown or greenish hue. Melanomacrophages may accumulate in the liver, kidneys and spleen, particularly with age, and impart a grey or black hue or fine speckling to the organs (Figure 30.6c). The liver should be inspected for evidence of embolic showering of infectious organisms from the blood, which manifests as multiple pale or caseous foci scattered throughout the parenchyma (Figure 30.6d). In bacterial septicaemia, the liver may be friable and irregularly mottled brown and pale red (Figure 30.6Ee). As in other organs, neoplastic masses in the liver may be single or multiple and often appear pale and raised, replacing normal tissue (Figure 30.6f). The gall bladder may be enlarged if the reptile has been anorexic or if there is blockage due to choleliths (Figure 30.6c).

Urinary System

The kidneys are relatively easy to locate in snakes, being obvious elongate normally red-brown lobulated organs in the caudal body cavity. However, in lizards, crocodilians and turtles, kidney location may be more obscure, lying dorsally inside the pelvic girdle and covered by adipose tissue and the peritoneal lining of the body cavity (Figure 30.7a). As with other organs, pallor can be suggestive of either fibrosis (Figure 30.7b) or cellular infiltration (Figure 30.7c). Fine pale streaking following the lines of renal tubules or ducts may indicate pyelonephritis (Figure 30.7b) or urate tophi (Figures 30.7c,d). In extreme cases of urate nephrosis, the kidneys may appear diffusely white (Figure 30.7e). If present, the bladder should be located and mucosa inspected.

Reproductive System

In reproductive females, check for yolk peritonitis and egg binding and open the oviduct to inspect the mucosa for reddening, ulceration or exudate. The activity status of gonads can be estimated grossly by the size of the testes and degree of development of the ova.

Haematopoietic and Lymphoid Tissues

The reptilian spleen varies from round to ovoid or elongate, depending on species, and is generally located in the vicinity of the gastroduodenal junction, near the gallbladder, often closely approximated to the pancreas. Normal splenic size and colour can vary considerably depending on the species (some species have primarily white pulp while others have white and red pulp), degree of congestion (enlarged and darker red when congested) and activity (may be enlarged, brown and meaty with lymphoid aggregates visible as indistinct pale foci when very active). Inspect the spleen and liver for evidence of embolic showering of infectious organisms. Bone marrow is relatively uncommonly examined in reptiles, either grossly or histologically, therefore there is little known regarding interpretation. However, if there is a suggestion from the clinical history or other necropsy findings that there may be abnormalities of bone marrow, bone marrow sampling for histological examination should be considered. Bone marrow in reptiles is typically interspersed with bone trabeculae at the metaphyses of long bones (or a rib in snakes). To obtain a sample for histology, rongeurs or a saw can be used to expose the marrow and either the entire end of the bone or a section of the metaphysis placed in formalin.

Gastrointestinal System

It is best to leave this relatively heavily contaminated system until other internal organs have been examined and sampled. Use scissors

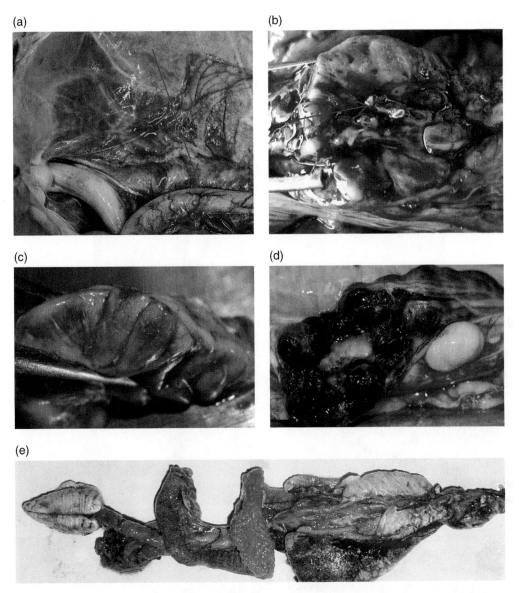

Figure 30.7 Urinary system. (a) Juvenile sea turtle showing inconspicuous retroperitoneal location of normal kidney (arrows) adjacent to the colon, underlying the immature ovary and oviduct. (b) Transverse section through kidney showing pallor from fibrosis surrounding caseous exudate in collecting ducts (arrows) in a sea turtle with pyelonephritis. (c) Multiple fine, white, pinpoint foci and streaks visible on the renal surface in a crocodile with visceral gout. There was also marked renal interstitial lymphoid proliferation, imparting the diffusely pale pink colour. (d) End-stage kidneys in an aged snake. There are pinpoint tan foci representing urate tophi surrounded by granulomas in collecting tubules. Histologically, generalized interstitial fibrosis was also present, although the gross pallor typical of fibrosis is obscured by marked renal infiltration by macrophages containing brown ceroid/lipofuscin (aging pigment). (e) Chalky, white, serosal and renal urate deposits in a lizard with severe visceral gout. The heart is to the right of the image, the kidneys to the left.

or rongeurs to cut through the angle of the jaw to expose the oral cavity. Incise the oesophagus down to the stomach, inspecting for ulcers, haemorrhages or other lesions. When examining gastrointestinal mucosa, lightly scrape mucus and sloughed cells from the surface so that the mucosa can be carefully scrutinized (Figures 30.8a,b). Intestinal lesions can often be appreciated by running the loops through fingers to detect irregularities, adhesions (Figure 30.8c) or haemorrhage (Figure 30.8d). Cuts should be made in several segments along the length of the intestine and the mucosa examined.

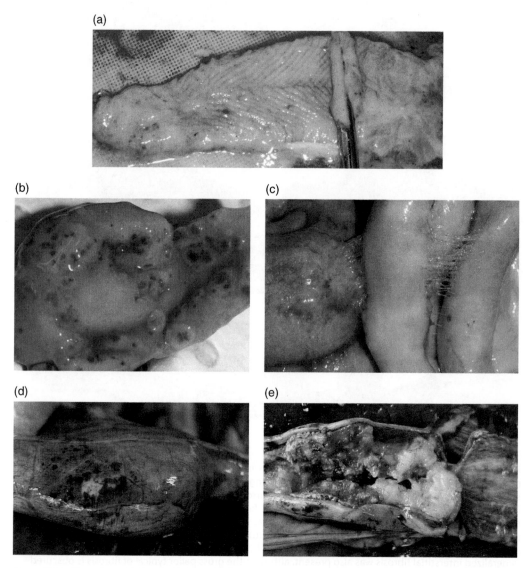

Figure 30.8 Gastrointestinal tract. (a) Normal pale, pink, shiny, smooth mucosa of lizard duodenum revealed by gently wiping the luminal mucus and sloughed cells from the surface. (b) Multiple red gastric ulcers overlying areas of mucosa that are raised and pale in a crocodile with lymphoproliferative disease. (c) Serosal reddening, thickening and light fibrous adhesions between intestinal loops in a crocodile with transmural coccidiosis. (d) Segmental enlargement and serosal haemorrhage in a sea turtle with severe bacterial enteritis. (e) Intestine from previous figure opened to reveal mucosal necrosis and copious caseous exudate. Note normal, partially pigmented intestinal mucosa to the right of the affected segment.

Musculoskeletal System

Comparison of the shape of bones and joints of the left and right sides of the body is useful to determine whether abnormal asymmetries exist. Particularly in young reptiles, bone density should be assessed by manually attempting to bend bones without having them break, which is suggestive of metabolic bone disease, and may occur in the absence of visible bone deformity (Figure 30.9a). If abnormalities of the vertebral column are suspected, good visualization of the ventral vertebral column can be achieved by removal of all the viscera and inspection from inside the body cavity (Figure 30.9b). A few joints should be opened and examined for exudate or bone irregularities (Figure 30.9c). Muscle in reptiles is generally white to pale pink and can be examined grossly by cutting through large muscle groups and inspecting them for variations in colour or texture (Figure 30.9d).

Nervous System

Although gross examination of the brain is typically unrewarding in reptiles, the brain should be exposed or removed and submitted for histological examination, particularly if the necropsy has been otherwise completed and a diagnosis has not yet been reached (Figure 30.10a,b). If neurological

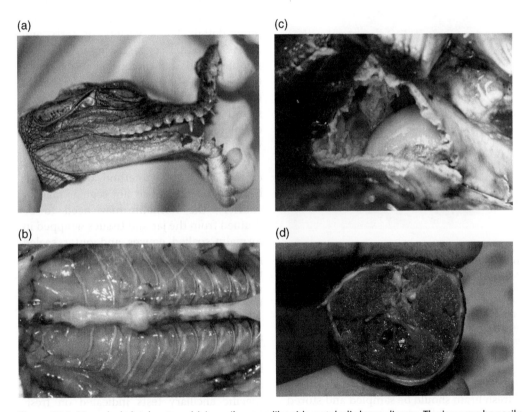

(a) (b) (c) (d)

Figure 30.9 Musculoskeletal system. (a) Juvenile crocodile with metabolic bone disease. The jaws can be easily bent without breaking. (b) Viscera removed from juvenile crocodile with metabolic bone disease to reveal a fibrous callous (arrow) and haemorrhage of ventral vertebral bodies due to pathological fractures. (c) Fibrinocaseous exudate in the shoulder joint of sea turtle with septic arthritis. (d) Transverse section of the proximal tail of a snake with red-brown discoloration of muscle, connective tissue and the hemipenes due to the combined effects of heterophil infiltration, coagulation and liquefactive necrosis and bacterial overgrowth in necrotic tissue. The primary pathogenesis was suspected to be septic thrombosis.

(a)

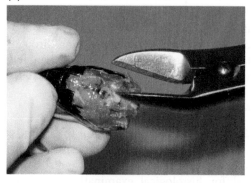

(b)

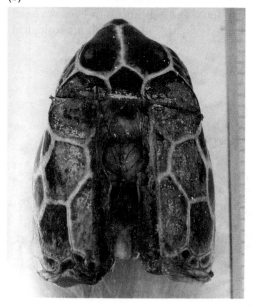

Figure 30.10 Brain removal. (a) Use of fine, sharp, pointed rongeurs for careful dissection of the head to expose the brain in a small snake. Once the calvarium is removed, the brain can be fixed in situ in formalin. (b) Brain of a sea turtle exposed using three cuts with a hacksaw. The head is then tilted so the brain gently 'spills out' under gravity as the ventral attachments are carefully cut.

disease is suspected, a parasagittal section of fresh brain should be sampled and stored frozen for possible other ancillary testing. If clinical signs specifically referable to the spinal cord were present, use rongeurs or a saw to either remove entire 1–2 cm sections of vertebral column (small reptiles) or to dissect out segments of spinal cord (large reptiles) for formalin fixation and histology.

Sample Collection and Submission to the Laboratory for Ancillary Testing

A definitive diagnosis is not usually reached from gross examination but rather a refined list of differential diagnoses is obtained, which then necessitates more definitive ancillary testing. The appropriateness and quality of samples taken at necropsy will directly influence the value of laboratory results obtained. Table 30.2 provides sampling details for a variety of tests and Box 30.1 gives a suggested minimal list of samples to take routinely during a diagnostic necropsy. Particular tests performed at the laboratory and test results may vary significantly depending on the amount of detailed information about the case provided to the laboratory.

For transport of formalin fixed samples, depending on the method of transport being used (ground or air, regular mail or courier), the formalin may need to be drained from the jar and tissues wrapped in formalin-soaked gauzes and outer sealed plastic bag used to prevent leakage during transport. If this procedure is used, it is essential that the tissues are thoroughly fixed prior to transport.

Fresh (refrigerated or frozen) samples need to be transported to the laboratory in a small cooler with ice bricks, with transport time less than 24–48 hours (depending on the ambient temperature). In many cases, the specific ancillary tests indicated on fresh samples are unknown before histological examination, in which case, the samples can remain frozen at the clinic until a decision on further testing is made.

Table 30.2 Sampling for various types of ancillary necropsy testing.

Test	General comments	Specific sampling notes
Histology	Primary routine ancillary testing. Submit a standard broad range of tissues, even if they appear grossly normal. Sample any lesions and describe them to the pathologist. Sample any margins of lesions with normal tissue.	Preserve tissues in formalin (10% phosphate buffered) at 1 : 10 tissue to formalin ratio. Tissues may be mixed in one jar. Tissues should generally not exceed 1 cm in diameter. For small reptiles, entire 'pluck' of tissues in body cavity can be removed as one piece and placed in formalin. For very small reptiles (< 1 cm body diameter), after opening body cavity, whole carcase can be placed in formalin. Inject formalin into unopened intestine and eyes. Store formalin-fixed samples at room temperature.
Cytology	Not routinely performed when necropsy tissues for histological evaluation are available. Organ impressions may be useful in conjunction with histology to provide cellular detail or detect organisms. In some cases, cytology performed by the clinician may provide sufficient diagnostic information.	Slides are fixed in methanol and usually stained with Wright's type rapid stain Additional diagnostic potential can be obtained by use of Gram's stain for bacteria and periodic acid-Schiff stain for fungi. Smears are destroyed by formalin fumes (keep separate).
Bacterial and fungal culture	Minimize contamination as it will influence culture results or confound interpretation. Some bacteria (e.g. *Mycoplasma* spp.) require specialized storage media and culture conditions (contact laboratory). Accurate anaerobic culture requires use of specialized swabs or immediate transport of sample to laboratory. For fungal culture, tissue samples are generally better than swabs. If you have sampled a heavily contaminated site (mouth, intestine), advise the laboratory of the bacterial species of interest. If *Salmonella* spp. is suspected, request specific culture.	Aseptically sample filtering organs as soon as the body cavity is opened (liver, kidney, lung and spleen). Sterilize instruments with flame before taking samples. Sample 1-cm or larger pieces of tissue into individual sterile vials. Moisten small (< 5 mm) pieces of tissue with normal saline. Use swabs in bacterial transport medium for exudates. Store refrigerated (a few days) or frozen.
Molecular testing	Polymerase chain reaction and/or genetic sequencing. Commonly used for detecting reptile viruses. May also be used for fastidious bacteria and fungi. Tests are specialized and may only be available at research laboratories.	Generally, fresh tissues or plain swabs can be used (contact laboratory). Moisten small (< 5 mm) pieces of tissue and swabs with 0.9% saline solution. Store refrigerated (a few days) or frozen. Testing of formalin-fixed, paraffin embedded tissues may be possible but is not ideal.
Virus isolation	Specialized testing, usually requiring reptilian cell lines. May take weeks or months. Isolates require further testing for identification. Generally pursued only by researchers looking for novel viruses.	Generally, fresh tissues or plain swabs can be used. Moisten small (< 5 mm) pieces of tissue and swabs with 0.9% saline solution (or specialized viral transport medium if available). Store refrigerated (a few days) or frozen.
Serology	Testing for antibodies to a specific disease. Not commonly used due to poor or unreliable reptilian humoral response. Limited availability for only a few diseases (contact laboratory).	Useful serum or plasma may be obtained from carcase blood after death (as long as there is minimal decomposition). Store refrigerated (a few days) or frozen.

(Continued)

Table 30.2 (Continued)

Test	General comments	Specific sampling notes
Parasitology	Identification of parasites may be by morphological or molecular means. Availability of testing may be poor (contact laboratory).	Preserve helminths and arthropods in 70% ethanol. Gross examination and faecal flotation for eggs are generally more sensitive for identification of helminth infections than histology. Histology is more useful for detecting protozoal infections. Make a blood or lung impression smear if haemoparasitism is suspected.
Toxicology	Specialized testing by referral laboratories. Laboratory needs to be advised which toxin(s) to test for. Interpretation of significance of results may be difficult.	Sample type required depends on toxin suspected. Common samples are liver, kidney and stomach contents. 1–5 g of tissue or material may be required. Store frozen.
Haematology and clinical chemistry	May be useful under some necropsy circumstances to clarify gross or histological findings (e.g. hypocalcaemia, anaemia, hepatic necrosis).	Only samples taken prior to euthanasia or from carcase within minutes of death can be used. Lithium heparin anticoagulated blood sample can usually be used for both haematology and clinical chemistry. Store whole blood under refrigeration. Store serum and plasma refrigerated (few days) or frozen.

Box 30.1 Suggested minimal routine diagnostic necropsy samples.

For Histological Examination

(fixed in 10% formalin, stored at room temperature)
Essential:

- lung
- heart
- liver
- spleen
- kidney
- brain
- any grossly abnormal tissues or lesions.

Plus, if the carcase is fresh:

- stomach
- pancreas
- duodenum
- jejunum
- colon.

Plus, depending on suspected disease:

- reproductive organs
- segments of spinal cord
- bone (metaphysis with marrow and growth zone).

For other ancillary testing

(stored under refrigeration for a few days, otherwise frozen)

- A 1-cm^2 piece (or as large as available) of:
- liver
- kidney
- lung
- spleen
- pieces or swabs of any abnormal tissues or lesions.

Reference

Johnson-Delaney, C. (2006) Zoonoses and threats to public health, in *Reptile Medicine and Surgery*,.), 2nd ed. (D.R. Mader, ed). Elsevier Saunders, St. Louis, MO, pp. 1017–1030.

31

Reptile Parasitology in Health and Disease

Jan Šlapeta, David Modrý and Robert Johnson

Introduction to Parasites

Internal and external parasites occur commonly in captive and free-living reptiles and a parasitological examination should be part of every clinical examination. Once a parasite is identified, determine whether the parasite requires elimination, management or no treatment. Parasites are associated with a diverse range of clinical signs, including anorexia, pica, prolapse, regurgitation, diarrhoea, constipation, lethargy, weight loss and death. A thorough parasitological examination is paramount to the formulation of a diagnosis and treatment plan.

Practical In-Clinic Diagnostics

A routine parasitological examination should address the three most commonly affected systems, the gastrointestinal tract, the respiratory tract and the skin. In the case of large collections, inspecting all individuals may not be possible. Animals with obvious clinical signs should undergo a thorough clinical examination. Gastrointestinal parasites are routinely detected by examination of a fresh faecal sample. Parasites from the respiratory system may also be observed in faeces due to migration from the pharynx into the gastrointestinal tract.

The gastrointestinal system is commonly inhabited by a variety of parasites (Figures 31.1–31.6). Similar to birds, reptiles have a cloaca through which the faecal sample is expelled together with urates and urine. Reptile owners should be instructed to collect only the moist part of the faecal matter. Faeces should be stored in a disposable container or small Ziplock® bags. All containers should be labelled with the reptile's identification and date of collection. A sample size of 1–2 g is sufficient for most parasitological tests, but repeated testing is recommended to rule out false negative result due to shedding intermittency. If multiple reptiles are housed together and individual identification is not possible, a collection of pooled faecal samples over several days should be collected into a single container. If an individual is to be examined, it should be separated temporarily and placed either into a clean enclosure or a linen bag for defecation. Faeces should be stored at 10–20 °C and examined within 48 hours. Refrigeration is usually not required.

For a routine respiratory examination, a pharyngeal swab for detecting parasites should be carried out on any animal that has been recently introduced to the collection, quarantined or is showing respiratory signs. Pharyngeal swabs will aid in differentiating lungworms (*Rhabdias* spp.), causing a respiratory infection, from *Strongyloides* species,

Reptile Medicine and Surgery in Clinical Practice, First Edition. Edited by Bob Doneley, Deborah Monks, Robert Johnson and Brendan Carmel.
© 2018 John Wiley & Sons Ltd. Published 2018 by John Wiley & Sons Ltd.

(a)

(b)

(c)

(d)

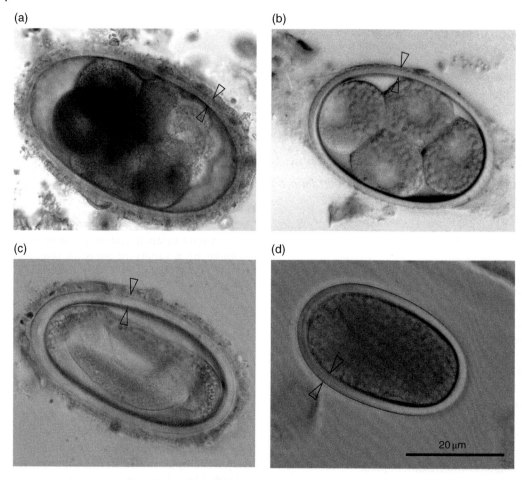

20 μm

Figure 31.1 Nematode eggs commonly encountered in faecal samples of reptiles I. Ascarid egg from *Heosemys spinosa* (a) and from *Morelia viridis* (b). Heterakid egg from *Agama finchi* (c) and from *Goniurosaurus huuliensis* (d). Note the smooth outer egg wall surface of heterakid eggs compared with the ascarid eggs (arrowhead). Heterakids are typically in lizards such as geckoes and agamas.

detected in the faeces, that may be causing intestinal disease.

Blood parasitism is relatively frequent in animals from the wild, but the clinical significance is low. Blood parasites found in blood smears are usually considered an incidental finding.

Ectoparasitism is relatively easy to diagnose if heavy burdens are present; low burdens are much harder to detect (Figure 31.7). Mites are photophobic and consequently favour hiding under scales, in skin folds, heat sensing pits and around the periorbital conjunctivae. Detection is aided by the use of a magnifying glass or otoscope.

Necropsy may reveal previously undiagnosed or subclinical parasitic infections, in particular *Cryptosporidium* and *Entamoeba*.

Gross lesions, such as thickening of the gastric rugae, suggest gastric cryptosporidiosis; similarly, ulceration and necrosis of the liver and intestine suggest amoebiasis. Fresh tissue samples, including liver, stomach and intestine, placed in buffered 10% formalin, should be submitted for histopathological examination. Fresh tissue from affected organs should also be collected and immediately frozen in case molecular diagnostic testing is required (i.e. DNA isolation and diagnostic polymerase chain reaction, PCR).

Some parasites are not detected at gross examination; these include tissue protozoans (*Sarcocystis*), larval stages of helminths (plerocercoids/spargana, acanthocephalans, spirurid larvae, pentastomids) and filaria

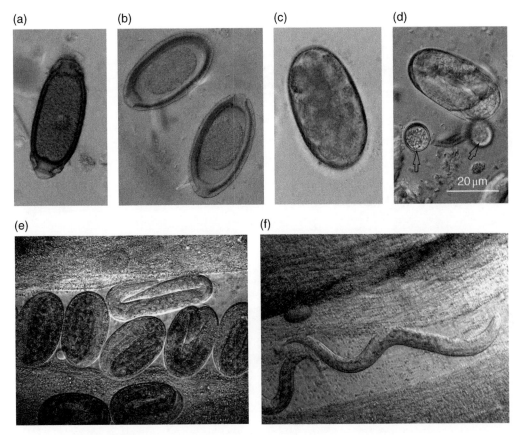

Figure 31.2 Nematode eggs commonly encountered in faecal samples of reptiles II. *Capillaria* eggs from *Acanthosaura nataliae* (a) and *Python regius* (b). Note the typical barrel-shaped eggs with polar plugs of capillaria eggs. Strongylid eggs from *Goniurosaurus huuliensis* (c) and *Corallus caninus* (d). Note the presence of unsporulated *Caryospora* species oocysts (arrow, D). Mucus from the mouth with eggs (e) and larvae (f) of *Rhabdias* species from *Pantherophis obsoletus*. (images E and F courtesy of Dr Frank Mutschmann, Exomed, Berlin, Germany).

that are present on the serosa of pleuroperitoneal cavity (Figure 31.8).

Overview of Faecal Sample Diagnostic Techniques

A direct microscopic examination of a faecal smear is a simple and efficacious diagnostic test for detecting moderate to heavy parasite burdens: most nematode eggs (10× objective); coccidia, *Strongyloides*/*Rhabdias* eggs (20×); *Cryptosporidium* and flagellates (40×). Flotation is a concentration technique and in the case of low burdens may detect parasites not revealed in direct smears.

Test samples may need to be submitted for specific parasites, e.g. *Entamoeba* and *Cryptosporidium*. Some commercial laboratories offer reptile parasite specific PCR, although the use of a domestic animal PCR panel may be suitable for *Giardia* and *Cryptosporidium*, as they are often not species specific and may amplify reptile specific species. Alternatively, direct fluorescence antibody testing for *Cryptosporidium* of humans, which is based on monoclonal antibodies, commonly recognizes antigen on reptile parasites. Veterinary diagnostic laboratories should be contacted to enquire about the availability of testing, including *Entamoeba* (*E. invadens*) diagnostics, which are particularly problematic, with specific PCR being the most reliable option.

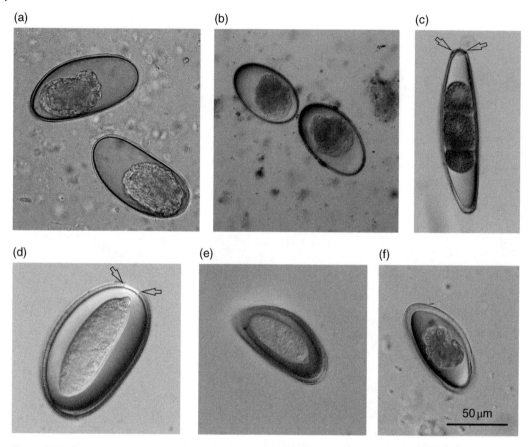

Figure 31.3 Nematode eggs commonly encountered in faecal samples of reptiles III. Pinworm/oxyurid eggs from *Iguana iguana* (a), *Testudo hermanni* (b), *Goniurosaurus huuliensis* (c), *Uromastyx acanthinura* (d), *Agama finchi* (e) and *Eublepharis macularius* (f). Pinworms are highly species specific and their eggs possess a smooth wall and one side is more concave than the other. Operculum is often visible (arrows).

Sedimentation may be requested for heavy eggs but is rarely required in clinical settings. If the veterinary practice is not confident in performing sedimentation, it is best to contact the local diagnostic service.

What to do With Parasitological Results?

Microscopical examination should aim to identify the principal structure and features of parasitic stages. Identification to species or genus level will be, in most cases, impossible or even unnecessary. The common parasitic stages and parasites are demonstrated in Figures 31.1–31.8. For parasites and eggs in faeces, note the size, colour and organization of the wall to guide identification. It is important to note the frequency and load of the parasites. For microscopic specimens, noting less than 10 (+),10 to less than 50 (++) and over 100 (+++) per field of view at 10-times magnification would be a suitable approach to rank parasite load. At least annual monitoring and recording of parasite loads is recommended.

Determine whether the structures observed are true parasites causing harm to the animal or harmless parasites from a prey item. Insectivorous and carnivorous reptiles will excrete intact parasite stages originating from the insect or animal fed to the reptile. These parasites are specific to the prey and are termed pseudoparasites (Figure 31.9). A negative test result in a sample collected 24–48 hours

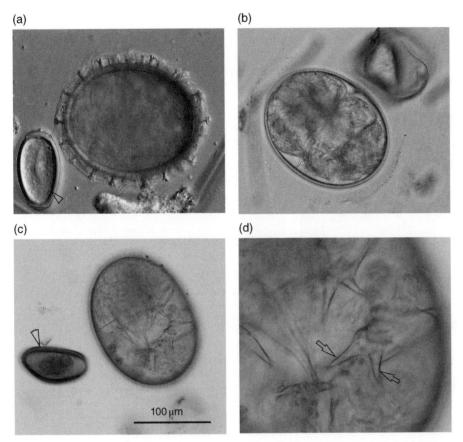

(a) (b) (c) (d)

100 μm

Figure 31.4 Pentastomid (tongue worms) eggs of reptiles. Pentastomid and spirurid (arrowhead) in *Varanus* species (a). Pentastomid eggs from *Goniurosaurus huuliensis* (b). Pentastomid and oxyurid (arrowhead) eggs in *Goniurosaurus luii* (c). Detail of the pentastomid larvae within the eggs with the typical four pair of V-shaped claws (arrows; d).

later from the same animal would confirm transitory status. Pollen and plant material as well as chitin-based structures of insects may also be confused with parasites. Faecal samples should be fresh, since samples in contact with the enclosure substrate may be quickly contaminated with free-living non-parasitic nematodes and their larvae, complicating the accurate identification of strongylid and rhabditid nematode parasites.

Questions to Ask the Client

- What is the animal fed?
  This question is asked to rule out the possibility of pseudoparasitism and whether the diet is the source of the parasites. Examination of faeces of the prey (e.g. rodents, insects) may reveal coccidia that appear in the faeces of the snake or lizard, as they are not digested. Similarly, rodent mites and their eggs may appear in faeces of snakes.
- Where does the animal live?

- Is the animal housed with other reptiles?
- Does the enclosure have any contact with potential sources of parasites or the outside environment?

Also consider:
- Is the parasite capable of causing the clinical signs?
- Is the parasite capable of completing its life cycle within its enclosure or captive environment?

(a)

(b)

(c)

(d)

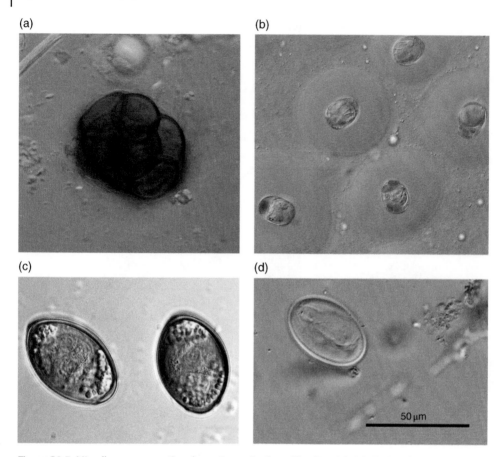

50 µm

Figure 31.5 Miscellaneous eggs. *Capulotaenia* species from *Morelia viridis* (a). *Oochoristica* species from *Iguana iguana* (b). Operculated trematode eggs from *Furcifer pardalis* (c). Spirurid egg with coiled larva inside (*Abbreviata* sp.) from *Uromastyx* species (d).

Parasites Associated with Disease

Parasites of reptiles are numerous; nevertheless, only a handful of parasite groups and parasite species attract veterinary attention Table 31.1 outlines the biology and the significance of the major parasites of reptiles. Other parasites not listed represent those that are only rarely associated with disease. Flagellates and ciliates (*Nyctotherus* spp.) are commonly encountered; however, they probably play only a secondary role to a primary disease process.

Gastric and Intestinal *Cryptosporidium* Species

Cryptosporidium species (Apicomplexa) are protozoan parasites, which in acute cases cause regurgitation and diarrhoea and in chronic cases regurgitation and anorexia. In snakes, postprandial regurgitation is a frequent sign of gastric cryptosporidiosis caused by *C. serpentis*. Lizards are more frequently clinically affected by intestinal cryptosporidiosis caused by *C. varanii* (syn. *C. saurophilum*). Infected reptiles will shed resistant oocysts. Transmission is via the faecal and oral route, specifically by the ingestion of oocysts. Many chronically infected reptiles will shed oocysts for life.

Gross lesions associated with gastric cryptosporidiosis typically include marked thickening of the gastric rugae, while intestinal cryptosporidiosis is less pronounced. Ante mortem diagnostics aim to detect oocysts in the faeces, in gastric contents sampled by

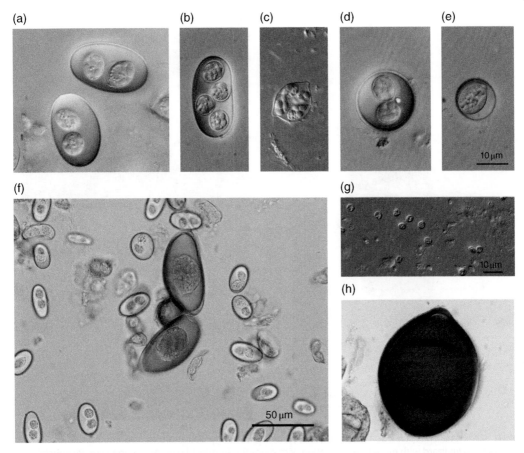

Figure 31.6 Protozoa shed in reptile faeces. Sporulated oocysts of *Isospora jaracimrmani* each with two sporocysts, from *Chamaeleo calyptratus* (a). Sporulated oocyst of *Choleoeimeria* species with four sporocysts, from *Hemidactylus brooki* (b). Sporulated oocyst of *Eimeria* species with four sporocysts, from *Heosemys depressa* (c). *Isospora* species from *Nactus* species (d). Sporulated oocyst of *Caryospora* species with a single sporocyst, from *Naja haje* (e). Size comparison of sporulating oocysts of *I. jaracimrmani* and two oxyurid eggs, from *Chamaeleo calyptratus* (f). Oocysts of *Cryptosporidium* species from *Goniurosaurus luii* (g). Cyst for of a ciliate *Nyctotherus* species from *Uromastyx* species (h).

gastric lavage or in a surgical biopsy. Reptile species are distinct from those affecting humans, nevertheless they share the same oocyst epitopes and tests for human cryptosporidiosis based on fluorescently labelled antibodies binding to the oocyst wall are suitable for detection. Veterinary diagnostic laboratories frequently offer tests based on antibody labelling of *Cryptosporidium* oocysts. Alternatively, species specific PCR for reptile cryptosporidia and multiplex PCR may also be used. As there is no effective cure, euthanasia of clinically affected reptiles is recommended. Quarantine and repeated testing are recommended for newly acquired reptiles. No effective household disinfectant is effective against *Cryptosporidium*, although oocysts are highly susceptible to heat and drying.

Intestinal and Biliary Coccidiosis

Coccidiosis is caused by multiple different genera including *Isospora*, *Eimeria*, *Choleoeimeria*, *Caryospora* and *Sarcocystis* (Figure 31.6). Coccidia (Apicomplexa) commonly develop in the gastrointestinal tract of reptiles (e.g. *Isospora*). Some species affect the gallbladder and associated bile ducts (e.g. *Choleoeimeria*). Coccidia are very common

(a)

(b)

(c)

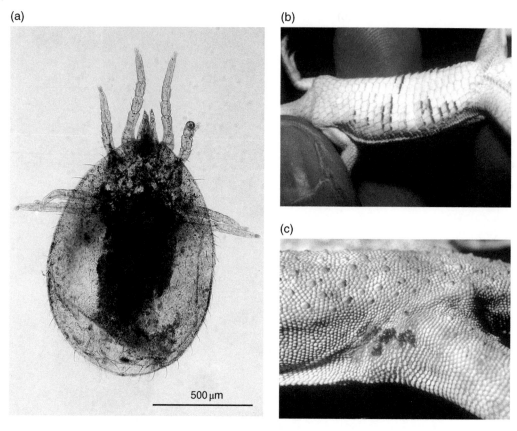

Figure 31.7 Mites on reptiles. Snake mite (*Ophionyssus natricis*) engorged adult (a). Abdomen of *Acanthodactylus* lizard with moderate infestation with mites (b). Trombiculid mites (chiggers) on *Ptyodactylus* gecko (c).

parasites and oocysts are found on direct smear or faecal floats of lizards and snakes. Oocysts of *Isospora, Eimeria, Caryospora* are environmentally resilient and shed unsporulated, requiring several days to sporulate in moist faeces. They can directly infect the same host species. Differentiation to genus level in the unsporulated state is unreliable. The only oocysts to be shed already sporulated are those belonging to *Choleoeimeria* and *Sarcocystis*, a genus of coccidia which cycles between predator and prey (indirect lifecycle) and thus do not complete their lifecycle in captive environments.

Detection of oocysts does not immediately indicate the presence of disease. Coccidiosis can be a serious problem in intensively reared reptiles such as bearded dragons and chameleons.

Young animals will often present emaciated. Separation of the adult reservoirs from younger animals is recommended. Treatment with toltrazuril or sulfa-drugs can be considered; however, in chronically infected animals treatment is less effective because of the high probability of reinfection.

Intestinal and Liver Amoebiosis Caused by *Entamoeba invadens*

The protozoan parasite *Entamoeba invadens* (Amoebozoa) causes severe vomiting, anorexia and diarrhoea. Snakes are more susceptible than other reptiles. In large snakes, amoebiasis can quickly reach epidemic proportions if not diagnosed early. Transmission is faecal and oral, by the ingestion of the environmentally

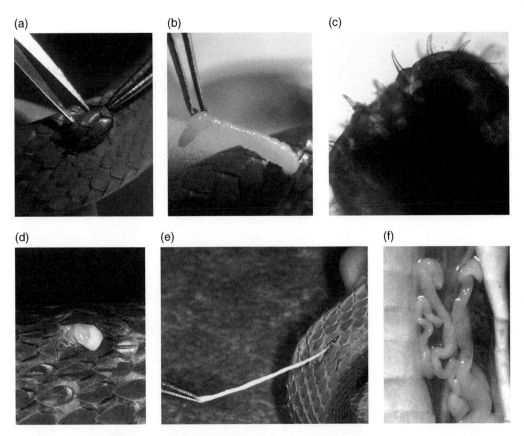

Figure 31.8 Skin nodules with parasitic stages. Larval stages of helminths as seen on the skin of snakes. Extraction of an acanthocephalan (thorny headed worm) (a, b) and microscopic image of the extracted parasite anterior 'thorny' part confirming its identity (c). Extraction of a tapeworm larval stage: plerocercoid (spargana) through snake skin (d, e) and a necropsy image of spargana in the pleuroperitoneal cavity of a snake (f).

resistant cyst form. Importantly, turtles and some herbivorous reptiles often remain asymptomatic carriers and reservoirs of *E. invadens*. The general recommendation is to separate turtles from snakes.

Lesions caused by *E. invadens* are confined to the liver and the gastrointestinal tract. Ulceration, necrosis and haemorrhage may extend from the stomach to the cloaca. Chronic cases of amoebiasis may involve multifocal abscessation of the liver. Ante mortem diagnosis may be difficult as routine diagnostic tests are not available. Trophozoites and *E. invadens* cysts may be difficult to observe in direct faecal smears. *E. invadens* may be detected using the emerging multiplex PCR technology on faecal samples. Diagnosis

should be promptly followed by treatment with metronidazole. Strict hygiene and quarantine measures must be observed. Testing asymptomatic reptiles is recommended.

Anaemia and Emaciation Caused by Hookworms and Roundworms (Strongylid and Ascarid Nematodes)

Roundworms (Ascarididae) and hookworms (Strongylidae) are significant parasites of the gastrointestinal tract of snakes and lizards. Heavy burdens may lead to gastrointestinal inflammation, haemorrhagic ulceration and death. *Ophidascaris* species (Ascarididae) and *Kalicephalus* species (Strongylidae) are

(a)

(b)

(c)

(d)

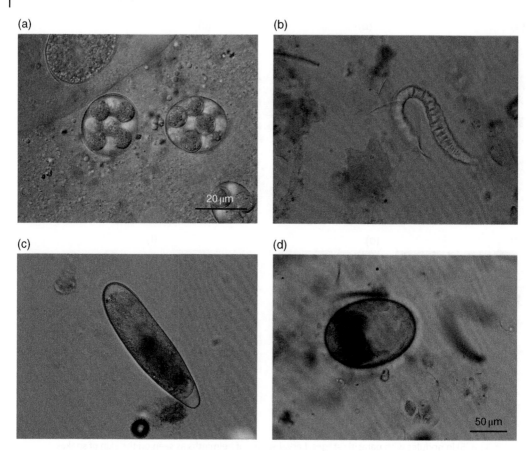

20 µm

50 µm

Figure 31.9 Pseudoparasites encountered in reptile faeces. Coccidia of insects can pass through the intestinal tract of reptiles, typical insect coccidian oocysts possess eight round sporocysts, *Adelina grylli* frequently parasitizes common cricket (*Gryllus* sp.) fed to lizards (a). Faeces of reptiles are a rich source of nutrients for free-living nematodes that rapidly invade faeces that is left on the enclosure substrate. In such faeces, the presence of free-living nematodes needs to be ruled out. A free-living nematode crumbled in the flotation solution (b). Rodents from pet stores are often parasitized by mites. Their exoskeletons and eggs will pass in faeces intact and need to be recognized as parasites of the prey, not as parasites of the reptile (c, d).

frequently found in reptiles. Several other genera are also present such as *Angusticaecus* in tortoises (*Testudo*). In clinical practice, identification to genus level is usually not required. Most ascarid eggs are elongated, brownish yellow and have a thick wall (Figure 31.1). Hookworm eggs are more elongated, often colourless and thin walled, containing either blastomeres or (later) coiled larva (Figure 31.2). The life cycle of hookworms is usually direct with the potential to build up heavy burdens within the enclosure.

Even though some species of hookworm do have an indirect lifecycle, because of the difficulty of identification to a species level, it is recommended to consider that most have a direct lifecycle and low host specificity.

Management of roundworm and hookworm infestation involves frequent and complete removal of faeces from the enclosure and treatment of the affected reptiles using repeated doses of ivermectin or fenbendazole followed by retesting.

Table 31.1 Selection of important reptile parasites and parasite groups.

Parasite	Clinical significance	Life cycle	Pathology
Protozoa:			
Cryptosporidium spp.	★★★★	Direct	Failure to thrive, gastritis, enteritis
Coccidia (*Isospora*, *Eimeria*)	★★	Direct (need to sporulate outside the host)	Failure to thrive, enteritis
Entamoeba invadens	★★★★	Direct	Gastritis, ulceration
Nematodes:			
Rhabditida (*Rhabdias*)	★★★★	Direct (established free living population in soil)	Pneumonia
Rhabditida (*Strongyloides*)	★★	Direct (established free living population in soil)	Enteritis
Oxyurida (different genera, species)	★	Direct (need to embryonate outside the host)	Beneficial in herbivorous reptiles
Ascaridida (including ascarids and heterakids), Strongylida, Spirurida (different genera, species)	★★★	Direct or indirect	Failure to thrive, gastritis, enteritis
Acari:			
Pterygosoma spp.	★	Direct	None, dermatitis
Ophionyssus natricis	★★★★	Direct (development in the enclosure)	Anaemia, dermatitis
Pentastomida:			
'tongue worms'	★★	Indirect	None, zoonosis

Pneumonia Caused by *Rhabdias* Species and Differentiation from Intestinal *Strongyloides* Species

The nematode order Rhabditida is represented in reptiles by two genera: *Strongyloides* and *Rhabdias*. *Rhabdias* commonly parasitizes the lungs of snakes, causing a verminous pneumonia. Clinical signs include open mouth breathing and a frothy discharge from the nares. Severe cases may be complicated by a secondary bacterial pneumonia. *Strongyloides* parasitize the intestine, occasionally causing enteritis. Eggs of *Rhabdias* and *Strongyloides* are indistinguishable, so finding their eggs in faeces is not conclusive. Diagnosing verminous pneumonia is in most cases straightforward by the detection of larvae and eggs in a throat

swab (30 × 60 μm, thin walled with embryonated larva) of *Rhabdias* under a microscope (Figure 31.2).

Rhabditida are significant parasites of snakes because they complete their lifecycle in the reptile enclosures. Larvae shed into the environment and develop into free-living adults, which produce new eggs that hatch into larvae and subsequently penetrate the skin of the snake. Within the reptile host, the larvae will migrate either to the lung (*Rhabdias*) or intestine (*Strongyloides*) and develop into hermaphroditic females that will produce the next generation of eggs. Eggs and larvae of *Rhabdias* are moved up the trachea, swallowed and excreted with faeces. Rhabditida are highly fecund and can quickly produce a large free-living population within an enclosure, potentially spreading to neighbouring enclosures via shared equipment. Management of a rhabditid infection must include thorough and frequent cleaning of the enclosure. Snakes with verminous pneumonia require individual treatment (levamisole, ivermectin, fenbendazole) and housing in clean enclosures. A nonparticulate substrate, such as newspaper, is recommended to hamper maturation of the larval stage. Secondary, often anaerobic, bacterial infection needs to be managed simultaneously (metronidazole). All reptiles, especially new arrivals, should be checked for the presence of rhabditida.

Non-Pathogenic Pinworms (Oxyurid Nematodes) in Herbivorous Reptiles

Pinworms (Oxyurida) are frequently present in the lower gastrointestinal tract of herbivorous reptiles such as lizards and turtles (Figure 31.3). Their presence is considered beneficial to the host, improving the passage of ingesta through the intestinal tract. Consequently, their complete removal may negatively affect digestion. It is recommended that only heavy burdens are treated. Pinworms have a direct lifecycle and are host-species specific. Eggs are typically ovoid, with a yellowish egg wall that is thick and smooth and, typically, one side is more concave than the other. Eggs possess an operculum that may not always be clearly visible. In insectivorous reptiles, the presence of pinworms and effect on the host is poorly understood.

Anaemia and Emaciation Caused by Snake Mites

Ectoparasites are commonly found on captive reptiles and are a common reason for presentation for veterinary examination. The most significant ectoparasite of reptiles is the blood-sucking snake mite *Ophionyssus natricis* (Acari). Mite infestation may result in poor skin shedding (dysecdysis), failure to thrive, anaemia or even death. In captivity,

the snake mite is found on snakes more frequently than on lizards and rarely on chelonians. In suitable conditions, the snake mite will complete its life cycle in one to two weeks, quickly overwhelming the enclosure and the household.

The lifecycle of the mite is completed within the reptile enclosure, with larval and late nymph stages being free living. Early nymph and adult stages are parasitic, aggressive and highly motile blood feeders. The snake mites attach and feed underneath the scales, so a low burden can be difficult to diagnose. Careful inspection of the shed skin aids identification of mite infestation. During the week-long engorgement, the mites remain attached to the host and, after ingesting a blood meal, they turn red in colour. Engorged adults are approximately 1 mm in length. The eggs are laid in dark and moist crevices within the enclosure and require an ambient temperature above 20 °C and more than 85% humidity to hatch. Mites can be collected with the aid of a moistened cotton swab or sticky tape and are easily identified microscopically (Figure 31.7). Mites prefer dark and shaded areas, so the best chance of the reptile owner observing them is at night, as mites will quickly retract to dark places if exposed to light.

Infected reptiles may display unusual behaviour. Snakes may spend a long time in the water bowl or moving erratically within the enclosure. Preferred sites on the reptile for mite include the lower jaw, the heat-sensing pits, the periorbital region and the cloaca. Careful health monitoring of newly acquired reptiles and quarantine is mandatory in preventing infestation. Snake mites are easily spread within and between collections. The snake mite lifecycle can be very short, although the mites are hardy, remaining in the environment for up to three months. Temperatures above 50 °C and humidity less than 50% will kill mite stages; alternatively, mites can be easily drowned, so essential equipment and features within the enclosure can be fully immersed in water overnight.

Box 31.1 A mite management plan.

1) Isolate and treat reptiles within a simple hygienic enclosure where all components can be easily cleaned until the reptiles are deemed free of mites.
2) Clean, scrub and wash enclosures with water hotter than 50 °C and discard all substrates and non-essential cage furniture.
3) Thoroughly clean the room(s) where infected reptiles are housed, including any husbandry equipment, to minimize the potential presence of free-living mite stages.
4) Maintain isolation and quarantine for at least three months.

Drug treatment

- Drugs used for treatment of mites include fipronil and ivermectin.
- Caution should be exercised when attempting to use pyrethrins, pyrethroids, organophosphates and carbamates because of their high toxicity if overdosed.
- Acaricides can be highly toxic if inappropriately used by reptile owners.
- Refer to Appendix 1 for more detailed drug information.

Treatment of a mite infestation must address both mites on the host as well as all free-living stages. Free-living stages may remain outside the reptile enclosure and may serve as a reservoir for persistent reinfection. A management plan (Box 31.1) should include elimination of sources of reinfection both from the outside as well as inside the enclosures. The mite larvae can temporarily infest humans and cause skin irritation.

Other Noteworthy Parasites

Heterakid nematodes (Ascaridida: Anisakidae) occur in reptiles, sometimes in rather unusual locations (e.g. the ear of African agamids). *Capillaria* (Trichurida: Capillaridae) are common in reptiles from humid environments and easily identified in faecal smears from their typical barrel-shaped eggs with polar plugs (Figure 31.2). As the eggs are morphologically almost identical to those from rodents and birds, a determination should be made as to whether they are true parasites or pseudoparasites. Insectivorous reptiles are commonly infected with spirurid nematodes (Spirurida), localized usually to the stomach. The eggs have a smooth and relatively thick wall with coiled larva inside (Figure 31.5). Similarly, various species of filaria (Spirurida) do occur in the body cavity

and blood vessels of tropical reptiles (e.g. *Foleyella* in chameleons) and circulating larvae (microfilariae) can be detected in peripheral blood smears.

Occasionally, eggs of pentastomids (tongue worms, Pentastomida) are detected in the faeces of snakes, containing larva with diagnostically typical four pairs of claws (Figure 31.4). *Armillifer* and *Porocephalus* are both confirmed zoonotic pathogens. Control in reptiles with antiparasiticide (ivermectin) is not fully effective and reptiles often remain infected with the parasite residing in lungs for life.

Some snakes will be presented with skin nodules that harbour either acanthocephalans (thorny headed worms, Acanthocephala) or tapeworm (Cestoda) larval stages known as spargana (plerocercoid) that may be surgically removed (Figure 31.8). Snakes usually acquire spargana from eating wild prey such as frogs and rodents. Tapeworms of the genus *Oochoristica* are commonly found in the intestines of wild insectivorous and herbivorous reptiles (Figure 31.5). The lifecycle of *Oochoristica* species includes beetles and grasshoppers as intermediate hosts. *Oochoristica* species may, therefore, establish within and be transmitted within farmed reptiles, like green iguanas. Treatment of adult tapeworms is recommended (praziquantel).

Reptiles can be infected by a range of mites, some of which e.g. *Pterygosoma* can complete its lifecycle within the enclosure and potentially cause harm. Ticks can be encountered on reptiles that are exposed to the outside or that are recently imported from the wild. Interestingly, a tick, *Amblyomma komodoensis*, imported with Komodo dragons adapted to large terraria can now be found on captive monitors in zoos throughout the world.

Management of Parasite Infections

To manage and eliminate a parasite infection successfully, a thorough understanding of the parasite biology and environment of the captive reptiles is imperative (Figure 31.10). For each parasite present, developing a plan to eliminate environmental stages will be essential for successful parasite management. For example, the enclosure's soil needs to be completely removed if *Rhabdias/Strongyloides* are present, because they establish free-living population as the source of reinfective stages in the soil of the enclosure. Similarly thorough cleaning of the entire enclosure is imperative for eliminating *Ophionyssus* that has a great capacity to survive and live outside its hosts and hide.

Application of antiparasiticides must be in conjunction with the management of the parasitic stages outside the reptile. Antiparasiticides should be applied strategically and their effect assessed by re-testing. Common antiparasiticides and dose rates for reptiles are listed in the formulary. Ivermectin is an effective antiparasiticide for lizards and snakes but must not be used in chelonians because of its potential neurotoxicity. An integrated parasite management is the key to success and prevention of reinfection. In principle, it includes modification of the environment, use of antiparasiticides, regular testing and supportive care. In addition, regular health screening and quarantine of the collection is mandatory.

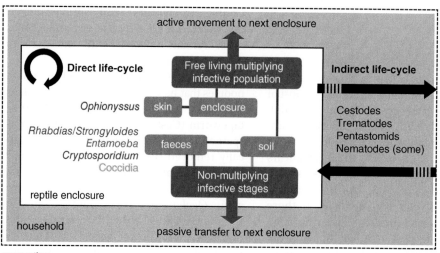

Figure 31.10 Parasite pathways within, in and outside an enclosure. Resident stages serving as reservoir pool are highlighted in red and arrows pointing out of the enclosure indicate potential for spread outside the enclosure. Locations of parasitic stages for principle parasite are colour coded for each direct lifecycle parasitic group. For parasites with an indirect lifecycle, the black arrows indicate either faecal contamination with parasitic stages (outwards arrow) or transmission via food serving as an intermediate host or transfer host (inwards arrow).

A reptile enclosure may appear to be a closed system but there remain opportunities for passive and even active movement of parasite stages from one enclosure to another (Figure 31.10), either through passive (fomites) movement of infective stages on cleaning equipment or cage furniture or from parasites actively moving to an adjacent enclosure (e.g. *Ophionyssus*).

Parasites with an indirect lifecycle have limited opportunity to parasitize captive reptiles. However, these parasites can be transmitted via feeding equipment or in food items, such as free-living rodents and birds, fish, amphibians and insects. Identification and elimination of the source is an integral component of the parasite management.

Prevention is fundamental and should be based on a knowledge of the diagnostics, differentiation of the clinically significant parasites from commensals and appropriate treatment plans and quarantine procedures. Veterinarians have the opportunity to play a significant role in eliminating the parasites before they enter the enclosure. Establishing standard operations, diagnostic testing and client education will demystify parasitology for reptile owners and improve reptile wellbeing. Routine parasitological examination and good record keeping will aid in the wellbeing of animals by either recognising association with disease or more importantly maintaining the balance between the host and its commensals within the reptile enclosure.

Further Reading

Mader, D. and Divers, S., eds (2014) *Current Therapy in Reptile Medicine and Surgery*. Elsevier Saunders, St Louis, MO.

Schneller, P,. and Pantchev, N. (2008) Parasitology in Snakes, Lizards and Chelonians: A Husbandry Guide. Edition Chimaira, Frankfurt am Main, Germany.

32

Nursing the Reptile Patient
Gary Fitzgerald and Emma Whitlock

Reception

Making an Appointment

The initial telephone call is the start of any diagnostic and treatment regimen, so it is wise to get as much information as possible in a clear and concise format. Questions to ask include:

- What are the patient's species and breed, age and sex?
- How long the client has owned the animal?
- What is the appointment for?
- Has the animal being seen by another vet and, if so, for what condition(s)?
- Is the animal receiving any medication?

Ask the client to bring detailed information about husbandry set-up, particularly the substrate, enclosure temperatures, diet form and feeding regimen, species interactions and so on. A concise history can take a significant amount of consult time; this can often be reduced by directing the client to an online form for the client to complete and bring with them to the appointment.

Digital photographs of the animal's enclosure are useful. If the patient is an aquatic species (e.g. a turtle), the client should bring a separate water sample (100 ml) from the enclosure. Any current medications should also be brought to the appointment.

This is also the time to give any pertinent information to the client about their appointment: timing and duration of appointments, transport recommendations and fasting periods if anaesthesia is likely.

Transportation

Reptiles should be kept at the preferred body temperature throughout transportation or at least immediately beforehand. Conversely, dangerous or particularly aggressive or agile reptiles may be easier to handle if they are slightly cool, but this should only be encouraged where deemed absolutely necessary (e.g. when dealing with highly venomous snakes).

Appropriate transport containers vary depending upon the animal and condition. Many reptiles are less stressed if carried in soft bags or pillow cases, especially in a soft (polystyrene) or cardboard box (Figures 32.1 and 32.2) Venomous snakes should be transported in a double, locked container. Aquatic turtles can be transported in a plastic bucket with a wet towel under them.

The Waiting Room

The reception area can create extreme stress for reptile patients if they are subjected to prey–predator interaction during the waiting

Reptile Medicine and Surgery in Clinical Practice, First Edition. Edited by Bob Doneley, Deborah Monks, Robert Johnson and Brendan Carmel.
© 2018 John Wiley & Sons Ltd. Published 2018 by John Wiley & Sons Ltd.

period. Prey species should not be able to see, hear or smell predator species so, ideally, a separate waiting area should be available. Alternatively, the client can wait in the consult room if necessary.

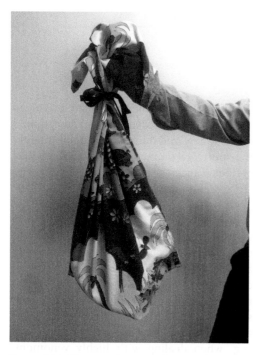

Figure 32.1 Transporting a reptile in a soft cloth bag.

Hospital Care

Reptile husbandry requirements can be very species specific, however for a temporary hospital stay most can be accommodated effectively and relatively cheaply. There are a few major factors to be considered.

Housing

The aim of housing reptile patients should be one of reducing stress during the hospital stay. Although most reptiles are predator species themselves, they often fall under the prey category when compared with the common small animal patients (dogs and cats). For this reason, it benefits all patients to house these species separately. Similarly, different species of reptiles should be kept separately. For example, housing a black-headed python (*Aspidites melanocephalus* – a reptile eater) in direct sight of a bearded dragon (*Pogona* spp.) would not benefit either party. Other steps that can be taken to reduce stress include:

- keeping the patient in an area with low human and animal traffic
- keeping the patient in a room with relatively stable temperature (but not overly cold air conditioning)
- encouraging normal behaviour by offering cage furnishings such as hides and branches.

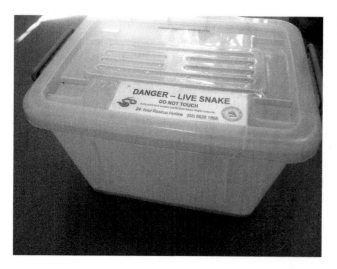

Figure 32.2 A polystyrene box for transporting a snake.

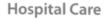

Hospital Enclosures

The design of the hospital enclosure is discussed in Chapter 9. Some summary points are:

- Materials should be nonporous and easy to clean. They should be able to retain heat to help with temperature control but still allow easy visualization of the patient.
- Heating can be achieved by many methods but the best method for hospital heating is the use of heat lamps controlled by a thermostat. Heating units such as heat rocks or mats produce localized heat in one area; a sick reptile is less able to regulate its own temperature and, unless closely monitored, may lie in an unheated part of the enclosure. Conversely, localized heating could also lead to burns if the patient does not move away from them.
- Lighting has a different function from heating, although some heat lamps can emit bright light. Considerations include:
  - Lighting will affect behaviour. Diurnal species (e.g. bearded dragon) require a day–night cycle of approximately 12 hours to encourage natural behaviour and for visualization of food items. In contrast, a nocturnal snake would require an infrared bulb, as constant white light would be stressful and prevent normal behaviour.
  - Ultraviolet B lighting should also be offered to diurnal and crepuscular reptiles.
- Humidity should replicate the natural environment of where the reptile is found. Humidity can be manipulated by:
  - Removal of water sources, increased ventilation and an absorptive substrate can lower humidity.
  - Increased water bowl size, placing the water bowl under the heat lamp, using a soaked sponge (increased surface area and evaporation), as well as misting from a spray bottle will increase humidity.

- Substrate helps the reptile move around while performing normal behaviour but it should be absorptive of waste, easy to clean, unlikely to be consumed and not adhere to a wound. Newspaper is an excellent choice for most hospital cages.
- Enclosure furniture should offer appropriate sized hides and, depending on the species, encourage normal behaviour (e.g. perches for arboreal species).
- Biosecurity makes it imperative that an excellent cleaning and disinfection regimen is maintained. A veterinary grade disinfectant should be used to clean the enclosure and all furnishings between patients. While the patient is in hospital, the enclosure should be cleaned daily and the substrate replaced.
- Diligent care should be taken to prevent the escape of reptile patients. Venomous or dangerous inpatients should be secured with a lock to prevent escape and appropriate signage to warn staff. The room should be secured and only trained staff should enter.

Daily Care

As with all hospitalized patients, reptiles must be monitored effectively throughout their stay. It is imperative that stress be minimized by not over-handling.

Weighing

Daily weighing should be performed before treatments are given, particularly where patients are very small, as it is easy to overdose even if only a very small amount of weight is lost over 24 hours (Figure 32.3). Recent feeding of large food items (e.g. rats) should be taken into account, as this will increase the animal's weight significantly but should not justify a change to dose rate until the food has been digested. The treating veterinarian should be notified of any changes to the reptile's weight.

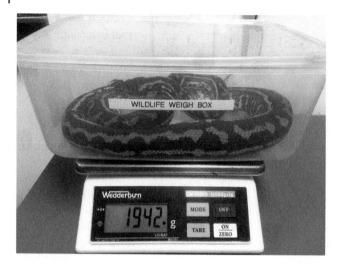

Figure 32.3 A lidded weigh box.

Handling

When handling a reptile, the safety of the patient and the handler is paramount. Handling techniques are described in Chapter 13 but the common factor in all techniques is that everything must be to hand before touching the patient. Not only does this minimize stress by ensuring any examinations or procedures are quick but it also increases handler safety (catch and release is the most dangerous time when handling a reptile).

Feeding

Before feeding reptilian patients, they should be hydrated to prevent the hypothesized condition 're-feeding syndrome', which occurs where chronically anorexic reptiles suffer a potentially life-threatening hypokalaemia following the ingestion of sudden excessive calories. The patient's current diet, even if not ideal, should be fed and any change should be gradual. Many pet reptiles may also be 'fussy' and only eat under certain circumstances (when the mouse is jiggled for example) or may only eat certain food items. If appropriate food items are not held in the clinic, ask the owners to provide it (Figure 32.4).

Observations and Record Keeping

Observations and record keeping go hand in hand and treatment charts should be tailor-made for reptile patients. Information that should be recorded includes:

- weight
- preferred body temperature for the species and the patient's actual temperature (usually measured by infrared thermometers
- enclosure temperature gradient – recommended and actual (daily)
- humidity requirement and readings (daily or more) and spray frequencies if misting of enclosure or body required
- feeding behaviour (attempted but did not swallow; not interested; interested but did not bite; fed but regurgitated etc.)
- lighting requirements (diurnal cycle and ultraviolet B)
- brumation requirements (gradient cooling, change to day length, food reduction, etc.)
- observations about shedding (opaque, shedding, shed etc.)
- defecation and urination
- any treatment given.

Medication

Handling should be kept to a minimum (to minimize patient stress) so where possible

Figure 32.4 Appropriate food should be provided.

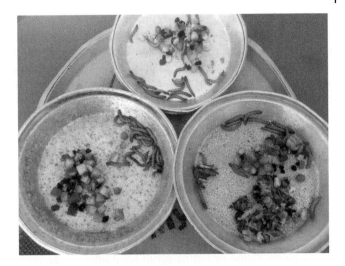

Figure 32.5 Recording the rotation of injection sites.

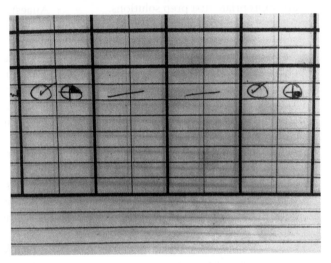

schedule medication administration to occur only once or twice daily. If injecting medication, ensure injection sites are rotated if multiple or repeated injections need to be given (Figure 32.5). If possible, oral medications can be offered in food to reduce stress and increase handler safety. Only offer medication in food if the whole dose can readily be taken as one dose and recorded as administered.

Anaesthesia and Surgical Nursing

The veterinary nurse or technician plays a vital role in the preparation for surgery and anaesthesia including preoperative, perioperative and post-operative monitoring and care. In many practices, it is common for the nurse or technician to monitor anaesthesia under the supervision of the clinician in charge.

Preoperative Nursing

Ensure that the reptile is in a heated enclosure so the patient is at its preferred body temperature (and this may take some time depending on the patient's size). As temperature has a dramatic effect on the reptile metabolism, the patient should be examined once it is at its preferred body temperature and before sedation, to record the base parameters such as the heart rate, respiratory rate and respiratory effort. The clinician and nurse should discuss pre-anaesthetic pathology testing, pain scoring and hydration status.

While the patient is warming up, the operating theatre can be prepared for the surgical procedure. The patient will rapidly cool down once removed from the heated enclosure, so delays should be minimized.

Surgical and Anaesthetic Equipment

The following equipment and supplies will be needed:

- Patient prep solution (warmed):
  - Chlorhexidine or iodine scrub solution are appropriate first prep solutions.
  - Alcohol-based second and third prep solutions may cause rapid cooling of the small patients. In these cases, aqueous chlorhexidine solutions are used as the final skin prep.
- Sterile surgical kit: choice of surgical instruments will come from the clinician but often ophthalmic instruments are used on small patients.
- Sterile patient drapes:
  - Clear sterile drapes are often used to allow visual monitoring of the patient during procedure.
  - Cloth or disposable paper drapes may be used especially in larger patients, at the surgeon's discretion
- Patient positioning equipment: sandbags, foam blocks and other support may be required for some patients.
- Patient heating: can be provided through the use of heated air blankets, heat mats, heat lamps and 'hotties' (warmed fluid bags). Care should always be taken not to burn the patient, particularly if using a heat mat. A thermostat probe should be placed in between the mat and patient to ensure that it does not overheat. The heated air and HotDog® patient warming systems are controlled by an internal thermostat and are considered the safest patient warming systems. Monitoring of patient temperature is recommended.

Normal rectal thermometers for small animals will not read as low as the average reptile body temperature. Electric probe thermometers, available from most hardware stores, can be used instead.

- Endotracheal tubes: a range of non-cuffed endotracheal tubes appropriate to the patient size should be ready at hand.
  Tip: for very small patients, intravenous catheters can be used with the connector from the 3.5 mm endotracheal tube.
- Tape and tongue depressor: use tape and a tongue depressor to secure the endotracheal tube to the patient to prevent the patient extubating itself if it moves during anaesthesia.
- Anaesthetic machine:
  - Anaesthetic machines should be set up and checked for leaks before every procedure. Access to medical air and oxygen is preferable, as reptiles will often have to be ventilated on air during recovery to initiate spontaneous ventilation.
  - The vaporizer should be filled. Isoflurane or sevoflurane are two common choices of gaseous maintenance anaesthesia.
- Breathing system/ventilator:
  - A breathing system should be chosen and attached to the machine and checked for leaks. Most reptile patients under 5 kg would use a non-rebreathing system (e.g. a T-piece or Bain breathing system). Larger species can be maintained on a rebreathing system such as a paediatric Y-system with a soda lime absorber to remove expired carbon dioxide.
  - Expect that all anaesthetized reptiles will become apnoeic and be prepared to manually or mechanically ventilate the patient for the entire procedure until the patient spontaneously ventilates on recovery. Ventilation pressure is usually 5 cm H_2O for reptiles under 5 kg and 10 cm H_2O for patients over 5 kg. The rate of ventilation is 2–10 breaths per minute.

Tip: use the base parameters to replicate normal resting ventilation for the patient, aiming for the same respiratory rate and respiratory movement.

- Anaesthesia record: a legal document and should begin with your base parameters and end when the patient has recovered. Record all medications, time, effect and route of administration and five-minute interval records taken.
- Monitoring equipment:
  - The most useful piece of monitoring equipment for reptile anaesthesia is the Doppler. It allows the user to listen to the heart rate and rhythm pulse of the patient in real time, where it would be very difficult to do so with a stethoscope alone. A Doppler will also accurately pick up a heartbeat from very small patients.
  - Other monitoring equipment can be of use: capnography, electrocardiography (ECG), pulse oximetry and blood pressure monitoring can help you to assess your patient's status during anaesthesia.

Monitoring the Anaesthesia

Anaesthesia monitoring is discussed in detail in Chapter 27 (Anaesthesia and analgesia). Commonly used monitoring equipment includes:

- Capnography will not give an accurate reading of true endotracheal CO_2 but trends can be evaluated. On average endotracheal CO_2 readings within the range of 10–30 should be expected.

As small endotracheal tubes are often used, assessing the capnogram can help to determine whether there are leaks around the tube, or semi- or full obstruction of the tube because of mucous plugs.

- A Doppler unit can be used to auscultate the heartbeat of the patient and to monitor systolic blood pressure in lizards.
- ECG can be difficult due to the ridged scales of the skin but alcohol or ultrasound gel can be used to increase conductivity.
  Tip: ECG Alligator clips can be quite traumatic to reptile skin; flattening the teeth will reduce trauma.
- Pulse oximetry can be used to monitor pulse rate and oxygenation. Because reptile skin is thick, with often highly pigmented and nucleated blood cells, readings can be difficult and inaccurate; however, trends can be followed.
- Monitoring of the depth of the anaesthesia can be difficult in reptiles but some reflexes prove useful (Table 32.1).

Patient Support

Patient support during anaesthesia is discussed in Chapter 27. There are a few points of note for the nurse or technician supporting a patient under anaesthesia.

- Positive pressure ventilation will be required at surgical planes of anaesthesia. As reptile ventilation is controlled by skeletal muscle, spontaneous respiration is lost at a surgical plane of anaesthesia.

Table 32.1 Reptile reflexes.

Reflex	Light Plane	Surgical Plane	Deep Plane
Righting	Present	Absent	Absent
Tail toe pinch	Present	Absent	Absent
Jaw tone	Increased	Decreased	Absent
Palpebral	Present	Absent	Absent
Corneal	Present	Present	Absent
Tongue retraction	Present	Absent	Absent

- Maintaining the patient's body temperature is paramount.
- Cardiovascular support can be achieved with perioperative intravenous or intraosseous fluids at a rate of 1 ml/kg/hour. If this is not achievable, subcutaneous or intracoelomic fluids can be given at 20–30 ml/kg/24 hours. **Tip**: Administering adequate pain relief will reduce the gaseous anaesthetic requirement during the procedure, which will in turn reduce the dose-dependent effects of vasodilation on the body.

Recovery

Recovery is the most dangerous period of a reptile anaesthetic procedure. The patent airway should be closely monitored and maintained until the patient is spontaneously ventilating and starting to move. Maintaining optimal body temperature is important during this time to allow the rapid excretion of anaesthetic drugs. The recovery period can vary from a few minutes to many hours. Ventilation with medical (or even room) air with a reduced inspired oxygen percentage will stimulate spontaneous ventilation, as stimulation to breath come from decreasing oxygen levels rather than increasing carbon dioxide levels.

Once the patient is spontaneously ventilating and starting to move, it can be extubated. The patient must be monitored to ensure that the airway remains patent and the patient continues to breathe. If not, the patient should be reintubated and ventilation continued. Once the patient is stable, it can be moved back to its heated enclosure and monitoring reduced to 5–10-minute intervals until it is behaving normally.

Further Reading

Ballard, B. and Cheek, R. (2010) *Exotic Animal Medicine for the Veterinary Technician*, 2nd ed. Wiley-Blackwell, Oxford.

Girling, S. (2003) *Veterinary Nursing of Exotic Pets*. Blackwell Publishing, Oxford.

Maclean, B. and Raiti, P. (2004) Emergency Care, in *BSAVA Manual of Reptiles*, 2nd ed. (S. Girling and P. Raiti, eds) BSAVA Publications, Gloucester, pp. 63–70.

Mader, D. (2005) *Reptile Medicine and Surgery*, 2nd ed. Elsevier Saunders, St. Louis, MO.

Meredith, A. and Johnson-Delaney, C. (2010) *BSAVA Manual of Exotic Pets*, 5th ed. BSAVA Publications, Gloucester.

Martinez-Jiminez, D. and Hernandez-Divers, S.J. (2007) Emergency Care of Reptiles. *Veterinary Clinics of North America: Exotic Animal Practice*, 11, 551–567.

Mitchell, M.A. (2006) Therapeutics, in *Reptile Medicine and Surgery*, 2nd ed. (D.M. Mader, ed.). Elsevier Saunders, St. Louis, MO, pp. 631–664.

Mitchell, M.A. and Tully, T.N. Jr (2009) *Manual of Exotic Pet Practice*. Elsevier Saunders, St Louis, MO.

Rendle, M. and Cracknell, J. (2012) Reptiles: biology and husbandry, in *BSAVA Manual of Exotic Pet and Wildlife Nursing* (M. Varga, R. Lumbis and L. Gott, eds). BSAVA Publications, Gloucester, pp. 80–108.

Rees Davis R. and Klingengberg, R.J. (2004) Therapeutics and medicine, in *BSAVA Manual of Reptiles*, 2nd ed. (S. Girling and P. Raiti, eds). BSAVA Publications, Gloucester, pp. 115–130.

33

Euthanasia
Tim Hyndman

Introduction

The euthanasia of animals should be smooth and painless; reptiles should not be an exception to this expectation. The clinician should be aware that it is difficult to achieve humane euthanasia of reptiles that is both rapid and palatable to most owners. For this reason, it is not recommended that reptile euthanasias are booked during busy consulting hours. The owner should be made aware that there are important differences in how a reptile is euthanized compared with how their dog or cat would be euthanized. Most notably, the time to complete the procedure can be very different.

Methods of Euthanasia

Instantaneous Brain Destruction

As the name suggests, instantaneous brain destruction involves the rapid and total obliteration of the brain, usually by blunt force trauma. While it can be argued that this method is rapid and humane, it will rarely be acceptable to an owner. It will destroy the brain as a necropsy sample and, if performed incorrectly, the results can be catastrophic.

Decapitation

Decapitation is an equally simple method of euthanasia but the reptilian brain has a remarkable capacity to function in an anoxic environment and therefore it is assumed that the perception of pain can continue for at least several minutes after the animal's head has been removed.

Freezing

Freezing a reptile (with or without prior refrigeration) is another simple method of euthanasia but the progressive freezing and rupture of cells means that this method is considered by most to be unacceptably painful. Freezing will also destroy the integrity of necropsy samples intended for histological examination. There is continuing debate as to whether freezing reptiles (after prior refrigeration) is ethical and humane. The clinician is therefore encouraged to remain abreast with advances in research which attempt to clarify this issue.

Pentobarbitone

Injecting pentobarbitone into the body cavity or the muscle of an animal (as opposed to intravenously) has been criticized because

Reptile Medicine and Surgery in Clinical Practice, First Edition. Edited by Bob Doneley, Deborah Monks, Robert Johnson and Brendan Carmel.
© 2018 John Wiley & Sons Ltd. Published 2018 by John Wiley & Sons Ltd.

preparations of this drug are necessarily alkaline (pH 9–10.5) so the acidic drug does not precipitate. It is therefore assumed by many that this injection will cause an unacceptable level of pain in the conscious animal. Some veterinarians will address this problem by diluting pentobarbitone in isotonic saline. In theory, this may not influence the pH of the preparation by much, considering that the pH scale is logarithmic. Anecdotally, however, many practitioners believe that this dilution significantly reduces the pain associated with this injection.

Using an acidic solution, such as isotonic saline, as the diluent will decrease the alkaline pH more than solutions which are either pH neutral or close to it (e.g. water for injection, Hartmann's solution or lactated Ringer's solution). An alternative practice to attenuate the pain associated with this injection is to mix the pentobarbitone with lignocaine. This has been shown to decrease (but not eliminate) the pain associated with intraperitoneal injections of pentobarbitone in mice.

The administration of undiluted pentobarbitone into the alimentary tract of reptiles is another method used by some veterinarians. Barbiturates have high oral bioavailability and so drug can reach the brain quite quickly. Moreover, the concern over the alkaline pH of the preparation becomes less important when the drug is instilled into the alimentary tract. This method, if used, is typically reserved for small lizards and chelonians.

Analgesia

Modern recommendations for the euthanasia of reptiles consist of two stages. The first stage involves anaesthetizing the animal or at least deeply sedating it with analgesia. It is important to note that an animal that is deeply sedated without analgesia (i.e. through the use of benzodiazepines, acepromazine and/or subanaesthetic doses of barbiturates or propofol) will still be able to perceive pain, even if they have lost their capacity to react to it. Once the animal has been deeply sedated with analgesia or has been anaesthetized, the perception of pain should be reduced, if not totally eliminated. The neurosteroid alfaxalone is a good choice to anaesthetize a reptile and doses of 5 mg/kg intravenously or 10 mg/kg intramuscularly are advocated. The dissociative and benzodiazepine combination of tiletamine–zolazepam can also work well.

Gas

Some clinicians will induce anaesthesia using gas but this process may not be practical for snakes and breath-holding species such as chelonians.

Confirming Death

Once the patient is deeply sedated or anaesthetized, as defined by diminished or absent righting and tail/toe reflexes, intracardiac pentobarbitone is recommended. A Doppler probe can be of great help in locating the heart and also in confirming the absence of a heartbeat (Figure 33.1). Typical doses of pentobarbitone are 160 mg/kg. Using higher doses can cause tissue artefacts that may affect a pathologist's interpretation of histological lesions (see Chapter 30). Once spontaneous breathing and a heartbeat have ceased and all reflexes have stopped (which can sometimes take minutes), the animal is considered dead.

If a necropsy is then performed on the reptile, the clinician will sometimes be faced with a beating heart (especially in snakes) and this can be alarming to see. The leaky electrolyte channels in the pacemaker cells allow the heart to beat independently to the nervous system. It can take several minutes following death, even if the heart is resected from the animal, before the heart has exhausted all of its energy stores and stops beating. The presence of a heart beat seen at necropsy should not be automatically interpreted to mean that the animal was not euthanized.

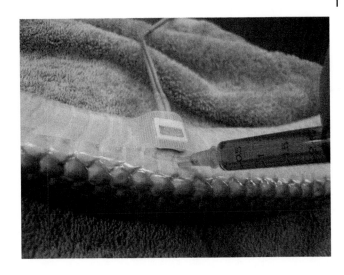

Figure 33.1 A Doppler probe can be used to confirm the absence of a heartbeat.

Redundancy

Some clinicians choose to add layers of redundancy into their euthanasia protocols. For example, once the reptile has been deeply sedated or anaesthetized and after pentobarbitone has been injected into its heart, some clinicians will choose to decapitate the animal and, even then, pithing of the cranial spinal cord in the decapitated head is sometimes performed. As before, this is because of a reptile's remarkable ability to maintain brain function in anoxic environments. Pithing is performed by placing a needle into the cranial spinal cord of the decapitated head and then advancing it cranially, with agitation, through the foramen magnum. It goes without saying that many owners will be shocked to see their pet decapitated and pithed and so this practice is usually reserved for non-pet reptiles (e.g. wildlife or zoo animals) or the animals belonging to highly experienced reptile owners.

If the owner elects to take their reptile home, it is imperative that the clinician is certain that the animal has been euthanized. It is also the duty of the veterinarian to address the unpleasant subject of what will happen to the animal when it is returned home. If an animal is to be buried, the owner needs to be made aware that the drug residues remaining in their reptile could be toxic (and potentially fatal) to other animals that may dig up and ingest the deceased reptile.

Further Reading

American Veterinary Medical Association (2013) *AVMA Guidelines for the Euthanasia of Animals: 2013 Edition*. AVMA, Schaumburg, IL.

Appendix 1

Formulary

KEY

The following abbreviations are used in the tables in this formulary:

CSF	cerebrospinal fluid
CNS	central nervous system
GI	gastrointestinal
IM	intramuscularly
IV	intravenously
PO	orally
q	every
SC	subcutaneously
spp.	species

Tables

- Table A1.1 Emergency drugs
- Table A1.2 Antibiotics
- Table A1.3 Anti-fungal drugs
- Table A1.4 Antiviral drugs
- Table A1.5 Anti-protozoal drugs
- Table A1.6 Internal parasiticides
- Table A1.7 External parasiticides
- Table A1.8 Hormonal therapies
- Table A1.9 Drugs used to treat liver disease
- Table A1.10 Drugs used to treat kidney disease
- Table A1.11 Drugs used to treat cardiovascular disease
- Table A1.12 Gastrointestinal drugs
- Table A1.13 Anaesthesia and sedatives
- Table A1.14 Analgesia
- Table A1.15 Nutritional support

Reptile Medicine and Surgery in Clinical Practice, First Edition. Edited by Bob Doneley, Deborah Monks, Robert Johnson and Brendan Carmel.
© 2018 John Wiley & Sons Ltd. Published 2018 by John Wiley & Sons Ltd.

Table A1.1 Emergency drugs.

Class	Drug	Dose and route	Comments
Anti-muscarinic agent: • Used to treat bradycardia	Atropine	0.01–0.2 mg/kg IM or IV	May thicken respiratory secretions.
	Glycopyrrolate	0.01 mg/kg IV	
Alpha- and beta-adrenergic agonist agent: • Used systemically for treating anaphylaxis and cardiac resuscitation	Adrenaline (epinephrine)	0.1 mg/kg IV	Care with hypovolaemic patients (not a substitute for adequate volume replacement).
Opiate antagonist	Naloxone	0.01–0.04 mg/kg IV q 2–3 minutes to effect	At reversal dosages, naloxone can negate opioid analgesic effects. The reversal effect may last for a shorter time than opioid effect, so repeated dosing may be needed.
Benzodiazepine	Diazepam	0.5 mg/kg IM, IV	Seizure control.
	Midazolam	1–2 mg/kg IM, IV	
Benzodiazepine antagonist	Flumazenil	0.05–0.1 mg/kg IV or IM	Flumazenil is used for the reversal of benzodiazepine after overdoses or toxicity. The reversal effect may last for a shorter time than benzodiazepine effect, so repeated dosing may be needed.
Fluids (shock)	Crystalloid fluids (0.9% saline)	10 ml/kg IV bolus	See Chapter 13 for maintenance fluids.
Fluids (shock)	Colloid fluids	5 ml/kg IV bolus	See Chapter 13 for maintenance fluids.

Table A1.2 Antibiotics.

Class	Drug	Dose and route	Comments
Penicillins:			
• Bactericidal	Amoxicillin	10 mg/kg q 24 hours IM 22 mg/kg q 12–24 hours PO	Effective against Gram-positive bacteria, especially *Staphylococcus*; many Gram-negative bacteria are resistant. Often combined with an aminoglycoside. Pharmacokinetic studies in reptiles are lacking.
• Well distributed in extracellular spaces especially in inflamed tissues	Ampicillin	3–6 mg/Kg IM, PO, SC q 12–24 hours	
• Do not readily penetrate the eye and CNS			
• Excreted by the kidneys, largely unchanged, therefore high concentrations can be found in the urine	Amoxicillin–clavulanic acid	15 mg/kg q 24hours IM 30 mg/kg q 12–24 hours PO	Clavulanic acid is added to inhibit beta-lactamase.
• Potentially synergistic in combination with aminoglycosides	Carbenicillin	400 mg/kg IM q 48 hours	Improved spectrum against *Pseudomonas* and other Gram-negative bacteria. Oral form has poor bioavailability.
	Piperacillin Piperacillin with tazobactam	100 mg/kg IM q 48 hours	Good activity against most Gram-negative bacteria including *Pseudomonas*, *Klebsiella* and *Enterobacter*. Piperacillin with tazobactam is commonly used to overcome beta-lactamase-producing bacteria. Parenteral administration only. Reconstituted drug should be used within 24 hours or 7 days if refrigerated.
	Penicillin, benzathine	10,000–20,000 units/kg (6.25–12.5 mg/kg) IM q 48–96 hours	Infrequently used
	Penicillin G	10,000–20,000 units/kg (6–12 mg/kg) SC, IM, IV q 8–12 hours	
	Ticarcillin	50 mg/kg IM q 24 hours	Similar to carbenicillin; much more active against *Pseudomonas*. Also found in combination with clavulanic acid and used at the same dose. Parenteral administration only.

(Continued)

Table A1.2 (Continued)

Class	Drug	Dose and route	Comments
Cephalosporins:			
• Three generations; effective against both gram Gram-positive and -negative bacteria	Cephalothin	20–40 mg/kg IM q 12hours	First generation cephalosporin: Effective against most Gram-positive cocci, many
• Well distributed in extracellular spaces	Cephalexin	20–40 mg/kg PO q 12hours	Gram-negatives and some anaerobes.
• Do not readily penetrate eye and CNS, except for cefotaxime and ceftazidime	Ceftazidime	20–40 mg/kg IM q 72hours	Third generation. Penetrates CSF. Excreted through the kidneys. Dose should be reduced in renally
• Synergistic with aminoglycosides			impaired patients. Following reconstitution, solution is stable for 18 hours at room temperature, 7 days if refrigerated or 3 months if frozen at −20 °C. Once thawed, it should not be refrozen and thawed solutions are stable for 8 hours if refrigerated and 4 hours at room temperature.
	Ceftiofur	5–15 mg/kg IM q 12 hours	Third generation with activity against *Pasteurella, E. coli, Streptococcus, Staphylococcus* and *Salmonella* spp.
	Cefotaxime	20–40 mg/kg IM q 24 hours	Third generation: expanded Gram-negative spectrum. Penetrates CSF.
Chloramphenicol:			
• Bacteriostatic	Chloramphenicol succinate (injectable)	20–40 mg/kg IM or PO q 12–72hours	Broad spectrum against *Chlamydia, Mycoplasma,* Gram-positive and Gram-negative bacteria and some protozoa.
• Highly lipid soluble, so good tissue penetration, including CNS and eye; tissue concentrations often exceed serum levels			
• Anaemia and CNS depression			
• Caution needed in handling the drug			

Aminoglycosides:

- Bactericidal
- Synergistic with penicillins and cephalosporins
- Excellent spectrum against Gram-positive and -negative bacteria
- Ineffective against anaerobic bacteria and in proteinaceous environments such as abscesses and exudates
- Poor penetration into CNS and eye
- Nephrotoxic, especially in snakes, dehydrated reptiles or those with compromised renal function (the dose should be reduced or a less toxic drug selected)

Drug	Dose	Comments
Amikacin	2.5–5 mg/kg IM q 48–72 hours	Greater activity against Gram-negatives, including some resistant to gentamycin and tobramycin. Achieves higher serum concentrations than gentamycin but is less toxic so levels are better tolerated. Fewer toxic adverse effects.
Gentamycin	2.5 mg/kg q 72 hours	Dose > 5 mg/kg may be toxic. Not generally recommended owing to narrow margin of safety.
Tobramycin	2.5 mg/kg q 24 hours	Pharmacology is similar to gentamycin but has greater activity against *Pseudomonas*. Neurotoxicity and nephrotoxicity may develop.

Quinolones:

- Bactericidal
- Most Gram-negative pathogens, some Gram-positive pathogens, most *Mycoplasma* and possibly *Chlamydia* are sensitive
- Limited efficacy against anaerobes
- Achieve high levels, especially in the liver and urinary tract; **tissue** concentrations may exceed serum concentrations
- Use with caution in juveniles; may cause permanent articular defects
- IM injection causes pain and necrosis at the site of injections

Drug	Dose	Comments
Enrofloxacin	5–10 mg/kg IM q 48 hours	Excellent activity against *Mycoplasma*, some Gram-positive and most Gram-negative bacteria. However, *Pseudomonas* resistance is common. Unsuitable for anaerobic infections. Diluted with saline before injection as repeated injections cause significant bruising and muscle necrosis. Alternatively, switch to oral dosing if gut is motile.
Ciprofloxacin	10 mg/kg PO q 48 hours	Antibacterial spectrum similar to enrofloxacin.
Marbofloxacin	2 mg/kg IM, IV q 24 hours; 10 mg/kg PO q 48 hours	

(Continued)

Table A1.2 (Continued)

Class	Drug	Dose and route	Comments
Trimethoprim–sulfa derivatives: • Bactericidal • Moderate Gram-positive and -negative spectrum • *Pseudomonas* and some strains of *Enterobacteriaceae* are resistant • May be effective against some coccidia • Wide extracellular distribution • Sulfas are excreted via the same pathway as uric acid; in dehydrated reptiles and those with compromised renal function sulfas may form crystals and damage renal glomeruli	Trimethoprim–sulfadiazine	30 mg/kg PO q 24 hours for 2 days, then q 48 hours or 20–30 mg/kg IM q 24–48 hours	

Tetracyclines:
• Bacteriostatic
• Spectrum includes many Gram-positive organisms; poor efficacy against most Gram-negative isolates
• Used for *Chlamydia* and *Mycoplasma*
• Wide volume of distribution
• Adverse effects:
  o Anorexia, vomiting, diarrhoea
  o Immunosuppression
  o Hepatotoxicity (rare)
  o Localized tissue reactions to doxycycline injections formulations
  o Alteration of gut flora, especially yeast overgrowths and secondary bacterial infections
  o Chelates calcium in gut and bone; dietary calcium interferes with the oral uptake of tetracyclines; use cautiously if needed for extended periods of time
	Oxytetracycline
	
	Chlortetracycline
		10–80 mg/kg IM q 4 hours
		
		200 mg/kg PO q 24 hours
			Poorly absorbed when given orally, oral formulations are not recommended. IM well absorbed and widely distributed but will cause necrosis at the injection site.
			
			Better oral absorption than oxytetracycline

Drug	Dosage	Notes
		More lipophilic than other tetracyclines; absorbed better and faster through the GI tract and greater bioavailability.
Doxycycline	5–10 mg/kg PO q 24 hours or 50 mg /kg IM once then 25 mg/kg IM q72 hours	

Macrolides and lincosamides:

- Bacteriostatic
- Indicated for *Pasteurella*, *Bordetella*, some *Mycoplasma*, *Campylobacter* spp. and *Clostridia* spp. and obligate anaerobic bacteria
- Often used for susceptible upper respiratory tract infections and osteomyelitis
- Active against Gram-positive organisms and anaerobes but virtually all aerobic Gram-negative bacteria are resistant

Drug	Dosage	Notes
Clarithromycin	15 mg/kg PO q 3.5 days	Excreted through the kidneys. Effective against a variety of Gram-positive and -negative bacteria as well as *Mycobacterium avium* complex bacteria, *Chlamydia* and *Mycoplasma*. It may also be effective against some anaerobic bacteria.
Clindamycin	5 mg/kg PO q 12 hours	Used occasionally to treat osteomyelitis caused by susceptible Gram-positive pathogens.
Lincomycin	5 mg/kg q 24 hours	It has been used to treat respiratory and GI infections caused by Gram-positive bacteria and *Mycoplasma*.
Azithromycin	10 mg/kg PO q 3–7 days	New generation macrolide; it appears to be active against intracellular infections including *Chlamydia*, *Toxoplasma*, *Plasmodium* and *Cryptosporidium*, as well as a number of Gram-positive and -negative bacteria. It is excreted through the liver and may be hepatotoxic. May cause a reversible anaemia in some reptiles.
Tylosin	5 mg/kg IM 24 hours	Used predominantly for suspected *Mycoplasma* infections. Intramuscular injections can be very irritating.

Nitroimidazoles:

- Bactericidal
- Effective against many Gram-positive and most Gram-negative obligate anaerobes
- Ineffective against aerobic bacteria
- Highly effective against many motile protozoa
- well absorbed from GI tract
- highly lipophilic and penetrates bones, CNS and abscesses

Drug	Dosage	Notes
Metronidazole	20 mg/kg PO q 24–48 hours	Frequently used for anaerobic infections, (including clostridial infections) and motile protozoa.

Table A1.3 Anti-fungal drugs.

Class	Drug	Dose and route	Comments
Azoles:			
• Inhibit ergosterol synthesis, increasing cellular membrane permeability; also causes secondary metabolic effects and growth inhibition	Ketoconazole	15–30 mg/kg PO q 24 hours for 10–30 days Administer with food.	For *Candida* infections. Probably not as effective with *Aspergillus* infections as other azoles. Widely distributed to tissues but is highly protein-bound and does not penetrate CNS or eye fluids. Water insoluble unless dissolved in acid first.
• Fungistatic, so months of therapy are often required	Fluconazole	5 mg/kg PO q 24 hours	Effective against *Candida* (especially mycelial form), *Aspergillus* and *Cryptococcus*. Penetrates eye, CNS and CSF. Best safety margin of the azoles.
• Take several days to reach steady-state concentrations	Itraconazole	5–10 mg/kg PO q 24 hours given with food for at least one month after signs have resolved	Some hepatotoxicity noted Can cause anorexia and weight loss Has been used for skin infections with *Chrysosporium* anamorph of *Nannizziopsis vriesii* (CANV)
	Voriconazole	5–10 mg/kg PO q 24 hours at least 1 month after signs have resolved	High oral bioavailability Can cross into the CNS Used for CANV infections
Allylamines:			
• Inhibit squalene epoxidase, which is critical for fungal sterol and cell wall synthesis	Terbinafine	5–10 mg/kg PO q 24 hours Can also be applied topically.	Aspergillus and dermatophytes Good oral absorption; distributed well to fat and skin
Polyenes:			
• Act by binding to sterols (primarily ergosterol) in the cell membrane and alters the permeability of the membrane, allowing the loss of intracellular potassium and other cellular constituents	Amphotericin B	0.5 mg/kg IV q24–72 hours for 14–28days or Intra-tracheally 1 mg/kg (diluted in saline) q 24 hours or Nebulize at 0.3–1 mg/ml for 60 minutes q 24 hours	Fungicidal. Active against both yeast and fungal hyphae. Not absorbed orally; for aspergillosis, drug must be administered IV, topically or by nebulization. Widely distributed when given IV but only minor systemic absorption with aerosol or topical administration. Nephrotoxic.
	Nystatin	100,000 iu/kg PO q 24 hours	For yeast infections of the gut.

Table A1.4 Antiviral drugs.

Class	Drug	Dose and route	Comments
Purine analogues:			
Used for treating outbreaks of herpesvirus infection in tortoises	Aciclovir	80 mg/kg PO q 8 hours for a minimum of 7 days	Poor oral absorption. Efficacy uncertain.
	Valaciclovir	40 mg/kg PO q 24 hours	

Table A1.5 Anti-protozoal drugs.

Class	Drug	Dose and route	Comments
Nitroimidazoles:			
Used against motile protozoa (*Trichomonas, Giardia, Cochlosoma, Spironucleus, Histomonas*)	Metronidazole	20–50 mg/kg PO q 24–48 hours	Frequently used for motile protozoa (*Trichomonas and amoeba*).
Sulfonamides:			
• Used to treat coccidia	Sulfadimethoxine	50 mg/kg PO q 24 hours for 3–5 days	Be careful using this in a patient with dehydration, liver disease, renal disease. Treatment periods greater than 2 weeks may require supplementation with folic acid. All treatments should be repeated after 5 days to allow for the prepatent period of coccidia.
	Sulfamethazine	25–50 mg/kg PO q 24 hours for 3 days on, 3 days off	
Benzeneacetonitrile derivatives:			
• Used to treat coccidia	Ponazuril	30 mg/kg PO q 48 hours for 2 treatments	
• All treatments should be repeated after 5 days to allow for the prepatent period of coccidia	Toltrazuril	7–15 mg/kg PO q 24 hours for 3 days or 25 mg/kg PO for 1 dose	
Quinacrine HCl			
• Used for haemaprotozoa	Quinacrine HCl	19–100 mg/kg PO q 48 hours 14–21 days	Overdosage may cause hepatotoxicity.
Chloroquine:			
• Used for haemaprotozoa	Chloroquine	125 mg/kg PO q 48 hours for 3 treatments	Use in conjunction with primaquine.

Table A1.6 Internal parasiticides.

Class	Drug	Dose and route	Comments
Fumarate reductase inhibitors:			
• Benzimidazole derivatives	Albendazole	50 mg/kg PO for 1 dose	Can be used for treating *Microsporidia*, as well as some nematodes.
• Used mainly for treating nematodes	Fenbendazole	25–100 mg/kg q 14 days for 1–4 treatments or 50 mg/kg/day for 3 days	May also be effective against some cestodes, trematodes and *Giardia*. Can be toxic to bone marrow, causing leucopenia.
• Interfere with parasite microtubules and sugar metabolism			
• Usually require several days of treatment, although single high doses can be effective	Oxfendazole	68 mg/kg PO for one dose; repeat in 14 days	
• Can affect haematopoietic cells and intestinal epithelium			
• Toxicity varies with species and drug			
Gamma amino butyric acid-interfering drugs:			
• Macrocyclic lactones	Ivermectin	200–400 µg/kg PO or IM for one dose	DO NOT use in chelonians, skinks, crocodilians or indigo snakes.
• Used against Ascarids and other nematodes; bloodsucking external parasites	Moxidectin (2.5%) + imidacloprid (10%)	0.2 ml/kg, applied topically, q 14 days for 3 treatments	Used for nematodes. Only tested in a small number of agamid lizards. DO NOT use in chelonians, skinks, crocodilians or indigo snakes.
• Toxicity is low, except in chelonians, but overdosing and idiosyncratic reactions include severe depression, inactivity, excessive sleeping and neurological signs			
Octadepsipeptides:			
• Induce paralysis of the parasites	Emodepside (1.98%) + praziquantel (7.94%)	1.12 ml/kg applied topically	Used for nematodes and cestodes in many species; aquatic turtles must be kept dry for 48 hours after application.
Miscellaneous drugs:	Praziquantel	5–10 mg/kg PO or IM for 1 dose, repeat in 14 days	Used for treating cestodes and trematodes. Very unpalatable.
	Pyrantel tartrate Pyrantel pamoate Pyrantel embonate	5–25 mg/kg PO for 1 dose, repeat in 14 days	Used for nematodes. Poorly absorbed from the GI tract and so only suitable for gut parasites. Good safety margin.
	Paromomycin	100 mg/kg PO q 24 hours for 7 days, then every 2 weeks for 3 months	Used for treating *Cryptosporidia*. Does not eliminate the organism.

Table A1.7 External parasiticides.

Class	Drug	Dose and route	Comments
Pyrethrins and synthetic pyrethroids:			
	Pyrethrin	Spray or wash	All are potentially neurotoxic: Do not leave on the animal – wipe off after application. Do not use on animals that are shedding. Caution when applying to juveniles.
	Permethrin	Spray or wash	
Piperonyl butoxide	Usually combined with a pyrethrin or permethrin		
Broad-spectrum insecticides	Fipronil	Spray or wipe on then wash off in 5 minutes, Repeat every 7–10days as required	Potentially neurotoxic Beware of inhalation or dermal absorption of the alcohol base
Organophosphates	Carbaryl	Lightly dust animal and environment; rinse after 1 hour; repeat in 7 days	Carbamate flea powder. Use is illegal in many countries. Narrow therapeutic index. Safer products are available.
Macrocyclic lactones: • Used against reptile mites • Toxicity is low except in chelonians but overdosing and idiosyncratic reactions include severe depression, inactivity, excessive sleeping, and neurological signs	Ivermectin	5–10 mg/l water topical spray q 3–5 days for up to 28 days for mites.	DO NOT use in chelonians, crocodilians, skinks and indigo snakes. Spray on skin and in newly cleaned cage, then allow to dry before replacing water dish.

Table A1.8 Hormonal therapies.

Class	Drug	Dose and route	Comments
Reproductive hormones:			
	Arginine vasotocin	0.01–1 µg/kg IV, SC q 12–24 hours for 2–3 treatments	No commercial preparations available. Must be purchased from chemical suppliers. Used for dystocia; give 30–60 minutes after parenteral calcium.
	Deslorelin	4.7 mg implant SC	Gonadotrophin-releasing hormone agonist, shown to suppress follicular development and steroidogenesis in female iguanas.
	Leuprolide acetate	0.4 mg/kg IM	Gonadotrophin-releasing hormone agonist. Trialled in iguanas for aggression without effect.
	Oxytocin	1–10 units/kg IM q 4–6 hours for 1–3 treatments	Used to stimulate oviductal contractions but is not naturally occurring in most reptiles and may not be effective. Works well in chelonians, less so in snakes and lizards. Use is contraindicated if uterovaginal sphincter is not dilated. Should be used in conjunction with calcium gluconate injections: give 1 hour after calcium administration.
	Prostaglandin E2	0.02–0.1 mg/kg applied topically into the cloaca	Used to induce egg laying in dystocic reptiles; simultaneously relaxes uterovaginal sphincter while contracting oviduct.
	Prostaglandin F₂α (dinoprost)	50–200 µg/kg SC	Contracts the oviduct but does not relax uterovaginal sphincter. Use concurrently with prostaglandin E2.
Thyroxine	Levothyroxine	0.02 mg/kg PO q 48 hours	Stimulates feeding in debilitated tortoises.
Insulin:			
• Used for treating hyperglycaemia • More research is needed	Regular insulin	Lizards and crocodilians: 5–10 iu/kg body weight IM q 24 hours Snakes and chelonians: 1–5 iu/kg body weight IM every 24–72 hours	These doses are empirical, and should be adjusted based on response to therapy and continued serial sampling of blood glucose
Other hormones:			
• Calcium regulation • Used for treating hypercalcaemia and hyperparathyroidism	Calcitonin	1.5 units/kg SC q 8 hours for 14–21 days as needed or 50 units/kg IM, repeat in 14 days	Administer after calcium; avoid if hypocalcaemic. Inhibits calcium absorption by the intestines. Inhibits osteoclast activity in bones. Stimulates osteoblastic activity in bones. Inhibits renal tubular cell reabsorption of calcium allowing it to be excreted in the urine.

Table A1.9 Drugs used to treat liver disease.

Class	Drug	Dose and route	Comments
• Anti-inflammatory • Anti-fibrotic	Colchicine	0.04–0.2 mg/kg PO q 24 hours	Overdose can lead to dehydration and electrolyte abnormalities. As reptile kidneys lack a Loop of Henle, efficacy is uncertain.
Diuretics: • Reduce ascites	Furosemide (frusemide)	2–5 mg/kg PO, IM, IV q 12–24 hours	Monitor hydration status.
	Hydrochlorothiazide	1 mg/kg q 24–72 hours	
Laxatives: • Reduce intestinal ammonia absorption • Decrease the pH of the intestinal lumen creating an 'acidic sink' that will decrease ammonia levels; also promotes an osmotic catharsis. • Best results are seen in carnivorous reptiles, as vegetable protein lacks many encephalopathic precursors	Lactulose	150–650 mg/kg PO q 24 hours	Can cause diarrhoea.
Antioxidants: • Unproven remedy that offers promise in reptile medicine as a hepatoprotectant • Enhances protein synthesis and hepatocellular regeneration • Suppresses fibrogenesis • Promotes fibrinolysis	Silibinin (active component of silymarin, extract of milk thistle)	4–15 mg/kg PO q 8–12hours	Use a low-alcohol or alcohol-free base.
Hepatoprotective drugs:	Ursodeoxycholic acid	10–15 mg/kg PO q 24 hours	Bile acid. Cytoprotective. Reduces involvement of hepatocytes and biliary epithelium in inflammatory process. Changes mix of bile acids to eliminate toxic bile acids from liver.

Table A1.10 Drugs used to treat kidney disease.

Class	Drug	Dose and route	Comments
Drugs acting on uric acid:			
• Decrease production of uric acid	Allopurinol	10–20 mg/kg PO q 24 hours	Long-term therapy; tortoises may respond best.
		25 mg/kg PO q 24 hours	Green iguanas.
		50 mg/kg PO q 24 hours for 30 days, then q 72 hours	Used in chelonians with hyperuricaemia
• Increase excretion of uric acid	Probenecid	250 mg/kg PO q 12 hours	
• Reduce inflammation associated with articular gout	Colchicine	0.04–0.2 mg/kg PO q 24 hours	
• Phosphate binders	Aluminium hydroxide	100 mg/kg PO q 12–24 hours	Decreases intestinal absorption of phosphorus. Use cautiously in patients with gastric outlet obstruction.
	Calcium carbonate and chitosan (Ipakitine®)	1 g diluted in 9 ml water; give 1 ml/500 g PO q 12 hours	

Table A1.11 Drugs used to treat cardiovascular disease.

Class	Drug	Dose and route	Comments
Positive Inotrope	Pimobendan	0.2 mg/kg PO q 24 hours	Similar in effect to digoxin but with lower risk of adverse effects.
Diuretics:			
• May reduce ascites associated with liver disease or congestive heart failure	Frusemide	2–5 mg/kg PO, IM, IV q 12–24 hours	Overdose can lead to dehydration and electrolyte abnormalities. As reptile kidneys lack a loop of Henle, efficacy is uncertain.
	Hydrochlorothiazide	1 mg/kg q 24–72 hours	Monitor hydration status.

Table A1.12 Gastrointestinal drugs.

Class	Drug	Dose and route	Comments
Intestinal motility modifiers:			
● Used for GI motility disorders	Metoclopramide	0.06 mg/kg PO q 24 hours for 7 days	Increases force and frequency of gastric contractions, relaxes pyloric sphincter, and promotes peristalsis in the duodenum and jejunum. Usually only effective if given with IV fluids as a constant rate infusion.
	Cisapride	0.5–2 mg/kg PO q 8–12 hours	Stimulates GI motility.
Gastrointestinal protectants:			
● Used when gastric ulceration is present	Cimetidine	4 mg/kg PO, IM q 8–12 hours	Reduces gastric secretion of HCl and pepsin. May impair the metabolism of concurrently administered drugs. Gastric and duodenal ulceration; oesophagitis; gastroesophageal reflux; may use in renal failure to increase phosphate loss.
	Sucralfate	500–1000 mg/kg PO q 6–8 hours	A complex disaccharide that reacts with stomach acid to form a complex that binds to proteins associated with an ulcer and produces a protective layer that protects the ulcerated mucosa from gastric acids and microbial pathogens.
Laxatives and cathartics:			
	Dioctyl sodium sulfosuccinate	1–5 mg/kg PO	Use 1 : 20 dilution.
	Mineral oil (paraffin oil)	20–30 ml (50 : 50 with electrolyte solution)/kg PO q 24 hours	Acts unchanged as an emollient laxative. Care must be taken to prevent aspiration.
	Methylcellulose	1–3 ml/100 g	Absorbs water and swells. Care must be taken not to mix too thickly or give too much, as it can absorb enough water to block the GI tract.
	Lactulose	150–650 mg/kg PO q 24 hours	Has a laxative effect through osmotic catharsis.

Table A1.13 Anaesthesia and sedatives.

Class	Drug	Dose and route	Comments
Benzodiazepines: • Sedation or pre-medication for anaesthesia • Used in seizures • Often used in conjunction with an opioid	Diazepam Midazolam	0.2–1 mg/kg IM 1–3 mg/kg IM	Can be used as a pre-medication prior to anaesthesia if given 10–20 minutes before induction. Onset of action 10–20 minutes when given IM. At sedative doses, there are minimal effects on blood pressure and heart rate.
Local anaesthesia: • Techniques for local and regional anaesthesia, including epidural anaesthesia, have not been described in reptiles • Indications for use of local anaesthetic techniques are similar to those in domestic animals	Lignocaine Bupivacaine	2–4 mg/kg SC 1–2 mg/kg SC	
Injectable anaesthesia: See Chapter 27	Alfaxalone	2–4 mg/kg IM (front leg) 5 mg/kg IV 10 mg/kg IM 2–4 mg/kg IV	Sedation for chelonians. IV induction most species. IM induction in most species. IV induction small crocodiles.
	Ketamine	20–50 mg/kg IM, IV	Ketamine alone is not recommended for anaesthesia. Inadequate analgesia and muscle relaxation. Associated with spontaneous movements and muscular rigidity. Violent and/or prolonged recoveries. Lack of coordination.
	Xylazine	0.1–1.25 mg/kg IM, IV	Does not usually produce adequate surgical immobilization. Reversible with yohimbine 0.11–0.27 mg/kg IM.

Agent	Dose	Notes
Ketamine(K) with butorphanol (B)	(K) 10–30 mg/kg + (B) 0.5–1.5 mg/kg IM	Minor surgical procedures.
Ketamine with diazepam (D)	(K) 60–80 mg/kg + (D) 0.2–1 mg/kg IM	Improved muscle relaxation.
Ketamine with medetomidine (Me)	(K) 10 mg/kg + (Me) 0.1–0.3 mg/kg IM (or half this dose if giving IV)	Medetomidine may no longer be commercially available in some countries. If not, use dexmedetomidine at half the dose of medetomidine. Reverse with atipamezole.
Ketamine with midazolam (Mi)	(K) 20–40 mg/kg + (Mi) 1–2 mg/kg IM	
Propofol	5–10 mg/kg IV, IO or Constant rate infusion at 0.3–0.5 mg/kg/min IV, IO or 0.5–1 mg/kg IV, IO periodic bolus	Causes pronounced cardiopulmonary depressant effects in reptiles, so should be titrated to effect. Apnoea is common following rapid IV induction. Intubation and IPPV are recommended.
Tiletamine–zolazepam	4–5 mg/kg IM for noninvasive procedures or 5–10 mg/kg IM for more invasive procedures	Variable results – sedation or anaesthesia. Severe respiratory depression; possible may require IPPV. Prolonged induction and recovery times. Lower dose in larger patients.

Table A1.14 Analgesia.

Class	Drug	Dose and route	Comments
Opioids	Buprenorphine	0.005–0.02 mg/kg IM q 24–48 hours	Studies have called into question use in providing analgesia in reptiles, including red-eared sliders, ball pythons, bearded dragons and green iguanas (for further information see Chapter 27). Adverse effects include depression, nausea and vomiting, bradycardia and constipation.
	Butorphanol	0.5–2 mg/kg IM	
	Morphine	1.0–5.0 mg/kg IM, SC	Evidence of analgesic efficacy in red-eared sliders and some lizards.
	Methadone	3–5 mg/kg IM, SC	Evidence of analgesic efficacy in red-eared sliders and anecdotally in some lizards.
	Tramadol	5–10 mg/kg IM, PO q 48–72 hours	Evidence of long duration of action in chelonians.
Non-steroidal anti-inflammatory drugs: • Indicated when tissue damage and inflammation are the source of the pain • Have the potential to cause renal damage and GI ulceration	Carprofen	1–4 mg/kg PO, SC, IM, IV q 24 hours, follow with half the dose q 24–72 hours	
	Flunixin	0.1–2 mg/kg IM, PO q 12–24 hours	
	Ketoprofen	2 mg/kg IM q 24–48 hours	
	Meloxicam	0.2–0.3 mg/kg IM, PO q 24 hours	Choose higher doses for chelonians.

Table A1.15 Nutritional support.

Class	Drug	Dose and route	Comments
Calcium: • Used to treat hypocalcaemic diseases, including hypocalcaemic tetany, dystocia, metabolic/nutritional bone disease	Calcium borogluconate	10–50 mg/kg IM q 12–24 hours as needed	Oral supplement.
	Calcium glubionate	10–100 mg/kg PO q 12–24 hours as needed	For hypocalcaemia or dystocia.
	Calcium gluconate	10–50 mg/kg IM	
		100–200 mg/kg IM, SC q 8 hours	For nutritional secondary hyperparathyroidism, hypocalcaemic muscle tremors and seizures or flaccid paresis in lizards. When patient is stable, switch to oral calcium.
Iodine	Lugol's iodine	2–4 mg/kg PO q 24 hours for 2–3 weeks, then weekly	Used in herbivorous species maintained on goitrogenic diet. Alternatively, can use balanced vitamin–mineral mixture or iodized salt (0.5% of feed).
Iron	Iron dextran	12 mg/kg IM q 72 hours for 45 days	Used for treating anaemia, although not used as frequently as it once was.
Vitamins: • Vitamin D3: nutritional secondary hyperparathyroidism and hypocalcaemia	Vitamin A	1000–5000 iu/kg IM q 7–10 days for 4 treatments	Hypovitaminosis A; may have value in infectious stomatitis. Overdose may cause epidermal sloughing.
	Vitamin B1 (thiamine)	25 mg/kg PO q 24 hours as needed or 30 g/kg feed fish PO	Used in piscivorus species, e.g. crocodilians.
	Vitamin B12	0.05 mg/kg SC, IM	May cause orange/pink urine and urates. Used as an appetite stimulant.
	Vitamin C	10–20 mg/kg SC, IM q 24 hours	Supportive therapy for bacterial infections; higher doses (i.e. 100 mg/kg) may be used for severe burns.
		100–250 mg/kg PO q 24 hours	Infectious stomatitis.
	Vitamin D3	200 iu/kg IM q 4 weeks or 1000 iu/kg IM, repeat in 1 week	See Chapter 6 for details on providing adequate ultraviolet B lighting. Beware of oversupplementation. Herbivores are sensitive to excess. Excessive supplementation may result in soft-tissue calcification.
		200 iu/kg PO q 7 days	
	Vitamin E	25 mg/kg IM weekly	Dietary sources include green plants. Low in whole prey (rodents and fish).
	Vitamin K1	0.25–0.50 mg/kg IM	Hypovitaminosis K1; coagulopathies.

Appendix 2

Reference Intervals for Commonly Kept Reptile Species

Unless otherwise stated, reference intervals are adapted from *Reptile Medicine and Surgery*, 2nd ed. (D.R. Mader, ed., Elsevier, 2006, pp. 1103–1118) and *Current Therapy in Reptile Medicine and Surgery* (D.R. Mader and S.J. Divers, eds, Elsevier, 2014, pp. 382–410).

Tables

- Table A2.1 Lizards
- Table A2.2 Snakes
- Table A2.3 Chelonians

KEY
The following abbreviations are used in the tables in this formulary:
AST   aspartate aminotransferase BUN   blood urea nitrogen CK   Creatine kinase LDH   lactate dehydrogenase PCV   packed cell volume WBC   whole blood count

Reptile Medicine and Surgery in Clinical Practice, First Edition. Edited by Bob Doneley, Deborah Monks, Robert Johnson and Brendan Carmel.
© 2018 John Wiley & Sons Ltd. Published 2018 by John Wiley & Sons Ltd.

Table A2.1 Lizards.

Measure	Units	Bearded dragon (*Pogona vitticeps*)	Blue-tongued skink (*Tiliqua scincoides*)	Tokay gecko (*Gekko gecko*)[1]	Crested gecko (*Correlophus ciliatus*)	Chinese water dragon (*Physignathus cocincinus*)	Panther chameleon (*Furcifer pardalis*)	Green iguana (*Iguana iguana*)	Lace monitor (*Varanus varius*)[2]	Savannah monitor (*Varanus exanthematicus*)
Haematology										
PCV	%	30	31	30	26–34	35	27	38.5	35	31.2
	(range)	(19–40)	(22–46)	(25–34)		(32–40)	(16–35)	(25–38)	(29–43)	(21–51)
WBC	×10⁹/l	5.07	7.3	10.3	8–23	19.4	0.47–18.6	11.26	22.4	5.07
	(range)	(1.2–11.3)	(2.2–19.6)	(4.2–20.3)		(16–23)		(7–14)	(0.6–63.8)	(1.2–11.3)
Heterophils	×10⁹/l	1.95	2.45	2.2	–	5.1	1.57	0.35–5.2	6.39	1.95
	(range)	(0.38–4.06)	(0.54–6.24)	(0.8–4.4)		(3.9–6.9)	(0.09–4.17)		(0.33–26.72)	(0.38–4.06)
	%	17–43	25–32		3–39	26–50	55–72	43–69	12–81	–
Lymphocytes	×10⁹/l	2.12	2.75	4.8	5–15	7.2	2.96	0.5–5.5	11.1	2.12
	(range)	(0.43–5.25)	(0.32–10.9)	(1.6–10.1)		(5.6–9.5)	(0.21–9.67)		(0.13–32.3)	(0.43–5.25)
	%	47–69	15–56			22–65	22–31	31–55	2–68	–
Monocytes	×10⁹/l	1.64	0.84	0.84	–	1.1	–	0–0.1	4.14	1.64
	(range)	(0.06–2.72)	(0.35–1.49)	(0.15–3.0)		(0.4–1.9)			(0.07–12)	(0.06–6.67)
	%	0–4	7–16		6–33	0–2	5–18	0–8	7–57	
Azurophils	×10⁹/l	0.54	0.34	0.77	–	0	1.25	0–1.7	–	0.11
	(range)	(0.04–1.84)	(0–1.08)	(0.2–1.6)		(0–0.6)	(0.08–3.74)			
	%	0–9	0–5					0–2	–	–
Eosinophils	×10⁹/l	0.15	1.5	0.07	–	0.2	–	0–1	–	–
	(range)	(0.06–0.27)	(0.03–2.96)	(0.05–1.0)		(0.1–0.3)				
	%	<1	1–2		0–2	0–1	–	0–3	–	–
Basophils	×10⁹/l	0.15	0.98	2.2	–	0.5	0.1	0–0.5	–	0.15
	(range)	(0.07–0.28)	(0.11–2.24)	(0.3–9.4)		(0.2–0.8)	(0.07–0.13)			(0.07–0.28)
	%	<1	1–2		0–12	0–2	0–2	0–3	–	–

Biochemistry

	units									
AST	units /l (range)	15–447	7–106	9–146	9–127	4–60	0–31	12–84	11–36	22 (1–78)
CK	units/l (range)	59–7000	73–35832	117	58–3905	19–6630	331– >1000	150–450	50–809	764 (150–3048)
Bile acids	µmol/l	–	–	–	35–89	–	–	1–13	–	–
LDH	units/l (range)	35–628	364–1106	189	–	–	–	12–95	–	427 (29–3699)
Uric acid	µmol/l	95–680	41–506	80–700	48–684	78–450	238–958	113–653	123–925	71.4–1070
Calcium	mmol/l	4.3–13.5	2.6–5.15	4.3–4.5	2.9–5	2.4–3.7	2.2–2.9	2.25–3.99	2.67–3.74	3.0–4.4
Phosphorous	mmol/l	0.9–4.9	0.9–2.5	0.9–2.5	1.3–3.1	1.1–2.7	1.8–3.2	1.7–2.5	0.81–2.76	1.0–2.4
BUN	mmol/l	0.4–2.5	0.0–0.7	–	–	–	0.36	–	–	0.0–1.8
Glucose	mmol/l	7.7–16.1	3.5–8.9	5.8–9.6	4.1–7.7	3.3–10.1	3.5–8.9	5–8.33	5–18.3	5–9
Cholesterol	mmol/l	5.9–23.3	1.9–11.1	–	–	–	–	4.2–6.6	–	1.3–6
Triglyceride	mmol/l	1–5	–	–	–	–	–	–	–	0.2–5.4
Protein	g/l	36–64	53–76	–	60–66	66–75	47–78	49–78	58–96	42–86
Sodium	mmol/l	137–190	142–158	158	134–150	147–153	145	157–163	143–169	149–165
Potassium	mmol/l	1–6.5	43–86	–	1.1–6.5	3.8–4.5	5.1	3.6–4	3.9–6.7	3.2–5.7
Chloride	mmol/l	104–160	111–115	119	–	–	113	119–121	–	105–124

[1] Values provided by CTDS Ltd, UK.
[2] From: Scheelings, T. and Jessop, T.S. (2011) Influence of capture method, habitat quality and individual traits on blood parameters of free–ranging lace monitors (*Varanus varius*). Australian Veterinary Journal, 89 (9), 360–365.

Table A2.2 Snakes.

	Units	Carpet python (*Morelia* spp.)	Green python (*Morelia viridis*)	Black-headed python (*Aspidites melanocephalus*)	Boa (*Boa constrictor constrictor*)	Rainbow boa (*Epicrates cenchria*)	Ball (royal) python (*Python regius*)	Corn snake (*Pantherophis guttatus*)
Haematology								
PCV	%	25	17	24	29	28	22	32
	(range)	(10–46)	(8–27)	(20–29)	(10–45)	(11–40)	(10–30)	(21–52)
WBC	×10^9/l	11.9	11.3	11.8	4.35	8	9.74	11.3
	(range)	(2–34)	(3.5–22.1)	(2–24)	(0.4–10.6)	(1–35.2)	(1–26)	(1.0–31.4)
Heterophils	×10^9/l	2.8	3.89	1.3	1.6	2.85	2.86	2.7
	(range)	(0.3–11.3)	(0.86–6.63)	(0.14–3.1)	(0.2–5.4)	(0.03–10)	(0.37–10.8)	(0.2–8.35)
	%	38–68	–	–	20–65	–	56–67	–
Lymphocytes	×10^9/l	6.11	3.44	8.2	2.5	3.9	4.2	5.6
	(range)	(0.9–19.7)	(0.2–11.2)	(1.2–16.2)	(0.14–8.3)	(0.1–32.4)	(0.13–14.1)	(0.4–22.9)
	%	35–51	–	–	10–60	–	7–21	–
Monocytes	×10^9/l	2.2	0.74	0.4	0.45	0.9	1	0.93
	(range)	(0.06–8.8)	(0.04–2.35)	(0.1–0.5)	(0.06–2.1)	(0.03–3.1)	(0.01–3.2)	(0.04–1.8)
	%	0–1	–	–	0–6	–	12–22	–
Azurophils	×10^9/l	3.46	5.42	2.1	0.7	1.1	3.4	2
	(range)	(0.1–18)	(0.97–13.9)	(0.05–7.6)	(0.1–1.84)	(0.11–4.4)	(0.3–13.3)	(0.15–5.3)
	%	0–5	–	–	–	–	–	–
Eosinophils	×10^9/l	0.2	0.16	0.2	0.07	0.1	0.25	0.1
	(range)	(0.08–0.34)	(0.1–0.2)		(0.06–0.1)	(0.04–0.2)	(0.12–0.37)	(0.08–0.1)
	%	0–1	–	–	0–18	–	–	–
Basophils	×10^9/l	0.26	0.55	0.5	0.07	0.1	0.55	0.55
	(range)	(0.05–1.76)	(0.07–1.8)	(0.16–0.9)	(0.03–0.14)	(0.02–0.3)	(0.07–1.8)	(0.07–1.4)
	%	0–3	–	–	0–20	–	0–2	–

Biochemistry

AST	units/l	5–46	11–75	3–184	3–331	9–136	2–118	10–224
CK	units/l	27–1350	600	162–336	53–1728	31–745	93–3108	91–2460
LDH	units/l	48–547	206	57–270	16–877	141–661	77–787	48–444
Uric acid	μmol/l	81–333	60–1213	200–1095	0–708	125–1647	190–245	167–1184
Calcium	mmol/l	3.2–4.1	5.8	2.9–3.6	2.3–6.8	2.8–4.8	2.7–5.5	3.4–4.9
Phosphorous	mmol/l	0.9–1.1	0.4–0.9	1.0–2.1	0.8–3.8	1.2–2.5	0.3–2.7	0.9–1.8
BUN	mmol/l	0–1	0.7–1	0.36–1.1	1.8	0.4–1	0–1	0–2
Glucose	mmol/l	0.5–3	0.3–12	0.7–2	0.5–4.7	0.1–2.6	0.1–2.4	1.8–4.9
Cholesterol	mmol/l	6-8–10	3–9.3	7.4–15.7	0.9–8.1	3.6–8.1	0.6–7.8	8.1–14.8
Triglyceride	mmol/L	–	–	1.2	0.04–5.2	0.7–1.1	–	0.5–1.3
Protein	g/L	56–105	39–69	54–87	43–108	37–80	50–56	46–108
Sodium	mmol/L	135–158	157–163	153	130–171	137–163	138–173	154–174
Potassium	mmol/L	4.2–5.5	3.4–5	4.3	3–10	1.2–5	2.1–9	3.3–16.6
Chloride	mmol/L	109–123	119–130	115	108–139	94–128	109–130	109–137

Table A2.3 Chelonians.

	Units	Long-necked turtles (*Chelodina* spp)[1]	Short-necked turtles (*Emydura* spp)[1]	Red-eared slider (*Trachemys scripta elegans*)	Painted turtle (*Chrysemys picta*)	Mediterranean tortoises (*Testudo* spp)	Sulcata (*Centrochelys sulcata*)	Box turtles (*Terrapene* spp)	Star tortoise (*Geochelone elegans*)
Haematology									
PCV	%	22	24	29	22	23	28	22	21
	(range)	(16–26)	(18–30)	(16–47)	(24–30)	(22–34)	(9–48)	(7–35)	(12–31)
WBC	$\times 10^9$/l	14.6	6.5	13	5.5	8.5	8	7	11
	(range)	(6–35.9)	(2.4–9.5)	(3.5–25.5)	(0.4–13)	(5–12.5)	(1.2–25.6)	(1.7–16)	(0.75–31)
Heterophils	$\times 10^9$/l			5	2.2	3.7	3.44	4.8	4.1
	(range)			(0.95–14)	(0.17–4.3)	(1.3–4.6)	(0.32–9.64)	(1.7–9)	(0.7–14.9)
	%	9–58	18–69	–	–	–	–	11	–
Lymphocytes	$\times 10^9$/l			3.3	1.6	4.7	3.68	4.9	5.14
	(range)			(0.25–7.9)	(0.23–3.46)	(3.6–7.6)	(0.19–13.7)	(2.6–8.2)	(0.16–17.6)
	%	29–82	12–63	–	–	–	–	56	–
Monocytes	$\times 10^9$/l			0.24	0.26	0.01	0.64	0.11	0.38
	(range)	–	–	(0.14–0.38)		(0–0.02)	(0.06–2.25)	(0–0.4)	(0.02–1.35)
	%	2–19	1–18	–	–	–	–	9.4	–
Azurophils	$\times 10^9$/l			0.58	0.51	0.05	0.25	–	0.72
	(range)	–	–	(0.23–1.33)	(0.25–0.8)	(0.03–0.12)	(0.02–0.54)		(0.08–1.73)
	%	–	–	–	–	–	–	–	–
Eosinophils	$\times 10^9$/l			1.53	0.55	0.05	0.35	0.02	0.96
	(range)	–	–	(0.17–5.9)	(0.1–1.03)	(0.02–0.06)	(0.03–1.41)	(0–0.1)	(0.08–2.24)
	%	4–10	1–24	–	–	–	–	–	–
Basophils	$\times 10^9$/l	0	0	3.8	2.17	0.05	0.3	0.21	0.76
	(range)			(0.31–8)	(0.04–4.86)	(0.02–0.08)	(0.02–0.54)	(0–0.4)	(0.04–3)
	%	0–4	0	–	–	–	–	8	–

Biochemistry

AST	units/l	25–91	54–181	0–522	62–380	12–32	34–401	2–620	12–296
CK	units/l	17–390	100–1360	108–4856	35–355	6–344	103–6205	37–898	144–8518
Bile acids	µmol/l	–	–	–	0.1	–	34–401	–	–
LDH	units/l	–	–	371–5763	412–1035	111–313	258–1980	–	12–863
Uric acid	µmol/l	390–890	4200–790	18–190	12–130	48–232	125–625	29.8–185	60–482
Calcium	mmol/l	3.3–5	2–4	2.5–4.5	1.4–4.8	2.5–4.9	1.6–5	1.6–6.6	2.3–4.4
Phosphorous	mmol/l	0.9–1.8	1.1–2.8	1.2–2.4	0.8–1.3	0.4–1.3	1.2–2.8	0.5–2.7	1.3–1.9
BUN	mmol/l	–	–	1.4–19.3	7–30	1.4–6.1	0–2.1	7–36	0–3.9
Glucose	mmol/l	5–10.4	3.5–8.4	1.1–7.7	3.8–9.8	2.2–4.8	4.4–4.5	1.8–8.5	2.2–11
Cholesterol	mmol/l	–	–	2.9–5.9	–	0.7–5.4	1.5–10.5	1.7–13	2–6.5
Protein	g/l	37–53	25–42	28–66	19–65	25–46	6–20	25–47	30–60
Sodium	mmol/l	124–136	128–135	124–144	126–137	131–149	121–155	138–149	122–150
Potassium	mmol/l	2.9–4.3	2.8–4.2	3.5–9.1	2.6–3.2	1.9–7.2	1.6–7	3–9.7	1.5–3.1
Chloride	mmol/l	–	–	97–107	88–99	95–100	69–394	101–112	90–112

[1] Scheelings, T.F. and Rafferty, A.R. (2012) Hematologic and serum biochemical values of gravid freshwater Australian chelonians. *Journal of Wildlife Diseases*, 48, 314–321.

Index

Note: Page numbers followed by "*b, f* and *t*" refer to "boxes, figures and tables" respectively.

Reptile Medicine and Surgery in Clinical Practice, First Edition. Edited by Bob Doneley, Deborah Monks,
Robert Johnson and Brendan Carmel.
© 2018 John Wiley & Sons Ltd. Published 2018 by John Wiley & Sons Ltd.

Printed and bound by CPI Group (UK) Ltd, Croydon, CR0 4YY

16/04/2025

14658503-0005